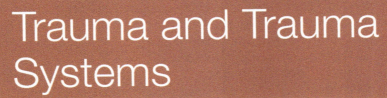

Trauma and Trauma Systems

Robert S. Porter, MA, EMT-P

STANDARD
Trauma (Trauma Overview)

COMPETENCY
Integrates assessment findings with principles of epidemiology and pathophysiology to formulate a field impression to implement a comprehensive treatment/disposition plan for an acutely injured patient.

OBJECTIVES

Terminal Performance Objective
After reading this chapter you should be able to describe the operation of a functional trauma care system and discuss the roles and responsibilities of paramedics within a trauma care system.

Enabling Objectives
To accomplish the terminal performance objective, you should be able to:

1. Define key terms introduced in this chapter.
2. Describe the epidemiology of trauma in general, and with respect to trauma that results in requests for emergency medical care.
3. Compare the role of a paramedic caring for a patient with life-threatening injuries to the role of a paramedic caring for a patient with non-life-threatening injuries.
4. Apply the five-step public health model to injury prevention.
5. Describe the capabilities of the various levels of designated trauma centers.
6. Given a variety of scenarios, conduct trauma assessments that result in categorization of patients as critical, unstable, potentially unstable, or stable.
7. Discuss the role of time to definitive care in the outcomes of trauma patients.
8. Apply trauma triage criteria to identify patients who should be transported to a trauma center.
9. Describe the purposes of data collection in injury prevention, the trauma registry, and quality improvement.

KEY TERMS

blunt trauma
epidemiology
Golden Period
Haddon Matrix

index of suspicion
mechanism of injury
 (MOI)
penetrating trauma

trauma
trauma center
trauma registry
trauma triage criteria

On a sunny and warm midsummer day, the annunciator sounds and requests that the quick response vehicle with paramedic Earl Antak and the Hamilton Area Volunteer Ambulance respond to a bicycle/auto collision 3 miles south of Amble Corners. It is a 10-minute trip for Earl, and about the same for the volunteer ambulance service. While the vehicles are en route, the dispatcher radios that the sheriff's department is on scene and that they have reported an unresponsive bicyclist.

Arriving at the collision scene, Earl notes that sheriff's deputies have secured the scene and are directing traffic. As he begins his scene size-up, Earl notices that several cars are parked along the highway's shoulder. Earl also sees a bicycle with a mangled front wheel resting against the open door of one of the cars. A deputy is attending to a young adult who is lying on the roadside about 45 feet in front of the car. As Earl studies the scene more closely, he observes that the car's open door has been bent forward and that glass from the car door is strewn along the highway.

The deputy tells Earl that the person he is attending to is named John. He reports that John was unresponsive when the deputy arrived but is now responsive, though somewhat confused. Earl's general impression is that the patient is a thin but well-developed male in his early 20s. He is wearing a bicycle helmet, shorts, and a T-shirt. He has several abrasions to his right shoulder, arm, and forearm, as well as to his right thigh. His helmet is badly scraped and deformed. Earl asks the deputy to continue holding manual head immobilization while Earl applies a cervical collar.

Earl's primary assessment suggests possible spine injury from the mechanism of injury and reveals that John is responsive and oriented to person but not to place or time. A witness reports that John was riding along at about 20 miles per hour when "this lady opened her door right in front of me." John flew through the door window and onto the pavement. Now John asks, "How's my bike?" His radial pulse is strong with a rate of about 100 and his respirations are about 22 and full. Both lung fields are clear, and his skin is warm and very wet. Earl asks the deputy to continue stabilizing the head and neck while he applies oxygen via nonrebreather mask at 15 liters per minute. At the end of the primary assessment, Earl categorizes John as U (unstable) on the basis of his period of unconsciousness, will expedite further assessment and care, and plans to transport John to the regional trauma center with neurosurgical capability.

The rapid trauma assessment reveals a small deformity just medial to the right upper anterior shoulder and some crepitus and pain with any movement of the right upper extremity. There is a large abrasion to the right thigh. Extremity evaluation reveals limited sensation to touch and limited strength in all limbs, pain on motion with the right upper limb (suspected clavicle fracture), but otherwise equal and strong pulses with good capillary refill and all limbs warm to the touch. There are no signs of soft-tissue injuries to the head and John denies any pain other than to his right shoulder and thigh, a "twinge of pain" in his neck, and a sensation of "pins and needles" in his extremities. When vital signs are taken, John's pulse is still strong at 100, his respirations remain 22 and unlabored, and his blood pressure is 132/84.

As the volunteer ambulance arrives, Earl uses his cell phone to contact medical direction for trauma center assignment. He is directed to Mercy Hospital, the regional trauma center, and speaks to the trauma triage nurse. Earl tells the nurse that John meets the system's trauma triage criteria—initial unresponsiveness and a serious mechanism of injury—and relates his assessment findings, Glasgow Coma Score, and patient's vital signs. Since ground transport time is projected to be 45 minutes, and because the mechanism of injury puts this patient within the guidelines for air transport, he requests a helicopter intercept.

After about 8 minutes at the patient's side, Earl and the EMTs from the volunteer ambulance have immobilized John to a spine board and loaded him into the ambulance.

As transport begins, Earl establishes a 16-gauge IV access site, begins to administer normal saline at a to-keep-open rate, and continues to provide frequent reassessments. He notices that John can no longer remember what happened to him or the name of the paramedic. John then begins to mumble incoherently.

Earl and the ambulance intercept with a Central State Medevac helicopter at a predesignated landing zone, a parking lot at the county community college. The flight paramedic greets Earl, takes his report, and quickly begins her assessment. She readies John for flight and Earl helps load him into the helicopter. Within minutes of the ambulance's arrival, the helicopter takes off for Mercy Hospital.

Later that day, Earl gets a follow-up phone call from the flight paramedic thanking him for providing good care for the patient and an informative patient report. She says that the patient had a fracture of the right clavicle, an epidural hemorrhage which required emergency surgery, and a C2 and C3 fracture managed by immobilization. Because of the patient's age and excellent physical condition, he is expected to recover quickly.

INTRODUCTION TO TRAUMA AND TRAUMA CARE

Trauma is a physical injury or wound caused by external force or violence. It is the third leading cause of death in the United States today behind cardiovascular disease and cancer. It is, however, the leading killer of persons under age 44. As such, trauma steals the greatest number of productive years from its victims. It also may be the most expensive medical problem because of the lost productivity it causes its victims and the high cost of initial care, rehabilitation, and often lifelong maintenance of those victims.

Trauma accounts for about 177,000 deaths per year, with auto crashes responsible for about 34,500 and gunshot wounds for another 31,500.[1] Despite reductions in auto-crash and violence-related death rates, the overall trauma and injury mortality rates have been inching steadily upward over the past decade. This is due in part to an aging population that is more vulnerable to the effects of injury and in part to rising rates from other forms of injury. Other trauma deaths can be attributed to falls, blasts, burns, stabbing, crush injuries, drowning, and sports injuries. In addition to the great death toll from trauma, many more of its victims are injured and carry lifelong physical reminders of their experiences with it.

Trauma accounts for approximately 30 percent of requests for prehospital emergency medical service. Of these requests, 47 percent are for falls, 28 percent are for on-the-roadway vehicle collisions, 13 percent are for other blunt trauma, 3 percent are for off-the-road vehicle collisions, and 2 percent are for intentional lacerations/stabbings. Other requests for EMS responses that account for less than 1 percent each are pedestrian/vehicle collisions, unintentional lacerations/stabbings, and intentional and unintentional firearm injuries.[2]

Your role in trauma care, as a member of the emergency medical services team, is to understand the design and purpose of the trauma care system, to promote injury prevention, and to provide seriously injured trauma patients with proper

assessment, aggressive care, and rapid transport to the most appropriate facility. The remainder of this chapter will help you with these responsibilities as it further defines trauma, explains components of trauma care systems, identifies differing trauma center capabilities, and more fully defines your role in assessment and care as a prehospital provider in the trauma system.

TRAUMA

The nature and severity of trauma can range from slight abrasions resulting from a slide into first base to fatal, multiple-system injuries that might result from a high-speed automobile-versus-pedestrian collision. Trauma is broken down into two major categories, blunt and penetrating. Penetrating trauma occurs when an arrow, bullet, knife, or other object enters the body and exchanges energy directly with human tissue, thereby causing injury. Blunt trauma is injury that occurs as energy and collision forces associated with an object—not the object itself—enter the body and damage tissue.

Although trauma poses a serious threat to life, its presentation often masks a patient's true condition. Extremity injuries,

CONTENT REVIEW

▶ Trauma as a Disease: The Public Health Model

- Surveillance
- Risk analysis
- Intervention development
- Implementation
- Evaluation

for example, infrequently cause death. Yet they are often obvious and can be grotesque (Figure 1 ●). Life-threatening problems such as internal bleeding and shock may occur with only subtle signs and symptoms. When assessing a trauma patient, you must look beyond obvious injuries for evidence that suggests a life-threatening condition. When such evidence is found, you must ensure aggressive care and rapid access to the trauma system for your patient.

Serious and life-threatening injury occurs in fewer than 10 percent of trauma patients. In most patients with life-threatening trauma, injury is internal and is likely to involve the head, physical injury, or hemorrhage into the body cavity (chest, abdomen, or pelvis). Prehospital care can neither properly nor definitively stabilize these patients and their injuries in the field. The best care you as a paramedic can offer is to immobilize the cervical spine, secure the airway, ensure adequate ventilation, control any significant external hemorrhage, and rapidly transport the patient to definitive trauma care. Definitive trauma care is only available at a specialized treatment facility with rapid access to surgery—a trauma center.

Some 90 percent of trauma patients do not have serious, life-threatening injuries.[2] You can best care for these patients by providing thorough on-scene assessment and care followed by conservative transport to the nearest general hospital or other appropriate health care facility.

During your assessment, it is essential that you determine the difference between trauma patients with serious, life-threatening conditions and those less seriously injured. You will be aided in making this determination by using guidelines known as trauma triage criteria, which will be discussed in

detail later in this chapter. These criteria involve consideration of physical or clinical findings that indicate internal injury and mechanisms by which patients are injured. Using the trauma triage guidelines will help ensure that you properly direct patients as they enter the trauma care system.

TRAUMA AS A DISEASE

Modern-day emergency medical services began with the white paper "Accidental Death and Disability: The Neglected Disease of Modern Society" and subsequent passage of the Highway Safety Act of 1966. Despite plaguing humanity from the beginning of time, it is only since the publication of the white paper that trauma has been viewed—and managed—as a disease. Modern medicine uses a five-step approach to prevent or reduce the impact of disease. Often known as the public health care model, the five steps are surveillance, risk identification, intervention development, implementation, and evaluation. Note that a major focus of medicine is prevention, since it is often easier to prevent a disease (such as trauma) than to treat it.

Surveillance

Surveillance is the collection of data to identify the existence, significance, and characteristics of disease. (The study of disease based on such surveillance is called **epidemiology**). For example, we know that trauma is the number-one cause of mortality between the ages of 1 and 44, accounting for 177,000 deaths annually. We also know that for every death (mortality), another two persons will survive with a significant disability (morbidity), and another 20 will require an emergency medical service response and emergency department care. Further, we know that more than 123,000 persons die yearly because of unintentional injury, with 34,500 of those deaths resulting from auto crashes alone. Falls account for another 24,000 unintentional deaths, drowning 4,000, and burns 4,000. Intentional death accounts for 30,000 lives lost from suicide and about 20,000 from homicide. About 60 percent of these intentional deaths are caused by firearms, most commonly the handgun (Figure 2 ●). Thirty percent of EMS responses are to trauma calls.[3]

Risk Analysis

Risk analysis looks at disease and determines various factors that impact its development, course, and consequences. Males, for example, account for more than 65 percent of all trauma deaths and 75 percent of trauma mortality between the ages of 16 and 24. Alcohol is related to around 50 percent of traffic fatalities and is also considered a major contributing factor in off-road vehicle and boating crashes, falls, drownings, and homicide/suicide. Clearly, behavior plays an important role in trauma. The high number of young male deaths might be attributed to risk-taking behavior, alcohol consumption, and a general disregard for safety.

A helpful tool to identify risk elements associated with trauma is the **Haddon Matrix** (Figure 3 ●). The Haddon Matrix for identifying risk elements for disease is often constructed

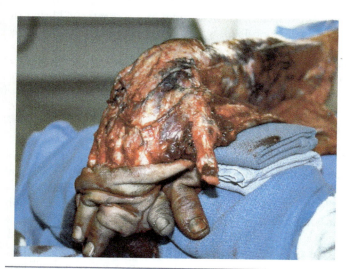

● **Figure 1**   In prehospital care, it is essential that gruesome, non-life-threatening injuries do not distract you from more subtle, life-threatening problems. (*© Edward T. Dickinson, MD*)

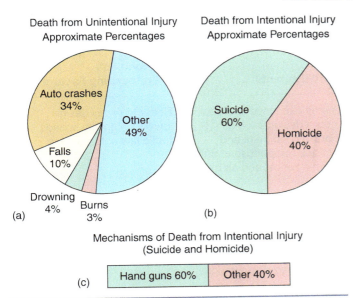

Death from Unintentional Injury
Approximate Percentages

Auto crashes
34%

Other
49%

Falls
10%

Drowning
4%

Burns
3%

(a)

Death from Intentional Injury
Approximate Percentages

Suicide
60%

Homicide
40%

(b)

Mechanisms of Death from Intentional Injury
(Suicide and Homicide)

Hand guns 60% | Other 40%

(c)

● **Figure 2** Causes of trauma deaths by approximate percentage. (a) Deaths from unintentional injury. (b) Deaths from intentional injury. (c) Mechanisms of death from intentional injury.

as a three-by-three matrix. When applied to trauma, it segregates causative and contributive elements and helps us identify factors we can modify to reduce trauma incidence, severity, and outcome. The Haddon Matrix identifies elements occurring before the incident (pre-event), during the incident (event), and after the incident (post event). It also looks at the victim (host), causative elements (agent), and factors surrounding the incident (environment). In motor vehicle collision, the event is the collision, the host is the driver and other vehicle occupants, the agent is the kinetic energy exchange between the automobile interior and its occupants, and the environment is the roadway and weather and lighting conditions.[4]

Pre-event factors are those things that happen well before the collision and cause, influence, or prevent the outcome (injury). Pre-event host factors include defensive driver training, traffic law compliance, and behaviors regarding drinking and driving and using safety equipment (seat belts or helmets). Pre-event host factors also include the patient's general health (age, preexisting disease(s), medications, and physical conditioning), state of alertness, and absence of distractions. The agent, which is really kinetic energy exchange, is reduced before the collision by better auto design such as anti-lock brakes, lap belts and shoulder straps, proper use of child seats, and crumple zones and air bags. The environment is improved by better highway design (improved traffic flow patterns, keeping high-speed oncoming traffic separated,

lines painted on the roadway, increased intersection visibility, appropriate and clear signage, and better barrier engineering), lowered highway speeds, and traffic law enforcement.

Event factors exist during the crash. Host-related event factors include the occupant's health at crash time, rest state and alertness, any influence of alcohol or other drugs, and seat belt use. The agent (impact) is reduced by lower vehicle speeds, better pre-impact braking (including the beneficial effects of anti-lock brakes), the effectiveness of crumple zones, seat belt use, and air bag deployment. Environmental event considerations include such things as crash barriers deflecting an auto away from a bridge abutment, open space between lanes preventing the auto from crossing into oncoming traffic, and weather that may reduce visibility, reduce vehicle control, and extend stopping distances.

Post-event factors are those that either worsen or improve the victim's outcome after the energy exchange. For the host, they include his knowledge of what to do after the crash: first aid, not to move if he has spinal symptoms or pain, and how to access the EMS system (cell phone, 911, OnStar). Post-event host elements also include the victim's ability physiologically to deal with blood loss and shock as influenced by the person's general health and conditioning and the effects of medications such as beta-blockers and anticoagulants. Potential agent effects are reduced by fire-resistant fuel systems and advanced automatic collision notification (AACN) systems such as OnStar. Post-crash environmental factors include video surveillance of high traffic and frequent crash areas and priority dispatch to ensure the right resources arrive quickly at the scene. Post-event environmental factors also include the EMS system and trauma system responses and possibly a teachable moment (future incident prevention). Finally, post-event environmental factors include the effects adverse weather (cold, heat, wind, and precipitation) now have on collision victims (Figure 4 ●).

Intervention Development

Intervention development creates or modifies programs to reduce both the incidence and the seriousness of trauma. In an auto crash, we can see preventative opportunities in almost all components of the Haddon Matrix. Safer highway design like barriers that deflect traffic or absorb impact energy; autos that have better braking systems, crumple zones, and passive restraint systems; and programs that encourage drivers to use their seat belts and to drive rested and distraction-free, not to drink and drive, and to drive defensively—all reduce the number and seriousness of collisions and resulting injuries. Emergency medical services was, in fact, a post-event intervention that was

● **Figure 3** A Haddon Matrix for risks and preventive measures regarding disease (including trauma) often assumes a three-by-three construction.

Haddon Matrix

	Host	Agent	Environment
Pre-event			
Event			
Post-event			

Haddon Matrix for a Vehicle Collision:
Analysis of Factors that May Ameliorate or Exacerbate the Event

	Host: Driver/Occupants	Agent: Causative Elements	Environment: Surrounding Factors
Pre-event: Before the collision	Defensive driver training, traffic law compliance, behaviors regarding drinking and driving and using safety equipment (seat belts or helmets), general health, alertness, absence of distractions.	Kinetic energy exchange reduced by better auto design such as anti-lock brakes, lap belts and shoulder straps, proper use of child seats, crumple zones, and air bags.	Better highway design, lowered highway speeds, traffic law enforcement.
Event: The collision	Effects on occupant influenced by health at crash time, rest state, alertness, influence of alcohol or other drugs, seat belt use, air bag deployment.	Impact reduced by lower vehicle speeds, better pre-impact braking (including anti-lock brakes), effectiveness of crumple zones, seat belt use, and air bag deployment.	Environmental considerations include presence of crash barriers, lane spacing, and weather.
Post-event: After the collision	Outcome after crash worsened or improved by knowledge of what to do: first aid, not moving, accessing EMS, physiological ability to deal with blood loss and shock based on health, condition, and medications.	Effects reduced by fire-resistant fuel systems, advanced automatic collision notification (AACN) systems, video surveillance of crash area, priority dispatch of right resources, and speed of reaching the scene.	EMS and trauma system responses, use made of teachable moment, effect of weather on collision victims after the crash.

● **Figure 4**   A Haddon Matrix identifying preventive elements for motor vehicle collisions.

developed through this health care approach to provide better care for injured patients once trauma has occurred.

As technology progresses, more accurate information regarding auto crash dynamics is available through General Motors' OnStar, Ford's SYNC, BMW's Assist, and other advanced automatic collision notification (AACN) systems. These devices, located within modern vehicles, send data that identify the vehicle's initial speed; strength of gravitational equivalent forces (G-forces) from frontal, side, rear, and rollover impact sensors; and denote air bag deployment and vehicle GPS (global positioning system) position. This information helps public-safety dispatch direct the needed services to the collision scene and can also help responders anticipate the degree of injury and better prepare for patient assessment and care.

Implementation

Implementation is putting an intervention into practice. It may be enforcing traffic laws, reducing speed limits in hazardous areas, rebuilding highways to be safer, building safer autos, gun safety programs, workplace safety codes, behavior change and safety education, or continuing to improve our emergency medical services system. As health care providers, we bear responsibility to promote, teach, and teach by example—all actions that help reduce trauma. We are also responsible to identify ways to provide better trauma patient care.

An important and very effective intervention for trauma is the use of a "teachable moment." We often treat individuals who have come to harm because of carelessness or a disregard for safety. In a supportive, nonjudgmental manner, we can suggest that a modest and positive behavior change can prevent an event

like this from repeating itself. We all learn from our mistakes and using a teachable moment can reduce the likelihood of another similar trauma event.

Evaluation

Evaluation is repeating the surveillance that took place before an intervention to identify benefits of the intervention. For example, we know that the highway death toll has dropped from 56,000 per year when the Highway Safety Act was passed (in 1968) to just under 36,000 in recent times—this despite more people, traveling farther, at faster speeds. This significant reduction in motor vehicle collision (MVC) mortality demonstrates intervention effectiveness over the past four decades. However, people still die as a result of drunk driving, failure to wear seat belts, falling asleep at the wheel, excessive speed, distraction by cell phone use, and other modifiable risk factors and behaviors. Using the public health care model, we must continue to search out risk factors, develop and implement interventions, and evaluate our system's performance. We also need to apply the public health care model to other types of trauma: falls, gunshot wounds, burns, sports injuries, recreational injuries, and others.

Injury prevention is an evolving role of the modern EMS system.

THE TRAUMA CARE SYSTEM

Development of the modern-day trauma care system mirrors the development of the public health care model just discussed. In the mid to late 1960s, several medically oriented groups investigated the death toll on U.S. highways. Their studies revealed that vehicle collision victims suffered not only from their crash-related injuries but also from the lack of an organized approach to bringing these victims into the health care system. Studies also demonstrated that most hospitals at that time were inadequately equipped and staffed to care for crash victims.

More than two decades later, the American College of Surgeons recognized that the system caring for severely injured trauma victims was still inadequate and successfully worked to achieve passage of the Trauma Care Systems Planning and Development Act of 1990. This act helped establish guidelines, funding, and state-level leadership and support for trauma systems.

Recent statistics show that for the most common type of trauma system activation—a patient with a blunt trauma mechanism—fewer than 1.5 percent of adult cases and less than 0.1 percent of pediatric cases require urgent surgical intervention. (In penetrating trauma, the surgical intervention rates are considerably higher.)

The overall rate of surgical intervention for trauma may be low, but the injuries that do require an operation (internal hemorrhage sites, for example) are often difficult to identify in the field and, once identified, can be complex and require a skilled and experienced trauma surgical team. This means that proper hospital care for serious trauma should include the immediate availability of skilled surgical intervention. Although patients with life-threatening injuries account for less than 10 percent of all trauma patients, and although even fewer need emergent surgery, immediate surgical care remains important for some patients and can drastically reduce trauma mortality and morbidity in selected circumstances.

Care for seriously injured trauma patients is expensive and complicated. A well-designed EMS system allocates trauma resources in a way that provides these patients with the most efficient and effective care. Such a system utilizes hospitals with special resources and a commitment to trauma patient care. These hospitals are designated as trauma centers.

TRAUMA CENTER DESIGNATION

The current model for a trauma system includes three **trauma center** levels, with a differing ability and commitment to provide trauma care at each level, with Level I centers offering the highest level of care (Table 1).

A Level I, or regional, trauma center is a hospital, usually a medical university teaching center, prepared and committed to handle all types of specialty trauma (Figure 5 ●). These

---

TABLE 1 | Criteria for Trauma Center Designation

Level I—Regional Trauma Center

Commits resources to address all types of specialty trauma 24 hours a day, 7 days a week.

Level II—Area Trauma Center

Commits the resources to address the most common trauma emergencies with surgical capability available 24 hours a day, 7 days a week; will stabilize and transport specialty cases to the regional trauma center.

Level III—Community Trauma Center

Commits to special emergency department training and has some surgical capability, but will usually stabilize and transfer seriously injured trauma patients to a higher level trauma center as needed.

Level IV—Trauma Facility

In remote areas, a small community hospital or medical care facility may be designated a trauma receiving facility, meaning that it will stabilize and prepare seriously injured trauma patients for transport to a higher level facility.

---

centers provide neurosurgery, often provide microsurgery (limb replantation), and care for multisystem trauma. They also provide leadership and resource support to other trauma center levels within the regional trauma system through system coordination, data collection, research, and continuing medical and public education programs. When population density or available resources do not permit a commitment to Level I trauma center requirements, a Level II trauma center may act as a regional trauma center.

A Level II, or area, trauma center has a high commitment to trauma care but not as great as a Level I facility. It has surgical care capability available at all times for incoming trauma patients. Level II centers can handle all but the most seriously

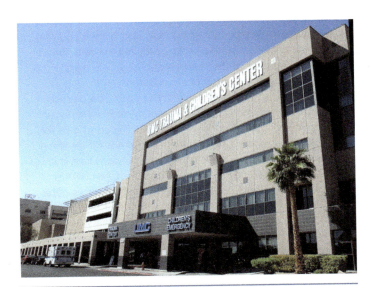

● **Figure 5** University Medical Center in Las Vegas, Nevada. As a level 1 trauma center, it provides trauma care for a large geographic area. (© Dr. Bryan E. Bledsoe)

injured specialty and multisystem trauma patients. (Some of these services may be on-call rather than in-house.) Staff at these facilities can stabilize those patients in preparation for transport to a Level I trauma center.

A Level III, or community, trauma center is a general hospital with a commitment to special staff training and resource allocation for trauma patients. These centers are located in smaller communities situated in generally rural areas. They are well prepared to care for most trauma victims and to stabilize and triage more seriously injured ones for transport to higher-level trauma centers.

There is provision for an additional trauma-patient destination level in some remote areas, designated as a Level IV trauma facility. Here, seriously injured trauma patients may be taken for stabilization and care before transport, often by helicopter, to a more distant, higher-level trauma center. In these areas, trauma incidence does not support resource allocation great enough to meet the requirements of a trauma center, so, by default, some other type of health care facility is identified as a trauma transport destination.

Trauma system design should be flexible enough to meet regional needs. In urban and suburban areas, there are just a few trauma centers to ensure that each receives adequate patient volume to maintain staff proficiency and to ensure that resources are being used effectively. In rural regions, a Level III center may act as a regional trauma center because the incidence of serious trauma does not support any greater commitment. In some areas, a Level IV facility may be all that is available and thus becomes the default destination for seriously injured trauma patients. Consult your EMS system plan and protocols to ensure you follow the intended patient flow patterns in your region.

Specialty Centers

Beyond classification as trauma centers, certain medical facilities may be designated as specialty centers, such as neurocenters, burn centers, pediatric trauma centers, and centers specializing in hand and limb replantation by microsurgery. One other specialty service is hyperbaric oxygenation, which is important in the treatment of carbon monoxide poisoning and problems associated with scuba diving.

Specialty centers have made a commitment of trained personnel, equipment, and other resources to provide services not usually available at a general or trauma hospital. These centers are also more likely to provide specialized intensive care and state-of-the-art injury management that your patient would not find at other facilities. Be aware of specialty services available in your system as well as protocols defining when patients should be directed to them.

YOUR ROLE AS A PARAMEDIC

As a paramedic, your tasks in the trauma system are likely to begin with an appropriate patient assessment and then triage of trauma patients against standards established by your medical direction system (trauma triage criteria), followed by expeditious patient care and then transport to the closest appropriate medical facility (Figure 6 ●). For those patients who meet trauma triage criteria, the appropriate facility is the nearest trauma center.

Trauma Assessment

Trauma patient assessment follows the general patient assessment format for all patients but differs from medical patient assessment in some very important ways. These include addressing

---

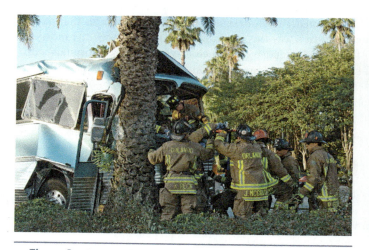

● **Figure 6** Your role as a paramedic attending a trauma patient is to ensure the ABCs and prepare the patient for rapid transport. (© *Craig Jackson/In the Dark Photography*)

an increased likelihood of scene hazards, analyzing the mechanism of injury, considering the impact the environment may have on your patients and their assessment and care, establishing scene oversight, applying trauma triage guidelines, and determining an appropriate patient destination. In trauma assessment you often treat patients with serious and/or life-threatening injury (necessitating a rapid trauma assessment) or ones with limited injury to a specific body area (such as an isolated forearm fracture and necessitating only a focused trauma assessment). In spite of its special aspects, trauma assessment proceeds much as it does for the medical patient. Its steps include the scene survey, primary assessment, secondary assessment (rapid or focused trauma assessment), and periodic reassessments.

Scene Survey

The scene survey focuses your attention on scene safety and scene evaluation, elements that set the stage for scene oversight and efficient delivery of assessment and care. Critical scene survey elements are scene safety (including Standard Precautions), mechanism of injury evaluation, environment impact consideration, and scene oversight.

Scene Safety

Because trauma scenes often involve the outdoors, industry, or machinery, the environment is more likely to have associated hazards such as traffic hazards from oncoming vehicles; electrocution from disrupted electrical lines; laceration hazards from jagged metal and broken glass; toxic substance exposure from smoke and spilled fluids such as battery acid; confined space (adverse atmosphere) as in silos and tanks; rough unstable terrain; slippery surfaces from spilled oil, radiator fluid, or transmission fluid; and violence as with weapons, violent patients, or hostile bystanders. Scene safety is of paramount importance for you, your crew, your patient, and bystanders. Many scene hazards will go unnoticed unless you look for them and rule them out. If the scene is not safe and you cannot make it so, do not enter; instead, protect others from the hazards. Request needed resources to ensure a safe scene and then await their arrival.[5]

Mechanism of Injury Analysis

To help determine the **mechanism of injury (MOI)**, mentally re-create the incident from evidence available at the scene. You should attempt to identify the strength of the forces involved in the incident, the direction from which they came, and areas of the patient's body most likely to have been affected by these forces. In an automobile collision, for example, the mechanism of injury includes the energy exchange process between the auto and what it struck, between the patient and the auto's interior, and among various tissues and organs as they collide with one another within the patient. Close inspection of the collision site and the mangled auto reveals evidence about the collision and the forces at work within it.

Information you gather during your consideration of the mechanism of injury suggests an **index of suspicion** for possible injuries. This index is a mental summation of anticipated injuries based on your event analysis. For example, an adult pedestrian struck by a car can be expected to have lower extremity fractures. Further, if the auto was moving at 20 miles per hour, fracture severity would be less than if it was moving at 55 miles per hour. Also, the probability of internal injury at lower speeds is less than it would be at higher speeds. By evaluating the strength and nature of the impact, you can anticipate body structures and organs that received damage and the degree of that damage.

In addition to examining the mechanism of injury, you will also examine trauma patients for signs of physical injury, during both the primary and the secondary (rapid or focused) trauma assessment. Current research suggests mechanism of injury alone is not as good a trauma severity predictor as was once thought. At best, the mechanism of injury is only an indirect indicator of energy transmission. For example, modern vehicle design and restraint systems are better able to absorb the energy from violent auto collisions, and patients often survive with only limited injuries. So it is important to look carefully at patient signs and symptoms, vital signs, Glasgow Coma Scale score, and level of consciousness for abnormal findings as well as analyzing the mechanism of injury.

Physical signs that suggest serious trauma include signs and symptoms of shock and those of internal head injury. Because shock and head injury cause the greatest trauma mortality, be watchful for the earliest evidence of their existence. It is important to note that the body compensates well for internal blood loss and hides serious injury signs until late in the shock process. If you have any reason to suspect that a patient has sustained serious internal injury, including head injury, carefully monitor the vital signs and level of consciousness and enter that patient rapidly into the trauma system. Otherwise, provide frequent reassessments to ensure you discover progressing signs of shock and head injury as early as possible.

Environmental Impact Consideration

It is important to anticipate the impact environmental extremes may have on assessment and care. Adverse weather, as with a severe thunderstorm, may expose both you and the patient to wind, precipitation, and cold. It may be beneficial to have the fire department provide tarps and wind screens to protect you and your patient. Some conditions, like a blizzard or extreme heat, may merit moving the patient to the ambulance earlier in assessment and care than you would normally consider. Carefully evaluate any extreme of heat or cold, precipitation (snow, sleet, rain), or adverse wind or strong direct sunlight for any possible adverse impact on your assessment and care or on your patient's condition. Identify the resources needed to address environmental hazards and to ensure a scene that is not environmentally hostile for you and your patient.

Scene Oversight

Overall scene organization is critical to effective scene safety and patient access, disentanglement, assessment, care, extrication, and transport. If you are first on the scene, establish scene oversight and report your scene findings to dispatch. Relinquish oversight duties and begin assessment and care as soon as a fire or rescue service representative arrives. If scene oversight is already established, report your arrival and begin your scene survey and patient assessment and care.

Primary Assessment

Primary assessment of a trauma patient varies slightly from that of a medical patient. The primary assessment of a trauma patient includes forming a patient impression; ruling out the need for spinal precautions; evaluating and securing your patient's airway, breathing, and circulation; and identifying patient priority for care and transport. As with a medical patient, quickly determine your patient's orientation and responsiveness, chief complaint or complaints, and anxiety level. This information will form the basis of your general patient impression, an impression that will gain in depth and specificity as you continue assessment of your patient.

The need to exclude the risk of spinal injury is specific to trauma patient assessment, requiring that you have determined the patient is a reliable reporter of spinal symptoms and reports none. Unreliable reporters are patients who have an altered level of consciousness (due either to injury or to the effects of alcohol or drugs), have a significant distracting injury, or are elderly or very young.

Assessing and securing the airway, breathing, and circulation mirror medical patient assessments, although looking for significant hemorrhage is more involved than with a medical patient. Note that you should assess circulation first if you suspect the patient is in cardiac arrest (the American Heart Association's C-A-B formulation).

At the end of the primary assessment, you will assign the patient a preliminary priority for further assessment, care, and transport. Those patients who do not make it out of the primary assessment (you are unable to secure the airway, breathing, or circulation) are considered critical (C). Those who present with limited injuries and are breathing well and have strong pulses are stable (S). Those in between are either unstable (U) or potentially unstable (P). These are the familiar CUPS categorizations of patient severity: Critical, Unstable, Potentially unstable, or Stable.

Secondary Assessment

Stable patients receive a focused trauma assessment. This is simply an application of the elements of a detailed patient assessment looking only at the area of suspected injury and/or chief complaint. There you will confirm injury and provide the limited care it requires. Reassessments will monitor vital signs and level of consciousness to ensure your patient does not deteriorate as a result of any unrecognized pathology.

Potentially unstable or unstable patients receive a rapid trauma assessment that includes a quick evaluation of major body regions (a quick head-to-toe exam) and focused assessments where the mechanism of injury, patient complaint, or finding from the rapid trauma assessment suggests injury. A degree of emphasis is placed on the Glasgow Coma Score (GCS) as it is an element for predicting the severity of patient injury, yet it requires training and practice to employ accurately and consistently. The GCS, along with other factors, is used to help make the priority determination for patient care and transport.

Reassessment

Periodic reassessments permit you to trend any patient improvement or deterioration. They include any primary and secondary assessment elements that revealed signs or symptoms

and a set of vital signs every 15 minutes for the stable patient and every 5 minutes for all others.

The Golden Period

Time is a critical consideration for the survival of a seriously injured trauma patient. Research has demonstrated that, for certain patients, survival rates increase dramatically as time from a trauma incident to surgery decreases. The current goal for incident-to-surgery time is about 1 hour, often referred to as the **Golden Period**. The Golden Period used to be called the Golden Hour, but the name has evolved to reflect the fact that the science behind the 1-hour designation has not been substantiated; for most trauma patients, minutes or even a few hours do not change survival rates. However, because at least a few trauma patients will require urgent surgical intervention, it is good EMS practice to minimize scene and transport times in trauma cases.

Factors such as response time and the time needed to access a patient, to extricate a patient (in some cases), to assess and care for a patient, and to transport a patient to the trauma center all consume a portion of the Golden Period. Many of these time-consuming factors are beyond your control; for that reason, it is vital to keep to a minimum time spent on factors over which you do have control.[6] Ideally, you should provide the primary and secondary assessments, emergency stabilization, patient packaging, and initiation of transport in less than 10 minutes. When distances or traffic conditions present prolonged ground transport times, consider reducing these by calling for an air medical service, if available, and if your patient's condition falls within the guidelines for air transport.[7]

Air medical service, usually provided by helicopter, has added a tool to the race against time for the seriously injured trauma patient (Figure 7 ●). Helicopters travel much faster than ground transport and in a straight line from the crash site to the trauma center. Recognize, however, that helicopters normally serve a greater geographic area than ground-based EMS, are often further from the trauma scene, and take some time to prepare for takeoff. Measure your request for air medical service

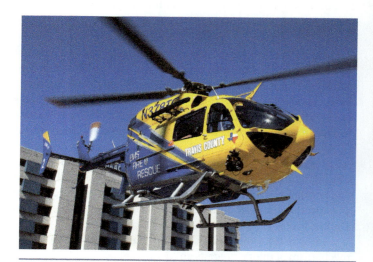

● **Figure 7**   An air medical services helicopter can sometimes reduce transport time from the accident scene to the trauma center. (© *Austin/Travis County STAR Flight*)

with their normal response times to the crash scene to ensure their use will decrease patient transport time to the hospital.[8]

Be aware, also, that air medical transport is not appropriate in many cases. A trauma patient must be in relatively stable condition for air transport to be utilized. This is because the limited space within the aircraft and its associated engine noise make in-flight care difficult. Further, a combative patient may endanger flight crew and aircraft safety. Adverse weather conditions can also limit the use of air medical transport. In many cases, ground transport is as fast or faster. Finally, air medical transport services are very expensive and can be used most effectively only as part of a comprehensive EMS trauma system. The utilization of air medical services is evolving with a trend toward tightening the medical criteria for which flights are authorized. Follow local protocols about when and how to request and utilize air medical transport.[9]

The Decision to Transport

The Centers for Disease Control has introduced revised criteria for prioritizing trauma patients for care and transport: 2011 Guidelines for Field Triage of Injured Patients[10] (Figure 8 ●). These criteria, often known as trauma triage criteria, identify the Glasgow Coma Scale, physical findings (vital signs), and the anatomy of the injury as elements of the trauma care and transport decision tree, followed by mechanism of injury and special considerations such as age.

As mentioned earlier, the mechanism of injury (MOI) (at least as related to auto collisions) is not as good a predictor as one might think. Modern vehicle design sacrifices vehicle structure to protect the occupants. Consequently, vehicle damage may suggest the degree of energy absorption rather than injury production. During the primary assessment (scene survey), however, mechanism of injury remains the first element of patient assessment to suggest trauma patient acuity. Since the Glasgow Coma Scale and vital sign evaluation are performed during the secondary assessment, MOI often provides preliminary information necessary to determine patient priority (CUPS) at the conclusion of the primary assessment. As noted earlier, CUPS is the acronym for categories of patient severity: Critical, Unstable, Potentially unstable, and Stable.

The decision to either transport a trauma patient immediately or attempt more extensive on-scene care is among the most difficult you must make. Trauma triage criteria are designed to help you with this decision. As a rule, you should transport patients who display key clinical and anatomic findings or experience certain mechanisms of injury quickly, with intravenous access, endotracheal intubation, and other time-consuming procedures attempted en route. The 2011 Guidelines for Field Triage of Injured Patients (review Figure 8) lists the indicators for immediate transport.[11]

When applying trauma triage criteria, it is best to err on the side of caution. Even if a patient does not meet the stated physical findings for rapid transport, be suspicious. Remember, you often arrive at a patient's side only minutes after the collision. The patient may not yet have lost enough blood internally to exhibit signs of shock or progressive head injury. If in doubt, consider rapid transport to a trauma center, and frequently reassess vital signs and level of consciousness.

The criteria listed in the Trauma Triage Protocol are, by design, sensitive for injury and thus may lead to "over-triaging" trauma patients. The criteria ensure that patients with significant and serious injuries but with very subtle signs and symptoms are not missed during assessment. Application of these criteria may cause you to transport some patients to trauma centers who ultimately will be determined not to require this high level of service. However, transporting a patient to a trauma center who may not need their resources is far better than not transporting a patient who truly does needs those services.

Injury Prevention

Prevention is our best, and most cost-effective, way to reduce trauma morbidity and mortality. It is easier and much less costly to reduce the number of intoxicated drivers on the highway than to care for them and their victims after they are injured in crashes. This is especially true when you consider the loss of life associated with drunk driving and the cost of rehabilitation for its victims.

Programs promoting defensive driving, seat belt use, undistracted driving, and use of designated drivers encourage teenagers and adults to drive more safely and responsibly. Other programs, like "Let's not meet by accident" and "Shattered Dreams" (Figure 9 ●), increase society's awareness of trauma systems as well as an appreciation for safety-oriented behaviors.[12] Safety programs for off-road vehicle, boat, and firearm users also raise safety awareness and promote injury prevention. The EMS system has a responsibility to support such programs and to promote their development where they do not exist. As an EMS provider, you should participate in these programs and encourage your peers to take part in them as well.[13]

Technical developments such as better highway design, air bag restraint systems, and vehicles constructed to absorb crash energy have also played major roles in reducing the yearly highway death toll. Paramedics have a responsibility to support such development and use of new designs and technologies as a way of further reducing trauma deaths and injuries.[14]

Data and the Trauma Registry

As discussed earlier in this chapter, and as with all emergency medical services, surveillance is the only way to recognize those trauma care practices and procedures that benefit patients and those that do not. In trauma systems, there is a health care surveillance process called the trauma registry. It is a uniform and standard set of data collected by regional trauma centers. These data are analyzed to describe the types of patients and injuries we respond to, determine how well the system is performing, and identify factors that may either lessen or increase patient survival.

It is important to support the trauma registry and research efforts by ensuring that your prehospital care reports accurately and completely describe your assessment findings, patient care, reassessment results, and times associated with calls. You should also consider taking part in and supporting prehospital research projects. Research can help establish the value of existing and new field techniques and equipment and can ultimately help reduce patient morbidity and mortality.

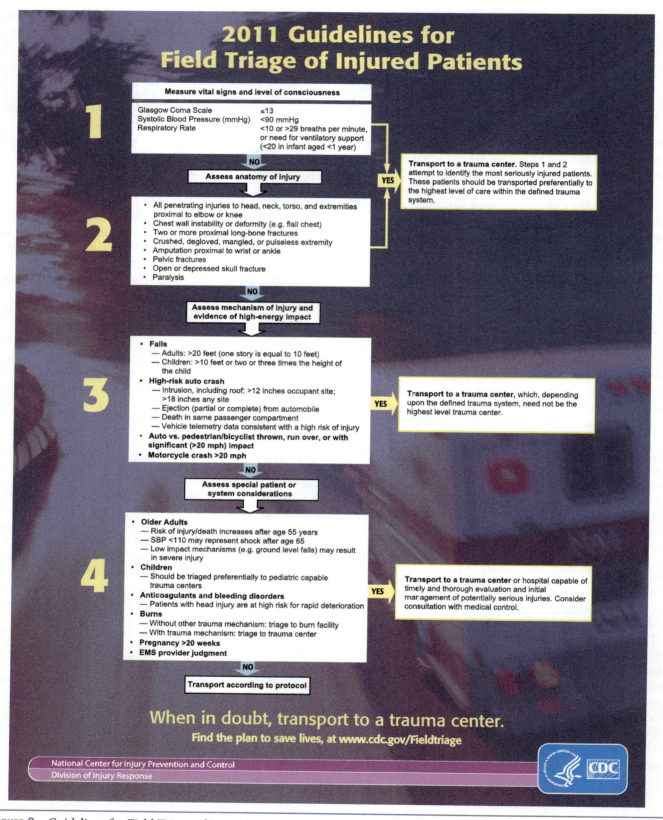

Figure 8 Guidelines for Field Triage of Injured Patients, Centers for Disease Control, 2011.

Quality Improvement

Trauma system Quality Improvement (QI), or Quality Management (QM), is another way of examining system performance with the aim of providing better patient care. In the QI process, committees look at selected care modalities (called indicators) to determine if designated system care standards are being met. For trauma system QI, committees study trauma triage criteria application; field skill performance; time spent in various aspects of response, assessment, care, and transport; and the appropriateness of trauma patient destinations. QI committees may also look at select calls to determine if documentation accurately reflects assessment results and care given. If system standards are not being met, committees may suggest such steps as continuing education programs, EMS equipment modifications, or protocol revisions. *True QI is not punitive and does not look to identify fault with individual providers.* QI is an effective method to assess system quality and provide for its improvement. As a prehospital trauma system member, you should become actively involved in, and encourage peer participation in, these or similar programs.

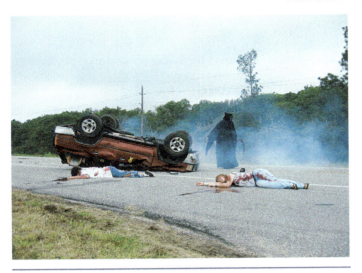

● **Figure 9** Public education programs such as the "Shattered Dreams" program can increase people's awareness of the role of the EMS system and of the importance of safe behaviors. (© *Austin County, Texas, EMS*)

SUMMARY

Trauma remains one of modern society's greatest tragedies. It accounts for frequent death and disabling injuries and often affects those who have their most productive years before them. A well-designed and well-implemented trauma system offers a way of lessening the incidence and impact of these traumas. Such a system consists of several levels of trauma centers possessing increasing levels of commitment to immediate and intensive trauma care. The well-designed and well-implemented trauma system also has prevention programs that encourage safe practices and behaviors. Finally, such a system has trauma triage protocols that guide paramedics in prioritizing and transporting trauma patients.

As a paramedic, you are a part of the trauma care system. You are charged with evaluating trauma patients by comparing their mental status, physical signs of injury, vital signs, and injury mechanisms to preestablished trauma triage criteria. This comparison helps you determine which patients should enter the trauma system and which could be best cared for with less emergent care and transport. In the presence of severe, life-threatening trauma, you must ensure rapid trauma assessment, time-critical on-scene care, and expedited transport to an appropriate facility, a trauma center, to provide your patients the best chances for survival.

YOU MAKE THE CALL

Just as you are about to move a seriously injured 12-year-old patient who has been in a bicycle/auto collision, her mother, Janet, emerges from the crowd. She is quite distraught and becomes even more so when you tell her that you'll be transporting her daughter to the Great Meadows Trauma Center on the far side of town. Janet informs you that she is a "lab tech" at Livingston Community Hospital just a few minutes from your location and wants her child transported there.

1. What authority does Janet have regarding the decision to transport her daughter?

2. What will you tell her regarding your choice for a hospital destination?

See Suggested Responses at the back of this chapter.

REVIEW QUESTIONS

1. The leading killer of persons under age 44 in the United States is _____.
   a. cancer
   b. stroke
   c. trauma
   d. cardiovascular disease

2. The best care you, as a paramedic, can offer a trauma patient is to immobilize the cervical spine, secure the airway, and _____.
   a. ensure adequate respirations
   b. control any significant external hemorrhage
   c. rapidly transport the patient to definitive trauma care
   d. all of the above

3. Certain trauma centers located in smaller communities situated in generally rural areas commit to special emergency department training and have a degree of surgical capability but usually stabilize and transfer seriously injured patients. These centers are designated _____.
   a. Level II   c. Level IV
   b. Level I   d. Level III

4. One specialty service important in the treatment of carbon monoxide poisoning and problems related to scuba diving is the _____.
   a. neurocenter
   b. hyperbaric oxygenation center
   c. burn center
   d. pediatric trauma center

5. When determining the mechanism of injury, you will identify the _____.
   a. forces involved in the collision
   b. person who caused the collision
   c. number of patients
   d. need for additional resources

6. You will begin your consideration of the mechanism of injury _____.
   a. during the scene size-up
   b. during the rapid trauma assessment
   c. during the focused trauma assessment
   d. during reassessments

7. The goal of EMS when dealing with the serious trauma patient is to get the patient quickly to definitive care. The objective time frame, describing the period from the incident to the patient's arrival at surgery, is the _____.
   a. Platinum 10 minutes
   b. Golden Period
   c. chronological limit
   d. maximum time of run

8. In the ideal scenario, you should provide the primary and rapid trauma assessments, emergency stabilization, patient packaging, and initiation of transport in under _____ minutes.
   a. 15   c. 10
   b. 20   d. 12

9. Limitations of air medical transport include all of the following except _____.
   a. limited space within the aircraft
   b. associated engine noise
   c. indirect route of travel
   d. inability to handle combative patients

10. In the Quality Improvement process, committees look at selected care modalities to determine if designated standards of care are being met. These modalities are also called _____.
    a. tips   c. indicators
    b. pointers   d. suggestions

See Answers to Review Questions at the back of this chapter.

REFERENCES

1. Centers for Disease Control and Prevention. Deaths: Final Data for 2009, table 18. [Available at www.cdc.gov/nchs/fastats/injury.htm]

2. National EMS Information System. "Report: Frequency of Injury Related to EMS Encounter by Cause." 2012. [Available at www.nemsis.org]

3. Centers for Disease Control and Prevention. "10 Leading Causes of Deaths, United States—2008." Atlanta, GA, 2010. [Available at www.cdc.gov]

4. Laraque, D., B. Barlow, and M. Durkin. "Prevention of Youth Injuries." *J Nat Med Assoc* 91(10) (1999): 557–571.

5. Reichard, A. A., S. M. Marsh, and P. H. Moore. "Fatal and Nonfatal Injuries among Emergency Medical Technicians and Paramedics." *Prehosp Emerg Care* 15(4) (Oct–Dec 2011): 511–517.

6. Gonzalez, R. P., et al. "On-Scene Intravenous Line Insertions Adversely Impacts Prehospital Time in Rural Vehicle Trauma." *Am Surg* 74(11) (Nov 2008): 1083–1087.

7. Ringburg, A. N., et al. "Helicopter Emergency Medical Services (HEMS): Impact on On-Scene Times." *J Trauma* 63(2) (Aug 2007): 258–262.

8. Sullivent, E. E., M. Faul, and M. M. Wald. "Reduced Mortality in Injured Adults Transported by Helicopter Emergency Medical Services." *Prehosp Emerg Care* 15(3) (Jul–Sep 2011): 295–302.

9. Talving, P., et al. "Helicopter Evacuation of Trauma Victims in Los Angeles: Does It Improve Survival?" *World J Surg* 33(11) (Nov 2009): 2469–2476.

10. National Center for Injury Prevention and Control. "Guidelines for Field Triage of Injured Patients." 2011. [Available at www.cdc.gov/fieldtriage]

11. Smith, R. M. and A. K. Conn. "Prehospital—Scoop and Run or Stay and Play?" *Injury* 40 Suppl 4 (Nov 2009): S23–S26.

12. City of Frisco Police Department. "Shattered Dreams." Texas 2012. [Available at www.ci.frisco .tx.us/departments/police]

13. Sleet, D. A. "Reducing Motor Vehicle Trauma through Health Promotion Programming." *Health Educ Q* 11(2) (Summer 1984): 113–125.

14. Rasouli, M. R., et al. "Preventing Motor Vehicle Crash-Related Spine Injuries in Children." *World J Pediatr* 7(4) (Nov 2011): 311–317.

FURTHER READING

American College of Surgeons, Committee on Trauma. *Advanced Trauma Life Support for Doctors: Student Course Manual.* Chicago: American College of Surgeons, 2008.

American College of Surgeons, Committee on Trauma. *Resources for Optimal Care of the Injured Patient.* Chicago: American College of Surgeons, 2006.

Legome, Eric, and Lee W. Shockley, eds. *Trauma: A Comprehensive Emergency Medicine Approach.* Cambridge, England: The Cambridge University Press, 2011.

SUGGESTED RESPONSES TO "YOU MAKE THE CALL"

The following are suggested responses to the "You Make the Call" scenarios presented in this chapter. Each represents an acceptable response to the scenario but should not be interpreted as the only correct response.

1. What authority does Janet have regarding the decision to transport her daughter?

Janet is the mother and legal authority over her child. She has full authority to make decisions for the child. In the case where parents or guardians are present, they are capable of making the decisions for the patient as if they were the patient.

2. What will you tell her regarding your choice for a hospital destination?

Explain to the mother your concern for the injuries and the need for specialized treatment that the trauma center can provide. By explaining your rationale and letting the mother know that this is what you feel is truly in the best interest of the patient, you should be able to persuade the mother and get her to agree to transport to the trauma center.

ANSWERS TO REVIEW QUESTIONS

1. c
2. d
3. d
4. b
5. a

6. a
7. b
8. c
9. c
10. c

GLOSSARY

blunt trauma injury caused by the collision of an object with the body in which the object does not enter the body.

epidemiology the study of disease to determine its prevalence, course, and seriousness.

Golden Period the 60-minute period after a severe injury; it is the maximum acceptable time between the injury and initiation of surgery for the seriously injured trauma patient.

Haddon Matrix   a framework for classifying factors associated with injury, death, or events that may cause injury or death. The matrix is used to identify factors that can be modified and interventions that can be taken to prevent or reduce the severity of such events.

index of suspicion   the anticipation of injury to a body region, organ, or structure based on analysis of the mechanism of injury.

mechanism of injury (MOI)   the processes and forces that cause trauma.

penetrating trauma   injury caused by an object breaking the skin and entering the body.

trauma   a physical injury or wound caused by external force or violence.

trauma center   a hospital that has the capability of caring for acutely injured patients; trauma centers must meet strict criteria to use this designation.

trauma registry   a data retrieval system for trauma patient information, which is used to evaluate and improve the trauma system.

trauma triage criteria   guidelines to aid prehospital personnel in determining which trauma patients require urgent transportation to a trauma center.

Special Considerations in Trauma

Robert S. Porter, MA, EMT-P

STANDARD
Trauma (Trauma Overview; Multisystem Trauma)

COMPETENCY
Integrates assessment findings with principles of epidemiology and pathophysiology to formulate a field impression to implement a comprehensive treatment/disposition plan for an acutely injured patient.

OBJECTIVES

Terminal Performance Objective
After reading this chapter you should be able to integrate principles of trauma management, injury prevention, and care of special patient populations into professional decision making to impact trauma morbidity and mortality.

Enabling Objectives
To accomplish the terminal performance objective, you should be able to:

1. Define key terms introduced in this chapter.
2. Describe the importance of an organized system of trauma care to reducing trauma morbidity and mortality.
3. Describe the potential impact of full engagement of EMS in injury prevention initiatives.
4. Describe the key actions and decisions in each phase of trauma assessment.
5. Given a variety of trauma patient scenarios, identify signs and symptoms of injury.
6. Given a variety of trauma patient scenarios, demonstrate assessment-based decision making, including treatment and transport decisions.
7. Recognize the need for immediate lifesaving interventions, including airway management, ensuring adequate oxygenation and ventilation, controlling external hemorrhage, providing appropriate fluid resuscitation, and performing pleural decompression.
8. Describe the importance of recognizing, preventing, and treating hypothermia in trauma patients.
9. Describe the differences in anatomy, physiology, pathophysiology, assessment, and management of pediatric trauma patients.
10. Describe the differences in anatomy, physiology, pathophysiology, assessment, and management of pregnant trauma patients.
11. Describe the differences in anatomy, physiology, pathophysiology, assessment, and management of bariatric trauma patients.
12. Describe the differences in anatomy, physiology, pathophysiology, assessment, and management of geriatric trauma patients.

From Chapter 13 of *Paramedic Care: Principles & Practice, Volume 5,* Fourth Edition. Bryan Bledsoe, Robert Porter, and Richard Cherry. Copyright © 2013 by Pearson Education, Inc. All rights reserved.

hypoperfusion   hypothermia   hypovolemia
hypotension

CASE STUDY

At 2:30 A.M., County Dispatch calls ALS 21 to the scene of an auto collision on Highway 192. Once en route ALS 21, and paramedic Alex Dalburg, receive an update on the crash. An OnStar dispatcher reports a serious frontal impact with air bag deployment at the GPS coordinates of Highway 192, one mile south of Bronson Road. The OnStar dispatcher is unable to communicate with the vehicle occupants. County Dispatch also reports that Emmerson Police, Fire Rescue, and their BLS Ambulance units are responding as well.

As ALS 21 arrives at the scene, Alex notes the police and fire services have secured the scene and have routed traffic safely around the collision site. There are two vehicles that have collided head-on in the northbound lane of the divided highway. A sedan and a pickup truck have sustained severe front-end damage, the front windows are broken out, and it appears the air bags have deployed. An EMT from the Emmerson Fire Department Ambulance reports the driver of the pickup truck is conscious, alert, and apparently uninjured. The driver of the sedan appears unconscious. Both drivers wore lap and shoulder belts.

Alex reports to the sedan to find an early twenties female unresponsive to his initial introduction and his query "Are you OK?" He directs the EMT to enter the vehicle from the other side and initiate spinal precautions. Alex notes some snoring airway sounds that clear as the EMT brings her head and neck from flexion to the neutral position. A quick check of her radial pulse reveals a rapid and strong pulse but no response as he asks the woman to grasp his fingers. Capillary refill is at about 3 seconds. Alex places his hand on her upper chest and notes modest chest rise at a slightly rapid rate. Further examination of the passenger compartment reveals the steering wheel and dash have been pushed inward and are trapping the woman against the seat. Alex categorizes her as unstable because of her unresponsiveness and asks fire rescue to extricate her quickly.

While they prepare the equipment, Alex begins a rapid trauma assessment. Using a penlight to illuminate the woman's face, neck, and left arm, Alex notices a bit of air bag dust but the facial features and assessment are otherwise unremarkable. Her skin is slightly pale in color. The left pupil is slowly reactive to light and Alex cannot access the right pupil. The neck appears symmetrical with flat jugular veins. Palpation of the upper chest notes a "crackling like" feeling with skin that moves under his fingers and quick auscultation picks up only very quiet breath sounds on the right and somewhat louder sounds on the left. Alex notes that her respiratory rate appears to have increased and is now about 26 breaths per minute. Alex cannot continue his rapid trauma assessment while the woman remains trapped in the car.

Emmerson Fire Rescue has their equipment ready and begins disentanglement. After about 45 seconds, they have removed the roof and have pushed the dash forward and seat back, freeing the woman. Rapid extrication ensues and the woman is moved to the awaiting stretcher, where a cervical collar is applied and she is firmly secured. A quick look at the abdomen defines that this women is pregnant and probably in the late second or early third trimester. Both lower extremities appear distorted and Alex suspects bilateral femur fractures and a possible pelvic fracture. Alex continues his assessment while the EMTs place a splint between the patient's legs and firmly immobilize the lower extremities. Alex notices a grating feeling as he compresses the ribs inward (probable rib fractures) and confirms reduced breath sounds over the entire left thorax. The left thorax is hyperresonant to percussion.

An EMT reports the blood pressure is 66 by palpation and the pulse is at a rate greater than 140. Pulse oximetry intermittently reads about 84 percent and displays a pulse rate of about 146. Alex calls for high-concentration oxygen via nonrebreather mask and prepares for needle decompression of the chest. Chest decompression appears to release some air and the woman's breathing rate slows and depth increases. Alex decides to rapidly transport the patient to the ambulance, then to the trauma center with IVs started en route.

Once in the ambulance, Alex tilts the entire spine board 15 degrees, elevating the right side. Alex starts one IV with normal saline, a nonrestrictive three-way valve, and trauma tubing. He administers a quick 500 mL bolus of fluid and rechecks vital signs. The automatic BP cuff displays 72/46 and a pulse rate of 148. Oxygen saturation is 92 and the pregnant woman does not respond to painful stimuli as Alex squeezes the fleshy skin between the thumb and first finger. Alex reassesses respiration and notes breath sounds on the left and right are now equal. Because of the pregnancy and the MOI, Alex inspects for vaginal bleeding and finds a small amount of hemorrhage.

On arrival at the emergency department the trauma team takes Alex's report and performs a quick assessment. They place a chest tube in the fifth intercostal space along the left midaxillary line and then arrange for a CT scan of the head, neck, chest, and abdomen and an ultrasound of the uterus and fetus. While waiting for the scans, the emergency department staff administers packed red blood cells and more fluids, the blood pressure rises to 86/62, and the pulse slows some. Fetal heart tones are not found by auscultation or by Doppler.

Shortly after returning to quarters, ALS 21 receives a call from the trauma center. The woman had an apparent placental abruption and miscarried about 30 minutes after arrival. She has regained consciousness from an apparent concussion and is in serious condition but expected to recover.

INTRODUCTION TO SHOCK TRAUMA RESUSCITATION

In the mid-1960s, trauma was identified as the neglected disease of a modern society. At that time, more than 150,000 persons died each year from trauma, while even greater numbers suffered some level of disability. Health care leaders, recognizing that no organized system existed to care for these victims, took the first steps toward forming what has grown into today's emergency medical services system. Forty-five years later, EMS has become a highly sophisticated system, yet 177,000 lives are still lost yearly to trauma (Figure 1 ●).[1] Most of these lives are taken, not at the end of a progressive disease in the later years of life, but from young and active members of society. Today, research has indicated that the skills that have been mainstays of prehospital trauma care often do not affect patient outcome and, worse, they occasionally increase patient mortality and morbidity.

As professionals in the field of prehospital emergency care, we need to look carefully and honestly at our actions and ensure that they best serve our patients. We must do several things to secure a future for prehospital emergency care and to ensure that our patients receive the best chances for survival. We must help strike at trauma at its source by supporting and promoting injury prevention in our society. We need to ensure that our

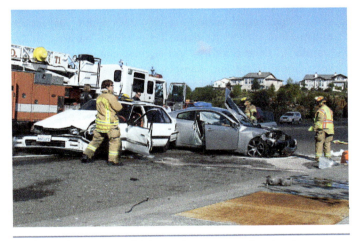

● **Figure 1**   Motor vehicle crashes account for about 30 percent of trauma fatalities in the United States. (© *Joshua Menzies*)

practices are current and truly benefit those who receive our care. Finally, we need to function as an integrated component of the health care system serving our patients and our communities. To help accomplish these objectives, this chapter examines injury prevention, trauma assessment, shock/multisystem trauma resuscitation, care for special patients (pediatric, pregnant, bariatric, geriatric, and cognitively impaired), care provider interaction, air medical service, and trauma research.

INJURY PREVENTION

Of all the care procedures and advanced interventions available to treat the trauma patient, none has more promise for reducing mortality and morbidity than prevention. Here, we in emergency medical services can learn a great deal from the fire service. The efforts of the fire service in encouraging smoke and carbon monoxide detector use, promoting more rigorous fire codes and inspections, and educating the public—especially children—about both the dangers of fire and the techniques to preserve life during fire are credited with greatly decreasing fire incidence, morbidity, and mortality. These fire service efforts are a valuable model for programs aimed at reducing death and disability from trauma.

If EMS is to maintain a leadership role in prehospital emergency care, we must place a new and continuing emphasis on injury prevention. The "Let's Not Meet by Accident" program, developed jointly by a trauma system and prehospital providers, is just one example of a prevention program. It aims both to acquaint high school students with EMS and to alert them to trauma hazards in our society. Other citizen groups have formed to help increase public awareness of social behaviors that lead to trauma. One such group, Mothers Against Drunk Driving (MADD), draws attention to the highway death toll associated with driving while alcohol or substance impaired. The EMS system must encourage or conduct programs like these with active participation from prehospital care providers to fulfill its responsibilities to the community.

A new program, sponsored by EMS and modeled after the fire service approach to prevention, is the home inspection (Figure 2 ●). After a significant event, such as the birth of a child, local EMS personnel perform a voluntary home inspection. The inspectors survey the home for potential hazards, notify the family of their findings, and suggest changes that would increase home safety. For example, inspectors might check the temperature of the hot water tank (and suggest lowering it when necessary) to prevent scalding injury to children; examine infant cribs to ensure the slats are close enough to prevent strangulation and other injuries; and test child auto seats for proper fit and instruct parents in their proper use. They might also check for ground fault outlets in bathrooms, overloaded electrical sockets or circuits, electrical cords under rugs, and other improper electrical connections. The inspectors can recommend installation of railings or replacement of treads on stairways, porches, and other potential fall locations. While in the home the crew also ensures there are adequate smoke and carbon monoxide detectors with fresh batteries. While carrying on the inspection, the EMS crew can also promote other safe practices such as the use of helmets and other protective equipment for motorcycling, skateboarding, in-line skating, and bicycling. In addition, they can instruct the family on the best way to access police, fire, and medical services in the event of emergency. Widespread adoption of programs like these carries a tremendous potential to reduce trauma mortality and morbidity by reducing trauma in the home. These programs also introduce family members to the EMS team before an emergency strikes, thus helping to foster a good public image for the EMS system.

Currently, the Occupational Safety and Health Administration (OSHA) and other governmental agencies have developed and are enforcing workplace safety standards. Their efforts ensure that the workplace is reasonably safe and that workers are provided both with training in safe practices and with protective equipment appropriate to their work environment. The Department of Transportation is constantly improving motor vehicle safety through encouragement of better highway and vehicle design, testing, and inspection. These DOT programs ensure that the highways are safer and crashes are more survivable. Other governmental and quasigovernmental agencies monitor the safety of various products like children's toys, electronic equipment, and other consumer products.

An important consideration to keep in mind regarding any safety education program is the impact serious trauma has on the young male population. Males between 13 and 35 years of age account for about 27 percent of all serious trauma injuries and over 30 percent of all trauma deaths (Figure 3 ●).[2] At the same time, this group represents less than 20 percent of the total population. Thus, trauma among young males represents an epidemic of serious proportions. It is probable that the risk-taking nature of young males and an associated disregard for safe practices (like failure to use seat belts and motorcycle helmets and a willingness to drink and drive) contribute to this mortality. Encouraging behavioral changes in this population would likely have a marked effect on the overall incidence of trauma and the associated death and disability. Since many people entering EMS are of this gender and age group, we need to both speak to the problem and demonstrate safe practices by example to our peers.

TRAUMA ASSESSMENT

Trauma patient assessment is essential both to determining patient transport priority and identifying and prioritizing patient injuries for care. In this chapter, we review trauma assessment in a comprehensive way, much as you would when presented with a seriously injured trauma patient.

Trauma assessment progresses through the scene size-up, the primary assessment, the secondary assessment (either the rapid or focused trauma assessment), and is then followed by serial reassessments. However, your first opportunity to begin the assessment process is through a review of the dispatch information.

Dispatch Information

Dispatch information provides critical information that you can evaluate while responding to the scene. This information provides the nature of the call. Often, it specifies the mechanism of injury (like a fall, shooting, or auto crash) or the nature of the injury (like a broken leg, head injury, or deep laceration). This information permits you to prepare for patient care and to contemplate your

Welcome to the World Injury Prevention Survey
Orange County Emergency Medical Services
09/20/98

Family's Name	Phone Number
Address	City / Zipcode
Mother's Name	Mothers Age
Father's Name	Father's Age

EMS DATA:
Date | Paramedic Name/Number | Trip Number | IRV Number/Zone | Grid Number | On Scene Time | Back In Service Time

Individual Interviewed: ☐ Mother ☐ Father ☐ Other   Number of people living in home   Adults: ____   Children: ____

Childs Name	Date of Birth	Last Non-Sick MD Visit

Home Info

Building Type: ☐ Apartment ☐ Rented Room/Floor ☐ Mobile Home   Ownership: ☐ Public Housing
☐ Duplex ☐ Condominium ☐ Single Unit House   ☐ Rented ☐ Owned

Number of Stories (levels): 1 2 3 4   Interior Stairway: Yes No   No. of Doorway Exits: ____   Pool: Yes No   Latched Gate between House and Pool: Yes No

Fire Prevention and Safety

Smoke Detector 1 Location:	Ceiling Wall	Beep: Yes No	No. of Batteries Provided:
Smoke Detector 2 Location:	Ceiling Wall	Beep: Yes No	
Smoke Detector 3 Location:	Ceiling Wall	Beep: Yes No	Smoke Detector Provided: Yes No

Fire Extinguisher 1 Location: ____ Charged: Yes No   Fire Extinguisher 2 Location: ____ Charged: Yes No

Fire Exit Plan: Yes No   Have had Practice Drill: Yes No   If Yes to Drill, How often: Monthly Yearly Other _____

Space Heater 1 Location: ____ Type: Kerosene Electrical   Space Heater 2 Location: ____ Type: Kerosene Electrical

Are Woodstoves/Fireplaces used at this site: Yes No   If Yes, When was the Chimney last cleaned: ☐ < 1 Year ☐ > 1 Year

Education:
- Discuss Smoke Detector Pamphlet
- Discuss Fire Prevention and Emergency Exit Materials
- Advise to have Chimney cleaned if not done in the past 1 year.

First Aid

First Aid Kit in home: Yes No   First Aid Kit provided: Yes No   Emergency Numbers posted in visible place near phone: Yes No

Medications out of Reach: Yes No   Medications Locked up: Yes No   Poison Control Center Number posted visibly near phone: Yes No

Cleaning Supplies out of Reach: Yes No   Cleaning Supplies Locked up: Yes No

Education: Discuss 911 and Poison Control Information

Firearms

Do you keep firearms locked up: Yes No   How many firearms in the home _____

Are any firearms loaded: Yes No   Are all firearms locked up: Yes No   If not locked up, are trigger locks used: Yes No

Education: Discuss Firearm Safety

AC

Are Electrical Outlets in Child's Bedroom and Playareas covered: Yes No   AC Outlet Covers provided: Yes No

Education: Discuss Electrical Risk

Water

Where do you bathe your child   ☐ Kitchen Sink   ☐ Bathroom Sink   ☐ Bathroom Tub

(Test 2 Locations)   Temperature _____   Temperature _____   Temperature _____

Education: Temperature should be < or = to 120 degrees

Crib

Crib railings spaced less than 2 3/8 inches apart: Yes No   Is Crib near any cords (ie window blinds): Yes No

Crib Mattress fits snugly (less than 2 fingers space between mattress and crib around all edges): Yes No

Education: Discuss Crib Safety and Strangulation Risk

Car Seats

Is there an infant car seat for the newborn: Yes No   Where does the **infant** ride in the car: ☐ Front ☐ Rear

Does the Vehicle have a passenger side air bag: Yes No   ☐ Rear Facing ☐ Forward Facing

Do Children over 40 lbs wear seatbelts: Yes No   Are car seats available for all other children under 40 lbs: Yes No

Education: Discuss Car Seat Safety Materials

W Bag/Referrals

Were the contents of the Welcome Bag reviewed with the parent: Yes No

Follow-up Visit or Referrals Requested:
☐ Smoke Detector / Batteries   ☐ Health Department-Health Services
☐ Rental Without Smoke Detector   ☐ Health Department-Safety Services
☐ Other _____   ☐ Health Department-Special Programs

Education: Record Details of Each Item in the Comment Area

Comments/Concerns

_____

Family contacted and declines visit ☐   Please Write Additional Comments or Concerns on the back of this form   Paramedic Signature: _____

Figure 2   A sample home safety inspection form.

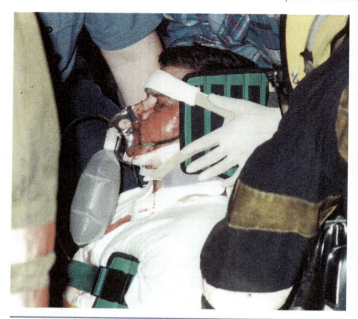

● **Figure 3** Young males account for a disproportionate representation of mortality and morbidity among trauma victims. (© Mark C. Ide)

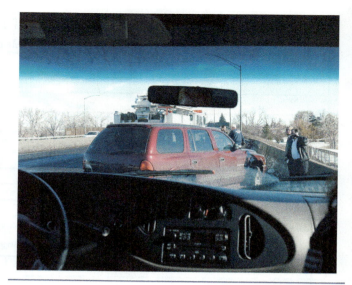

● **Figure 4** Assess the emergency scene quickly and carefully, looking for scene hazards, possible mechanisms of injury, the location of patients, and the possible need for additional resources. (© Jeff Forster)

approach to the scene. Occasionally, the dispatch information may suggest the scene is too dangerous to approach until it is secured by the police (such as cases of violence like shootings, stabbings, or domestic altercations with injuries). In such cases, you should remain at a distance from the scene until police arrive and notify you that it is safe to enter. At other times, dispatch information may alert you to potential hazards such as a toxic gas release or downed electrical wires for which you may need to request specialized response teams to secure the scene. This information also can cause you to be wary of the dangers as you approach the scene.

Use dispatch information to anticipate and prepare for your injury care. To speed your response at the scene, locate any equipment you will be likely to use. If appropriate, lay the equipment out on the stretcher so it can be taken immediately to the patient. (It is always easier to have a first responder or bystander return a piece of equipment to the ambulance than it is to ask them to go to the ambulance, find it, and bring it to the patient's side.) Inspect the equipment, check to see that it is working properly, and review its application and use. If you expect severe injuries, set up an IV bag and administration set in the ambulance for later use on the patient. This saves time that would otherwise be taken from patient care to assemble the administration equipment. Finally, review the assessment and care you intend to provide and, as necessary, review your protocols to ensure you are ready to respond to the emergency. These actions help you move quickly through the required care steps and to offer the optimum patient care in the shortest span of time.

Scene Size-Up

Trauma scene size-up involves several major elements (Figure 4 ●): identifying scene hazards including the need for Standard Precautions, determining the mechanism of injury, accounting for and locating all patients, requesting any

additional resources, identifying any environmental factors that might impact patient assessment and care, and establishing or linking up with scene oversight. The mechanism of injury analysis is also essential to help you anticipate and identify all scene hazards.

Mechanism of Injury Analysis

Analyze the mechanism of injury by re-creating the incident in your mind, and from that, anticipating the cause, nature, and severity of your patient's injuries (the index of suspicion). Take any evidence available to you as you arrive at, and first view, the scene, and use that evidence to determine exactly how the forces were expressed to the patient. If two autos came together, for example, determine what vehicle surfaces collided, from which direction the vehicles were traveling, and which patient surfaces were impacted (Figure 5 ●). Use the amount of

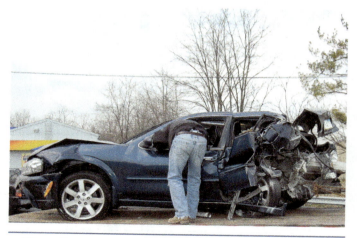

● **Figure 5** Analyze the forces of a vehicle collision and, based on that analysis, anticipate possible patient injuries. (© Edward T. Dickinson, MD)

internal compartment vehicular damage to approximate the impact energy delivered and then determine whether restraints or air bags were deployed that may have reduced the injury potential. Frontal and rear impacts afford the vehicle occupants the most protection, especially if seat belts are properly worn and air bags deploy. (Air bags deploy only in frontal and lateral impacts.) Lateral and rollover impacts are likely to cause the most serious injuries. (Remember, modern vehicle design has the ability to absorb great amounts of energy while protecting the patient. Confirm any suspicion of serious injury with the physical signs and symptoms gathered during the assessment.) In motorcycle, bicycle, and pedestrian-vs.-vehicle collisions, identify the relative speed of impact and appreciate the lack of protection afforded the victim. In other non-vehicular blunt trauma, examine the height of the fall or other indications of impact energy and the point of impact as well as the transmission path of those forces through the body.

When assessing the mechanism of injury for penetrating trauma, look at the relative velocity of the offending agent or projectile. Remember that an increase in mass directly increases the force's energy, while an increase in speed greatly increases (a squared relationship) the impact energy and the potential for serious patient injury. With gunshot wounds, identify the nature of the weapon (handgun, shotgun, or rifle), the relative power and profile (caliber), and then the distance and angle between the gun barrel and the impact point. Visualize the pathway taken by the bullet and its destructive power as it travels through human tissue. Head, central chest, and upper abdominal injuries are most lethal. Remember, however, that the bullet's path is frequently deflected from a straight line. In other penetrating trauma, mentally re-create the injury process and use kinetic energy principles to analyze the nature, process, and severity of the injury. Try to determine the object length and the depth and angle of insertion.

From your re-creation of the injury process, identify the individual organs affected and the extent of the injury to them. Approximate what significance their injury will have on the patient's condition and how it will affect him as time progresses. Assign each suspected injury a priority for both assessment and care. Finally, approximate the seriousness of your patient's overall condition and the potential need for either (1) rapid transport with most care provided en route or (2) on-scene care and then transport or (3) treatment and release (as permitted by protocol). Remember that patients with preexisting medical conditions, patients of advanced age, and the very young are at greatest risk when seriously injured. If there is more than one patient, identify the most seriously injured and order your patient assessment and care accordingly.

Hazard Identification

The mechanism of injury analysis helps you to identify many possible hazards at the scene. Search out all hazards and protect yourself, your patient, bystanders, and fellow rescuers from them. These hazards include the mechanism that injured your patient and may range from traffic associated with the auto crash to the assailant who is still holding a handgun. Search for additional sources of blunt and penetrating trauma such as the broken glass and jagged metal at an auto crash scene or moving machinery at an industrial injury site. Also search out and exclude any hazards from fire, heat, explosion, electricity, toxic chemicals, radiation, or deadly gas at each and every scene. It is important to rule out these hazards rather than just to note them when they are obvious. Otherwise you risk injury to yourself, fellow rescuers, the patient, and bystanders. Look for hazardous material placards. Your ambulance should carry the most current Department of Transportation's *Emergency Response Guidebook,* which will help you identify the type of material and the level of risk. (However, it is not the role of EMS to directly address the risks of hazardous materials. That responsibility lies with the hazardous material team or fire department.)

Be aware of the presence and mood of family members, bystanders, and crowds at the emergency scene. These people may welcome your assistance, obstruct your ability to assess and care, or possibly represent a serious threat of violence.

Analyze the scene carefully to identify each of these hazards and exclude them from the scene or be prepared to deal with each before you approach the patient. Your well-being and that of your patient depend on it.[3] If you are injured at the scene you will be less able to help your patient and may, in fact, yourself become a patient rather than a caregiver. For the paramedic, safety must be a lifestyle.

Standard Precautions

A special type of hazard existing at almost every emergency scene is the presence of body fluids and substances with the potential to spread infection (Figure 6 ●). Realize that infection risk extends to both you and your patient, especially when dealing with trauma. While a patient's open wound releases blood

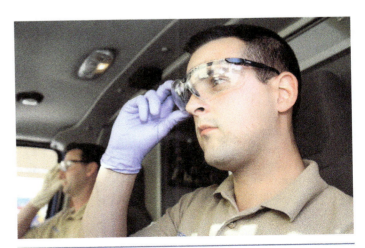

● **Figure 6** Use Standard Precautions at all scenes. (© *Dr. Bryan E. Bledsoe*)

that poses an infection threat to you and others, the open wound presents a pathway through which infection can enter your patient's body. The use of gloves and other Standard Precautions protects both you and your patient. Ensure that all rescuers who may come into contact with the patient also employ appropriate Standard Precautions as you prepare to approach the scene.

In all patient contacts, it is essential to don gloves in anticipation of contact with blood, saliva, mucus, urine, or fecal material. If the scene size-up reveals multiple patients, put on two or three sets of gloves, one over the other. Then peel gloves off as you move from one patient to another. If you prefer not to double glove, be sure to carry additional glove pairs and change them with each patient contact or at any time they become contaminated. Remember that body fluids from one patient are potentially as infectious to another patient as they are to you. Also remember that with any open wound the risk of infection transmission increases.

Your analysis of the mechanism of injury may also suggest airway or chest trauma or possible external arterial hemorrhage. These injuries may result in spurting blood or in blood or other fluids being propelled or coughed into the air. In such cases, wear both eye protection and splatter protection for your clothing. A mask may also be advisable. Consider wearing a mask if you have any type of respiratory infection, again to protect your patient. Ensure that all rescuers use the appropriate personal protective equipment (PPE). Once at the patient's side, your continuing patient evaluation may reveal the need for higher levels of protection than the scene size-up suggested; for this reason, always have goggles, gowns, masks, and additional gloves handy.

Accounting For and Locating All Patients

During your scene size-up, identify the number of likely patients and their locations around the emergency scene. During a collision, patients may be thrown from an auto or trapped within a twisted wreck and completely out of sight (this most frequently occurs with infants). A patient may also leave the vehicle and mill about the scene with bystanders, leave in an attempt to find help, or simply wander from the scene in confusion. Search for evidence that suggests the number and types of patients. Consider the number of vehicles involved in a crash; the number of spiderwebs on the windshields; purses or articles of clothing; and child seats, clothing, or toys. As you arrive at the scene, question the apparent patients and bystanders to better determine the number and locations of any additional patients.

Determining Resource Needs

Once you determine the likely number of patients and their injuries, estimate the type and nature of any other emergency medical resources that will be needed at the scene (Figure 7 ●). This may include additional ambulances, one for each seriously injured patient, and air medical service for patients who meet trauma triage criteria at a scene more than 45 minutes from the nearest trauma center (or as otherwise established by your system's protocols).

Also, determine the resources needed to control hazards identified in your scene analysis. These resources may include police for traffic control or for scene security with gathering

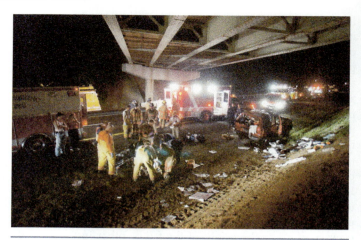

● **Figure 7** Assess the emergency scene to determine the need for any additional resources. (© *Mark C. Ide*)

crowds, a heavy rescue unit for extrication, the hazardous material team for fuel and oil spill cleanup, the power company for downed electrical lines, or the fire service for potential fire control at vehicle crashes. It is essential that you contact dispatch early so needed equipment and trained personnel are quickly en route to the scene. Waiting until later in the call delays their arrival and may hinder your ability to access and care for patients.

Environmental Considerations

Vehicle collisions and other trauma-causing events do not always occur on bright sunny days in 70-degree weather. View the scene and consciously note any impact weather might have on your ability to access, assess, care for, and move your patient. Rain-soaked grassy surfaces or those covered with ice or snow may make patient movement more risky. Weather extremes like excessive heat or cold may give you less time at the scene to assess and care. Wind and driving rain may make obtaining vital signs and bandaging and splinting less practical outside the ambulance. Evaluate the ambient lighting to determine any special needs for scene and patient lighting.

Scene Oversight

At the end of the scene size-up, you should have the information necessary to organize an overall incident response and determine the special focus of your assessment for each patient. Take a few seconds to organize how you will address the scene and coordinate additional resources as they arrive. Identify in your mind what you wish each respective service to accomplish and how these functions can best work together to meet your patient's needs. Then think through your primary assessment and what specific problems you might expect to find with each element of that evaluation for each patient (Figure 8 ●).

Also, define roles and assign tasks to the members of your crew. If you find you are responding to an incident that will require many different services (police, fire, rescue, and otherwise), ensure scene oversight or incident command is established. If not, do a scene walk-around, report your findings to dispatch and report yourself as incident command. (This will be temporary as your skills are best applied to assessment [or triage]

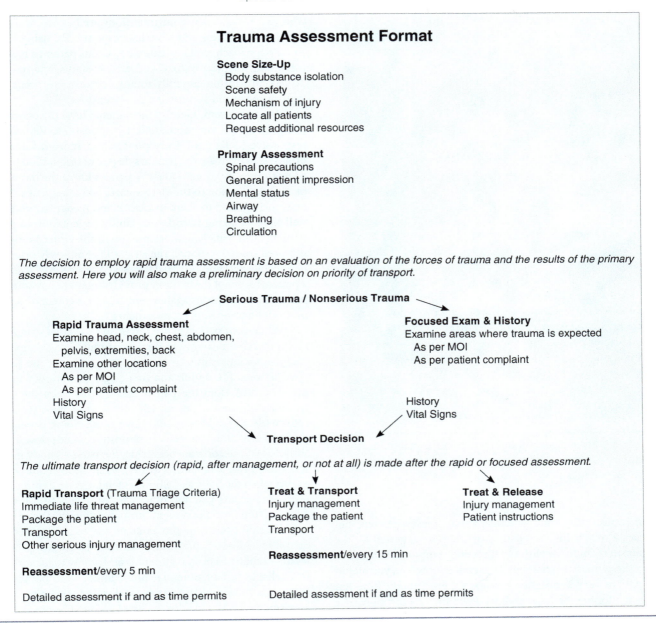

Trauma Assessment Format

Scene Size-Up
Body substance isolation
Scene safety
Mechanism of injury
Locate all patients
Request additional resources

Primary Assessment
Spinal precautions
General patient impression
Mental status
Airway
Breathing
Circulation

The decision to employ rapid trauma assessment is based on an evaluation of the forces of trauma and the results of the primary assessment. Here you will also make a preliminary decision on priority of transport.

Serious Trauma / Nonserious Trauma

Rapid Trauma Assessment
Examine head, neck, chest, abdomen,
 pelvis, extremities, back
Examine other locations
 As per MOI
 As per patient complaint
History
Vital Signs

Focused Exam & History
Examine areas where trauma is expected
 As per MOI
 As per patient complaint

History
Vital Signs

Transport Decision

The ultimate transport decision (rapid, after management, or not at all) is made after the rapid or focused assessment.

Rapid Transport (Trauma Triage Criteria)
Immediate life threat management
Package the patient
Transport
Other serious injury management

Reassessment/every 5 min

Detailed assessment if and as time permits

Treat & Transport
Injury management
Package the patient
Transport

Reassessment/every 15 min

Detailed assessment if and as time permits

Treat & Release
Injury management
Patient instructions

● **Figure 8**   A trauma assessment form can help you organize priorities at any emergency scene.

and patient care.) If incident command is established, ensure you integrate with it to report the number and seriousness of patient injuries and communicate your needs.

Primary Assessment

The primary assessment is intended to identify immediate patient life threats and correct them before a more detailed assessment continues. It consists of determining a general patient impression, applying spinal precautions when needed, and assessing the patient's airway, breathing, and circulatory status. If any serious or life-threatening problem is found, correct it immediately. As you carry out these steps, you add to the information you gathered during the scene size-up and continue to refine your general patient impression. Finally, you determine your patient's priority for assessment, care, and transport.

General Impression

The mechanism of injury analysis and the index of suspicion for injuries begin the development of a general patient impression. You continue to refine that impression as you arrive at your patient's side. Include any information you gather as you determine the need for spinal precautions and as you evaluate the patient's mental status, airway, breathing, and circulation. Add to it the general appearance and mental status you observe during these first few minutes at the patient's side. This general patient impression (Figure 9 ●) grows to include the seriousness of the patient's injuries and your patient's priority for care and transport. These determinations are very challenging to make early in your career; however, with experience, your level of comfort in judging patient severity and identifying the need for either rapid transport or on-scene care will grow.

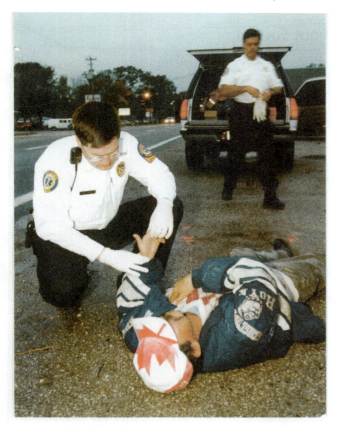

● **Figure 9** Form a general impression of the patient during the primary assessment and refine it during the rest of your time at the patient's side. (© *Craig Jackson/In the Dark Photography*)

In some cases, your general patient impression will not necessarily match the seriousness of trauma suggested by the mechanism of injury or with the signs and symptoms you gather during the primary assessment. Remember, however, you attend your patient very soon after trauma. Often, enough time has not passed for hemorrhage to draw down the blood supply. The body is not yet required to employ the most extreme compensatory mechanisms and does not yet display the most noticeable signs and symptoms of shock. Remain suspicious of developing hypovolemia and observe carefully for even the most subtle and early signs and symptoms of shock. On the other hand, the mechanism of injury may not reflect the actual injury severity and the patient may appear (and be) in a worse condition than expected. In all cases, base your patient management on the worst case scenario. As time and further assessment continue, modify your general patient impression and the care it suggests.

Mental Status

As you develop the general patient impression, evaluate the patient's mental status. Begin by introducing yourself, identifying your level of training, and explaining your desire to offer care to the patient. Extend your hand and offer to shake hands with the patient. While asking the patient what happened and what is bothering him the most, palpate the patient's radial pulse. This permits the patient to refuse care, ensures that he knows who you are and that your intentions are helpful, and calls for a physical reaction and a verbal response. By using this or a similar approach, you evaluate a conscious patient's mental status and airway, respiratory, and cardiac status, and in less than 30 seconds. Listen carefully to any responses as you continue your primary and secondary assessments.

At a minimum, identify the patient's level of consciousness using the AVPU mnemonic (*A*lert; responsive to *V*erbal stimuli; responsive to *P*ain; or *U*nresponsive). A more discerning approach is to evaluate the patient's degree of orientation by asking a few simple questions. Does the patient know the day and time of day (orientation to time); recognize what happened or where he is (orientation to event or place); and recognize who he is as well as recognizing friends and family (orientation to person)? (Patients will usually lose orientation in this order.) Orientation is scored from 3 to 0 with the alert and completely oriented patient being alert and oriented times 3 (A + O × 3). Determining a patient's level of orientation provides a baseline reading of the patient's mental status against which improvement or deterioration can be trended in reassessments.

When your patient is not responsive to verbal stimuli, check for the specific response to noxious stimuli. For example, if you apply a noxious stimulus (usually by squeezing the fleshy region between the thumb and first finger or trapezius muscle of the shoulder), does the patient move away from the stimulus (purposeful); move, but not effectively, away from the stimulus (purposeless); or does he not move at all? Some patients move toward a specific body position, or posture, in response to painful stimuli. With decorticate posturing, the patient's body moves toward extension with elbows flexing, while decerebrate posturing occurs when the body and elbows extend. Determining a baseline response permits you and other care providers to track patient deterioration or improvement throughout the course of care.

A helpful technique to evaluate the trauma patient is the Simplified Motor Score (SMS). It involves assessing only two factors—ability to obey commands and ability to localize pain—is a reliable test of potential brain injury and, because of its quickness and simplicity, can be performed during the primary assessment. Review the discussion of SMS in Chapter 11 and see the further discussion later in this chapter.

Spinal Precautions

Employ immediate spinal precautions in *any* of the following circumstances:

● The mechanism of injury suggests the possibility of spinal injury.

● You suspect any extreme of flexion/extension, lateral bending, axial loading, distraction, or rotation of the spine.

● The patient has any significant injury above the shoulders.

● The patient has a reduced level of consciousness (from injury, intoxication, or shock)

Consider discontinuing spinal precautions if you find *all* of the following:

● The patient is alert and fully oriented, has a Glasgow Coma Scale score of 15, is not significantly affected by the "fight-or-flight" response, and is not intoxicated or under the influence of drugs, including alcohol.

- The patient has no distracting injuries (e.g., serious long-bone fracture, other painful injury, shortness of breath, or other serious complaint).

- The patient does not complain of, nor does your assessment identify, any signs or symptoms of spinal injury (pain or tenderness along the midline of the cervical spine or any focal neurologic defects).

- The patient is not elderly or very young.

However, if you have an unreliable patient, significant distracting injuries, or any signs or symptoms of spinal injury, continue spinal precautions, including manual immobilization of the head and spine, application of a cervical collar, and full patient mechanical immobilization to a long spine board or full-body vacuum mattress.

When in doubt, err on the side of full spinal immobilization for your patient. In children and the elderly, signs and symptoms of spinal injury may not be as specific or obvious. Hence, maintain full spinal precautions, even if the previously listed criteria are met.

Airway

It is easy to evaluate the airway in the conscious patient by listening to him speak. If he can talk clearly, you know that the patient has control over an open airway, is breathing adequately enough to speak in full sentences, and has cerebral oxygenation enough to support conscious thought. If the speech is broken or forced, there are unusual airway sounds, or the statements are confused or unintelligible, suspect and further evaluate the airway and breathing for problems.

In the unconscious patient, watch to see if the chest rises and falls. Listen for the sound of air moving during respirations and feel for escaping air during exhalation. Reposition the patient's head and jaw with the head-tilt/chin-lift or the jaw thrust as needed. If repositioning improves air movement, then consider inserting an oral airway. If the patient does not have protective airway reflexes, consider early airway protection with an extraglottic airway or intubation, either now (if the airway is at immediate risk) or at the end of the primary assessment.

If you note airway sounds like stridor, snoring, gurgling, or wheezing, presume a partial airway obstruction that will get worse during assessment and care. Trauma to airway soft tissue will likely cause swelling and progressive airway restriction. Expect swelling to seriously obstruct respiration and again consider early airway protection.

Breathing

Apply a pulse oximeter and then administer only enough supplemental oxygen to maintain the SpO_2 above 96 percent. Avoid hyperoxia. Watch for symmetrical chest and abdominal movement with each breath. If necessary, expose the chest for a better assessment. Rule out flail chest or stabilize the flail segment and provide overdrive ventilation (bag-valve masking the breathing patient). Rule out diaphragmatic breathing (associated with cervical spine injury) or provide overdrive ventilation.

If the patient complains of dyspnea or if chest excursion or tidal volumes seem limited, auscultate the lung fields to identify unilateral diminished or absent breath sounds. Percuss the chest for resonance: A dull sound indicates blood in the pleural space, while hyperresonance indicates air, under pressure, in the pleural space. If you cannot rule out a building tension pneumothorax, consider needle decompression. If you note pneumothorax or decompress a tension pneumothorax, monitor the chest carefully for the development or redevelopment of tension pneumothorax.

If respirations are less than 10 per minute and/or the tidal volume appears less than a normal breath in the unconscious patient, consider overdrive ventilation. If the patient is breathing rapidly but ineffectively, you should also consider overdrive ventilation. If the patient is not breathing, ventilate at 10 to 12 times per minute with full breaths (500 mL) with high-concentration oxygen using the bag-valve mask and reservoir. Ensure good chest rise in the patient and maintain an oxygen saturation of greater than 96 percent. Use capnography to guide your ventilation (35 to 45 mmHg of carbon dioxide), especially in the head injury patient (30 to 40 mmHg of carbon dioxide) (Figure 10 ●).

Circulation

Quickly check the radial pulse for strength, regularity, and rate. A strong tachycardia suggests excitement, while a weak and thready pulse suggests shock compensation. If a radial pulse cannot be palpated, check for a carotid pulse. A rapid, weak carotid pulse suggests serious compensation for hypovolemia, the presence of severe hemorrhage (possibly internal), and the probable need for aggressive fluid resuscitation.

During the pulse check also note the patient's skin condition. Cool, clammy, ashen, or pale skin suggests shock compensation. Perform a capillary refill check. If refill takes more than 3 seconds, that finding supports a possible diagnosis of hypovolemia and compensation. (Please note that other conditions

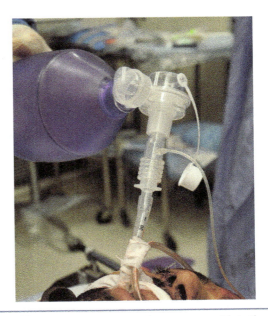

● **Figure 10** Monitor capnography as you ventilate the patient. (© Edward T. Dickinson, MD)

such as smoking, low ambient temperatures, preexisting disease, and use of medications may delay capillary refill as well. Using a central location to measure capillary refill and avoiding the extremities avoid the effects of these conditions.)

Make a quick visual sweep of the body, looking for any signs of serious and continuing hemorrhage. Using your mechanism of injury analysis, identify probable locations of bleeding and view them or, if the site is hidden from view, carefully pass a gloved hand under the area, looking for evidence of blood loss on your gloves. Also use the mechanism of injury analysis to identify likely locations of internal injury and any associated internal hemorrhage. Use this information to approximate the rate of probable blood loss and the priority for rapid transport.

A critical element of the primary assessment is detecting the earliest signs of shock. Remember that internal hemorrhage is the greatest killer of patients who survive the initial impact of trauma. Look carefully at your patient for any early signs of shock. These include a decreased level of consciousness or orientation, or increasing anxiety, restlessness, or combativeness. If the patient has consumed alcohol or is otherwise affected by drugs, be especially watchful and wary.

As internal hemorrhage continues, the body employs more drastic measures to compensate for the blood loss, and signs and symptoms become more obvious with the passage of time. The sooner the signs or symptoms develop, the more rapid the internal blood loss and the more quickly a patient is moving through compensated, then uncompensated, then irreversible shock. However, do not wait for signs and symptoms of later stages of shock to appear. At the first signs of hypovolemic compensation, prioritize the patient for immediate transport to the trauma center. If the patient demonstrates any early shock signs or the mechanism of injury suggests serious internal injury, initiate the steps of aggressive shock care that are described later in this chapter.

Concluding the Primary Assessment

As you complete the primary assessment, modify your mechanism of injury analysis based on additional evidence gained at the scene such as a bent steering wheel or intrusion into the passenger compartment. Continue to monitor the scene for safety, remaining alert to any alterations in conditions at the scene and ensuring that all providers, patients, and bystanders are protected from scene hazards (including the use of personal protective equipment).

At the conclusion of the primary assessment for the trauma patient, you must determine whether the patient merits a rapid trauma assessment or is best served by a focused trauma exam. The rapid trauma assessment aims to identify other life threats not revealed during the primary assessment, to provide appropriate rapid intervention, and to ensure that the seriously injured trauma patient receives quick transport to the trauma center. The focused physical exam is used for less seriously injured patients and focuses on the probable injury, or injuries, and their care. With both these categories of patients, you will

also make a preliminary decision about priority for transport. If the patient meets any of the trauma triage criteria, either a mechanism of injury recognized during the scene size-up, a recognized anatomic injury, or a physical condition identified during the primary assessment, consider the patient for rapid transport.

Blunt trauma patients found in cardiac arrest in the prehospital setting rarely, if ever, survive. This has prompted many EMS systems to institute trauma arrest protocols that permit paramedics to halt resuscitation when presented with a pulseless, nonbreathing blunt trauma patient who displays asystole on the ECG (in two leads). This action prevents the consumption of valuable resources by the EMS system and the generation of anxiety and expense for the family for what would be a fruitless effort. Consult your local protocols and medical director for your system's position on trauma arrest resuscitation.

Using the "CUPS" criteria, place your patient into the Critical, Unstable, Potentially unstable, or Stable category. Any patient who does not move out of the primary assessment because you cannot stabilize airway, breathing, or circulation is considered Critical. The unstable patient is one with signs and symptoms that suggest shock or has a potential problem with airway or breathing. A stable patient has relatively limited signs of injury, no major complaints, and no mechanism of injury to suggest serious injury. The potentially unstable patient is one who fits between stable and unstable. Early in your career, you will place a large majority of patients into the potentially unstable category. With experience, the number of patients you place in this category will shrink.

Finally make your preliminary decision regarding the patient's priority for care and transport, using the Centers for Disease Control Guidelines for Triage of Injured Patients, as discussed under "Transport Decision" later in this chapter.

Secondary Assessment

The secondary assessment employs the general examination techniques of questioning, inspection, palpation, auscultation, and percussion. It is either provided as the focused trauma assessment in which assessment is directed to a specific body area to assess a specific and isolated injury, or as the rapid trauma assessment in which assessment focuses where serious injuries are expected and to where serious injury might have occurred. Both the rapid and focused trauma assessments conclude with a quick, abbreviated patient history and the gathering of a set of baseline vital signs.

Questioning

Before you inspect or palpate a body region, question the patient about any symptoms. Symptoms may include sensations of discomfort, pain, pain on movement, tingling, a pins-and-needles sensation (paresthesia), numbness or lack of feeling (anesthesia), weakness, inability to move, or other unusual sensations. Also note the patient's response to the complaint. Patient complaints are subjective, and different people have different levels of pain tolerance. Watch how the patient responds to the pain and how easy it is to distract him from it. This gives you a good approximation of how significant the pain or sensation is to the patient. Report and record any patient complaint in the patient's own words.

Inspection

As you continue inspecting the patient, look first to the skin color. The skin of a Caucasian with normal circulation will appear light pink. Note any ashen (gray or dusky), cyanotic (bluish), or pale (very light pink or white) colorations. In people of color, look at the coloration of the lips, the conjunctiva of the eyes, the palms of the hands, or the soles of the feet. Any discoloration indicates a possible generalized problem like hypovolemia, hypoventilation, or hypothermia. Use the initial coloration you observe as a baseline when you examine specific regions of the body for injury. Look at those regions for erythema, a general reddening of the skin and the first sign of injury. The discoloration of ecchymosis (the "black and blue" normally associated with a contusion) is delayed because it takes the erythrocytes some time to migrate into injured tissue, lose their oxygen, and turn a deeper red or bluish color. A portion of a limb may also change color as a result of problems with distal circulation. The limb may turn pale (and cold) when arterial circulation is reduced or dark red, dusky, or ashen as circulation stagnates or venous return is halted.

The second element of inspection is looking for deformities. These become most recognizable if you carefully examine and compare limb to limb or one side of the body to the other. Deformity can be either an enlargement of the dimensions of a limb or body region or an abnormal angle or position of a limb or region. Enlargement is usually due to the accumulation of fluid—blood as in a hematoma or plasma and interstitial fluid (edema) as in inflammation associated with a contusion—but it may also be associated with the accumulation of air associated with subcutaneous emphysema. Angulation is the unusual positioning of a limb as with a bend in a bone where a bend would not be expected. Such a condition is most likely associated with a fracture. An unusual bend in a joint, meanwhile, suggests either a fracture or dislocation. Muscle spasm or abnormal retraction of a muscle caused by tendon rupture may also cause deformity. Compare any apparent deformity to the opposite limb to better determine the nature and extent of the variance from normal.

The third element of inspection is an examination for disruption of the skin (wounds). Examine for any abrasion of the skin's surface, any tearing of the skin (a laceration), or any signs of skin damage that may be associated with a burn, such as erythema, blistering or gross disruption of the skin, and discoloration. Also look for any penetrations and determine whether they are superficial or deep. Remember that deep wounds that close encourage infection and are often more serious than more grotesque superficial open wounds.

Palpation

After inspection, palpate any area for additional signs of injury. Gently touch the entire surface of the area being evaluated, feeling for general skin and muscle tone, any unusual or warm masses, any grating sensation, or the "Rice Krispies" feel of subcutaneous emphysema. You should also note any muscle spasm (guarding) or pain on palpation (tenderness) that may reflect injury. Determine if that pain is pain on touch (tenderness), pain on movement, or pain on rapid release of pressure (rebound tenderness). (Do not seek out rebound tenderness, but note it if it occurs during your assessment and care.) Also palpate for relative muscle tone—normal, flaccid, or in spasm.

Auscultation

Auscultate the chest carefully to evaluate for the presence and quality of breath sounds. Note side to side, upper lobe to lower lobe, anterior to posterior, or regional differences. Crackles may represent pulmonary edema most commonly related to pulmonary contusion and associated edema in trauma, while side-to-side inequality suggests pneumothorax or tension pneumothorax. Also listen for heart sounds, noting muffled sounds, as in pericardial tamponade. Abdominal auscultation is not merited in trauma because of the time required to adequately assess for bowel sounds and their poor correlation to injury.

Percussion

Percuss each lobe of the chest for resonance. A dull response suggests fluid or blood accumulating in the pleural space. Hyperresonant response suggests air under pressure in the pleural space.

Rapid Trauma Assessment

Use the rapid trauma assessment when you suspect a patient has a serious injury to the body and are inclined to transport him quickly to the trauma center. Such a patient is one who meets the trauma triage criteria: vital signs, anatomic signs of trauma, and mechanism of injury. Also consider consulting with medical direction regarding the transport of seriously injured patients to the trauma center if they are elderly (patients over 55 years); children; patients taking anticoagulants, with bleeding disorders or with end-stage kidney disease; patients with burns; patients in the later stages of pregnancy; or those who, in your judgment, need the services of a trauma center. During the rapid trauma assessment, quickly scan the body looking for hemorrhage or evidence of significant injury and examine the patient's head, neck, chest, abdomen, pelvis, extremities, and back. (Order your assessment to minimize the movement of the patient. For example, if the patient is found lying face down, quickly assess the back before turning the patient for further assessment and care.) Check the distal function in each limb by noting distal pulse strength, skin temperature and color, capillary refill time, and—as appropriate—sensation and grip strength. If you suspect specific injuries, provide a focused evaluation of the body region using the considerations for that region as specified in the detailed physical exam, discussed later in this chapter. Conclude the rapid trauma assessment by taking a quick patient history and a set of vital signs.

Focused Trauma Assessment

The focused trauma assessment is performed on a patient whom you suspect has limited injuries. This is unlikely to be a patient who meets trauma triage criteria. Direct your examination to the location of patient complaint or to any region of injury suggested by the mechanism of injury or by any signs and symptoms noted during the primary assessment. The actual focused trauma assessment uses the examination criteria for the body region as specified in the detailed exam. Like the rapid trauma assessment, it concludes with a quick patient history and vital signs.

Detailed Physical Exam

The detailed physical exam is a comprehensive examination of the entire body to locate and identify signs of injury. It is rarely used in the prehospital setting as seriously injured patients receive attention directed at their life-threatening injuries and time becomes a premium as they are rushed to a trauma center. The patient with moderate or minor injuries receives assessment and care directed just at those injuries (the focused trauma assessment). The only case where a complete detailed exam may be necessary is in a patient with an altered level of consciousness, limited apparent minor injuries, and a mechanism of injury that suggests possible multiple injury sites. Perform the detailed exam only after you have concluded the primary assessment and have stabilized or corrected any life-threatening conditions discovered during it.

The detailed physical exam is an organized and intensive evaluation of each body area: the head, neck, chest, abdomen, back, pelvis, and each extremity. When performing the detailed exam, use the physical assessment techniques of questioning, inspection, palpation, auscultation, and percussion discussed earlier in the chapter. (Using DCAP-BTLS or some other mnemonic or system may help you remember most of the important aspects of the evaluation of a body region.)

Head

When evaluating the head, inspect and palpate its entire surface looking for any deformity, asymmetry, or hemorrhage. In addition to looking for the obvious signs of trauma, direct special attention to the eyes, auditory canal, nose and mouth, and facial region.

Evaluate the eyes for pupillary response. Shade the eyes in a bright environment (or shine a light into them in a dark environment) and note their response. They should dilate (or constrict) briskly, equally, and consensually (together). Check eye movement by having the patient follow your finger as you trace an "H" pattern in front of him; any deficit in the patient's ability to follow your finger suggests either cranial nerve injury or orbital fracture and muscle entrapment.

Move your head to where you can visualize the length of the external auditory canal. The auditory canal should be clear of fluid and the tympanic membrane should be intact. The nose and mouth should be free of hemorrhage and physical obstruction. Any drainage of fluid from the mouth or nose endangers the airway, and nasal drainage suggests skull fracture and the possible leakage of cerebrospinal fluid. Notable signs of basilar skull fracture include bilateral periorbital ecchymosis (raccoon eyes) or retroauricular ecchymosis (Battle's sign), though both are late signs. (If you see them, suspect an earlier episode of trauma.) Gently palpate the upper jaw and feel for any crepitus or instability, indicative of a Le Fort-type fracture.

Neck

Evaluate the neck for signs of injury, for the position of the trachea, and for the status of the jugular veins. The trachea should be midline in the neck and not moving to one side or tugging with respiration. Displacement to one side suggests tension pneumothorax, although this is a very late sign and not as distinguishable as the other signs of the condition. The jugular veins should be distended in the supine, normovolemic patient and flatten as the patient's torso and head are raised to a 45-degree angle. Extremely distended jugular veins (or ones distended beyond 45 degrees) suggest tension pneumothorax, pericardial tamponade, or traumatic asphyxia. Flat jugular veins in the supine patient suggest hypovolemia. It may be helpful to shine a flashlight across the jugular veins to better visualize their state of fill. Examine the neck and head for the progressive distortion and crepitus associated with subcutaneous emphysema that may accompany tension pneumothorax. Examine for any open wounds, control any hemorrhage, and cover open wounds with occlusive dressings to prevent air embolism. Anticipate tracheal (airway) compromise that may result from swelling or hemorrhage and consider early extraglottic airway insertion, intubation, or possibly rapid sequence intubation if serious neck trauma is present.

Chest

In addition to the standard elements of the physical assessment, examine the chest for intercostal or suprasternal retractions, air moving through any open wounds, and paradoxical chest wall motion. Carefully observe the chest's surface for erythema mirroring the structure of the rib cage. When the skin is trapped between an impacting force and the ribs, it contuses and may demonstrate this sign. Auscultate all lung fields of the chest, both anteriorly and posteriorly. Also listen for heart sounds. If rib injury is not obvious and the patient does not complain of rib pain, apply pressure to the lateral aspect of the rib cage and direct it medially. This will help identify any fracture site along the ribs. The pressure flexes the ribs, moves the fracture site slightly, and creates local pain. You may feel a grating sensation (crepitus) that also suggests rib or sternal fracture. Palpation may reveal a crackling sensation associated with air under the skin (subcutaneous emphysema).

Abdomen

Observe the abdomen for any asymmetry or apparent pulsing masses. Also look for any indication of compression by the lap belt or other signs of impact. Palpate each quadrant, with one hand placing pressure on the other while you sense any unusual masses or muscle spasm (guarding). Quickly release the pressure of palpation to detect any rebound tenderness, only if no other sign of abdominal injury is present. Always palpate the quadrant with the suspected injury last. Finally, observe and palpate the flanks.

Pelvis

In the absence of any indication of pelvic fracture, evaluate the pelvis by placing firm pressure on the iliac crests directed medially and on the pubic bone directed downward. Suspect fracture and serious internal hemorrhage if you notice any crepitus and/or any instability of the pelvis. Examine the inguinal and buttock areas as these locations are often sites of serious injury and hemorrhage. It is essential that you expose these areas if the mechanism of injury suggests injury there because hemorrhage is frequently hidden in jeans or other articles of clothing. Examine the underwear or other clothing for blood staining often caused by urethral injury.

Extremities

Examine each extremity and evaluate its muscle tone, distal pulse, temperature, color, and capillary refill time. Also evaluate for motor response, sensory response, and limb strength. Compare your findings in one limb to those of the opposing limb.

Back

Examine the patient's back during your assessment or when using movement techniques such as a log roll. If spinal injury is suspected, be sure to maintain manual immobilization of the head and neck as you position the patient for examination. Examine the total surface of the back, and palpate the spinal column from top to bottom. Look carefully for any slight deformities, minor reddening, very subtle pain, or tenderness; these may be the only sign or symptom indicative of spinal column injury.

At the conclusion of the rapid trauma assessment, the focused trauma assessment, or the detailed assessment, mentally inventory all the suspected injuries you have found. Place them in descending order of priority for care and note the contribution they make to the patient's shock state.

Trauma Patient History

During the rapid trauma assessment or the focused trauma assessment (or, in some cases, the detailed physical exam), conduct an abbreviated patient history.

Signs and Symptoms

The elements of the *S* component of the SAMPLE history assessment, signs and symptoms, are extensively addressed as you perform the physical assessment. Gather the remaining elements of the SAMPLE history—*Allergies, Medications, Past medical history, Last oral intake,* and *Events* leading up to the incident—either while performing your physical examination of the patient or immediately after it.

Allergies

Question the patient about allergies, especially those to medications used commonly in emergency medicine. Such allergies include those to antibiotics, the "-caine" family, analgesics, and tetanus toxoid. If any of these are noted, pass this information on to the emergency department staff.

Medications

Investigate the patient's use of prescription and nonprescription medications as such use may impact response to care or suggest underlying medical problems or disease. For example, drugs such as beta-blockers reduce the heart's ability to respond to hypovolemia with an increased rate. Be especially watchful for use of aspirin and clopidogrel (Plavix), which interfere with clotting; anticoagulants like warfarin (Coumadin) and dabigatran (Pradaxa); and antibiotics.

CONTENT REVIEW

▶ Elements of a Trauma History

- Signs and symptoms
- Allergies
- Medications
- Past medical history
- Last oral intake
- Events leading to the incident

Past Medical History

Question the patient about any significant medical history that may impact either his response to shock, your care, or the medications the emergency department is likely to use during treatment. Current medical problems may limit the body's ability to compensate for shock from trauma and may affect the presentation of signs and symptoms. For example, a heart condition may limit the heart's ability to increase its rate in response to a reduced preload, confounding your assessment. A normally hypertensive patient may present with a normal blood pressure that, in fact, represents hypotension.

Last Oral Intake

The quantity and time since the patient's last fluid and solid oral intake should affect your index of suspicion for abdominal injury and the care a patient will receive in the emergency department. If the patient's bladder, stomach, or bowel was full and strong forces of deceleration or compression were directed to the abdomen, the risk of rupture and peritonitis is increased. You should be concerned if the trauma patient has recently had anything to eat or drink because vomiting and aspiration may complicate your prehospital airway care. Food and liquid in the stomach also pose serious risks should the patient need surgery. This is because anesthesia may precipitate vomiting, result in aspiration, and increase mortality and morbidity.

Events Leading Up to the Incident

The events immediately preceding the incident are very important. They may suggest that the patient's trauma was caused by a medical or other problem such as falling asleep while driving or becoming dizzy just before a fall. (Seeing no skid marks at a scene where an auto has collided with a tree is an important finding and suggests an intentional impact (attempted suicide) or some other contributing factor.)

Vital Signs

Complete the rapid trauma assessment or focused exam by collecting a baseline set of vital signs. You can do this either at the scene or during transport as the patient's condition and circumstances allow. These vital signs include pulse rate and quality, blood pressure, respiration rate and quality, and skin temperature and condition. Watch for increasing pulse rate and decreasing pulse strength, increasing respiratory rate and decreasing volume, decreasing pulse pressure, and the patient's skin becoming cool and clammy. These changes all suggest increasing compensation for blood loss and shock.[4]

Glasgow Coma Scale Score

At the end of the primary assessment or concurrent with the rapid trauma assessment or focused assessment and history, determine your patient's Glasgow Coma Scale score. Record the best eye opening, verbal response, and motor response individually (e.g., e4, v4, m6) along with the initial vital signs. Then track any changes during subsequent reassessments.

Researchis demonstrating that two components of the Glasgow Coma Scale—obeying verbal commands and localizing pain—are as reliable predictors of traumatic brain injury and patient severity as is the complete GCS. These two factors make up the Simplified Motor Score (SMS). If the patient obeys verbal commands (SMS 2) he is considered normal. If a patient cannot obey commands but can localize pain (SMS 1), the need for airway protection is indicated.[5] If the patient can neither obey commands nor localize pain, there is likely to be serious traumatic brain injury.

Transport Decision

The transport decision is made in a preliminary way at the end of the primary assessment and finalized at the end of the rapid or focused trauma assessment (Figure 11 ●). You will decide whether to provide rapid transport to the trauma center, treat at the scene and then transport to the nearest emergency department, or treat and release as permitted by local protocols.

The Centers for Disease Control and Prevention (CDC) has prepared a four-step process (trauma triage criteria) to make the final determination as to where the trauma patient should be transported. The CDC guidelines are shown in Figure 12 ●.) Step 1 considers the Glasgow Coma Scale score and vital signs, as they are the most dependable predictor of trauma seriousness and outcome. Step 2 examines anatomic signs of injury such as

evidence of penetrating trauma, serious extremity injuries, flail chest, or open or depressed skull fracture. Step 3 looks at mechanism of injury to identify those collisions or events that are most likely to produce serious injury. Finally, step 4 recognizes special patients who might be served by the services of a trauma center and those patients, who in the paramedic's judgment, are in serious condition when the other three steps of trauma triage criteria might not suggest it.

You will notice that the steps presented here do not mirror the assessment process defined in this text. Obviously you should not defer evaluating the mechanism of injury until after you have determined the vital signs. MOI assessment occurs, to some degree, even before you reach your patient, while vital signs are determined during the rapid trauma assessment. Note that MOI is not as dependable a determinant of injury severity as either vital signs or the physical signs of injury on the patient. The final decision as to where to transport a patient and the priority for that transport is made at the end of the rapid trauma assessment using the trauma triage criteria.

Rapid Transport

The decision to provide rapid transport to the trauma center is predicated on the trauma triage criteria. If any of the specified vital signs, anatomic signs of injury, or mechanisms of injury are present, the patient is a candidate for rapid transport. If the patient demonstrates a significant mechanism of injury but the signs and symptoms and the other results of your primary and rapid trauma assessment do not demonstrate the need for this level of transport, contact medical direction to possibly transport to a general hospital emergency department instead.

Revised Trauma Score

The revised trauma score is a numeric evaluation of the patient using the elements of the Glasgow Coma Scale (GCS) and the patient's respiratory rate and systolic blood pressure. Some EMS systems use this, or another trauma scoring system, to predict patient outcome and help make the decision on whether the patient requires rapid transport to a trauma center (Table 1). Consult your system's medical director and protocols to determine if the revised trauma score is in use in your jurisdiction and to learn what numerical score mandates rapid transport.

Treat and Transport

Provide on-scene care and then transport to the nearest emergency department any patient who does not meet the trauma triage criteria. Manage the patient's specific injuries on the scene, and transport once your care has stabilized the injuries and the patient is packaged so movement to the ambulance and hospital will not cause further harm. If at any time during your care the patient demonstrates any signs of more serious injury or shock compensation, consider rapid transport to the trauma center.[6]

Treat and Release

Some EMS systems permit care providers to treat patients with minor injuries and then release them to see their personal physician. Provide this service only to the patient with very minor and isolated injuries. Ensure that you carefully explain to the

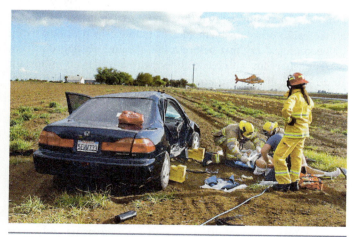

● **Figure 11** At the end of the rapid trauma assessment or the focused assessment, make the final decision on whether to provide stabilization on the scene or to expedite transport of the patient. (© *REACH Air Medical Services, Rick Roach*)

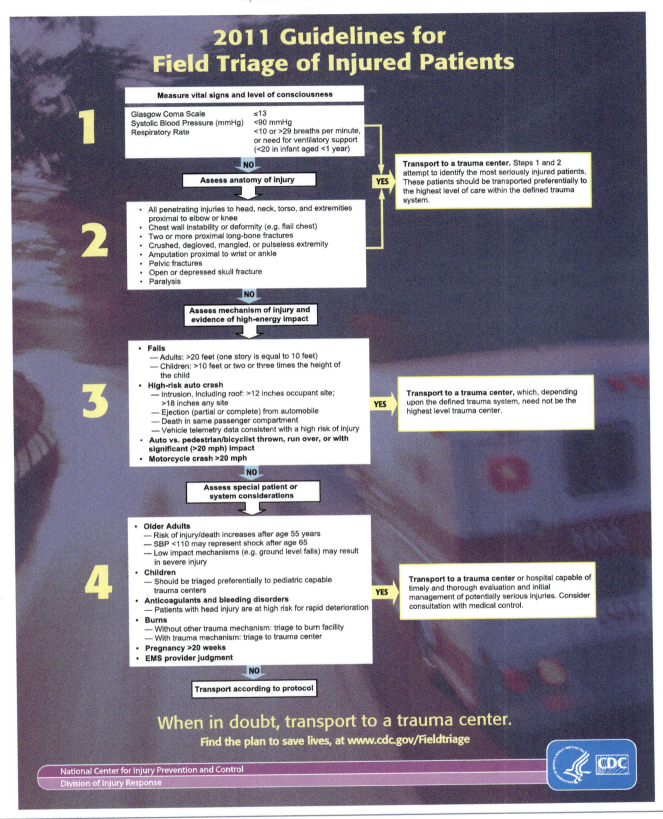

● **Figure 12** Centers for Disease Control and Prevention Guidelines for Field Triage of Injured Patients.

► Steps to Follow if a Patient Refuses Treatment

- Suggest strongly that the patient should receive assessment, care, and transport
- Warn the patient of the dangers of refusing assessment, care, and transport
- Suggest that the patient see a family physician
- Encourage the patient to contact EMS again if the problem persists or worsens

patient what care is needed for the injury. Describe the signs that may develop indicating that the injury requires immediate attention and advise the patient that he should call your service again if those signs appear. Finally, tell the patient that he should seek care from a family physician. If possible, provide this information in written form, approved by your system of medical direction, and have the patient acknowledge in writing the receipt of these instructions. If you have any questions about treatment or release of a patient, contact your medical direction physician.

Patient Care Refusals

Some patients suffering trauma will refuse assessment, care, and transport. While this is the patient's right, the situation represents a dilemma for prehospital care providers. The patient may not understand the significance of his injuries, and the early signs of trauma may not clearly reflect its nature or seriousness.

When confronted with a patient refusing care, advise the patient that serious injury may not present with overt or painful symptoms. Try to convince them to permit you to perform an assessment and provide on-scene care. If you are not successful, attempt to have the patient talk with the medical direction physician. Be sure the patient is an adult and is fully conscious, oriented, and able to make a rational decision. Try to use family members to help you encourage the patient to accept your assessment and care. If your attempts to convince the patient fail, suggest that they see a personal physician at the earliest opportunity. Stress that the patient should feel free to call for emergency medical service if additional signs or symptoms develop or existing ones worsen. Be sure to document the refusal thoroughly. Include your recommendation that the patient receive assessment, care, and transport; your warning of the dangers of refusing assessment, care, and transport; your suggestion that the patient see a family physician; and your recommendation to contact EMS again if the problem persists or worsens. Should the patient refuse to sign this documentation, have someone else review your documentation and sign to witness it.

TABLE 1 | Revised Trauma Score and Glasgow Coma Scale

Revised Trauma Score		Glasgow Coma Scale Score	
Respiratory Rate		**Eye Opening**	
10 to 29 breaths per minute	4	Spontaneous	4
Greater than 29 breaths per minute	3	To voice	3
6 to 9 breaths per minute	2	To pain	2
1 to 5 breaths per minute	1	None	1
No respiration	0	**Verbal Response**	
Systolic Blood Pressure		Oriented	5
Greater than 89 mmHg	4	Confused (cries, consolable)	4
76 to 89 mmHg	3	Inappropriate words (persistently irritable)	3
50 to 75 mmHg	2	Incomprehensible words (restless, agitated)	2
1 to 49 mmHg	1	None	1
No blood pressure	0	**Motor Response**	
Glasgow Coma Scale		Obeys commands	6
GCS score of 13 to 15	4	Localizes pain	5
GCS score of 9 to 12	3	Withdraws to pain	4
GCS score of 6 to 8	2	Flexes to pain	3
GCS score of 4 or 5	1	Extends to pain	2
GCS score of less than 4	0	None	1

Reassessment

Periodic trauma patient ___ ___ent is important to monitoring and guiding ___ ___vide. It is performed every
5 minutes wi___ ___injured patients and every
15 minut___ ___ perform a reassessment
whene___ ___ient's condition or you
instit___

bre___ ___e mental, airway,
m___ ___e primary assess-
c___ ___ the rapid or fo-
r___ ___blood pressure;
___ ___tory rate, vol-
___ ___ Coma Scale
___lse, capillary
___attention to
___ulse pres-
___ry volume,
___r consciousness
___rature, or increasing
___gns may indicate patient
___ each reassessment to baseline
___evious reassessments to identify any
___ovement in the patient's condition. Record
___ly so that trending of the patient's signs can con-
___ arrival at the emergency department.

[handwritten note: 3 H's / not reading / chest + abd / Hypovolemia]

SHOCK/MULTISYSTEM TRAUMA RESUSCITATION

Hypovolemia/Hypotension/Hypoperfusion

Three very important terms are used to describe the status of the
cardiovascular system in trauma. They are hypovolemia, hypotension, and hypoperfusion. **Hypovolemia** refers to a reduced
volume in the cardiovascular system, caused by hemorrhage,
by an excess of fluid loss against inadequate fluid intake, or by
losses into third spaces, as with plasma into burns. A relative
hypovolemia may occur as the vascular system expands (with
spinal injury) and the normal vascular volume is inadequate
to fill it. **Hypotension** simply refers to a reduction in blood
pressure caused by cardiac, vascular, neurogenic, or volume
problems to a level that is lower than normal for the patient.
Hypoperfusion is a low or inadequate distribution of blood to
body organs and tissues caused by cardiac, vascular, neurogenic,
or volume problems.

In serious trauma it is likely that more than one body system
will be involved. This multisystem trauma often involves the
central nervous, respiratory, and cardiovascular systems. Shock
trauma resuscitation is care for multisystem trauma to rapidly
support the seriously injured trauma patient while he is rushed
to the trauma center (Figure 13 ●). These include:

- Providing airway protection with extraglottic airway
  insertion, endotracheal intubation, or rapid sequence
  intubation

- Ensuring adequate
  oxygenation and
  ventilations

- Halting any serious
  external hemorrhage

- Providing appropriate
  fluid resuscitation with
  isotonic solution

- Performing pleural
  decompression

Whenever serious
trauma is expected or the
signs of shock compensa-
tion are evident, consider
protecting the airway with
an extraglottic airway. If that
is unsuccessful, consider introducing an endotracheal
tube using the orotracheal method of insertion. Anticipate that
the seriously injured patient will deteriorate and be prepared to
protect the airway early. Consider using rapid sequence intubation in the extremely agitated or combative patient when shock
is evident and the patient demonstrates a steady deterioration.
Recent studies are demonstrating that endotracheal intubation,
and especially rapid sequence intubation, are not without risks.
It may be prudent to focus on placing an extraglottic airway as
a first choice and only considering intubation when that airway
choice proves ineffective.[7]

If oxygen saturation is below 96 percent, apply supplemental oxygen immediately. Consider ventilating the patient (overdrive ventilation with bag-valve mask) if the respirations move
less than 500 mL of air or respirations occur less than 10 or more
than 29 times per minute. Rapidly control significant hemorrhage with direct pressure. Consider tourniquet use if you are
providing care in a hazardous environment or direct pressure
does not quickly control the bleeding.

Initiate a large-bore intravenous site in a large vein and
connect a nonrestrictive (either trauma or blood tubing)

CONTENT REVIEW

▶ Signs of Deterioration during
Reassessment

- Increasing pulse rate
- Decreasing pulse strength
- Narrowing pulse pressure
- Increasing respiratory rate
- Decreasing respiratory
  volume
- Increasing capillary
  refill time
- Decreasing level of
  consciousness or
  orientation
- Changes in skin color or
  temperature
- Increasing anxiety or
  restlessness

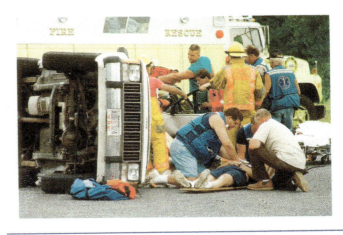

● **Figure 13** With a seriously injured trauma patient, employ
the aggressive care steps of shock trauma resuscitation.
(© *Craig Jackson/In the Dark Photography*)

CONTENT REVIEW

▶ Basic Steps of Shock
Trauma Resuscitation

- Providing airway protection
  with endotracheal
  intubation or rapid
  sequence intubation
- Ensuring adequate
  oxygenation and
  ventilations
- Providing rapid fluid
  resuscitation with isotonic
  solution
- Performing pleural
  decompression

administration set and a 1,000-mL bag of normal saline.[8] If traditional IV sites are not available, consider the humoral (or other) intraosseous site. If shock is present or expected, choose large veins for cannulation (the antecubital veins). Veins in the forearm or hand are secondary choices. Run the fluid at a to-keep-open rate as long as the patient maintains his blood pressure (pulse pressure) and pulse rate. Be ready to rapidly infuse fluids quickly should the patient begin to show increasing signs and symptoms of serious compensation and shock. Generally, the maximum prehospital fluid volume is 3,000 mL of isotonic solution administered in boluses. You may adjust this volume based on the size of the patient and the patient's response to infusion (slowing pulse, increasing pulse strength, increasing level of consciousness). Titrate your infusion rate to ensure a systolic blood pressure of 80 mmHg (or 90 mmHg for the suspected head injury patient). Auscultate the lung fields for signs of edema and halt or reduce the rate of fluid administration with the development of any crackles.[9]

Be sure to seek signs and symptoms of tension pneumothorax during your assessment. If the patient displays the appropriate signs and has significant dyspnea, decompress the affected side of the chest with a large-bore catheter inserted in the second or third intercostal space, midclavicular line. These steps of shock care are essential to maintain the patient until further, possibly invasive, procedures occur at the hospital.

There are several general considerations to keep in mind in shock/multisystem trauma resuscitation situations. These include preventing hypothermia, providing rapid body splinting, providing rapid transport, and reducing the effects of the fight-or-flight response.

Hypothermia

Hypothermia is a relatively unappreciated complication of serious trauma and shock. Lessons from the wars in Iraq and Afghanistan, however, have highlighted the need for attention to trauma-induced hypothermia and its consequences. Trauma often initiates the fight-or-flight response, which causes the body to direct its energy away from the internal organs and to the skeletal muscles. When a patient stops his flight (as during your care), the body's energy and heat production decrease dramatically. The problem is further compounded as the body directs its remaining blood volume to critical organs and not to temperature regulation activities. The result is a patient who is very susceptible to hypothermia (Figure 14 ●). Caregivers contribute to this problem when they provide rapid fluid resuscitation with fluids that are often at ambient, rather than body, temperature. The result is a rapid infusion of hypothermic fluid and a further lowering of the body's core temperature. In addition, care providers frequently disrobe patients during assessment and fail to re-cover them adequately with warm

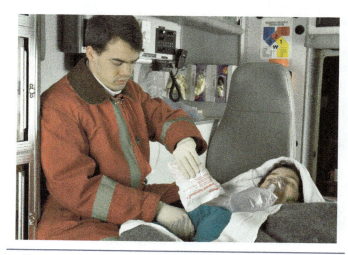

● **Figure 14** Hypothermia poses a serious threat to trauma patients. Ensure that your care helps the patient maintain his body temperature.

blankets. In all but the warmest environments, this behavior only compounds hypothermia.

Hypothermia can have several negative effects on a patient suffering from injury and shock. The body's natural response to heat loss is increased skeletal muscle activity, specifically shivering. This heat generation consumes the body's energy reserves and increases the impact of injury and shock. A decrease in body temperature also affects blood clotting by inhibiting the clotting cascade and prolonging clotting times. The colder temperature also causes the platelets to release a heparin-like anticoagulant agent that further slows the clotting process. Critical body enzymes, too, do not function efficiently at subnormal body temperature. This can disrupt oxygen utilization, decrease metabolism, and exacerbate acidosis.

It is essential to recognize the negative impact a lowering of body temperature has on the patient during shock. Always try to administer fluids that are as close to body temperature as possible, especially in colder environments. Use fluid warmers as necessary. Use more blankets to cover an injured patient than you would use with an uninjured patient in the same environmental conditions. A number of commercial high-efficiency passive and active external rewarming devices are available and should be considered for any lengthy transports or cold-weather operations. Keep your ambulance warmer than is comfortable for you with a target of 85 degrees Fahrenheit.

Body Splinting

The seriously injured trauma patient is likely to have suffered internal injury, life-threatening hemorrhage, and long-bone and possible spinal fractures. To ensure rapid transport to the trauma center while not compounding the patient's injuries, splinting must be effective yet must be done quickly. For the seriously injured trauma patient, you can best accomplish this splinting by gently aligning all the limbs and firmly securing the entire patient to a long spine board or orthopedic stretcher. Movement onto the movement device should occur in one coordinated move from the patient's initial location. Body splinting ensures that if there is any movement of the limbs while packaging, loading, or transporting the patient, the movement will be limited, thus reducing the chances of aggravating existing injuries.[10]

Rapid Transport

Research has clearly demonstrated that the best way to reduce trauma mortality is to bring the seriously injured patient to surgery as quickly as possible. This presumes that the greatest risk to life is from internal hemorrhage and the only definitive remedy for that risk may be surgical repair. Care providers can help meet this objective by providing rapid on-scene assessment, extrication, patient packaging, and transport while maintaining the patient through spinal, airway, ventilatory, and circulatory support. Make every effort to reduce the time at the emergency scene, and limit your actions there so that on-scene time is no more than 10 minutes ("platinum 10 minutes" of prehospital care). Perform procedures such as IV insertion while applying spinal precautions and mechanical immobilization, ensuring and supporting the airway and breathing, or controlling hemorrhage or while preparing to move the patient. Otherwise, carry out these procedures in the ambulance during transport. Using air medical service whenever it will substantially reduce transport time may be another way of speeding the patient to definitive care. Be sure to alert the trauma center of the nature of your patient's injuries, the mechanism of injury that caused those injuries, the care you are providing, the patient's response to that care, and any trending in vital signs you note. And always provide detailed and complete documentation of these items in your prehospital care report.

Fight-or-Flight Response

When a person is under extreme stress or in fear of bodily harm, the autonomic nervous system responds with a release of adrenaline and an increase in several body functions. These actions induce an increase in heart rate, stroke volume, blood pressure, respiratory rate and volume, and a release of glucose and insulin into the bloodstream. The result is a rapid expenditure of body resources that might be otherwise used for repair and recovery. To reduce the effect of the fight-or-flight response and to make the patient more comfortable with the emergency medical care, try to be calming and reassuring. Clearly tell the patient who you are and that you are there to help. Listen carefully to what the patient says, and describe what will happen during care and why. Let the patient see that you are confident in the care you are about to provide and that your sincere desire is to attend to his injuries. Maintain continuous communication with the patient and try to distract him from concerns over the injuries and the impact they may have on the patient's life. Doing these things will help reduce patient anxiety and the effects of the fight-or-flight response.

It should be noted that four critical factors are directly related to preventable trauma death. They are controllable airway obstruction, external hemorrhage, pneumothorax, and hypothermia. Ensure that any patient you are treating for serious injury and possible shock has a clear airway and no significant dyspnea. Ensure that all significant external hemorrhage is controlled. Rule out tension pneumothorax, and maintain the patient's body temperature.

Noncritical Patients

Patients needing the services of a trauma center represent only about 10 percent of all trauma patients.[11] While we "overtriage" around twice this number to ensure we do not miss individuals with subtle or concealed injuries, noncritical patients account for about 80 percent of trauma responses and receive the largest part of prehospital trauma care.[11] These are patients who do not demonstrate the vital signs, anatomic signs, or mechanisms of injury detailed in trauma triage criteria and who receive the focused trauma assessment.

Noncritical trauma patients receive care directed at their specific injuries. These patients normally require dressing, bandaging, and immobilization of the wound or skeletal injury site and comfortable (and slow) transport to the emergency department of their choice (within reason). With these patients, be careful to monitor distal sensation, motor function, pulses, temperature, and capillary refill to ensure there is no neurologic or vascular compromise from the injury or from the bandaging or splinting provided. Should you detect any deficit or any signs or symptoms of developing hypovolemia or shock, increase the patient's priority for transport and consider rerouting to the trauma center.

Special Patients

Two categories of trauma patients who require special attention are the very young and the old. The pediatric patient is small, growing, and somewhat different anatomically from the adult. The geriatric patient often has preexisting medical problems and body systems that are not as responsive to the effects of trauma as those of their younger adult counterparts. Three other categories of special patients are the pregnant, the bariatric (obese), and the cognitively impaired patients. These five categories of special patients respond differently to trauma than average adult patients and must be assessed, prioritized, and cared for accordingly.

Pediatric Patients

Pediatric patients are, in many ways, just small adults. They have the same basic anatomy and, for the most part, the same physiology. Because of their smaller size and the dynamics of their growth, however, the effects of trauma on pediatric patients are different from the effects on adults (Figure 15 ●). Further, damage to the child's rapidly growing body may have significant, long-lasting effects.

Trauma is the greatest cause of death and disability among pediatric patients after the first year of life. The pediatric patient is most likely to suffer blunt trauma. The most commonly experienced forms of blunt trauma in pediatric patients are auto impacts (including vehicle crashes and pedestrian-vs.-auto and bicycle-vs.-auto collisions), falls, and abuse (in that order). Penetrating trauma (gunshot and knife wounds) is also on the rise in the pediatric population over age 14.[12] Contributing factors to the mortality and morbidity of pediatric trauma are the child's limited life experience and undeveloped recognition of and respect for trauma hazards and their consequences.

The smaller size and weight of infants and children mean they have a larger ratio of body surface area to volume than

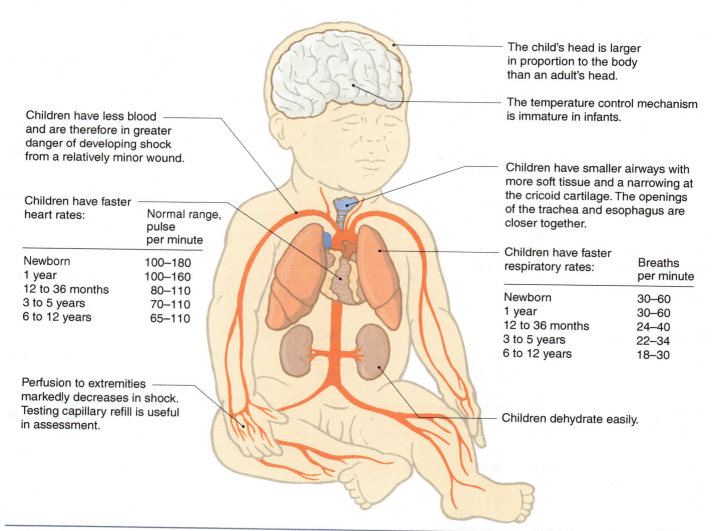

The child's head is larger in proportion to the body than an adult's head.

The temperature control mechanism is immature in infants.

Children have smaller airways with more soft tissue and a narrowing at the cricoid cartilage. The openings of the trachea and esophagus are closer together.

Children have less blood and are therefore in greater danger of developing shock from a relatively minor wound.

Children have faster heart rates:

	Normal range, pulse per minute
Newborn	100–180
1 year	100–160
12 to 36 months	80–110
3 to 5 years	70–110
6 to 12 years	65–110

Children have faster respiratory rates:

	Breaths per minute
Newborn	30–60
1 year	30–60
12 to 36 months	24–40
3 to 5 years	22–34
6 to 12 years	18–30

Perfusion to extremities markedly decreases in shock. Testing capillary refill is useful in assessment.

Children dehydrate easily.

● **Figure 15**   Anatomic and physiologic considerations with infant and child patients.

adults do. This means that infants and children lose or gain heat from the environment much more quickly than adults. Extensive body surface injuries (like abrasions and burns) become more devastating because of the proportionally greater fluid loss to the injury and the environment. Because of their smaller size, the organs of pediatric patients are closer together, and multisystem trauma is thus more frequent. In pediatric pedestrian-vs.-auto impacts, the energy causing injury is delivered higher on the anatomy. Initial impact is likely to affect the pelvis, abdomen, and chest, resulting in greater internal injuries and a smaller incidence of extremity trauma. The impact is also more likely to propel the child ahead of the car where he may be struck again by it or run over.

Some aspects of pediatric anatomy differ significantly from those of adults. The limbs are proportionally shorter than those of the mature adult and less able and effective in protecting children from trunk trauma. Infants and young children have less subcutaneous fat and less-developed muscle masses to protect the internal organs. The heads of infants and children are proportionally larger than those of adults, which results in a greater incidence of blunt head trauma and the application of proportionally greater forces to the neck during acceleration or deceleration. The increased head size also means that when infants or young children are supine the neck is flexed, which may contribute to airway obstruction. The tongues of infants and children fill more of the oral cavity and are more likely to obstruct the airway than in adults. The infant anatomy also means they must breathe through the nose (obligate nasal breathers), thus providing only one airway with no detour around its obstruction. The trachea in infants and children is shorter, more delicate, more prone to kinking, and more prone to intubation of the right mainstem bronchus and soft-tissue trauma. The mediastinum is more mobile in pediatric patients, which permits greater displacement during tension pneumothorax, resulting in an earlier development of the pathology and a greater restriction of venous return to the heart than in adults.

The pediatric skeletal system grows rapidly. It begins as cartilage and becomes more rigid and stronger with age. This development permits great flexibility and protects the skeleton from fracture. However, the energy of trauma is more easily transmitted through the rib cage, spine, and skull to injure the vital structures beneath. The soft and partial nature of the skull also permits a greater displacement of its contents with hemorrhage or edema and will present with bulging fontanelles with increased intracranial pressure in the child less than 18 months of age. This ability of the cranium to expand may also permit intracranial hemorrhage to substantially contribute to hypovolemia, though it, as the sole cause of shock, is very infrequent. The skeleton's flexibility also lessens the incidence, severity, and signs of soft-tissue injury. When injured, the long bones of the skeleton frequently resist fracture until just one side of the bone gives way. The resulting fracture, called a greenstick fracture, provides a relatively stable, though somewhat deformed, limb. However, this type of fracture promotes increased growth on the uninjured side, causing further angulation of the limb. For this reason, a surgeon sometimes completes a greenstick fracture later in the process of care. Long-bone injury is also likely to occur at the site of bone growth, the epiphyseal plate. This type of injury may damage the growth potential of the limb and create a lifelong disability.

The components of the cardiovascular systems of infants and children are much more vibrant than those in adults. They are very able to compensate for blood loss secondary to trauma and do not show overt signs of compensation as quickly. In fact, pediatric patients may lose up to 25 percent of their blood volume before any signs appear and may lose 50 percent of their blood volume before compensation fails. However, once pediatric patients can no longer compensate for blood loss, they move very quickly toward irreversible shock. The heart of a pediatric patient cannot increase its stroke volume as the heart of an adult does. In hypovolemia and shock, this results in an earlier and more pronounced tachycardia because an increase in heart rate is the only way to significantly increase cardiac output. Additionally, the respiratory system in a pediatric patient has less of a respiratory reserve, is less able to tolerate stress, and will tire more quickly than an adult's respiratory system.

Pediatric vital signs are very different from those of adults and change quickly during the developmental years (Table 2). As infants grow into toddlers, preschoolers, school-age children, and adolescents, their vital signs change, until, in the late teens, their ranges are very similar to those of adults. During these years, blood pressure levels rise and heart and respiratory rates fall. These changing vital signs make accurate assessment of pediatric patients more difficult because you must accurately determine the child's age and vital signs and then compare them to the normal rates for that age. It is helpful to keep a pediatric vital sign table handy when responding to a pediatric trauma emergency.

Psychologically and socially, pediatric patients respond very differently both to injury and to care providers than do adults. The responses also change dramatically with the child's growth and development.

As with adults, calculation of a trauma score can help to predict patient outcome and form transport decisions. However, the criteria for pediatric patients are different from the criteria for adults, as shown in Table 3.

Management of the Pediatric Patient Shock/multisystem trauma resuscitation for pediatric patients follows the same basic processes of assessment and care used with adults, but makes allowances for differences in pediatric anatomy and physiology. Maintain the airway in a neutral position with padding under the shoulders for an infant and limited or no padding under the shoulders or head of a child (depending on the child's anatomic size). This avoids kinking the relatively soft trachea, avoids blocking the airway, and helps align the structures of the posterior pharynx, the larynx, and the trachea to ease intubation. To secure the airway, use an appropriately sized oral airway or intubate. Insert the oral airway using a tongue blade, as the normal insertion technique with a 180-degree turn used in adults may injure the delicate soft tissue of the infant or very young child's oral pharynx. Be sure to keep the nasal passage clear in pediatric patients under six months of age as they are obligate nasal breathers. If intubation is considered, use a tube that approximates the diameter of the patient's little finger. Insert the tube gently and pass it only a couple of centimeters beyond the glottis because the

TABLE 2 | Normal Vital Signs

	Pulse (beats per minute)	Respiration (breaths per minute)	Blood Pressure (average mmHg)	Temperature	
Infancy					
At Birth	100–180	30–60	60–90 systolic	98°–100°F	36.7°–37.8°C
At 1 Year	100–160	30–60	87–105 systolic	98°–100°F	36.7°–37.8°C
Toddler (12 to 36 months)	80–110	24–40	95–105 systolic	96.8°–99.6°F	36.3°–37.9°C
Preschool Age (3 to 5 years)	70–110	22–34	95–110 systolic	96.8°–99.6°F	36.3°–37.9°C
School Age (6 to 12 years)	65–110	18–30	97–112 systolic	98.6°F	37°C
Adolescence (13 to 18 years)	60–90	12–26	112–128 systolic	98.6°F	37°C
Early Adulthood (19 to 40 years)	60–100	12–20	120/80	98.6°F	37°C
Middle Adulthood (41 to 60 years)	60–100	12–20	120/80	98.6°F	37°C
Late Adulthood (61 years and older)	+	+	+	98.6°F	37°C

+ *Depends on the individual's physical health status.*

pediatric patient is prone to soft-tissue injury and (because of the short trachea) to right mainstem bronchus intubation. Secure the endotracheal tube firmly and carefully monitor the tube's location and the breath sounds because uncuffed tubes, if used, may easily be dislodged from the very short trachea.

Initiate intravenous access as with an adult, and be certain to use catheters sized to the patient's veins because you will infuse reduced volumes of fluid. If you cannot obtain normal venous access, consider using the intraosseous site for administration of both medications and fluid (Figure 16 ●). Fluid boluses for volume replacement are usually given as 20 mL/kg boluses. Administer this volume sooner in the pediatric patient than you would in the adult. This is because infants and children compensate more effectively for fluid loss and you are likely to recognize hypovolemia late in its development. This bolus may be given up to three times for a total of 60 mL/kg.

Consider less significant mechanisms of injury and more minimal signs of injury than you would with adults as grounds for transporting pediatric patients to the trauma center. Pediatric patients have less protection for internal body organs and are

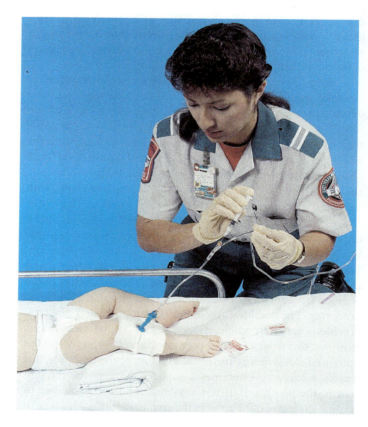

● **Figure 16** Consider intraosseous placement in the tibia when administering fluids and medications in children under age six if you cannot obtain normal intravenous access.

TABLE 3 | Pediatric Trauma Score and Glasgow Coma Scale Score

Pediatric Trauma Score

Score	+2	+1	−1
Weight	>44 lb (>20 kg)	22–44 lb (10–20 kg)	<22 lb (<10 kg)
Airway	Normal	Oral or nasal airway	Intubated, tracheostomy, invasive airway
Blood pressure	Pulse at wrist >90 mmHg	Carotid or femoral pulse palpable 50–90 mmHg	No palpable pulse or <50 mmHg
Level of consciousness	Completely awake	Obtunded or any loss of consciousness	Comatose
Open wound	None	Minor	Major or penetrating
Fractures	None	Closed fracture	Open or multiple fractures

Pediatric Glasgow Coma Scale

		>1 Year	<1 Year	
Eye opening	4	Spontaneous	Spontaneous	
	3	To verbal command	To shout	
	2	To pain	To pain	
	1	No response	No response	
		>1 Year	**<1 Year**	
Best motor response	6	Obeys		
	5	Localizes pain	Localizes pain	
	4	Flexion-withdrawal	Flexion-withdrawal	
	3	Flexion-abnormal (decorticate rigidity)	Flexion-abnormal (decorticate rigidity)	
	2	Extension (decerebrate rigidity)	Extension (decerebrate rigidity)	
	1	No response	No response	
		>5 Years	**2–5 Years**	**0–23 Months**
Best verbal response	5	Oriented and converses	Appropriate words and phrases	Smiles, coos, cries appropriately
	4	Disoriented and converses	Inappropriate words	Cries
	3	Inappropriate words	Cries and/or screams	Inappropriate crying and/or screaming
	2	Incomprehensible sounds	Grunts	Grunts
	1	No response	No response	No response

more likely to show fewer signs and symptoms of injury. They have a greater incidence of serious and multisystem trauma than adults. If possible, consider transport to a facility able to accommodate the special needs of pediatric trauma patients, the pediatric trauma center.

Pregnant Patients

Trauma in pregnancy represents an injury endangering the life and health of both the mother and developing fetus. Pregnancy represents physiologic changes to the mother that alter the way she responds to injury and blood loss. It also represents a second patient, the fetus. The fetus is completely dependent on the health of the mother and her ability to provide oxygen and nutrients and remove carbon dioxide and waste products from the fetal circulation through the placenta/uterine wall. This exchange is at risk early in the development of hypovolemia and shock in the mother. It is important for us to look at the incidence of trauma in pregnancy, physiologic changes to the mother during pregnancy, and factors that change the assessment and management of the pregnant female.

Trauma in pregnancy is the most common cause of both maternal and fetal mortality. Trauma in pregnancy is most frequently related to motor vehicle collisions, violence (most frequently domestic violence), and falls. Seat belt use is the most modifiable risk factor and has a significant influence on both maternal and fetal mortality and morbidity. Proper seat belt use for the pregnant mother should be a target of the EMS system's efforts at prevention.

Pregnant Physiology   The blood volume of a pregnant female increases throughout gestation to about 150 percent of normal (an increase of 50 percent). Most of this increased volume consists of increased plasma volume. Because red blood cell production does not match the vascular fluid increase, there is a relative anemia (that is, the number of red blood cells remains the same, but the plasma volume is increased). The heart rate increases by 10 to 15 beats per minute with an associated increase in cardiac output. Blood pressure falls by 5 to 15 mmHg during the second trimester but then returns to normal near term. Because of the size and placement of the near-term uterus, it may compress the inferior vena cava and result in supine hypotension. Displacement by the pregnant uterus can push the heart upward in the chest and may demonstrate a leftward 15-degree axis shift on the 12-lead ECG. Pregnancy induces an increased oxygen demand. To accommodate this increased demand, maternal tidal volume increases, resulting in a greater minute volume. The increased respiratory minute volume produces a slight hypocapnia at end of term.

The thickening uterus and developing fetus are well protected within the pelvic cavity during the first trimester. During the second trimester they are equally protected by the pelvic ring and the lower abdomen. However, by the third trimester the pregnant uterus is much thinner, the fetus much larger, and they displace the abdominal contents upward. This more directly exposes the uterus and fetus to direct trauma and places the abdominal contents much higher anatomically than they would be in the nonpregnant female.

Pregnant Pathophysiology   During gestation the developing fetus is well protected by the pelvic ring, the muscular uterine wall, and the amniotic fluid that surrounds it and fills the uterus. However, since the fetus receives its nourishment from the maternal circulation, through the placenta and umbilical cord, it is at risk whenever the mother is at risk. Any hypovolemia, shock, or hypoxia endangers the fetus well before it endangers the mother. It is said that the best fetal care is to care for the mother. The fetus is also at risk from blunt trauma that may occur as the mother strikes the auto dash during a

crash or when struck by an object like a baseball bat during an assault. These mechanisms may cause direct or indirect (contrecoup) injuries to the fetus or cause the placenta to shear and separate from the uterine wall—abruptio placentae.

The abdomen is dynamic as the pregnancy progresses. In the first trimester and early second trimester, the abdominal contents remain in their normal position and are subject to trauma as with those organs for the nonpregnant patient. As the pregnancy progresses, the increasing size of the pregnant uterus displaces most abdominal organs laterally and superiorly. This generally protects the organs and puts the uterus and developing fetus more at risk for injury. Pelvic fractures, when they occur in very late pregnancy (as when the head is engaged), may result in fetal head injury, but this is rare. Cardiac arrest occurs no more frequently in the pregnant mother than in nonpregnant women of the same age. When it does occur, it represents a threat to two lives and special energies toward resuscitation should be initiated. However, remember that arrest resulting from hypovolemia has a very poor prognosis.

Seat belts reduce the incidence of premature delivery, abruptio placentae, and fetal death. The use of a lap belt alone permits forward motion of the pregnant mother, compressing the uterus and its contents. This may lead to uterine rupture or abruptio placentae. A lap belt used alone and placed too high may compress the pregnant uterus and result in the same pathologies. The shoulder belt should be moved to the side of the pregnant uterus in the late pregnancy female.

Domestic violence is a major cause of trauma in pregnancy.[13] Be suspicious if you note the explanation of what happened does not fit with the injuries found, there is a series of unexplained injuries, the patient has a lowered self-image, or the domestic partner attempts to monopolize the conversation. Report any suspected abuse to the emergency department or as called for by your protocols or state statutes.

Assessment of the Pregnant Patient   Progress through your primary assessment as you would with any trauma patient observing the following differences for the pregnant female. During the general impression, ask the mother about the length of pregnancy and the trimester she is in. Visualize the abdomen and, from the size and placement of the uterus, approximate the gestational age. If spinal precautions are required, rotate the spine board at least 15 to 30 degrees to take the uterine weight off the vena cava. Ensure the airway is adequate and provide supplemental oxygen if needed to maintain an oxygen saturation of at least 96 percent. Remember, the fetus is often first affected by inadequate oxygen levels.

Quickly evaluate respiratory rate and depth. They should be slightly faster than normal and a bit deeper. If the respiratory rate is less than 20 it is possible that respirations are not adequate. Seek other respiratory signs and symptoms such as dyspnea and low oxygen saturation. Carefully look for signs of hemorrhage and be very watchful for signs of shock. They develop later in the blood loss process than for nonpregnant patients yet the fetus is at risk very early as shock develops. The third-trimester pregnancy patient may not display a significantly elevated pulse rate until late in the shock process. It is critical to stop bleeding early and stabilize the circulatory system with fluid resuscitation, as needed. If a late-term pregnancy patient is found in cardiac arrest, resuscitation efforts should be considered as the fetus may be viable. Note, however, that the heart may be displaced somewhat higher and to the left in the chest and the normal landmarks for CPR may not provide for proper hand positioning.

Categorize the pregnant patient one category more serious in the CUPS system at the end of the primary assessment. If you find your patient to be either U (unstable) or P (potentially unstable) perform the rapid trauma assessment. Otherwise, provide a focused trauma assessment while being watchful for any signs of maternal distress or early signs of shock.

If the patient is noticeably pregnant and a victim of a serious vehicle crash, and especially if a lap belt was worn without the shoulder strap, palpate the fundus of the uterus in the lower abdomen. It should be firm and round. If you feel significant irregularity, and any features of the fetus, suspect ruptured uterus. Also maintain a high index of suspicion for abruptio placentae with any significant blunt trauma to the abdomen. Examine for vaginal hemorrhage.

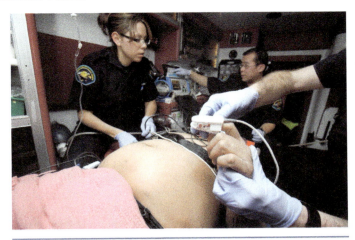

● **Figure 17** Obese trauma patients present numerous challenges for assessment and care. (© *Kevin Link*)

Management of the Pregnant Patient Management of the pregnant female subjected to trauma must place special emphases on ensuring an adequate airway, ventilation, and circulation. It is important to apply supplemental oxygen to ensure an oxygen saturation of at least 96 percent or higher. Remember that oxygen must travel through the mother's circulation to reach the uterine wall, then traverse the wall to the placenta and enter the fetal circulation. Then it must be circulated by the fetal circulation to the target tissues. Place a special emphasis on ensuring a good airway and ventilation for the mother because any hypoxia may have profound effects on the fetus.

The mother in late stages of pregnancy should not be positioned supine but in the left lateral recumbent position. If the patient is secured to a spine board, tilt the board 15 degrees. This prevents the uterus from compressing the inferior vena cava against the sacral spine, slowing venous return to the heart, and inducing hypotension. When blood loss is suspected consider aggressive fluid resuscitation. Remember that pregnancy increases the vascular volume and the pregnant mother may lose a great deal of blood and endanger the baby while displaying limited signs and symptoms of hypovolemia. A significant trauma risk to the mother and fetus is abruptio placentae. It should be considered when the patient complains of abdominal pain and there is any uterine bleeding (in about 70 percent of abruptio placentae cases).

Bariatric Patients

Society as a whole is getting heavier and it estimated that more than 25 percent of the population is obese. This is, in part, associated with greater access to higher caloric food and a more sedentary lifestyle. Thesepatients present problems to assessment and care when trauma is involved (Figure 17 ●).[14]

The obese patient is likely to have increased blood volume and increased cardiac output as a result of increased oxygen demand caused by an increase in body tissue. Over time, this can lead to systemic hypertension and myocardial

hypertrophy and a higher risk of arrhythmias, cardiac failure, and cardiac arrest. In trauma, it can leave the obese patient less able to accommodate the stresses of injury, hypovolemia, and shock. Obesity also increases the work of breathing as a result of increased intraabdominal pressure and increased chest wall resistance. Often the patient will exhibit reduced tidal volume, vital capacity, and total lung capacity. He may, however, have an increased respiratory rate and minute volume to accommodate increased metabolic needs. Obesity in trauma leads to an increase in multiple organ involvement, more serious pulmonary complications, and a mortality of up to six times greater than a normal-weight patient. Obese patients are more likely to suffer pulmonary contusions and pelvic, rib, and extremity fracture with slightly less incidence of head injury.[15] (Obese patients may also have multiple disease pathologies, such as diabetes, and may be on multiple medications—all of which may make assessment and care of the bariatric patient more complicated.)

The obese patient's primary assessment follows the standard primary assessment process and priorities. However, the patient's normal blood volume is more closely associated with ideal body weight and any hemorrhage is likely to be more severe than it appears. Carefully assess for shock and remember that the cardiovascular system is already stressed by the excess weight.

During the rapid trauma assessment, pay special attention to the thorax and pelvic ring because of the increased incidence of rib fractures, pulmonary contusions, and pelvic fractures. Carefully assess vital signs as they may be more difficult to palpate and hear because of greater body fat in the limbs and surrounding the chest cavity.

Management of the heavy patient presents hazards to the care provider. The increased weight makes lifting more hazardous and may stress equipment beyond its safe limits. Be careful to bring in enough people to provide a safe lift for you and your crew, and for the patient. Splinting equipment may need to be modified or used in innovative ways to accommodate obese patients with fractures. Be careful to plan all moves through hallways, narrow spaces, over rough terrain, and up or down stairways very carefully.

Geriatric Patients

The geriatric population is one of the fastest-growing demographics in the country. Healthier lifestyles and modern medicine advances are extending life and increasing the older population (Figure 18 ●). As this population grows over the next few decades, it will account for more and more trauma emergency responses. Currently trauma accounts for 25 percent of all geriatric mortality and, with the expected growth of this population, will become an even greater proportion of EMS responses.

The geriatric trauma patient often has coexisting problems associated with aging and chronic disease. Aging affects virtually every body system. Reduced reflexes, hearing, and eyesight result in more injuries in this population, while brittle bones produce fractures with less force. This is especially true of the cervical spine, where the vertebral column becomes more fragile and calcification narrows the spinal foramen, predisposing the geriatric patient to spinal injury. The brain loses mass after middle age and results in a greater incidence of injury because the brain is freer to move about within and impact the interior of the cranium. Smaller cardiac reserves leave older patients less able to respond to hypovolemia with increases in heart rate or cardiac stroke volume. Reduced fluid reserves limit the amount of fluid the cardiovascular system can draw from body tissues to compensate for fluid lost through burns or hemorrhage. The system also cannot accommodate great fluctuations in fluid volume and is more prone to problems of overhydration with resulting pulmonary edema. The vascular system, especially the venous system, is less able to constrict in response to hypovolemia and restore cardiac preload. In addition, reduced respiratory reserves reduce the ability of older patients to accommodate the problems of diaphragmatic respiration associated with spinal injury, of pneumothorax or tension pneumothorax, and of even the reduction in respiratory movement associated with the pain of rib fractures. A higher pain tolerance and reduced pain perception may also mask the symptoms of serious injury, and poorer temperature regulation may predispose the geriatric patient to hypothermia.

Preexisting diseases are more prevalent in the geriatric population and reduce these patients' abilities to handle the physiologic stress of trauma. Cardiovascular disease limits the heart's ability to assist with shock compensation. Chronic respiratory diseases (such as emphysema) increase the cardiac workload and reduce respiratory efficiency and reserves. Many other chronic diseases likewise affect geriatric patients by reducing their ability to compensate for hypovolemia and respond to the stresses of shock. Because of aging and chronic disease, geriatric patients are likely to move more quickly into compensation, then more quickly to uncompensated shock, and then to irreversible shock. They are less able to tolerate the shock state and experience a mortality rate from hypovolemia that is much greater than that of average adults.

Assessment of the geriatric patient is often difficult because the problem that led to the call to EMS is often masked or confused by signs and symptoms of preexisting disease or by a diminished response to pain. However, accurate assessment of these patients is critical because they are less able to tolerate hypovolemia and the stress of shock.

Management of the Geriatric Patient   Initiate shock care early with geriatric patients. Provide that care conservatively, however, to avoid the possibility of fluid overload. Intravenous catheters should be smaller than for normal adults as the catheters must be inserted through rather thin yet tough skin and then through veins that tend to be smaller and more delicate than normal adult veins and that also roll more. During any infusion, auscultate the chest frequently for breath sounds and halt fluid flow at the first signs of crackles. Keep the patient warm and watch carefully for any progression of the signs of shock. The use of ECG monitoring is indicated because hypovolemia and shock may initiate arrhythmias in patients with preexisting cardiac disease. Administer oxygen early to geriatric patients to increase the effectiveness of respirations. Artificial ventilation may be met with greater resistance because of lung stiffness, but excessive ventilation pressures are more likely to lead to pneumothorax. Carefully adjust the bag-valve-mask volume to obtain gentle chest rise. Remember that the elderly are prone to hypothermia, so ensure they are well covered in a cool or cold environment.

Cognitively Impaired Patients

Caring for the patient who has been subjected to trauma and is cognitively impaired presents some special challenges to prehospital assessment. These patients, by definition, have a lower intelligence quotient (IQ) and are less able to communicate and describe what has happened to them or how they feel. Often they have an atypical presentation of symptoms and a decreased threshold to pain. They are often unable to process information in a way that permits informed consent and may tend to be

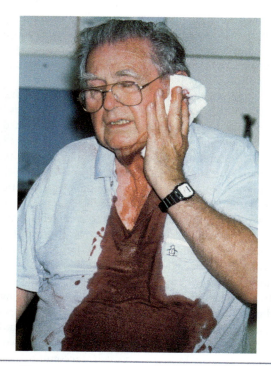

● **Figure 18**   Geriatric patients are one of the fastest-growing groups requiring emergency medical services.
(© *Science Photo Library/Custom Medical Stock Photos, Inc.*)

uncooperative. They may have anatomic abnormalities but are assessed and managed as most other trauma patients.

The cognitively impaired patient often has a lower developmental grade level than an individual of the same age without cognitive impairment. It may benefit your assessment to initially use simple, open-ended sentences to help you determine at what level you can communicate. Try to identify any caregiver and use them to reduce anxiety and increase communications. And be patient. Otherwise, prehospital care should follow that provided to other trauma patients.

Autism (autism spectrum disorder) is a prevalent subset of impaired patients. Incidence is about 1 in 100 and is 4 to 5 times more common in males.[16,17] The autism patient handles information differently than other patients and has difficulty in understanding information, resulting in abnormal social interactions, behavior, and communication. The autistic patient is treated as with any other trauma patient.

INTERACTION WITH OTHER CARE PROVIDERS

Emergency medical services often have a tiered structure consisting of progressive levels of care providers attending to the needs of patients. These care providers include the trained or untrained bystanders, certified Emergency Medical Responders, Emergency Medical Technicians, Advanced EMTs, and other Paramedics. Other members of the system include air medical personnel and the physicians, nurses, and technical personnel in the hospital emergency department, intensive care unit, or surgery. Appropriate interactions among all these members of the EMS system are essential to ensure a good continuum of care for the patient. Your interactions with these members also determine how you are perceived as a care provider and as a professional within the health care system. The information exchanged during these interactions is essential to an effective EMS system and, most importantly, to appropriate patient care (Figure 19 ●).

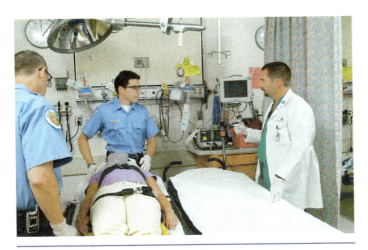

● **Figure 19**   It is essential that information exchange among care providers be rapid, thorough, and accurate.

The initial information you receive from emergency medical responders and EMTs about the patient's condition and the care he received as you assume assessment and care responsibilities is vital. This information is essential for developing your initial patient impression and then formulating a patient management plan. This information, supplemented by your assessment findings, is equally essential to the emergency department physician or nurse as he assumes responsibility for patient care from you. This information should include a description of the mechanism of injury, the results of your assessment, the interventions performed, and the results of those interventions.

Mechanism of Injury

Concisely describe the mechanism of injury with enough detail to identify the nature and severity of the energy exchange. An example might be "a high-speed frontal impact with severe vehicle deformity and passenger compartment intrusion of about 10 inches" or "a head-on collision while two football players were running full speed." Also indicate what the patient was doing when the incident occurred—for example, "was the driver." Give the approximate time of the incident (or time since the incident), if known.

Results of Assessment

Communicate the results of your assessment, describing the injuries and relating any abnormal or unusual history, vital signs, and other assessment findings to the emergency department staff. Describe any wounds covered by bandages or splints in significant detail so those items need not be removed for immediate assessment. Include in your statement all pertinent patient information such as the patient's age, sex, and weight. Also include any allergies, significant medications, significant medical history, last oral intake, and up-to-date vaccinations such as the last tetanus booster. Finally, identify the last set of vital signs, the Glasgow Coma Scale score, and any trends in patient condition noted from your serial ongoing assessments.

Interventions

Identify the care provided by others, then by you, and the results of that care on the patient's condition. Include the size of IV catheters and location of placement; the rate, volume, and type of fluid administered; the dosages, routes, and times of medications administered; and the size and depth of insertion of any advanced airway that has been used.

You should get this information from care providers as you accept responsibility for patient care. If necessary, question the care provider to obtain this information. This information exchange should take only a few moments, and rarely more than a minute. Use this same format and communicate this information to the receiving physician or nurse when you present your patient

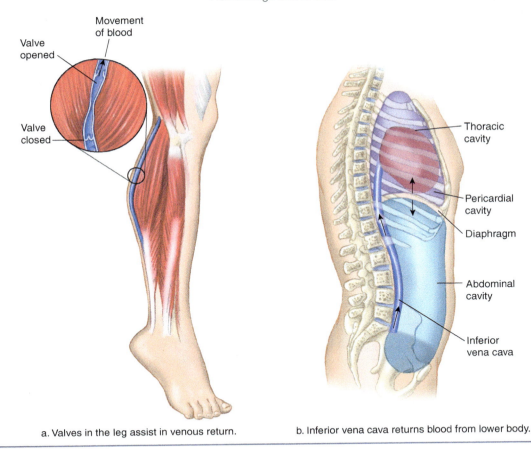

a. Valves in the leg assist in venous return.

b. Inferior vena cava returns blood from lower body.

Figure 11   Venous return.

cardiac output, arterial blood pressure, and, ultimately, the ability to direct blood flow to critical organs. This is the point at which the signs and symptoms of shock begin.

Cardiovascular System Regulation

Much of the human body is controlled by the autonomic nervous system. This system consists of two opposing subsystems that maintain equilibrium and help us respond to and recover from the stresses of daily life. These two systems act in balance, with the parasympathetic system inducing sleep and the sympathetic system responding to and controlling normal waking activity. When a stressor such as danger is perceived, the sympathetic nervous system prepares the organism either to combat or to physically flee the stressor. As just noted, this aggressive body response is termed the fight-or-flight response and is a deeply ingrained protective reflex. While many sympathetic nervous system activities are aimed at defending the organism, they can be detrimental once injury occurs and shock develops.

A system of receptors, autonomic centers, and nervous and hormonal interventions maintain control over the cardiovascular system (Figure 12 ●). **Baroreceptors** in the aortic arch and in the carotid sinuses monitor arterial blood pressure. **Chemoreceptors** in the carotid sinuses monitor carbon dioxide and, to a lesser degree, blood oxygen levels. (There are additional baroreceptors in the atria and chemoreceptors in the brain.)

These receptors send impulses to the cardiovascular centers located in the medulla oblongata. Hormones such as epinephrine, norepinephrine, antidiuretic hormone (ADH), angiotensin II, and aldosterone also influence cardiovascular system function. These agents enter the bloodstream at sympathetic nervous system command, in response to blood pressure fluctuations or by kidney perfusion changes.

Epinephrine and **norepinephrine** are sympathetic agents secreted by the adrenal medulla. They increase peripheral vascular resistance by causing arteriole constriction and by increasing heart rate and contractility. These two hormones, called catecholamines, cause the most rapid hormonal response to hemorrhage and cardiovascular insufficiency. Epinephrine and norepinephrine both have alpha-1 properties. Alpha-1 receptor stimulation causes vasoconstriction and increases both peripheral vascular resistance and cardiac afterload. Additionally, epinephrine has beta-1 and beta-2 properties. Beta-1 receptor stimulation results in an increase in heart rate (positive chronotropy), in cardiac contractile strength (positive inotropy), and in cardiac muscle conductivity (positive dromotropy). Beta-2 effects include bronchodilation and smooth muscle dilation in the bowel.

Antidiuretic hormone (ADH), also known as arginine vasopressin (AVP), is released by the posterior pituitary in response either to reduced blood pressure or increased osmotic pressure of the blood (dehydration). ADH induces an increase in peripheral vascular resistance and causes the kidneys to retain

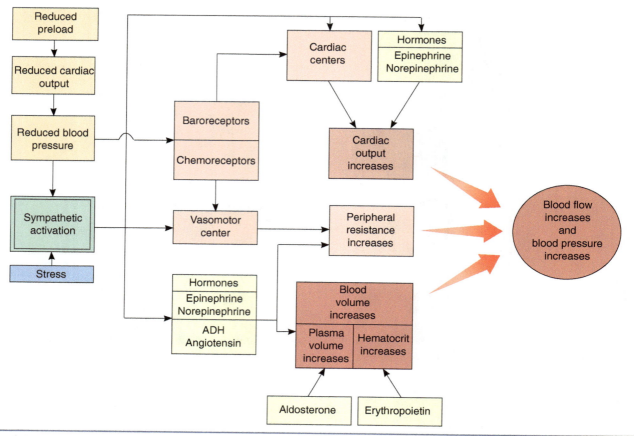

● Figure 12 The body's response to blood loss.

water, decreasing urine output. ADH also causes splenic vascular constriction, returning up to 200 mL of free blood to the circulatory system.

Angiotensin is created by the kidneys during lowered blood pressure and decreased perfusion. A chain reaction begins when specialized smooth cells in the renal venules release an enzyme, renin. Renin converts angiotensin (an inactive protein in the blood) to *angiotensin I*. Angiotensin I is further modified in the lungs by a converting enzyme into *angiotensin II*. This process usually takes about 20 minutes to become fully effective. Angiotensin II is a potent systemic vasoconstrictor that lasts up to an hour. It causes the release of ADH, aldosterone, and epinephrine and also stimulates thirst.

Angiotensin II stimulates **aldosterone** secretion by the adrenal cortex. Aldosterone stimulates kidney cells that maintain ion balance to retain sodium and water. It also reduces sodium and water losses through sweating and the digestive tract.

These nerve pathways and hormone response systems are the sympathetic and parasympathetic nervous systems' chief means of maintaining homeostasis when blood or blood volume is lost. Minor fluctuations in blood volume are regulated by small changes in peripheral vascular resistance, fluid movement to and from the interstitial space, contraction or dilation of the venous system, and increases or decreases in the heart rate and strength of contractions. The system works very well without our being aware of it. However, serious blood loss produces more intense, then more drastic, responses.

The Body's Response to Blood Loss

As hemorrhage causes blood to leave the cardiovascular system, the sympathetic nervous system (and the hormones it releases) begins the progressive responses described previously. As less blood reaches the heart, the ventricles do not completely engorge. Cardiac contractility therefore suffers as the ventricular myocardium does not stretch (Starling's law of the heart). Stroke volume drops, and there is an immediate drop in systolic blood pressure. This reduced pressure reduces the cardiovascular system's ability to drive blood through the capillary beds (tissue perfusion). Aortic and carotid baroreceptors recognize this blood pressure decrease and signal the cardiovascular center in the medulla oblongata. The vasomotor center increases peripheral vascular resistance and venous tone while the cardioacceleratory center increases heart rate. With reduced venous capacitance and an increase in heart rate and peripheral vascular resistance, blood pressure returns to normal and so does tissue perfusion. These actions normally compensate for small blood losses. Without further blood loss, the body reconstitutes the loss from interstitial fluid and replaces lost red blood cells gradually, without noticeable or ill effects.

Cellular Ischemia

If blood loss continues, the venous system constricts to its limits in order to maintain cardiac preload. However, it becomes more and more difficult for the venous system to compensate because its limited musculature tires and relaxes. Simultaneously, peripheral vascular resistance increases to maintain systolic blood pressure and ensure direction of blood flow to critical organs like the heart, brain, and kidneys. As it does, diastolic blood pressure rises, pulse pressure narrows, and the pulse weakens. Arteriole constriction results in less and less blood directed to noncritical organs, and these organs become hypoxic. The skin, the largest noncritical organ, receives reduced circulation and becomes cool, pale, and moist. If hemorrhage continues, some noncritical organ cells begin to starve for oxygen. Anaerobic metabolism is their only energy source, and lactic acid and other toxins begin to accumulate. Cellular hypoxia begins, followed by ischemia. The heart rate increases, but slowly, because other compensatory mechanisms are still effectively maintaining preload.

As blood loss increases, more and more body cells are deprived of their oxygen and nutrient supplies, and more and more waste products accumulate. The bloodstream becomes acidic, and the body's chemoreceptors stimulate an increase in the depth and rate of respiration. Hypoxia causes alterations in the level of consciousness, and circulating catecholamines cause the patient to become anxious, restless, and possibly combative. Hypoxia and ischemia now begin to affect arterioles. These vessels, which also require oxygen, relax. Meanwhile, coronary arteries provide a decreasing amount of oxygenated blood to the laboring heart.

If blood loss stops, the cardiovascular system draws fluid from the interstitial space at a rate of up to 1 L per hour to restore its volume, and erythropoietin accelerates red blood cell production. Kidneys reduce urine output to conserve water and electrolytes, and a period of thirst provides a stimulus to drink liquids and replace lost fluid volume on a more permanent basis. Transfusion with whole blood may be required at this point. While some signs of circulatory compromise and fatigue are present, the patient's recovery is probable with a period of rest.

Capillary Microcirculation

If blood loss continues, sympathetic stimulation and reduced kidney, pancreas, and liver perfusion cause hormone release. Angiotensin II further increases peripheral vascular resistance and reduces blood flow to more tissues. As hemorrhage continues, circulation is further limited to only those organs most critical to life. This further decrease in circulation leads to an increase in cellular hypoxia in noncritical tissues, and more cells begin to use anaerobic metabolism for energy in a desperate attempt to survive. The buildup of lactic acid and carbon dioxide relaxes precapillary sphincters. Circulating blood volume is further diminished both by continued hemorrhage and by fluid loss as capillary beds engorge. Postcapillary sphincters remain closed, forcing fluids into interstitial spaces by hydrostatic pressure. The circulatory crisis worsens as compensatory mechanisms begin to fail. Interstitial edema further reduces capillary ability to provide oxygen and nutrients to and remove carbon dioxide and other waste products from cells. Capillary walls and cell membranes also begin to break down. Red blood cells begin to clump together, or agglutinate, in hypoxic and stagnant capillaries forming columns of coagulated erythrocytes called rouleaux formation.

Capillary Washout

Building acidosis from accumulating lactic acid and carbon dioxide (which rapidly converts in the blood to carbonic acid) finally causes postcapillary sphincter relaxation. With relaxation, these by-products, along with potassium (released by the cells to maintain a neutral environment in the presence of building acidosis) and rouleaux, are dumped into the venous circulation. This capillary washout causes profound metabolic acidosis and microscopic emboli. Cardiac output drops toward zero. Peripheral vascular resistance drops toward zero. Blood pressure drops toward zero. Cellular perfusion, even to the most critical organs, drops toward zero. The body moves quickly and then irreversibly toward death.

Stages of Shock

The shock process, as previously described, can be divided into three stages based on the body's ability to compensate and presenting signs and symptoms. These stages are progressively more serious and include compensated, decompensated, and irreversible shock (Table 2).

Compensated Shock

Compensated shock is the initial shock state. In this stage, the body is capable of meeting its critical metabolic needs through a series of progressive compensating actions (Figure 13 ●). This progressive compensation creates a series of signs and symptoms that range from subtle to obvious. Compensated shock ends with a precipitous drop in blood pressure. This is the shock stage in which prehospital interventions and rapid transport are most likely to meet with success.

A patient's first recognizable response to serious blood loss is an increase in pulse rate. However, this may be difficult to differentiate from tachycardia caused by pain, excitement, and the fight-or-flight response. The first sign reliably attributable to shock is a narrowing pulse pressure as cardiac output drops and peripheral vascular resistance increases to maintain circulation. Here the pulse weakens and its rate increases. With initial hypovolemia, the patient may complain of thirst. As blood loss continues and becomes more serious, vasoconstriction causes the patient's skin to become pale, cyanotic, or ashen as blood is directed away from skin and toward more critical organs. The skin becomes cool and moist (clammy), and capillary refill times lengthen. Respiratory rate increases slowly and becomes more labored. As compensation continues and becomes more acute, victims become anxious, restless, or combative and complain of increasing thirst and weakness. Near the end of the compensated shock stage, the patient may experience air hunger and tachypnea.

Decompensated Shock

Decompensated shock begins as compensatory mechanisms become unable to respond to a continuing blood loss. Mechanisms that initially compensated for blood loss now fail, and the body moves quickly toward complete collapse. Entry into

CONTENT REVIEW

▶ Stages of Shock

- • Compensated
- • Decompensated
- • Irreversible

TABLE 2 | The Stages of Shock

Compensated Shock
Initial stage of shock in which the body progressively compensates for continuing blood loss.

- Pulse rate increases
- Pulse strength decreases
- Skin becomes cool and clammy
- Progressing anxiety, restlessness, combativeness
- Thirst, weakness, eventual air hunger

Decompensated Shock
Begins when the body's compensatory mechanisms can no longer maintain preload.

- Pulse becomes unpalpable
- Blood pressure drops precipitously
- Patient becomes unconscious
- Respirations slow or cease

Irreversible Shock
Shortly after the patient enters decompensated shock, the lack of circulation begins to have profound effects on body cells. As they are irreversibly damaged, the cells die, tissues dysfunction, organs dysfunction, and the patient dies.

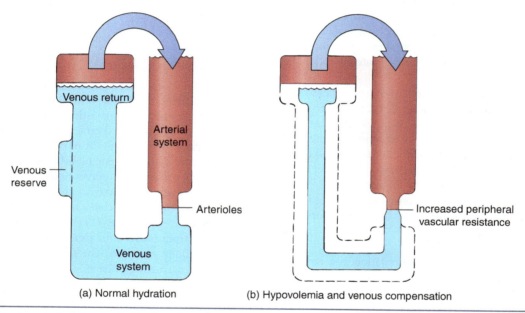

● **Figure 13**   In compensated shock, the body reduces venous capacitance in response to blood loss.

decompensated shock is heralded by the inability of peripheral vascular resistance to maintain blood pressure. This results in a precipitous drop in blood pressure. As all compensatory mechanisms fail, venous return is inadequate, and the heart no longer has enough returning blood volume to pump. Even extreme tachycardia produces little additional cardiac output. No amount of vascular resistance can maintain blood pressure and circulation. Even the most critical organs of the body are hypoperfused. The heart, already hypoxic because of poor perfusion and the increased oxygen demands created by tachycardia and increased contractility, begins to fail. In this stage, the brain is extremely hypoxic. This means that the patient displays a rapidly dropping level of responsiveness. The brain's control over bodily functions, including respiration, diminishes, and the body takes on a death-like appearance.

Irreversible Shock

Irreversible shock exists when the body's cells are so badly injured and die in such quantities that organs cannot carry out their normal functions. While aggressive resuscitation may restore blood pressure and a pulse, organ failure ultimately results in organism failure. The transition between decompensated and irreversible shock is a clinical one and impossible to differentiate using signs or symptoms. Clearly, the longer a patient is in decompensated shock, the more likely it is that he has moved to irreversible shock.

Etiology of Shock

The shock discussion to this point has focused on blood loss and its effects on the cardiovascular system. However, shock can have many causes, and a common way of classifying types of shock is based on its origins: hypovolemic, cardiogenic, neurogenic, anaphylactic, and septic. Despite a variety of origins, patients suffering from different types of shock present with similar signs and symptoms; go through the same compensated, decompensated, and irreversible shock stages; and suffer similar systemic complications.

Hypovolemic Shock

Hypovolemic shock, which we have already discussed in detail, is caused by any significant reduction in the volume of the cardiovascular system. While hemorrhage is a common cause, fluid loss from other pathologies can occur. Plasma losses may result from severe and extensive burns or possibly from granulating (seeping) wounds. Fluid and electrolyte losses such as those that occur with protracted vomiting, diarrhea, sweating, and urination also diminish the body's vascular fluids and may result in hypovolemia. Hypovolemic shock may also result from "third space" losses such as fluid shifts into various body compartments as occurs in severe pancreatitis. Hemorrhagic shock is a specific subset of hypovolemia caused by blood loss.

Cardiogenic Shock

Cardiogenic shock results from cardiac insufficiency. Because of the heart's essential function, any cardiac pathology has a profound impact on circulation. If cardiac artery blockage deprives a portion of the heart muscle of oxygenated circulation, it becomes hypoxic, then ischemic, and then necrotic. During infarct evolution, there can be cardiac electrical system disturbances, cardiac valve failure, cardiac rupture, or reduced cardiac pumping action. Any of these problems reduces cardiac output, which cannot be compensated for by some other body system. If cardiac output falls below what the body requires, cardiogenic shock ensues. Cardiogenic shock may present with the signs and symptoms of myocardial infarction or pulmonary edema and with the classic signs and symptoms of shock. The prognosis for cardiogenic shock is very poor, with an 80 percent mortality rate.

Neurogenic Shock

Neurogenic shock results from an interruption in the communication pathway between the central nervous system and the body. A spinal injury or, in some cases, a head injury, either temporary or permanent, disrupts nervous (generally sympathetic nervous) system control over vasculature distal to the injury. Arterioles dilate, the vascular container expands, and fluid is driven into the interstitial space. The body's compensatory mechanisms are often affected, and tachycardia and rising diastolic blood pressure expected with shock states may not occur. In these cases, the patient's skin below the nervous system injury is warm and pink while the skin above it displays more classic signs of shock: pallor, coolness, and clamminess.

Anaphylactic Shock

In **anaphylactic shock**, the introduction of a foreign substance into the body causes a massive histamine release. This, in turn, causes general vasodilation, precapillary sphincter dilation, capillary engorgement, and fluid movement into the interstitial compartment.

Septic Shock

Septic shock results from massive infection releasing toxins that adversely affect the vascular system's ability to control blood vessels and distribute blood.

CONTENT REVIEW

▶ Types of Shock

- Hypovolemic
- Cardiogenic
- Neurogenic
- Anaphylactic
- Septic

HEMORRHAGE AND SHOCK ASSESSMENT

As we have already emphasized, because shock is the transition between normal life and trauma death, its discovery and treatment are essential trauma skills. The early signs of shock are subtle and not easy to recognize unless you are specifically looking for them. Hence, shock assessment and discovery becomes an important primary paramedic skill. Trauma assessment for hemorrhage and shock begins with the scene size-up and continues throughout transport and care.

Scene Size-Up

Remember that Standard Precautions are essential during trauma patient assessment. A patient's blood and other body fluids may contain pathogens capable of transmitting HIV, hepatitis, and other diseases. Conversely, you may transmit infectious agents to your patient, through their wounds, as you assess and care for them. In fact, the risk of your transmitting disease or infection to patients with open wounds or burns is much greater than the risk that they will transmit disease or infection to you. For these reasons, observe Standard Precautions with all trauma patients. These precautions include using gloves and a mask when you inspect or palpate any injured area, especially one with open wounds (Figure 14 ●). If blood is spurting, as with arterial hemorrhage; if a patient is combative; or if there is

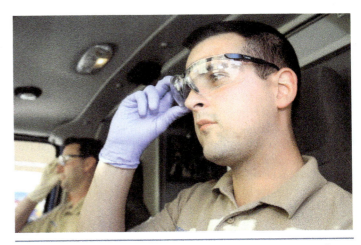

● **Figure 14**   When caring for a hemorrhaging patient, employ appropriate Standard Precautions. (© Dr. Bryan E. Bledsoe)

airway trauma with or without bleeding, also wear eye protection and a disposable gown (to protect your clothing).

Search for and rule out other scene hazards such as traffic; electrocution; sharp objects; fire and explosion; hot objects; toxic substances; confined spaces; structural instability; rough, slippery, or unstable terrain; environmental extremes; and violence. If you cannot rule out these hazards or make the scene safe, do not enter the scene. Also, ensure the safety of fellow rescuers, your patient (or patients), and bystanders.

Examine the weather conditions affecting the emergency scene. It will impact both how you and your patient respond to the incident. Be mindful that extremes of heat and cold can provide additional stress to the patient who is subject to hemorrhage and shock compensation. Environmental conditions can also impact your ability to determine vital signs and perform a physical assessment. Anticipate these effects and do what you can to compensate for them. And, keep the hemorrhage and shock patient warm.

When scene hazards have been taken care of, continue with scene size-up. Evaluate the mechanism of injury to anticipate where external and internal hemorrhage might be found. Anticipating external hemorrhage sites directs your subsequent assessment and, possibly, care, while anticipating internal hemorrhage affects your decision on whether to provide rapid transport or more extensive scene care.

When evaluating mechanism of injury (MOI), also attempt to determine the time elapsed between injury and your patient evaluation. Knowing this time period is essential to determine the amount and rate of blood loss. For example, if a patient is losing about 150 mL of blood per minute and you arrive on a scene 3 minutes after an injury-producing incident, the patient has lost 450 mL of blood. You would not expect this patient to display signs and symptoms of class I hemorrhage. If, however, you arrive 10 minutes after the incident, the same patient, losing blood at the same rate, will have lost 1,500 mL of blood and is likely to have reached class III hemorrhage and to display frank signs of shock. In both these cases, the patient is suffering serious, life-threatening hemorrhage. Good assessment techniques and early hemorrhage severity recognition ensure you will provide a proper course of care. However, the earlier you arrive at the patient, the harder it is to identify serious hemorrhage. For this reason, you must be aware of and appreciate the progressive effects of blood loss. Consider the time since an incident and the patient's presentation to help you determine the seriousness of hemorrhage and the potential for shock. Remember, the sooner signs of severe hemorrhage appear, the greater the rate and volume of blood loss and the more serious the patient's condition. Anticipate shock during the scene size-up. Look especially for injury mechanisms that might result in serious internal chest, abdominal, or pelvic injuries or in external hemorrhage from the head, neck, and extremities. This information will guide your later assessment. With serious trauma forces subjected to the body, carry a high index of suspicion for shock and remember it is the most frequent cause of trauma death.

Finally, complete the remaining elements of the scene size-up. Be sure to identify and locate all possible patients and determine what effect, if any, environmental conditions will have on patient assessment, care, and transport. Lastly, ensure there is scene oversight. In a limited event, assign roles to the members of your team. In a large event or one where there are several or many services involved, employ a more involved system of incident management.

Primary Assessment

The primary assessment directs your attention to body systems and patient priorities that present the earliest signs of shock. As you begin the primary assessment, form a general patient impression and assess the patient's initial mental status to determine alertness, orientation, and responsiveness. Be alert for any signs of anxiety, confusion, or combativeness. Any mental status deficit may be secondary to hemorrhage, hypovolemia, and shock, so be suspicious. Also look for facial expression and any signs of fear that might suggest how they perceive their condition. Carefully observe the patient's body surface and be quick to anticipate shock, either as a cause of or a contributing factor to the patient's condition. Look to the patient's general skin condition. It should be warm, pink, and dry. If it is cyanotic, gray, ashen, pale, and cool and moist (clammy), suspect peripheral vasoconstriction, which is an early sign of shock. With this information you form a preliminary patient impression that continues to evolve during all of your assessment and care. If it appears your patient is in cardiac arrest, begin the C-A-B of Advanced Cardiac Life Support in which cardiovascular care precedes airway and breathing care. Otherwise continue with the A-B-C approach to primary assessment and care as well as secondary assessment and trauma care.

If you cannot rule out spinal injury, provide spinal precautions. (Apply manual immobilization but delay cervical collar application until you assess the neck during the rapid trauma assessment.)

As you assess for airway patency and breathing adequacy, apply high-concentration oxygen as needed to ensure an oxygen saturation of at least 96 percent. Ensure that injuries do not interfere with airway control and that the patient is fully able to protect his airway. If the airway is not under the patient's control, consider an extraglottic airway or endotracheal intubation.

Carefully visualize the chest and observe the patient's respiratory effort and chest excursion. Watch for tachypnea and air hunger, which are late signs of shock. Continue to monitor oxygen saturation and keep it at least 96 percent, if possible. If it falls below 90 percent, consider ventilating the patient. As shock compensation increases and pulse pressure diminishes, the pulse oximeter has a more difficult time recognizing pulsing arterial blood. Thus, its readings will become more and more erratic. Should this occur, suspect increasing cardiovascular compensation and progressing shock as the reason.

Capnography can be a valuable assessment tool during trauma patient resuscitation and is now a standard of care. Waveform end-tidal CO_2 ($ETCO_2$) analysis helps ensure proper initial and continuing endotracheal tube placement and guides artificial ventilation. The capnograph measures CO_2 partial pressures in exhaled air, reflecting both ventilation and circulation status. Decreased $ETCO_2$ levels reflect cardiac arrest, shock, pulmonary embolism, or incomplete airway obstruction (bronchospasm, mucus plugging). Increased $ETCO_2$ levels reflect hypoventilation, respiratory depression, or hyperthermia. $ETCO_2$ readings above 40 mmHg suggest the need for increased ventilatory support. Readings below 30 mmHg suggest hyperventilation or the need for circulatory support. Capnography may not signal intubation of a mainstem bronchus, so ensure that breath sounds are bilaterally equal while an endotracheal tube is in place.

Capnography is especially important in head-injured patients who are intubated, as abnormally low alveolar CO_2 levels (hyperventilation) may produce severe cerebral vasoconstriction. Normal expiratory CO_2 levels are between 35 and 40 mmHg and should not drop below 30 mmHg, especially in head trauma patients. An expiratory CO_2 level above 40 mmHg suggests hypoventilation and the need for faster and/or deeper ventilations.

When assessing circulation, note heart rate and pulse strength. A heart rate above 100 in an adult (tachycardia) suggests hypovolemia or excitement. Baseline rates suggestive of tachycardia are about 160 in the infant, 140 in the preschooler, and 120 in the school-age child. An increase of 20 beats per minute above any of these rates suggests a significant blood loss. Pay special attention to pulse pressure. Remember that it narrows well before systolic pressure begins to drop. A fast—and especially a fast, weak (thready)—pulse may be the first noticeable sign of serious internal blood loss, hypovolemia, and shock. Note also skin color and condition. As the body begins its compensation for blood loss, it constricts the peripheral arterioles and reduces blood flow to and through the skin. Pale or mottled skin is an early sign of shock, as is cool and clammy skin.

Complete the primary assessment by establishing patient priorities, using the CUPS acronym. A patient who, because of serious and life-threatening injury, does not make it out of the primary assessment (you cannot stabilize the airway, breathing, or circulation) is considered critical (C). Otherwise, categorize the patient as unstable (U), potentially unstable (P), or stable (S). Decide, based on your findings to this point, whether the patient is to receive a rapid trauma assessment, quick care, and rapid transport (the unstable and potentially unstable patient) or a focused trauma assessment (the stable patient) and more traditional care and transport. If any sign or symptom suggests serious internal hemorrhage or uncontrolled external hemorrhage, and shock, ensure rapid trauma assessment and then immediate patient transport.

Secondary Assessment

Critical patients do not receive a secondary assessment because, by definition, you are unable to stabilize the airway, breathing, or circulation during the primary assessment. For the critical patient, you will continue primary assessment and the associated interventions. Unstable and potentially unstable patients receive a rapid trauma assessment. Stable patients (and generally ones with a single isolated injury) receive a focused trauma assessment.

Rapid Trauma Assessment

For trauma patients with serious injury signs and/or a significant MOI, you will perform a rapid trauma assessment, quickly inspecting and palpating the patient from head to toe. Pay particular attention to areas where critical trauma may have occurred and areas where the MOI suggests forces were focused. If you notice any significant hemorrhage, control it immediately. Quickly put a dressing and bandage over the wound and apply direct pressure. Provide more complete hemorrhage control after you finish the secondary assessment and attend to any injuries with a higher priority for care.

Carefully and quickly observe the head for serious bleeding. Internal head injury rarely accounts for classic signs of shock (except in the very young patient). However, the scalp bleeds profusely because vessels there are large and lack ability to constrict (at least as well as other peripheral vessels can). If any external bleeding appears serious, halt it immediately. Look at the facial region to rule out an injury that might compromise the airway or be a source of serious hemorrhage.

Next, examine the neck. In the supine, normovolemic patient, the jugular veins should be fully distended. If they are flat, you should suspect hypovolemia. The carotid arteries and jugular veins are large blood vessels located close to the anterior and lateral surfaces of the neck and their injury can produce rapid and fatal exsanguination. An added danger is air aspiration directly into an open jugular vein. At times, jugular venous pressure, as a result of gravity and deep inspiration, may be less than atmospheric pressure. Air may then be drawn into the vein, traveling to the heart and forming air (gas) emboli, which then may lodge in the pulmonary circulation. Quickly control any serious hemorrhage from neck wounds with a sterile occlusive dressing. If spinal injury is suspected, apply a rigid cervical collar when neck assessment is complete, but maintain manual spinal immobilization until the patient is secured to a vest-type immobilization device, spine board, or rigid scoop (orthopedic) stretcher.

Visualize the anterior and lateral chest and abdomen (presuming the patient is supine) for any serious external hemorrhage, though such external bleeding is uncommon there. You are more likely to note signs of blunt or penetrating trauma, suggesting injury and hemorrhage within. Look at the abdomen for signs of soft-tissue injury, contusions, abrasions, rigidity, guarding, and tenderness that suggest internal injury. Note that the dramatic discoloration of a contusion is unlikely to develop by the time of your arrival. Simple erythema (skin reddening) may be the only indicator of serious blunt trauma to either the chest or abdomen.

During your rapid trauma assessment, rule out the possibility of obstructive shock. Assess the chest to identify any tension pneumothorax. Look for dyspnea, a hyperinflated chest, asymmetrical chest movement, distended jugular veins, resonant percussion, diminished or absent breath sounds on the affected side, lower tracheal shift to the opposite side (a late sign), and any subcutaneous emphysema. Consider pleural decompression if the signs suggest tension pneumothorax. Also suspect pericardial tamponade with penetrating central

▶ Signs and Symptoms of Internal Hemorrhage

Early

- Pain, tenderness, swelling, or discoloration of suspected injury site
- Bleeding from mouth, rectum, vagina, or other orifice
- Vomiting of bright red blood
- Tender, rigid, and/or distended abdomen

Late

- Anxiety, restlessness, combativeness, or altered mental status
- Weakness, faintness, or dizziness
- Vomiting of blood the color of dark coffee grounds
- Thirst
- Melena
- Shallow, rapid breathing
- Rapid, weak pulse
- Pale, cool, clammy skin
- Capillary refill greater than 2 seconds (most reliable in infants and children under 6)
- Dropping blood pressure
- Dilated pupils sluggish in responding to light
- Nausea and vomiting

chest trauma. Look for distended jugular veins, muffled or distant heart tones, tachycardia, and progressive and extreme hypotension. Pericardial tamponade is treated with IV fluids in the field and requires immediate and rapid transport to a trauma center. If the patient received significant anterior chest trauma, you should suspect myocardial contusion. Apply an ECG monitor and analyze the cardiac rhythm.

Quickly examine the pelvic and groin region. Test pelvic ring integrity by pressing gently on the iliac crests. If you already suspect pelvic fracture, do not compress the iliac crests or otherwise manipulate the pelvis. Remember that pelvic fractures can account for blood loss of more than 2,000 mL. Lacerations to the male genitalia may also account for serious external hemorrhage.

Assess extremities to identify the presence of femur, tibia/fibula, or humerus fractures. Keep in mind that a femur fracture can account for up to 1,500 mL of blood loss, while each tibia/fibula or humerus fracture may contribute an additional 500 to 750 mL of blood loss. Hematomas and large contusions may account for up to 500 mL of blood loss in the larger muscle masses. Quickly check distal pulse strength, capillary refill, muscle tone, and sensation in each extremity, comparing findings in the opposing extremities.

Be sure to carefully examine body areas where the mechanism of injury and your index of suspicion suggest serious injury. Examine these areas carefully because signs and symptoms of serious internal injury may be difficult to recognize. Remember, minor skin reddening may be the only sign of a developing contusion and serious internal injury. Remember also that classic signs of shock take time to develop.

Finally, sweep all body regions hidden from your view for external hemorrhage that may have gone unnoticed during your examination to this point. Remember to assess these areas as they become accessible during patient movement or further patient care.

During assessment, be alert to problems other than hemorrhagic shock affecting your patient. Conditions such as stroke, epilepsy, or heart attack can lead to auto crashes and other trauma events. Be careful to rule out cardiogenic shock by questioning

the patient about chest pain and looking for pulmonary edema, jugular vein distention, and cardiac arrhythmias. Also suspect and check for neurogenic shock. Ask about neck or back pain and evaluate for tenderness along the spine or any numbness or tingling sensations. Look for the presence of pink and warm skin below a nervous system injury, while skin above the injury is pale, cool, and clammy. Other shock states such as anaphylactic, septic, and diabetic shock are not likely unless the patient history suggests them.

At the end of the rapid trauma assessment, assess patient vital signs, determine a Glasgow Coma Scale score, complete a patient medical history as time permits, and inventory injuries you have found that may contribute to shock. Revise your patient's priority for transport and for injury care, as necessary. If any sign or symptom suggests serious internal or uncontrolled external hemorrhage, consider rapid transport for the patient. Approximate the probable volume of blood lost to fractures, large contusions, and hematomas. Also note the probable locations of internal hemorrhage and attempt to approximate blood loss from them. Identify all significant injuries and assign each a priority for care. While you may not complete care for all injuries, setting priorities ensures that you quickly address those injuries most likely to contribute to patient hypovolemia and shock. As the patient displays more and more signs of shock compensation, increase his priority for transport and care. Be sure to record your assessment results carefully. Compare these results with signs and symptoms you discover during reassessments to identify trends in the patient's condition.

Focused Trauma Assessment

Employ a focused trauma assessment for patients without signs or symptoms of serious injury or blood loss—for example, a patient who has lacerated her finger with a knife. You can control hemorrhage for this patient at the scene when the MOI and primary assessment do not suggest additional problems (CUPS – Stable patient). With patients like this, focus your exam on the area injured. Inspect and palpate the area thoroughly, looking for additional injuries beyond the one that you initially saw. Obtain baseline vital signs and a patient history, and prepare and transport the patient.

In some cases, you may wish to perform a rapid trauma assessment, even though the patient does not have significant signs of injury. This would be the case, for example, if you suspect a patient has more injuries than he complains of, if his general condition appears worse than his injuries would cause, you discover vital signs that suggest injuries that are worse than you have found, or if his condition suddenly begins to deteriorate.

Additional Assessment Considerations

In trauma or medical patients showing signs and symptoms of blood loss and shock, it is important to search for evidence of internal hemorrhage. This evidence may be frank blood or other material suggestive of blood loss. Bright red blood from the mouth, nose, rectum, or other orifice suggests direct and active bleeding. Coffee-grounds-appearing emesis is often associated with slow hemorrhage into the stomach. Stool with frank blood in it (hematochezia) reflects active bleeding in the colon or rectum. A black, tarry stool (melena) suggests blood has remained in the bowel for some time. During your rapid trauma assessment be sure to examine all body orifices for signs of hemorrhage.

In patients with nonspecific complaints—general ill feeling, anxiousness, restlessness—or a lowered level of responsiveness, suspect and look for other signs of internal hemorrhage. Watch your patient for an increasing pulse rate, weakening pulse strength (rising diastolic blood pressure and narrowing blood pressure), and cool and clammy skin.

Also observe for dizziness or syncope when a patient moves from a supine to a sitting or standing position. This diagnostic sign is called orthostatic hypotension and suggests a blood volume loss, possibly attributable to internal hemorrhage. This phenomenon is the basis of the tilt test, which you can employ to determine blood or fluid loss and the body's reduced ability to compensate for normal positional change. Perform this test only on patients who do not already display signs and symptoms of shock. Prepare for the test by obtaining blood pressure and pulse rates from the patient in a supine or seated position. Then have the supine patient move to a seated position or the seated patient stand up and obtain another quick blood pressure and pulse rate. If the systolic blood pressure drops more than 20 mmHg, the pulse rate rises by more than 20 beats per minute, or the patient experiences light-headedness, the test is considered positive and indicates hypovolemia.[3]

Patient Medical History

During the rapid or focused trauma assessment, question your patient regarding the chief complaint and his past medical history. Listen to any patient complaints of weakness, thirst, or nausea, which may be further signs of shock. Pay close attention to evidence your questioning reveals because preexisting medical problems, medications, last oral intake, and other medical information can identify just how your patient will respond to the stress of blood loss and shock compensation. Aspirin and other anticoagulants (e.g., warfarin, dabigatran, and enoxaparin) can prolong or worsen hemorrhage. Beta-blockers can reduce tachycardia associated with reduced venous blood return and hypotension. Any significant preexisting medical condition can reduce the patient's ability to tolerate and compensate for hemorrhage and shock.

Detailed Physical Exam

Consider performing a detailed physical exam on a potential shock patient only after all priorities have been addressed and the patient is either en route to the trauma center or circumstances, such as a prolonged extrication, prevent immediate transport. If you have time, assess the patient from head to toe and look for any additional signs of injury. Remember that your early arrival at the patient's side may mean that ecchymosis (black-and-blue discoloration) associated with injuries has not had time to develop. Therefore, very carefully look for reddening (erythema) and areas of local warmth, suggestive of trauma.

Reassessment

After completing the primary assessment, rapid or focused trauma assessment, and all appropriate lifesaving care, perform serial reassessments. Perform these reassessments frequently—at least every 5 minutes with critical, unstable, or potentially unstable patients and every 15 minutes with stable ones. Reevaluate your patient's general impression; reassess his mental status, airway, breathing, and circulation; obtain an additional set of vital signs and Glasgow Coma Scale score; and note oximetry and capnography readings. Compare each finding with earlier ones to determine if the patient's condition is stable, deteriorating, or improving. Pay particular attention to pulse rate and pulse pressure. If the pulse rate is increasing and the difference between diastolic and systolic pressures is decreasing, suspect increasing compensation and worsening shock. Also pay particular attention to changes in your patient's other symptoms or mental status, noting any increasing confusion, anxiety, or restlessness. Perform a focused assessment for any changes in symptoms the patient reports. Also, check the adequacy and effectiveness of any interventions you have performed.

HEMORRHAGE AND SHOCK MANAGEMENT

Hemorrhage management is an integral part of trauma patient care that begins during the primary assessment and is shaped by findings of the rapid or focused trauma assessment. A patient who is hemorrhaging may not need further shock care if bleeding can be controlled early and effectively. Otherwise, shock care will be essential. We will address the care for the patient with active bleeding first (Hemorrhage Management), then discuss hemorrhagic shock care (Shock Management).

Hemorrhage Management

First, ensure that the airway is patent and breathing is adequate or establish and maintain the airway and provide the necessary ventilatory support. Administer high-concentration oxygen as needed and use pulse-oximetry, capnography, and patient signs and symptoms to guide ventilation depth and rate.

During primary assessment, care for serious (arterial and heavy venous) hemorrhage immediately after you correct airway and breathing problems. Quickly apply dressings, held firmly in place by self-adherent bandage material or cravats. Return to provide better hemorrhage control and bandaging after you complete the primary and rapid trauma assessments. Then set your priorities for care of wound sites and other trauma you discover. If the patient displays early signs of shock, consider initiating one or two large-bore IVs as long as the procedure does not delay transport. If IV initiation is likely to delay transport of a critical or unstable patient, provide it during transport.

Once you complete the rapid trauma assessment, begin caring for injuries, including hemorrhage, in the priority order you have established. As you work down your injury priority list and come to a wound, inspect the site to identify the type and exact location of bleeding. This helps you apply pressure—either digitally or with dressings and bandages—to most effectively halt blood loss. Carefully describe the wound's nature as part of your prehospital care report. If you document and convey this information clearly to emergency department staff, you reduce any need for others to remove the dressing (thus disrupting the clotting process) to identify the injury's nature.

Direct Pressure

Direct pressure controls all but the most persistent hemorrhage. Although systolic blood pressure drives arterial hemorrhage, you can stop such a hemorrhage with simple finger pressure properly applied to the bleeding source. If a wound looks as though it may pose a problem, insert a wad of dressing material over the heaviest bleeding site and apply a firm bandage over the dressing. This focuses pressure on the site and away from the surrounding area. If bleeding saturates the dressing, cover it with another dressing and apply another bandage to keep pressure on the wound. Removing the soaked bandage and dressing disrupts the clotting process and prolongs hemorrhage. If, however, the wound continues to bleed through your dressing and bandage layers, consider removing all dressing materials to visualize the exact site of bleeding. Then reapply a wad of dressing and firm direct pressure to the precise hemorrhage site. Often, when blood loss control is ineffective, direct pressure has not been applied to the hemorrhage source.

There are three anatomic sites where firm digital pressure to control bleeding must be performed with precision to avoid damaging nearby or underlying tissues. These are the head, the eye orbits, and the neck. When a head wound is associated with an open fracture and possible brain injury (e.g., brain tissue is exposed), do not place pressure directly on the fractured skull or brain, neither of which contribute much bleeding. Instead, apply digital pressure to the scalp edges. When serious bleeding arises from the eye orbits, avoid placing pressure directly on the globe of the eye, which is sensitive to pressure and may be permanently damaged if severely compressed. The neck contains many large blood vessels that can bleed profusely if lacerated. Firm digital pressure may be critical to stanching hemorrhage. However, avoid pressure on the trachea, larynx, and other airway structures as this may lead to airway constriction and hypoxia.

Other techniques that can aid in hemorrhage control include limb splinting and the use of pneumatic splints. Splinting helps maintain wound site stability and does not disturb clot development. Splinting may also protect the site from movement and injury that might occur if the patient is jostled as you assess and care for other wounds or during extrication and transport. Pneumatic splints immobilize and apply direct pressure, circumferentially, to an injured limb.

Elevation and Pressure Points

Elevation and pressure point application have been used in the past to augment direct pressure and hemorrhage control. Research has put into question just how effective these techniques are. Elevation also causes you to move a patient's injured limb while pressure point application requires a care provider to maintain the pressure once applied (limiting any additional care he is able to apply). Consult your instructor, protocols,

and system medical director about using elevation and pressure points in your EMS system.

If direct pressure alone does not halt minor-to-moderate extremity hemorrhage, consider elevation. Elevation reduces the systolic blood pressure because the heart has to push the blood against gravity and up the limb. Use elevation only when there is an isolated bleeding wound on a limb and movement will not aggravate any other injuries. Remember, however that direct pressure is the most effective hemorrhage control procedure.

If bleeding still persists, find an arterial pulse point proximal to the wound and apply firm pressure there. This further reduces blood pressure within the limb and may reduce the hemorrhage rate. Keep in mind that such pressure must be maintained once applied.

Topical Hemostatic Agents

A recent development in hemorrhage care is the introduction of hemostatic dressings and agents (Figure 15 ●). These materials are FDA approved and are applied directly or indirectly to active hemorrhage. They use various methods to support blood coagulation and help control further blood loss. Agents either are in dust or powder form applied directly to the wound, contained within a fabric pouch, or are impregnated into dressings that are then applied directly to the wound. Some hemostatic agents are made from the shells of shrimp, crabs, and other crustaceas (e.g., Chitosan). When moistened by blood, they become adherent, collect red blood cells, and stop the hemorrhage. These agents are also somewhat antibacterial and hypoallergenic. Another class of hemostatic agents is made from chemically altered volcanic rock (e.g., Zeolite). When poured on fresh blood it reacts, creating heat (an exothermic reaction) and drawing water from the blood. The heat and dehydration concentrate the blood and enhance coagulation. A final hemostatic agent is a

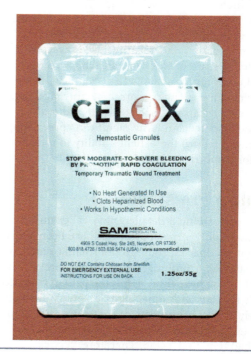

● **Figure 15**   Topical hemostatic agents such as Celox™ are a new development in wound care. (© *Dr. Bryan E. Bledsoe*)

starch-based powder derived from plants. It is dusted over the wound with a small bellows device and causes its action by drawing up water and dehydrating the clotting blood.[4,5,6]

Tourniquets

Consider using a tourniquet only as a last resort when hemorrhage is prolonged and persistent (Figure 16 ●). Tourniquet use may be necessary in crush injury where it is very hard to locate the exact location of blood loss. It is also suggested that deep penetrating trauma might provide a wound with hemorrhage that is difficult to control. However, as mentioned earlier, there are hazards associated with tourniquet use. Apply a commercial tourniquet just proximal to the hemorrhage site and firmly secure it. If you use a blood pressure cuff, inflate it to a pressure of 20 to 30 mmHg greater than the systolic blood pressure. Ensure bleeding does not continue after you apply the tourniquet. If hemorrhage does continue, increase the pressure in the blood pressure cuff or tighten the commercial device. Be sure that emergency department personnel are aware of the use of a tourniquet.[7,8,9]

With the increasing incidence of gunshot wounds and acts of terrorism, care-under-fire in emergency medical services is becoming a reality. Both the use of hemostatic agents and tourniquets provide quick solutions to hemorrhage control and may be indicated when the patient's and your life are in danger during patient care.

Specific Wound Considerations

Several wound types require special attention for hemorrhage control. They include head wounds, neck wounds, large gaping wounds, and crush injuries (Figure 17 ●).

Head injuries raise some special concerns regarding hemorrhage control. These include controlling hemorrhage associated with a skull fracture, bleeding or fluids leaking from the ears and nose, and facial injuries threatening the airway. Head wounds may be associated with both severe hemorrhage and loss of skull integrity (fracture). Attempts at applying direct pressure to control hemorrhage may risk displacing unstable skull fracture fragments into the brain tissue. Control bleeding very carefully when you suspect such a wound, using direct pressure on the scalp and around the wound site and against the stable skull.

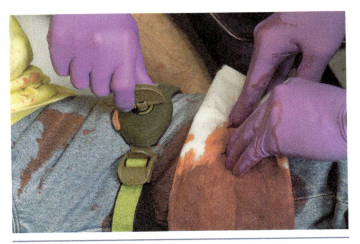

● **Figure 16**   Use a tourniquet as a last resort when hemorrhage is prolonged and persistent.

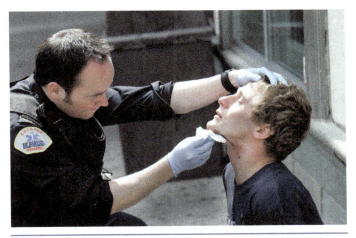

● **Figure 17**   Potential shock-inducing injuries to the head, neck, and torso require special attention. *(© Kevin Link)*

Fluid drainage from the ears and nose may be secondary to skull fracture. Cerebrospinal fluid, as it escapes the cranial vault, relieves any building intracranial pressure. Halting fluid flow would end this relief mechanism and compound any increasing intracranial pressure. In addition, stopping the flow may provide an easier pathway for pathogens to enter the meninges and cause serious infection (meningitis). Cerebrospinal fluid will quickly regenerate as the injury heals. Thus, if there is hemorrhage from either the nose or ear canal, simply cover the area with a soft, porous dressing (such as a gauze 4 × 4), bandage it loosely in place, and permit some blood to flow from the wound.

Wounds associated with the eye orbits can be controlled with digital pressure. However, avoid compressing the globe because it is sensitive to pressure and may be damaged by prolonged or high pressure. If ruptured, the globe can lose irreplaceable vitreous contents even if only gently compressed. Apply pressure only to the intact and stable bony orbital rim.

Neck wounds carry the risk of air being drawn into the venous circulation with life-threatening consequences. Cover any open neck wound with an occlusive dressing, covered by a soft dressing and held firmly in place with bandaging. Do not employ circumferential bandages to create direct pressure with neck wounds. Digital pressure controls most, if not all, neck bleeding. Avoid compressing the trachea, larynx, and other structures as this may cause airway compromise. It may be necessary to apply and maintain continuous manual pressure during the patient's prehospital care and transport.

Gaping wounds often present hemorrhage control problems. With such wounds, bleeding originates from multiple sites and their open nature prevents application of uniform direct pressure. To manage bleeding from such a wound, create a mass of dressing material approximating the volume and shape of the wound. Place the material with the sterile, nonadherent side down into the wound and bandage it firmly in place.

Controlling hemorrhage associated with crush injuries can be particularly challenging. Frequently, the hemorrhage source is difficult to locate, and the nature of vessel damage prevents normal clotting mechanisms from being effective. Here you should place a dressing around and over the crushed tissue, place a pneumatic splint over the dressing, and inflate to a pressure that holds the dressing firmly in place and controls the bleeding. If bleeding is heavy and persistent, consider using a tourniquet but keep in mind the precautions associated with its use.

Transport Considerations

Consider rapid transport for any patient who experiences serious external hemorrhage that you cannot control and for any patient with suspected serious internal hemorrhage. Be vigilant for any blood loss compensation signs and for the early shock signs. Monitor your patient's mental status, Glasgow Coma Scale score, pulse rate, respiratory rate, and blood pressure (for narrowing pulse pressure). When in doubt, transport.

Understand that serious hemorrhage can have a significant psychological impact on patients. Stress triggers the fight-or-flight response, increases heart rate and blood pressure, increases the body's metabolic demands, works against the body's hemorrhage control mechanisms, and contributes to the development of shock. Do what you can to ease the anxieties of patients with significant hemorrhage. Communicate often with them, and explain what care measures you are taking and why. Be especially alert to their comfort needs and address them as appropriate. If possible, keep these patients from seeing their injuries or the serious injuries affecting friends and other event victims.

Shock Management
Airway and Breathing Management

Shock patient management begins with corrective actions taken during primary assessment. One of the primary principles of shock care is to ensure the best possible chance for tissue oxygenation and carbon dioxide offload. Accomplish this by ensuring or providing a secure and patent airway and good ventilations with supplemental high-concentration oxygen guided by oximetry to maintain a saturation of at least 96 percent.

As necessary, protect the airway with an oral airway, nasal airway, or possibly an endotracheal tube (or other advanced airway adjunct). If the patient is unresponsive or somewhat unresponsive and unable to protect the airway, be ready with suction and consider intubation. Shock patients frequently vomit, and gastric aspiration presents a serious, possibly fatal, consequence. If endotracheal intubation is chosen, capnography is used to ensure its proper placement, guide your ventilatory rate and volume, and confirm tube placement in the trachea. Rapid sequence intubation (RSI) may be considered; however, research is suggesting this approach may not be as beneficial as first thought. If RSI is not immediately successful, the airway is in danger and the patient cannot breathe on his own.

If the patient is moving air ineffectively (at a breathing rate less than 8/minute or with inadequate respiratory volume), provide positive-pressure ventilations.[10] Positive-pressure ventilation for the breathing patient, called **overdrive respiration**, is coordinated with the patient's breathing attempts, if possible (Figure 18 ●). However, ensure that the ventilations provide both a good respiratory volume (500 mL) and an adequate respiratory rate (at 10 to 12 per minute). Overdrive respiration may be indicated in patients with rib fractures, flail chest, spinal

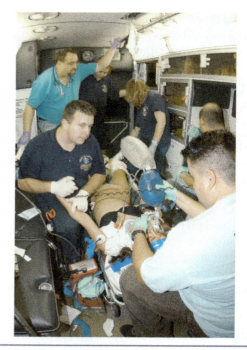

● **Figure 18**   Ensure that the potential shock patient receives adequate ventilation. (© Craig Jackson/In the Dark Photography)

injury with diaphragmatic respirations, head injury, or any condition in which the patient, because of bellows system or respiratory control failure, is not breathing adequately.

Two techniques to improve ventilation are positive end-expiratory pressure (PEEP) and continuous positive airway pressure (CPAP). PEEP uses a restrictive valve on an endotracheal tube or mask of the bag-valve unit. There, it resists exhalation, maintaining a positive pressure and keeping the patient's airways open longer during exhalation. CPAP uses special ventilation equipment to increase pressure during both inspiration and expiration. This keeps the airway open during more of the respiratory cycle, increases the partial pressure of oxygen, and may push fluid (in cases of pulmonary edema) back into the capillary circulation.[11]

If there is any sign of tension pneumothorax, confirm it and provide pleural decompression at the second intercostal space, midclavicular line. Continue to monitor the patient, because it is common for the catheter to clog and tension pneumothorax to reappear. Insert another needle close to the first to relieve any subsequent pressure buildup.

Ensure that an unconscious and unresponsive patient has a palpable carotid pulse. If not, initiate CPR, attach a monitor-defibrillator, and employ advanced life support measures. Rule out pericardial tamponade and tension pneumothorax as possible causes of cardiac dysfunction. Understand that traumatic cardiac arrest carries an extremely poor prognosis, especially when it is due to hypovolemia. When resources are scarce, your efforts may be better utilized caring for other seriously injured but salvageable patients.

Hemorrhage Control

Provide rapid control of any significant external hemorrhage as explained earlier in this chapter.

Science vs. Dogma

For years the principal prehospital treatment of hypotension from trauma was the administration of large volumes of crystalloid solutions and rapid transport. However, research is starting to show that infusing massive quantities of crystalloids, without correcting the underlying problem, may be detrimental. Consider this: If large quantities of fluid are administered without the injury being repaired, blood loss will continue and the blood will become progressively more diluted. Thus, the number of red blood cells available to carry oxygen will begin to fall. In addition, as blood becomes diluted with IV fluids, the coagulation factors are diluted, and blood clotting becomes slower and less effective. For these reasons, some leading trauma researchers advocate limiting the amount of fluids administered prior to surgery.

Current research demonstrates that hypotension (within certain parameters) following trauma may actually be protective. In fact, some are calling for "permissive hypotension" where the systolic blood pressure is maintained between 70 to 85 mmHg instead of 100 mmHg or more. The theory behind this concept is straightforward. First, several protective mechanisms appear to be activated when the blood pressure is within this range. Second, increasing the blood pressure with fluids, PASG, or similar methods might lead to a more rapid blood loss. Thus, trying to maintain normal blood pressures may actually increase the rate of blood loss and may inhibit clot formation or may cause dislodgement of a clot that formed during periods of hypotension following trauma. This concept is being aggressively studied.

The information in this box is presented to introduce you to controversies and research in the field of trauma care. Despite this information, always follow the local protocols as established by your system and your medical director. *However, it is important to consider the ongoing research that may affect prehospital practice. EMS in the twenty-first century should be based on scientific evidence—not anecdotes or dogma.*

Fluid Resuscitation

The field treatment of choice for significant blood loss in trauma is whole blood. It has red blood cells to carry oxygen, clotting factors and platelets to assist in hemostasis, and remains in the bloodstream once it is infused. Whole blood, however, is almost never available in blood banks or hospitals. Most banked blood is concentrated and known as packed red blood cells. It must be refrigerated, typed, and cross-matched. (O-negative blood may be given in emergency circumstances.) Blood also has a short shelf-life, is costly, and is impractical for field use. The most practical fluid for prehospital administration is an isotonic crystalloid like normal saline. (Lactated Ringer's solution may be used in some systems.)

Hypertonic and synthetic solutions may have some applications for fluid resuscitation. None of these, however, have demonstrated superiority to isotonic electrolyte solutions for use in the civilian prehospital setting. Hypertonic crystalloid solutions can mobilize the interstitial and cellular fluid volumes to replace lost blood volume but, like other crystalloids, they are not able to carry either the oxygen or the clotting factors essential for hemorrhage control. The advantage of hypertonic solutions is their low volume and weight—an advantage in wilderness and military applications. Synthetic agents are now available that can carry oxygen. These agents, however, have not yet proven their efficacy in the emergency department or prehospital setting.

Isotonic Fluid Administration   Isotonic fluid administration is indicated for the patient with the classic signs and symptoms of shock and isolated but controlled external hemorrhage. Employ aggressive fluid resuscitation, using normal saline via one line running wide open until the systolic blood pressure returns to 100 mmHg and the level of consciousness increases. Use large-bore catheters (14 or 16 gauge) connected to trauma or blood tubing to ensure unimpeded flow and a non-flow-restrictive saline lock if your system so requires. If the patient has continuing (internal or uncontrolled external) hemorrhage with absent peripheral pulses or a systolic BP below 80 mmHg, run the infusion wide open until 250 to 500 mL of solution is infused. Then evaluate for the return of peripheral pulses or a rise in the systolic blood pressure to just under 80 mmHg—sometimes referred to as permissive hypotension. If the patient's condition or blood pressure does not improve, consider repeating the fluid bolus.[12]

Head injury patients (Glasgow Coma Scale [GCS] score of 8 or less) may require a slightly higher systolic blood pressure (100 mmHg) to ensure cerebral perfusion. Even brief periods of hypotension are detrimental to good outcomes in traumatic brain injury. Note, however, that prehospital fluid resuscitation is an area of much research and controversy. Consult with your medical director and local protocols to determine your system's parameters for prehospital fluid resuscitation of the shock patient with head injury.

In children, infuse 20 mL/kg of body weight rapidly when you see any signs and symptoms of shock. Administer a second fluid bolus if the vital signs do not improve after the first bolus or if, at some later time, the patient again begins to deteriorate. The objective of fluid resuscitation in the field is not the return of normal vital signs but the stabilization of vital signs until the patient reaches the trauma center.

When you are preparing to administer large volumes of fluid to a trauma patient, consider the internal lumen size of both the catheter and the administration set. Fluid flow is proportional to the fourth power of the internal diameter. This means that as you double the lumen's diameter, the same fluid under the same pressure will flow 16 times more quickly. Use the largest catheter you can introduce into the patient's vein and use a large-bore trauma or blood administration set (Figure 19 ●).

Catheter length and fluid pressure also influence fluid flow. The longer the catheter, the greater its resistance to fluid flow. The ideal catheter for the shock patient is relatively short, 1.5 inch or shorter. Likewise, an increase in fluid pressure increases flow. This means that the higher you position the bag or the greater the pressure differential between the solution and the venous system, the faster the fluid will flow. If you cannot elevate the fluid bag, position it under the patient with some of his weight on it or place it in a pressure infuser or a blood-pressure cuff inflated to 100 or 200 mmHg.

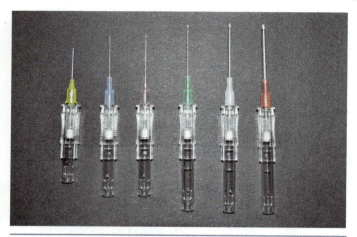

● **Figure 19** Catheter size greatly influences fluid flow. Shown here are catheters of various gauges.

During fluid resuscitation, cautiously control fluid volume, remembering that your goal is maintaining vital signs, not improving them. Increases in blood pressure can dislodge developing clots and disrupt the normal clotting processes. The result may be further hemorrhage with further dilution of clotting factors and hemoglobin. Closely monitor your patient's vital signs, and administer lactated Ringer's solution or normal saline to keep the patient's mental status and pulse pressure steady. Maintain the blood pressure at a steady level once it has dropped below 80 mmHg. Do not let the pressure drop below 50 mmHg or below 100 mmHg for head injury patients with a GCS of 8 or less.

Temperature Control

Trauma and blood loss deal serious blows to the mechanisms that normally adjust the body's core temperature. Reduced body activity reduces heat production to subnormal levels. Cutaneous vasoconstriction decreases the skin's ability to act as part of the body's temperature control system. The result is a patient highly susceptible to fluctuations in body temperature. In cases of trauma, patients commonly lose heat more rapidly than normal and heat production is low. At the same time, the heat-generating reflexes, like shivering, are ineffective and, in fact, are counterproductive to the shock care process. Shivering will consume oxygen and glucose when the body needs these materials to keep other cells alive. Hypothermia also reduces the effectiveness of the clotting mechanism and can worsen and prolong hemorrhage.

In all except the warmest environments, help conserve body temperature by covering the patient with a blanket and keeping the patient compartment of the ambulance very warm. If you infuse fluids, ensure that they are well above room temperature—ideally at body temperature or slightly above (no more than 104°F). Use fluid warmers or keep IV solutions in a compartment that is warmer than the rest of the ambulance. Be very sensitive to any patient complaints about being cold, and provide whatever assistance you can to ensure that heat loss is limited.

Pneumatic Anti-Shock Garment

The **pneumatic anti-shock garment (PASG)**, sometimes referred to as the medical anti-shock trouser (MAST), is a device designed to apply firm circumferential pressure around the lower extremities, pelvis, and lower abdomen (Procedure 1). The device is intended to compress the vascular space, thereby increasing peripheral vascular resistance, reducing vascular volume, and immobilizing the lower extremities and the pelvic region.

Research has determined that the garment is responsible for the return of a small volume of blood to the central circulation and probably reduces the venous capacitance by the same volume.[13] The PASG also does seem to increase the peripheral vascular resistance and blood pressure, although these actions may be detrimental to patients with uncontrolled internal hemorrhage.

Research has further revealed potential problems with PASG use. The abdominal component of the PASG pressurizes the abdominal cavity, increasing the work associated with breathing and, in some cases, reducing chest excursion. Garment application also increases mortality when used in cases of penetrating chest trauma. In light of this information, it is imperative that you understand the device's limitations and comply with your local protocols and medical direction when considering PASG use.

Pharmacological Intervention

In shock, pharmacological interventions are generally limited, especially in hypovolemic patients. The sympathetic nervous system efficiently compensates for low volume, and no agent has been shown effective in the prehospital setting, other than intravenous fluid and, in some cases, blood and blood products. For cardiogenic shock, fluid challenge, vasopressors like dopamine, and the other cardiac drugs are indicated. For spinal and obstructive shock, consider intravenous fluids like normal saline and lactated Ringer's solution. For distributive shock, consider IV fluids or a vasopressor.

The patient who has experienced trauma sufficient to induce hemorrhage and hypovolemia will be anxious and bewildered. As the care provider at the patient's side, it is your responsibility to be calm and reassuring, thus counteracting the natural fight-or-flight response (Figure 20 ●). By acting in this manner, you not only help your patient deal with the event's emotional trauma but also combat some of the negative effects of sympathetic stimulation.

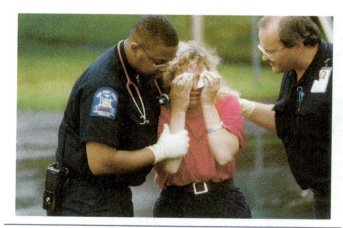

Figure 20 Emotional support for the seriously injured patient is an important part of shock patient care. (© Craig Jackson/In the Dark Photography)

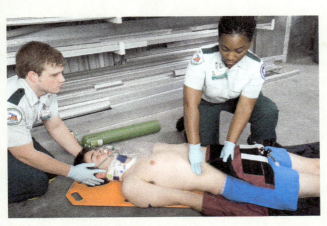

1a ● Place garment on spine board, then patient on garment. Position so top of garment is three finger widths below the rib cage.

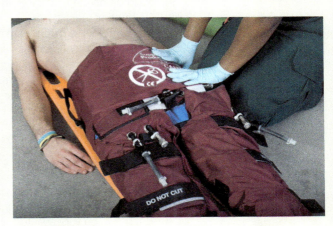

1b ● Apply the garment.

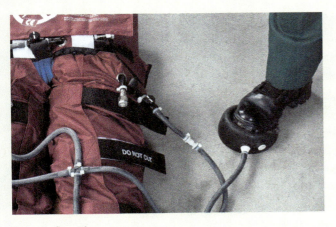

1c ● Inflate the garment.

The PASG should not be deflated in the prehospital setting.

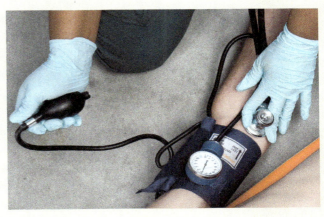

1d ● Monitor and record vital signs every 5 minutes. If the garment loses pressure, add air as needed.

SUMMARY

Significant hemorrhage and its serious consequence, shock, are genuine threats to the trauma patient's life. The signs of these threats are often subtle or hidden, especially if bleeding is internal. Only through careful analysis of the mechanism of injury during the scene size-up and careful evaluation of the patient during the assessment process can you recognize and then treat these life-threatening problems. Treatment often involves rapidly bringing the patient to the services of a trauma center and, while doing so, providing aggressive care—supplemental oxygen, positive pressure ventilations, and fluid resuscitation, as necessary—aimed at maintaining vital signs, not necessarily improving them. With this approach, you afford your patient the best chance for survival.

YOU MAKE THE CALL

A teenager working in the high school wood shop slips and runs his forearm into the running blade of a table saw. The blade cuts deeply into an artery, resulting in serious hemorrhage. On your arrival, you find the teenager to be very agitated and anxious. Your assessment reveals a blood pressure of 130/86, a pulse of 110, normal respirations at 24 breaths per minute, and skin that is cool and moist.

1. What signs suggest hypovolemia and early shock?
2. Does the blood pressure suggest shock? Why or why not?
3. What progressive steps would you take to control the hemorrhage?
4. What supportive care measures would you employ?

See Suggested Responses at the back of this chapter.

REVIEW QUESTIONS

1. Signs of compensated shock may include all of the following except _____.
   a. unconsciousness
   b. thirst
   c. combativeness
   d. weakness

2. You and your crew respond to a motor vehicle collision in which a 20-year-old female has received several cuts over her body. You determine that her airway is patent and she is breathing adequately. Her blood pressure is maintaining at a stable level, and you estimate that she has lost approximately 15 percent of her circulating blood volume. She is alert and oriented but seems a bit nervous. From these findings, you determine that your patient is in _____ hemorrhage.
   a. class IV
   b. class I
   c. class III
   d. class II

3. In a patient with no suspected trauma, and signs and symptoms of shock, you can perform the tilt test. This test is performed to determine _____.
   a. cardiogenic shock
   b. septic shock
   c. orthostatic hypertension
   d. orthostatic hypotension

4. The arterial blood pressure is monitored by receptors in the aortic arch and carotid sinuses. These receptors send signals to the medulla oblongata to help maintain a blood pressure that ensures adequate perfusion. These receptors are the _____.
   a. chemoreceptors
   b. baroreceptors
   c. cardioinhibitory centers
   d. cardioacceleratory centers

5. When the body is working to counteract the effects of hemorrhage and cardiovascular insufficiency, it constricts arterioles and increases the heart rate and contractility. The most rapid hormonal response occurs with the release of _____.
   a. angiotensin II   c. antidiuretic hormone
   b. glucocorticoids   d. catecholamines

6. You are called to the scene where a man is very nearly unconscious. His vital signs indicate a falling blood pressure and bradycardia as well as cool, clammy skin. Based on these assessment findings, you conclude that the patient is most likely in _____.
   a. neurogenic shock
   b. irreversible shock
   c. decompensated shock
   d. compensated shock

7. Rapid transport to a trauma facility is indicated in which of the following patients?
   a. a patient in class I hemorrhage
   b. a patient with suspected serious internal hemorrhage
   c. a patient who is vomiting coffee-ground material
   d. a patient with external hemorrhage that is controlled on the scene

8. PASG application has been found to increase mortality when used in which of the following situations?
   a. external hemorrhage from an extremity
   b. penetrating chest trauma
   c. pelvic fracture
   d. suspected internal abdominal hemorrhage

9. Your patient is determined to be in decompensated shock. Fluid therapy is indicated.

The most practical fluid for prehospital administration is _____.
   a. D_5W
   b. blood plasma
   c. normal saline
   d. D_5W in half normal saline

10. A patient develops shock secondary to hypovolemia. You understand that the reduced flow of oxygen to the cells leads to a buildup of lactic acid and other by-products. You further understand that _____ metabolism causes this process to occur.
    a. Krebs
    b. aerobic
    c. glycolysis
    d. anaerobic

See Answers to Review Questions at the back of this chapter.

REFERENCES

1. Haut, E. R., et al. "Prehospital Intravenous Fluid Administration Is Associated with Higher Mortality in Trauma Patients: A National Trauma Data Bank Analysis." *Ann Surg* 253(2) (Feb 2011): 371–377.

2. Frank, M., et al. "Proper Estimation of Blood Loss on Scene of Trauma: Tool or Tale?" *J Trauma* 69(5) (Nov 2010): 1191–1195.

3. Bates, Barbara and Peter G. Szilagyi. *A Guide to Physical Examination and History Taking.* 9th ed. Philadelphia: J. B. Lippincott, 2007.

4. Alam, H. B., et al. "Hemorrhage Control in the Battlefield: Role of the New Hemostatic Agents." *Mil Med* 170 (2005): 63–69.

5. Clay, J. G., J. K. Grayson, and D. Zierold. "Comparative Testing of New Hemostatic Agents in a Swine Model of Extremity Arterial and Venous Hemorrhage." *Mil Med* 175(4) (Apr 2010): 280–284.

6. Ran, Y., et al. "QuikClit Combat Gauze Use for Hemorrhage Control in Military Trauma: January 2009 Israel Defense Force Experience in the Gaza Strip—a Preliminary Report of 14 Cases." *Prehosp Emerg Med* 25(6) (Nov–Dec 2010): 584–588.

7. Taylor, D. M., G. M. Vater, and P. J. Parker. "An Evaluation of Two Tourniquet Systems for the Control of Prehospital Lower Limb Hemorrhage." *J Trauma* 71(3) (Sept 2011): 591–595.

8. Kragh, J. F., Jr., et al. "Survival with Emergency Tourniquet Use to Stop Bleeding in Major Limb Trauma." *Ann Surg* 249(1) (Jan 2009): 1–7.

9. Kragh, J. F., et al. "Battle Casualty Survival with Emergency Tourniquet Use to Stop Limb Bleeding." *J Emerg Med* 41(6) (Dec 2011): 590–597.

10. Stockinger, Z. T. and N. E. McSwain. "Prehospital Endotracheal Intubation for Trauma Does Not Improve Survival over Bag-Valve-Mask Ventilation." *J Trauma* 56(3) (2004): 531–536.

11. Stockinger, Z. T. and N. E. McSwain. "Prehospital Supplemental Oxygen in Trauma Patients." *Mil Med* 169 (Aug 2004): 609–612.

12. Merlin, M. A., et al. "Study of Placing a Second Intravenous Line in Trauma." *Prehosp Emerg Med* 15(2) (Apr–Jun 2011): 208–213.

13. Butman, Alexander M. and James L. Paturas. *Pre-Hospital Trauma Life Support.* Akron, Ohio: Emergency Training, 2007.

FURTHER READING

Bates, Barbara, and Peter G. Szilagyi. *A Guide to Physical Examination and History Taking.* 9th ed. Philadelphia: J. B. Lippincott, 2007.

Bledsoe, B. E., and D. Clayden. *Prehospital Emergency Pharmacology.* 7th ed. Upper Saddle River, NJ: Pearson/Prentice Hall, 2011.

Bledsoe, B. E., B. J. Colbert, and J. E. Ankney. *Essentials of A & P for Emergency Care.* Upper Saddle River, NJ: Pearson/Prentice Hall, 2010.

Martini, Frederic. *Fundamentals of Anatomy and Physiology.* 7th ed. San Francisco: Benjamin Cummings, 2011.

Rosen, P., and R. Barkin, eds. *Emergency Medicine: Concepts and Clinical Practice.* 7th ed. St. Louis: Mosby, 2009.

Tintinalli, J. E., ed. *Emergency Medicine: A Comprehensive Study Guide.* 7th ed. New York: McGraw-Hill, 2011.

SUGGESTED RESPONSES TO "YOU MAKE THE CALL"

The following are suggested responses to the "You Make the Call" scenarios presented in this chapter. Each represents an acceptable response to the scenario but should not be interpreted as the only correct response.

1. *What signs suggest hypovolemia and early shock?*

Agitation and anxiousness, cool and moist skin, and increased pulse rate.

2. *Does the blood pressure suggest shock? Why or why not?*

The blood pressure alone does not indicate shock. However, when coupled with all the other signs and symptoms, the pressure can be explained. The increased blood pressure indicates an excited state and is currently compensating well for the blood loss.

3. *What progressive steps would you take to control the hemorrhage?*

The first step is to firmly bandage a dressing over the wound. If this does not control the hemorrhage, include finger pressure through the dressing to the site of the leaking vessel. If the bleeding is persistent and life-threatening and cannot be controlled by direct pressure, as a last resort apply a commercial tourniquet or, if a commercial tourniquet is not available, a wide cravat, belt, or blood pressure cuff. Leave the tourniquet in place until the patient is in the emergency department or other facility where blood replacement is available and the negative effects of reperfusion can be addressed. Be sure to notify personnel at the receiving facility that a tourniquet has been applied.

4. *What supportive care measures would you employ?*

Provide oxygen therapy and IV therapy, maintain body temperature, and calm and reassure the patient.

ANSWERS TO REVIEW QUESTIONS

1. a
2. d
3. d
4. b
5. d

6. c
7. b
8. b
9. c
10. d

GLOSSARY

aerobic metabolism   the second stage of metabolism, requiring the presence of oxygen, in which the breakdown of glucose (in a process called the Krebs or citric acid cycle) yields a high amount of energy.

afterload   the resistance a contraction of the heart must overcome in order to eject blood; in cardiac physiology, defined as the tension of cardiac muscle during systole (contraction). Also called peripheral vascular resistance.

aggregate   to cluster or come together.

aldosterone   hormone secreted by the adrenal cortex that increases sodium reabsorption by the kidneys; it plays a part in the regulation of blood volume, blood pressure, and blood levels of potassium, chloride, and bicarbonate.

anaerobic   ability to live without oxygen.

anaerobic metabolism   the first stage of metabolism, which does not require oxygen, in which the breakdown of glucose (in a process called glycolysis) produces pyruvic acid and yields limited energy.

anaphylactic shock   form of shock in which histamine causes general vasodilation, precapillary sphincter dilation, capillary engorgement, and fluid movement into the interstitial compartment.

anemia   a reduction in the hemoglobin content in the blood to a point below that required to meet the oxygen requirements of the body.

angiotensin   a vasopressor hormone that causes contraction of the smooth muscles of arteries and arterioles, produced when renin is released from the kidneys; angiotensin I is a physiologically inactive form, while angiotensin II is an active form.

antidiuretic hormone (ADH) hormone released by the posterior pituitary that induces an increase in peripheral vascular resistance and causes the kidneys to retain water, decreasing urine output, and also causes splenic vascular constriction.

arteriole a small artery.

artery a vessel that carries blood from the heart to the body tissues.

baroreceptor sensory nerve ending, found in the walls of the atria of the heart, vena cava, aortic arch, and carotid sinus, that is stimulated by changes in pressure.

capillary one of the minute blood vessels that connects the ends of arterioles with the beginnings of venules; where oxygen is diffused to body tissue and products of metabolism enter the bloodstream.

capillary washout release of accumulated lactic acid, carbon dioxide (carbonic acid), potassium, and rouleaux into the venous circulation that occurs with relaxation of the post-capillary sphincters.

cardiac contractility the ability of the heart to contract; the strength of the heart's contractions.

cardiogenic shock shock resulting from failure to maintain the blood pressure because of inadequate cardiac output.

catecholamine a hormone, such as epinephrine or norepinephrine, that strongly affects the nervous and cardiovascular systems, metabolic rate, temperature, and smooth muscle.

chemoreceptor sense organ or sensory nerve ending located outside the central nervous system that is stimulated by and reacts to chemical stimuli.

citric acid cycle *see* Krebs cycle.

clotting factors proteins from damaged blood vessel walls and damaged platelets that, when released into the bloodstream, cause chemical reactions that result in the formation of clot-forming fibrin.

coagulation phase third step in the process of hemostasis, which involves the formation of a protein called fibrin that forms a network around a wound to stop bleeding, ward off infection, and lay a foundation for healing and repair of the wound.

compensated shock hemodynamic insult to the body in which the body responds effectively. Signs and symptoms are limited, and the human system continues to provide oxygenated circulation to most tissues.

decompensated shock continuing hemodynamic insult to the body in which the compensatory mechanisms break down. The signs and symptoms become very pronounced, and the patient moves rapidly toward death.

direct pressure method of hemorrhage control that relies on the application of pressure to the actual site of the bleeding.

epinephrine a hormone secreted along with norepinephrine by the adrenal medulla that, among other actions, causes arteriole constriction and increased heart rate and contractility.

epistaxis bleeding from the nose resulting from injury, disease, or environmental factors; a nosebleed.

erythrocyte peripheral blood cell that contains hemoglobin; responsible for transport of oxygen to the cells.

esophageal varices enlarged and tortuous esophageal veins.

external respiration the movement of oxygen from the alveolus to the red blood cell.

extrinsic pathway the activation of clotting factors from damaged blood vessel walls and surrounding tissue.

fascia a fibrous membrane that covers, supports, and separates muscles and may also unite the skin with underlying tissue.

fibrin protein fibers that trap red blood cells as part of the clotting process.

glycolysis the first stage of the process in which the cell breaks apart an energy source, commonly glucose, and releases a small amount of energy.

hematemesis vomiting of blood.

hematochezia passage of stools containing red blood.

hematocrit the percentage of the total blood volume consisting of the red blood cells, or erythrocytes.

hematoma collection of blood beneath the skin or trapped within a body compartment.

hemoglobin an iron-based compound found in red blood cells that binds with oxygen and transports it to body cells.

hemorrhage an abnormal internal or external discharge of blood.

hemostasis the body's three-step response to local hemorrhage, comprising a vascular phase that reduces blood flow, a platelet phase in which aggregating platelets form a weak clot, and a coagulation phase that results in the formation of fibrin, creating a strong clot.

homeostasis the natural tendency of the body to maintain a stable, steady, and normal internal environment.

hydrostatic pressure the pressure of liquids in equilibrium; the pressure exerted by or within liquids.

hypovolemic shock shock caused by loss of blood or body fluids.

internal respiration the movement of oxygen from the blood into the body cell.

interstitial space the space between cells.

intrinsic pathway the activation of clotting factors from damaged platelets within blood vessels.

irreversible shock final stage of shock in which organs and cells are so damaged that recovery is impossible.

ischemia a blockage in the delivery of oxygenated blood to the cells.

Krebs cycle process of aerobic metabolism that uses carbohydrates, proteins, and fats to release energy for the body; also known as the citric acid cycle.

lactic acid compound produced from pyruvic acid during anaerobic glycolysis.

melena black, tar-like feces due to gastrointestinal bleeding.

metabolism the total changes that take place in an organism during physiologic processes.

microcirculation blood flow in the arterioles, capillaries, and venules.

neurogenic shock type of shock resulting from an interruption in the communication pathway between the central nervous system and the rest of the body leading to decreased peripheral vascular resistance.

norepinephrine a hormone secreted along with epinephrine by the adrenal medulla that, among other actions, causes arteriole constriction and increased heart rate and contractility.

oncotic pressure the force exerted by large protein molecules in the plasma that tends to draw fluid into the capillaries, compensating for the loss of fluid that leaks out of capillaries because of hydrostatic pressure.

orthostatic hypotension a decrease in blood pressure that occurs when a person moves from a supine or sitting position to an upright position.

overdrive respiration positive-pressure ventilation supplied to a breathing patient.

peripheral vascular resistance the resistance of the vessels to the flow of blood; it increases when the vessels constrict and decreases when the vessels relax. Also called afterload.

platelet one of the fragments of cytoplasm that circulates in the blood and works with components of the coagulation system to promote blood clotting. Platelets also release serotonin, a vasoconstrictive substance.

platelet phase second step in the process of hemostasis in which platelets adhere to blood vessel walls and to each other.

pneumatic anti-shock garment (PASG) garment designed to produce uniform pressure on the lower extremities and abdomen; used with shock and hemorrhage patients in some EMS systems.

preload the pressure within the ventricles at the end of diastole; the volume of blood delivered to the atria prior to ventricular diastole.

pulse pressure difference between the systolic and diastolic blood pressures.

rouleaux group of red blood cells that are stuck together.

septic shock form of shock caused by massive infection in which toxins compromise the vascular system's ability to control blood vessels and distribute blood.

shock a state of inadequate tissue perfusion.

stroke volume the amount of blood ejected by the heart in one cardiac contraction.

tilt test drop in the systolic blood pressure of 20 mmHg or an increase in the pulse rate of 20 beats per minute when a patient is moved from a supine to a sitting position; a finding suggestive of a relative hypovolemia.

tourniquet a constrictor used on an extremity to apply circumferential pressure on all arteries to control bleeding.

vascular phase first step in the process of hemostasis, in which smooth blood vessel muscle contracts, reducing the vessel lumen and the flow of blood through it.

vein a blood vessel that carries blood toward the heart.

Soft-Tissue Trauma

From Chapter 5 of *Paramedic Care: Principles & Practice, Volume 5,* Fourth Edition. Bryan Bledsoe, Robert Porter, and Richard Cherry. Copyright © 2013 by Pearson Education, Inc. All rights reserved.

Soft-Tissue Trauma

Robert S. Porter, MA, EMT-P

STANDARD
Trauma (Soft-Tissue Trauma)

COMPETENCY
Integrates assessment findings with principles of epidemiology and pathophysiology to formulate a field impression to implement a comprehensive treatment/disposition plan for an acutely injured patient.

OBJECTIVES

Terminal Performance Objective
After reading this chapter you should be able to assess and manage patients with soft-tissue injuries.

Enabling Objectives
To accomplish the terminal performance objective, you should be able to:

1. Define key terms introduced in this chapter.
2. Describe the epidemiology of soft-tissue injuries.
3. Describe the anatomy and physiology of the skin and associated soft tissues.
4. Describe the pathophysiology of open and closed soft-tissue injuries.
5. Describe the process of wound healing.
6. Describe the pathophysiology and risk factors for soft-tissue injury complications, including:
   a. infection
   b. hemorrhage, impaired hemostasis, and rebleeding
   c. delayed healing
   d. compartment syndrome
   e. abnormal scarring
   f. complications associated with pressure injuries
   g. associated injuries
   h. crush syndrome
   i. injection injuries
7. Given a variety of scenarios, select appropriate dressing and bandaging materials and techniques.
8. Demonstrate the assessment of a variety of soft-tissue injuries.
9. Given a variety of scenarios, develop management plans for patients with open and closed soft-tissue injuries.
10. Reassess patients with soft-tissue injuries for complications of bandaging.

11. Describe special considerations in the management of the following injuries:

    a. amputations
    b. impaled objects
    c. crush syndrome
    d. compartment syndrome
    e. injuries to the face and neck
    f. injuries to the thorax
    g. injuries to the abdomen

12. Describe considerations in decisions to transport or treat and release patients with soft-tissue injuries.

KEY TERMS

abrasion
amputation
avulsion
chemotactic factors
collagen
compartment syndrome
contusion
crush injury
crush syndrome
degloving injury
dermis
ecchymosis
epidermis
epithelialization
erythema
fasciae

fibroblasts
gangrene
granulocytes
hematoma
hemostasis
hyperemia
impaled object
incision
inflammation
integumentary system
keloid
laceration
lumen
lymphangitis
lymphocyte
macrophages

necrosis
neovascularization
phagocytosis
puncture
remodeling
rhabdomyolysis
sebaceous glands
sebum
serous fluid
skeletal muscle
subcutaneous tissue
sudoriferous glands
tendons
tension lines
tetanus

CASE STUDY

Maria Gonza and Jon O'Sullivan, paramedics with University Medic 151, respond to an "axe injury." On arrival, they find an adult male standing next to a wood pile with a bloody axe at his feet. The man is holding a blood-soaked rag against his arm. Maria quickly ascertains from the patient and several bystanders that the wound is accidental and occurred while he was chopping wood. No other victims are present.

Maria and Jon proceed to help, donning disposable gloves and splash protection as they approach the patient. Primary assessment reveals the patient to be a healthy 42-year-old male, named Walter, who lacerated his left upper arm when an axe blade slipped during a chopping stroke. Walter states the wound is "deep" and there was "lots of blood" initially, but that he stopped the bleeding fairly easily by "putting this rag on it." Walter reports no other injuries or complaints. He is alert and oriented, standing upright, and shows no apparent distress. His airway is obviously open and his breathing is adequate, his skin is slightly pale, and his pulse rate is somewhat rapid.

Because Walter has an isolated injury and no significant mechanism of injury, Maria and Jon proceed with the focused trauma assessment at the scene. They perform an evaluation of the upper extremity, which reveals a large open and deep wound to the central upper arm just over the biceps muscle. Close inspection of the wound is not yet possible because the patient is holding a folded rag over the wound in an effort to control bleeding. Despite these efforts, a trickle of dark blood continues to flow. A small stain of dark blood is visible on the ground. Distal pulses and capillary refill are both present and equal to the opposite extremity. The patient can move all his fingers and his wrist, but cannot flex his elbow. Sensation appears intact, although Walter reports some vague tingling in the fingers.

To control the bleeding and better visualize the wound, Maria will need to remove the rag and inspect the wound. To prepare for this, she and Jon gather several bulky sterile dressings and have them ready. They then position Walter seated on the stretcher. In a coordinated fashion, they remove the rag (taking care to avoid dislodging clots) and simultaneously replace it with a bulky, sterile dressing. A quick look at the wound indicates that it measures approximately 8 cm long and extends deep through the skin and into subcutaneous tissue and muscle layers. There is no spurting or bright red blood, but a large amount of dark red blood flows from the uncovered wound. The new dressings and direct pressure applied with a bandage easily bring the bleeding under control.

While performing the focused assessment, the paramedics also gather a patient history. Walter reports no significant medical problems and says he takes no medications. He doesn't recall the date of his last tetanus booster. He reports no allergies and that his last meal was a large lunch 2 hours ago.

Following application of the dressings and bandage, distal pulse, motor function, sensation, and capillary refill in the extremity are unchanged. Maria and Jon then take a baseline set of vital signs: respirations—20 per minute and adequate; pulse—92; skin—warm, moist, and slightly pale; pupils—equal and reactive; blood pressure (obtained on the right arm)—134/78 mmHg.

Maria and Jon now transport Walter, with his bleeding under control, uneventfully to the hospital emergency department. In the hospital, the emergency physician examines Walter using local anesthetic and a pneumatic limb tourniquet to obtain a bloodless field. Using a combination of inspection under powerful exam lights and careful palpation with gloved fingers, the physician determines that the wound has not damaged any bones, arteries, nerves, or tendons, and that no foreign bodies have lodged in it. The wound does, however, extend into the muscle layer of the biceps. Using layered closure, the physician sutures the wound, and Walter receives a tetanus booster. The sutures will be removed after 10 to 14 days, by which time Walter should be well on his way to recovery.

INTRODUCTION TO SOFT-TISSUE TRAUMA

The skin is one of the largest, most important organs of the human body, accounting for 16 percent of total body weight. It provides a protective envelope that keeps invading pathogens out while containing body substances and fluids. It is also a key organ of sensation as well as a radiator of excess body heat in warm weather and a conservator of heat in cold conditions. Even as it accomplishes these various functions, the skin remains a durable, pliable, and accommodating tissue, and one that is very able to repair itself.

Known collectively as the integumentary system, the skin is the first tissue of the human body to experience the effects of trauma. Because skin covers the entire body surface, any penetrating injury or the kinetic forces of blunt injury must pass through it before impacting on other vital organs. Often, the signs of this energy transmission can only be recognized with very careful examination of the skin. Therefore, the skin is of great significance at all stages of the patient assessment process.

Trauma to the skin may present as open injuries—abrasions, lacerations, incisions, punctures, avulsions, and amputations—or as closed injuries—contusions, hematomas, and crush injuries. Although such injuries only infrequently pose direct threats to life, they may endanger blood vessels, nerves, connective tissue, and other important internal structures. Uncontrolled blood loss may lead to hypovolemia and shock, while the wound may provide a pathway for infection.

Epidemiology

Soft-tissue injuries are by far the most common form of trauma. Over 10 million patients present to emergency departments annually with soft-tissue wounds, many of which require closure. Most, but not all, open wounds require only simple care and limited suturing. A significant minority, however, damage arteries, nerves, or tendons and can lead to permanent disability. Uncontrolled external hemorrhage of an otherwise uncomplicated open wound is a very rare but completely preventable situation that sometimes occurs with this type of injury and can result in death. Of the open wounds presenting to emergency departments, up to 6.5 percent will eventually become infected, resulting in significant morbidity.

Closed wounds share a similar epidemiology, except that they are probably even more common than open injuries. Most minor "bumps and bruises" never reach the paramedic, as most patients elect to self-treat all but the most serious cases. Despite their frequency and usually minor nature, closed injuries *can* result in significant pain, suffering, and morbidity. Infection, however, is not usually a complication with closed wounds.

Risk factors for soft-tissue wounds include age (school-age children and the elderly are most prone), alcohol or drug abuse, and occupation. Laborers, machine operators, and others whose hands and body parts are exposed to heavy objects, machines, or tools are at great risk.

Simple measures can reduce risks and prevent soft-tissue injuries. For example, locating playgrounds on grass, sand, gravel, or other forgiving surfaces and padding the equipment in them can cut injury rates among children. In factories, machine guards, fail-safe switches, and similar engineering controls can reduce injuries. Protective clothing such as steel-toed boots and leather gloves also provide simple methods of reducing the incidence and severity of soft-tissue injuries. In Emergency Medical Services we need to establish a culture of safety: carefully ensuring scene safety, not entering an unsafe scene, wearing the appropriate protective clothing, properly disposing of sharps, carefully using patient movement devices to protect against pinch and back injuries, using restraint systems when in the ambulance, and driving responsibly, to just name a few.

CONTENT REVIEW

► Layers of the Skin

- Epidermis
- Dermis
- Subcutaneous tissue

ANATOMY AND PHYSIOLOGY OF THE SOFT TISSUES

The protective envelope we call the skin is a complex structure. Understanding how it is put together and how it functions will help you appreciate the importance of injuries to it and the value of their proper care.

Layers of the Skin

The epidermis, dermis, and subcutaneous tissue layers constitute what is commonly known as the skin (Figure 1 ●). Each of these layers performs functions essential to helping the body maintain homeostasis (maintenance of a stable, steady, and normal state), and each plays an important role in the wound repair process.

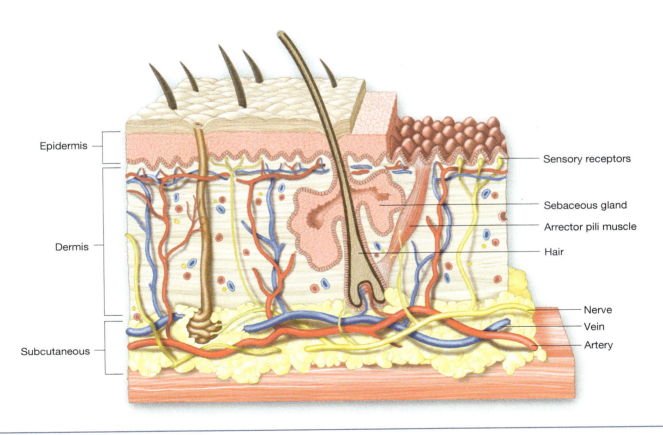

● **Figure 1**   Layers and major structures of the skin.

Epidermis

The outermost skin layer is the epidermis. It is generated by a layer of cells just above the dermis (stratum germinativum). These cells divide rapidly, generating a movement of cells upward toward the epidermal surface. As the epidermis contains no vasculature, the farther these cells are pushed away from the dermis, the less circulation they receive, and they eventually die. As they die, they flatten and interlock, providing a firm and secure barrier (stratum corneum) around the body. These cells contain a high percentage of the tough protein called keratin, the same substance that makes nails hard and hair strong and flexible. The outermost cells are eventually abraded or washed away and then replaced, allowing the epidermis to constantly refresh and maintain its thickness. It normally takes two weeks for a cell to move from the dermal border to the epidermal surface and another two to four weeks until it is abraded away. This outward movement of cells helps the body resist bacterial invasion.

A waxy substance called sebum lubricates the surface of the epidermis. This lubrication acts much like oil on leather. It keeps outer skin layers flexible, strong, and resistant to penetration by water. The epidermis is also responsible for pigmentation that protects the skin from harmful effects of ultraviolet radiation. The epidermal thickness varies greatly, depending on the amount of abrasion and pressure it receives. On the soles of the feet, it is very thick and strong, while over the eyelid it is very thin and delicate.

Dermis

Directly beneath the epidermis is the dermis, a connective tissue that helps contain the body and supports the functions of the epidermis. The upper dermal layer is the papillary layer, consisting of loose connective tissue, capillaries, and nerves supplying the epidermis. The reticular layer is the deeper dermal layer and is made up of strong connective tissue that integrates the dermis firmly with the subcutaneous layer below. The connective tissue in the dermis is rich in the protein collagen, the same fibers that give tendons and ligaments their great strength and flexibility.

The dermis contains blood vessels, nerve endings, glands, and other structures. It is here that sebaceous glands produce sebum and secrete it directly onto the skin's surface or into hair follicles. Sudoriferous glands secrete sweat to help move heat out of and away from the body through evaporation. Hair follicles produce hair that helps to reduce surface abrasion and conserve heat. The connective tissue within the dermis bonds it strongly to the subcutaneous tissue beneath and to the epidermis above. This tissue also holds the skin firmly around the body and permits stretching and flexibility necessary for articulation.

The dermis contains several resident body cells responsible for initiating the attack on invading organisms, foreign materials, and damaged cells, and for beginning the repair of damaged tissue. The macrophages and lymphocytes (types of white blood cells) begin the inflammation response by killing invading bodies and triggering a call for other, similar cells. Mast cells control the microcirculation to tissues and respond to the initial invasion, increasing capillary flow and permeability. Fibroblasts lay down and repair protein strands (collagen, mostly) to strengthen the wound site and begin restoring the skin's integrity.

Subcutaneous Tissue

Subcutaneous tissue is the body layer beneath the dermis. It is rich in fatty or adipose tissue, which helps it absorb the forces of trauma, protecting tissues and vital organs beneath. Because of its fatty content, heat moves outward through the subcutaneous tissue three times more slowly than through muscles or other layers of the skin; hence, it is of great value in conserving body temperature. The body directs blood below the subcutaneous tissue to conserve heat and above it through the dermis when it is necessary to radiate heat.

Blood Vessels

An important medium that moves through the dermis and subcutaneous layers of the skin is blood. Blood consists of water, electrolytes, proteins, and cells traveling through arteries, arterioles, capillaries, venules, and veins. Any soft-tissue wound can affect this blood flow; therefore, it is important to review the basic structure of blood vessels and actions the body takes once they are injured.

All blood vessels, except for the smallest—the capillaries, arterioles, and venules—are made up of three distinct layers: the tunica intima, the tunica media, and the tunica adventitia (Figure 2 ●).

The tunica intima is the blood vessel's smooth interior lining. It allows for free blood flow and prevents diffusion of nutrients and oxygen as well as waste products such as carbon dioxide.

The tunica media is the muscular component of the vessel. Its contraction or relaxation, as controlled by the central nervous system, determines a vessel's internal diameter, or lumen. The lumen size determines the extent of blood flow to a particular organ or extremity. Tunica media muscle fibers are found in two orientations. Most are wrapped around the vessel circumferentially and cause lumen constriction when they contract. Arterioles have the ability to vary their internal diameter by a factor of 5, permitting them to actively regulate blood flow to the tissues they precede. Other muscle fibers run lengthwise with the vessels, and their function is not well understood.

The outer blood vessel layer is the tunica adventitia. It consists of connective tissue (mostly strong collagen fibers) defining the maximum vessel lumen when the vessel's muscles relax (dilate).

The smallest blood vessels are the capillaries. Their walls are only one cell thick, allowing for easy diffusion of oxygen, carbon dioxide, nutrients, and waste products among the vascular, interstitial, and intracellular spaces. This ease of fluid flow, or permeability, through the capillary wall is a key factor in homeostasis and also plays an important role in a number of states of disease and damage, including localized swelling (edema), effusions, and pulmonary edema. The capillary wall structure also permits movement of disease-combating cells into the

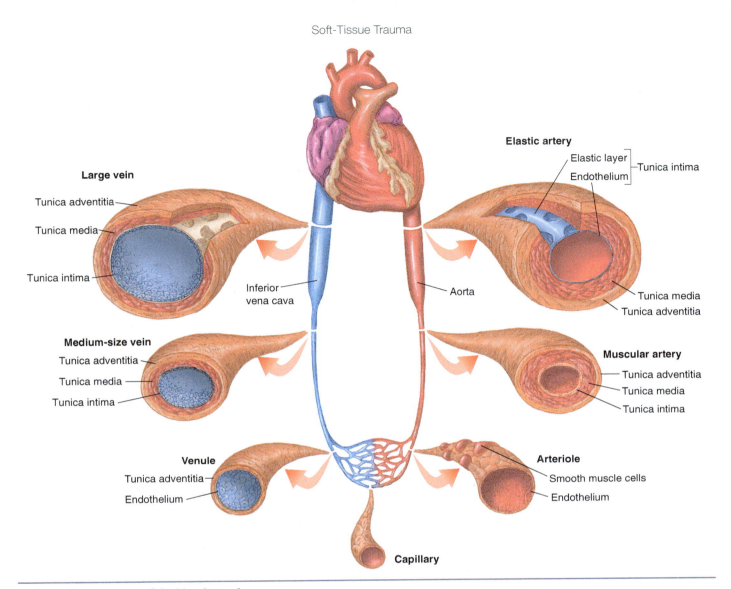

Elastic artery
Elastic layer
Endothelium ⎱ Tunica intima

Large vein
Tunica adventitia
Tunica media
Tunica intima

Inferior vena cava

Aorta

Tunica media
Tunica adventitia

Medium-size vein
Tunica adventitia
Tunica media
Tunica intima

Muscular artery
Tunica adventitia
Tunica media
Tunica intima

Venule
Tunica adventitia
Endothelium

Arteriole
Smooth muscle cells
Endothelium

Capillary

● **Figure 2**   Anatomy of the blood vessels.

interstitial space. Capillaries provide oxygenated circulation to virtually every cell of the body.

Not all fluids brought to the body cells are returned to the bloodstream directly. Some fluid is instead returned to the major veins by a system of channels and tissues called the lymphatic system. This system is especially important in carrying by-products of pathogen destruction to nodes where macrophages further break down the material. Lymph fluid is then directed to ducts just above the superior vena cava, where it is mixed with returning venous blood.

Muscles

Beneath the skin layers are the body's masses of **skeletal muscles**. They provide the power for movement and give the body its shape. They also produce much of the heat necessary to maintain body temperature. Muscles are strong contractile tissue, and their bulk helps protect vital organs, blood vessels, and nerves underneath. The muscle layer can be quite thick, as in the upper arms, shoulders, thighs and legs, and buttocks; or thin, as

in the forehead and hands. Muscles, which are connected to the skeleton by **tendons**, provide the driving force for the system of levers that moves the body and its appendages. Tendons are made up of almost pure collagen fibers arranged in a parallel fashion that gives them great tensile strength. Beneath the skeletal muscle layer lies the skeleton (the extremities, chest, and head) or the internal organs (the abdomen).

Fasciae

Fasciae are fibrous sheets that bundle skeletal muscle masses together and segregate them, one from another. The fasciae are made up of mostly collagen and can be very strong and thick, especially in the leg and upper arm. Within a limb, the fasciae define compartments with relatively fixed capacities and little room for expansion.

Tension Lines

The skin does not merely hang on the flesh but rather is spread over the body and attached to fit the contours of the underlying structures. This creates natural stretch or tension in the skin.

CONTENT REVIEW

▶ Types of Closed Wounds

- Contusions
- Hematomas
- Crush injuries

The orientation of tension in the skin is revealed in characteristic patterns called **tension lines** (Figure 3 ●). The effects of tension on the skin become evident when the skin is transected, as with a laceration. Lacerations cutting across tension lines have a tendency to be pulled apart and thus spread widely or gape. Lacerations parallel to tension lines tend to gape very little. An example of this is seen in the forehead where tension lines run across the forehead in a medial-lateral direction. Here, a vertically oriented laceration gapes widely while a horizontal laceration gapes less so. Wounds that spread widely tend to bleed more than those with minimal gaping. Large gaping wounds heal more slowly and are more likely to leave noticeable scars than wounds that spread less.

Tension represented by skin tension lines can be either static or dynamic. Static tension is noted in areas with limited movement of the tissue and structures beneath, as in the anterior abdomen or between joints in the extremities. Dynamic tension lines occur in areas subject to great movement, as in the skin over joints like the elbow, wrist, or knee. The increased motion in areas with dynamic skin tension lines means that clotting and tissue mending processes in these areas are more frequently interrupted, disrupting and complicating skin repair. It also explains why immobilizing a joint involved in a significant laceration can reduce blood loss and improve the formation of a clot.

PATHOPHYSIOLOGY OF SOFT-TISSUE INJURY

Although we often take the skin's functions for granted, soft-tissue injury can seriously affect health, causing severe blood and fluid loss, infection, hypothermia, and other problems. Therefore, as a paramedic, you need to become familiar with the pathophysiology of soft-tissue injuries.

Trauma is a violent transfer of energy that produces an open or closed wound to the skin and possible injury to the structures underneath. Wounds can be either blunt or penetrating. While all penetrating wounds are open, blunt trauma can, on occasion, create open wounds. Common soft-tissue injuries include closed wounds—contusions, hematomas, and crush injuries—and open wounds—abrasions, lacerations, incisions, punctures, avulsions, and amputations. Each type of wound is different and deserves special consideration.

Closed Wounds

Contusions

Contusions are blunt, nonpenetrating injuries that crush and damage small blood vessels (Figure 4 ●). Blood is drawn to the inflamed tissue, causing a reddening called **erythema**. Blood also leaks into the surrounding interstitial spaces through damaged vessels. As hemoglobin within the blood that flows into the interstitial space loses its oxygen, it becomes dark red and then bluish, resulting in the black-and-blue discoloration called **ecchymosis**. Because the development of ecchymosis is a progressive process, the discoloration may not be evident during prehospital care.

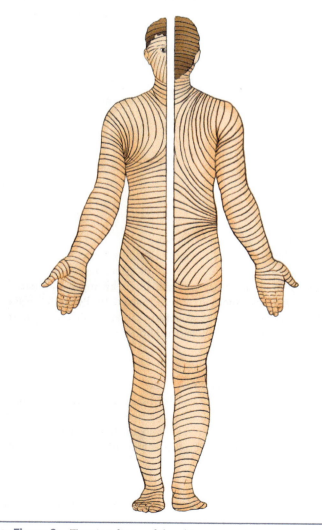

● **Figure 3**   Tension lines of the skin.

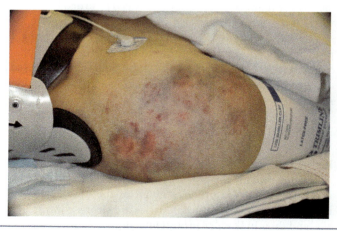

● **Figure 4**   A contusion. Note that the discoloration of a contusion is a delayed sign. (© *Edward T. Dickinson, MD*)

Contusions are more pronounced in areas where the mechanism causing the injury (for example, a steering wheel) and skeletal structures (such as the ribs or skull) trap the skin. Occasionally, a chest injury displays an erythematous or ecchymotic outline of the ribs and sternum, reflecting an impact with the auto dashboard or some other blunt object. The same effect can occasionally be seen when a hard object such as a belt buckle strikes the skin with the resulting outline of the object visible as an ecchymotic pattern in the skin. Early signs of such an injury may be difficult to identify, but they will become more evident as time passes and discoloration increases.

Hematomas

Soft-tissue bleeding can occur within tissue and at times can be quite significant. When the injury involves a larger blood vessel, most commonly an artery, blood can actually separate tissue and pool in a pocket. Such a trapped pool of blood is called a hematoma. These injuries are very visible in cases of head trauma because of the unyielding skull underneath. Hematomas tend to be less pronounced in other body areas, even though they can contain significant hemorrhage. If the hematoma is deep, it can be difficult to distinguish from the ordinary swelling and edema that occurs from blunt force injury. Severe hematomas to the thigh, leg, or arm may contribute significantly to hypovolemia. A hematoma in the thigh, for example, can contain a massive amount of blood before swelling becomes obvious.[1]

Crush Injuries

The term crush injury describes a collection of traumatic insults that includes both crush injury itself and crush syndrome. In crush injury, a body part that is compressed, possibly by a heavy object, sustains deep injury to the muscles, blood vessels, bones, and other internal structures (Figure 5 ●). Damage can be massive, despite minimal signs displayed on the skin itself. Crush syndrome is the term used to describe the systemic effects of a large crush injury. If the pressure that causes a crush injury remains in place for several hours, the resulting destruction of skeletal muscle cells leads to the accumulation of large quantities of myoglobin (a muscle protein), potassium, lactic acid, uric acid, and other toxins. When the pressure is released, these products enter the bloodstream. They circulate, causing a severe metabolic acidosis. These materials are also toxic to the kidneys and heart. Crush syndrome is thus a potentially life-threatening trauma event. It will be discussed in more detail later in this chapter.

Open Wounds

Abrasions

Abrasions are typically the most minor of injuries that violate the protective barrier of the skin. They involve a scraping or abrasive action that removes layers of the epidermis and the upper reaches of the dermis (Figure 6 ●). Bleeding from an abrasion can be persistent but is usually limited because the injury involves only superficial arterioles, venules, and capillaries. If the injury compromises a large area of the epidermis, it carries a danger of serious infection.

Lacerations

A laceration is an open wound that penetrates more deeply into the dermis than an abrasion (Figure 7 ●). A laceration tends to involve a smaller surface area, being limited to the tissue immediately surrounding the penetration. It endangers deeper and more significant vasculature—arteries, arterioles, venules, and veins—as well as nerves, muscles, tendons, ligaments, and perhaps some underlying organs. As with an abrasion, the injury breaks the skin's protective barrier and provides a pathway for infection. You should note a laceration's orientation to the skin tension lines during your patient assessment. If the orientation parallels those lines, the wound may remain closed. If it is perpendicular to them, the wound may gape open.

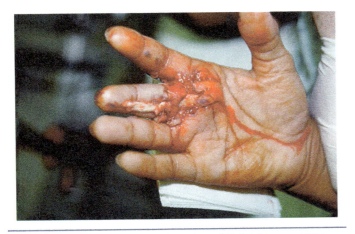

● **Figure 5** A crush injury. (© Edward T. Dickinson, MD)

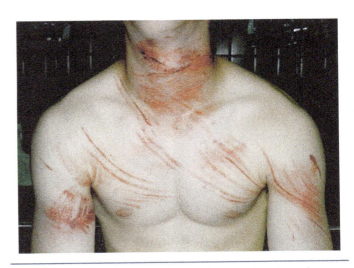

● **Figure 6** Abrasions. (© Charles Stewart, MD, MPH)

129

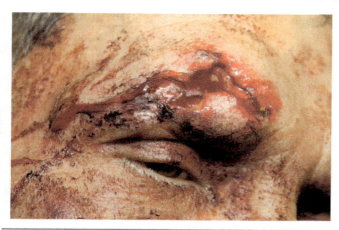

● **Figure 7**   Lacerations. (© *Dr. Bryan E. Bledsoe*)

Incisions

An **incision** is a surgically smooth laceration, often caused by a sharp instrument such as a knife, straight razor, or piece of glass. Such a wound tends to bleed freely. In all other ways, it is a laceration.

Punctures

Another special type of laceration is the **puncture**. It involves a small entrance wound with damage that extends into the body's interior (Figure 8 ●). The wound normally seals itself and presents in a way that does not reflect the actual extent of injury. If a puncture penetrates deeply, it may involve not just the skin but underlying muscles, nerves, bones, and organs.

A puncture additionally carries an increased danger of infection. A penetrating object introduces bacteria and other pathogens deep into a wound. There, the disrupted tissue and blood vessels, along with a reduced oxygen level, create a warm and moist environment that is ideal for the colonization of bacteria.

Impaled Objects

An **impaled object** is not a wound itself, but rather a wound complication often associated with a puncture or laceration. Impaled objects are important for the damage they may cause if withdrawn. Frequently, embedded objects are irregular in shape and may become entangled in important structures such as arteries, nerves, or tendons (Figure 9 ●). Their removal in the field can result in further damage. Perhaps more critically, the embedded object may have lacerated a large blood vessel and the object's presence temporarily blocks, or tamponades, blood loss. Object removal may cause an uncontrollable flow of blood. This situation is particularly dangerous when the object is impaled in the neck or trunk, where effective direct pressure application is difficult or impossible.

Avulsions

Avulsion occurs when a flap of skin, although torn or cut, is not torn completely loose from the body (Figure 10 ●). Avulsion is frequently seen with blunt trauma to the skull, where the scalp is torn and folds back. It may also occur with animal bites and machinery injuries. The seriousness of the avulsion depends on the area involved, the condition of the circulation to (and distal to) the injury site, and the degree of contamination.

A special type of avulsion is the **degloving injury**. In this wound, the mechanism of injury tears the skin off the underlying muscle, connective tissue, blood vessels, and bone. It is a particularly gruesome injury, occurring occasionally with farm and industrial machinery. The device pulls the skin off with great force as the skeletal tissue underneath is held stationary. The wound exposes a large area of tissue and is often severely contaminated. The injury carries with it a poor prognosis.

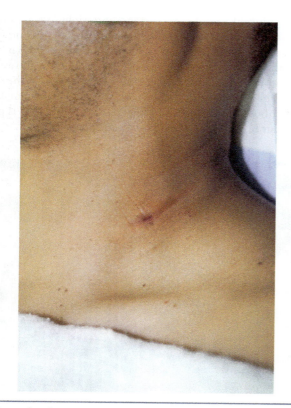

● **Figure 8**   A puncture wound. (© *Edward T. Dickinson, MD*)

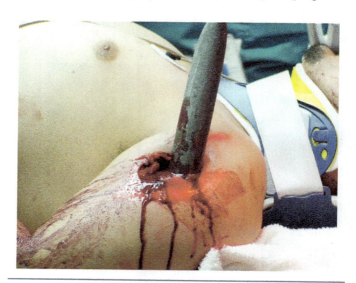

● **Figure 9**   An impaled object. (© *Michael Casey, MD*)

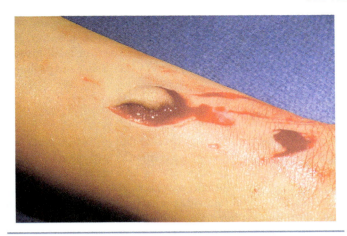

● **Figure 10**   An avulsion. *(© Dr. Bryan E. Bledsoe)*

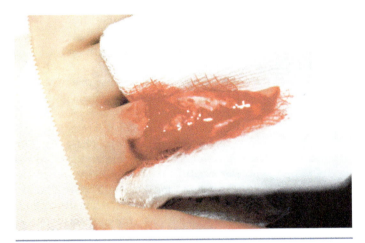

● **Figure 11**   A ring-type degloving injury.

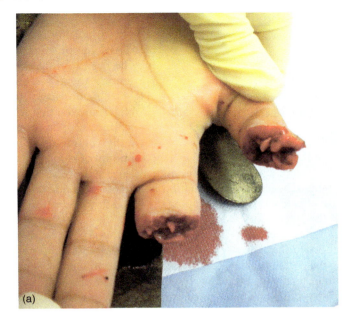

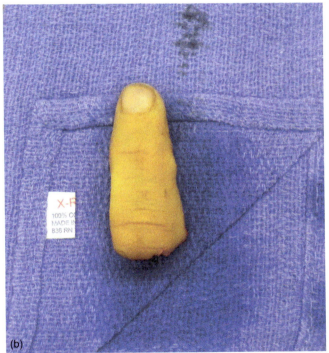

● **Figure 12**   (a) An amputation on the hand. (b) An amputated finger. *(Both: © Dr. John P. Brosious)*

If, however, the vasculature and innervation remain intact, there may be some hope for future use of the digit or extremity.

A variation of the degloving process is the ring injury (Figure 11 ●). As a person jumps or falls, the ring is caught, pulling the skin of the finger against the victim's weight. The force may tear the upper layers of tissue away from the phalanges, exposing the tendons, nerves, and blood vessels. Although the ring injury involves a smaller area, it is otherwise a degloving injury. The potential for degloving injuries is a reason for paramedics to not wear rings and other jewelry while on duty.

Amputations

The partial or complete severance of a digit or limb is an **amputation** (Figure 12 ●). It often results in the complete loss of the limb at the site of severance. The hemorrhage associated with the amputation may be limited if the limb or digit is cut cleanly or may be severe and continuing if the wound is a jagged or crushing one. The surgeon may attempt to replant the amputated part or use its skin for grafting as the remaining limb is repaired. If this skin is unavailable, the surgeon may have to cut the bone and musculature back further to close the wound. This reduces the limb length as well as its future usefulness. When amputation is undertaken, great care is used to ensure that the stump will be as functional as possible and suitable for prosthetic devices.

Hemorrhage

Soft-tissue injuries frequently cause blood loss, ranging in severity from inconsequential to life threatening. The loss can be arterial, venous, or capillary. Bleeding can be easy or almost impossible to control. Hemorrhage is usually dark red with venous injury, red with capillary injury, and bright red with arterial injury. The rate of hemorrhage also varies from

CONTENT REVIEW

▶ Stages of Wound Healing
- Hemostasis
- Inflammation
- Epithelialization
- Neovascularization
- Collagen synthesis

oozing capillary, to flowing venous, to pulsing arterial bleeding. In practice, it may be hard to differentiate among the types and origins of hemorrhage. Research has proven that it is very difficult to approximate the volume of blood loss at the scene. However, the relative amount of blood visible and the time since the injury event may suggest the relative rate of hemorrhage. This information helps you to decide on the most effective means of stopping the blood flow and prioritizing the patient for care and transport.

Often the nature of the soft-tissue wound may be more important than the size or type of vessel involved in determining the severity of the blood vessel injury. If a moderately sized vein or artery is cut cleanly, the muscles in the vessel wall will tend to contract. This constricts the vessel's lumen and retracts the severed vessel into the tissue. As the muscle is drawn back from the wound, it thickens and further restricts the lumen. This restricts blood flow, reduces the rate of loss, and assists

the clotting mechanisms. Therefore, clean lacerations and amputations generally do not bleed profusely. If, however, the vessel is not severed cleanly but is laid open instead, muscle contraction opens the wound, thereby increasing and prolonging blood loss.

Wound Healing

Wound healing is a complex process that begins immediately following injury and can take many months to complete. Wound healing is an essential component of homeostasis, the process whereby the body maintains a uniform environment for itself. Although it is useful to divide the wound healing process into stages or parts, it is important to note that these phases overlap considerably and are intertwined physiologically (Figure 13 ●).

Hemostasis

Arguably the most important aspect of wound healing is the body's ability to stop most bleeding on its own. This process is called **hemostasis**. Without hemostasis, even the most trivial nicks and scratches would continue to bleed, leading to life-threatening hemorrhage. Hemostasishas three major components: the vascular phase, the platelet phase, and the coagulation phase.

Hemostasis begins almost immediately following injury with the vascular phase. Arteries, arterioles, and some veins are endowed with a muscular layer that reflexively constricts the vessel in response to local injury. The longitudinal muscles, too, play a role by retracting the cut ends of larger vessels back into the contracted muscle, thus reducing flow. This immediate response usually reduces but does not entirely stop bleeding. Capillaries, which do not have a muscle layer, cannot contract and thus continue to bleed. This explains the continuing but minor bleeding associated with capillary wounds such as paper cuts and minor abrasions.

Platelets begin the clotting process (the platelet phase of hemostasis). The damaged vessel wall becomes "sticky," as do the platelets in the turbulent flow of the disrupted vessel. Platelets stick to the vessel wall and to one another. This forms a platelet plug, reducing blood flow or, in small vessels, stopping it altogether.

When a blood vessel is injured, the disrupted tunica intima exposes collagen and other structural proteins to the blood. In the coagulation phase of hemostasis, these proteins activate a complicated series of enzyme reactions that change certain blood proteins into long fibrin strands. These strands then entrap erythrocytes and produce a gelatinous mass that further occludes the bleeding vessel. This complex process, called coagulation, stops all but the most severe and persistent hemorrhage. With time, the clot

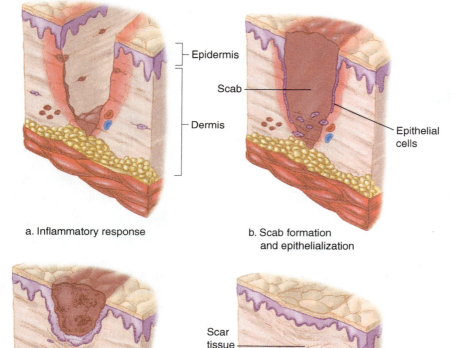

a. Inflammatory response

b. Scab formation and epithelialization

c. Scar tissue formation

d. Remodeling

● **Figure 13**   The wound healing process.

shrinks or contracts, bringing the wound margins closer together, further facilitating wound healing. When the clot is no longer needed, it is reabsorbed by the body and any superficial scab merely drops off.

Inflammation

Shortly after hemostasis begins, the body sets in motion a very complex process of healing called inflammation. The inflammatory process involves a host of elements including various kinds of white blood cells, proteins involved in immunity, and hormone-like chemicals that signal other cells to mobilize.

Cells damaged by direct trauma or by invading pathogens release a number of proteins and chemicals into the surrounding tissue and blood. These agents, called chemotactic factors, recruit cells responsible for consuming cellular debris, invading bacteria, or other foreign or damaged cells and for beginning the inflammatory process. The first cells to arrive are specialized white blood cells called granulocytes and macrophages. These cells (also called phagocytes) are capable of engulfing bacteria, debris, and foreign material, digesting them, and then releasing the by-products in a process called phagocytosis. Other white blood cells called lymphocytes, in combination with immunoglobulins or immune proteins, are also mobilized. Lymphocytes attack invading pathogens directly or through an antibody response.

The injury process, the material released from injured cells, and the debris released as the phagocytes destroy invading cells cause mast cells to release histamine. Histamine dilates precapillary blood vessels, increases capillary permeability, and increases blood flow into and through the injured or infected tissue. This is called hyperemia and is responsible for the reddish skin color, or erythema, associated with inflammation. The increased blood flow, along with increased capillary permeability, results in the transfer of protein and electrolyte-rich fluid into the surrounding tissues that is called edema. When edema is significant, it is manifest as swelling of the area. Hyperemia brings much-needed oxygen and more phagocytes to the injured area and draws away the by-products of cell destruction and repair. The increasing blood flow and local tissue metabolism also increase tissue temperature, which may in turn denature pathogen membranes. Overall, this response produces a swollen (edematous), reddened (erythematous), and warm region, characteristic of inflammation in response to local infection or injury. The result of the inflammation stage is the accumulation of fluid, heat, and immune and repair cells that enables the clearing away of dead and dying tissue, removal of bacteria and other foreign substances, and the preparation of the damaged area for rebuilding.

Epithelialization

Epithelialization is an early stage in wound healing in which epithelial cells migrate over the surface of the wound. The stratum germinativum cells rapidly divide and regenerate, thus restoring a uniform layer of skin cells along the edges of the healing wound. In clean, surgically prepared wounds, complete epithelialization may take place in as little as 48 hours. Except in minor, superficial wounds, the new epithelial layer is not a perfect facsimile of the original, undamaged skin. Instead, the new skin layer may be thinner, pigmented differently, and devoid of normal hair follicles. However, the new skin is usually quite functional and cosmetically similar to the original. If the wound is very large, epithelialization may be incomplete, and collagen will show through as a shiny, pinkish line of tissue called a scar.

Neovascularization

For healing to take place, new tissue must grow and regenerate. That requires blood rich in oxygen and nutrients. The body responds to this increased demand by generating new blood vessels in a process called neovascularization. These vessels bud from undamaged capillaries in the wound margins and then grow into the healing tissue. Neovascularized tissue is very fragile and has a tendency to bleed easily. It takes weeks to months for the newly formed blood vessels to become fully resistant to injury and for the surrounding tissue to strengthen enough to protect the new and delicate circulation.

Collagen Synthesis

Collagen is the body's main structural protein. It is a strong, tough fiber forming part of the hair, bones, and connective tissue. Scar tissue, cartilage, and tendons are almost entirely collagen. Specialized cells called fibroblasts are brought to the wound area and synthesize collagen as an important step in rebuilding damaged tissues. Collagen binds the wound margins together and strengthens the healing wound. It is important to note that as the wound heals, it is not "as good as new." Regenerated skin has only about 60 percent of the tensile strength of undamaged skin at four months, when the scar is fully mature. This accounts for the occasional reinjury and reopening of wounds weeks or months after healing. The fibroblasts continue to reshape scar tissue and shrink the wound for months after the scab falls off. This remodeling involves reorganizing collagen fibers into neat, parallel bands, strengthening the healing tissue still more. Remodeling can continue for up to 6 to 12 months after the initial injury, so the final cosmetic outcome of the healing process may not be evident until then.

Infection

Infection is the most common and, next to hemorrhage, the most serious complication of open wounds. Approximately 1 in 15 (6.5 percent of wounds seen at the emergency department) result in a wound infection. These infections delay healing. They may also spread to adjacent tissues and endanger cosmetic appearances. Occasionally, they cause widespread or systemic infection, called sepsis.

The common causes of skin and soft-tissue infections are the *Staphylococcus* and *Streptococcus* bacterial families. *Staphylococcus* and *Streptococcus* bacteria are gram-positive (based on Gram's method of staining, a procedure to differentiate between types of bacteria), aerobic, and very common in the environment. *Staphylococcus* bacteria frequently colonize on the surface of normal skin, so it is not surprising to find them driven into wounds by the forces of trauma. MRSA (methicillin-resistant *Staphylococcus aureus*) and VRSA (vancomycin-resistant *Staphylococcus aureus*) are staph infections resistant to the drugs normally used to combat them and are now a major cause of wound infections. Less commonly, wound infections are caused by other bacteria such as gram-negative rods, including *Pseudomonas aeruginosa* (diabetics and foot puncture wounds) and *Pasteurella multocida* (cat and dog bites).

It takes bacteria a few days to grow into numbers sufficient to cause noticeable signs or symptoms of infection. Infections appear at least two to three days following the initial wound and commonly present with pain, tenderness, erythema, and warmth. Infection earlier than that is very unusual. Pus, a collection of white blood cells, cellular debris, and dead bacteria, may be visible draining from the wound. The pus is usually thick, pale yellowish-to-greenish in color, and has a foul smell. Visible red streaks, or **lymphangitis**, may extend from the wound margins up the affected extremity proximally. These streaks represent lymph channel inflammation as a result of the infection. The patient may also complain of fever and malaise, especially if the infection has begun to spread systemically.

Infection Risk Factors

Risk factors for wound infections are related to the host's health, the wound type and location, any associated contamination, and the treatment provided. Diabetics, the infirm, the elderly, and individuals with serious chronic diseases such as chronic obstructive pulmonary disease are at greater risk for infection and heal more slowly and less efficiently than healthy individuals. Patients with any significant disease or preexisting medical problem such as cancer, anemia, hepatic failure, or cardiovascular disease have difficulty mobilizing the immune and tissue-repair response necessary for good wound healing. HIV and AIDS attack the body's immune system and seriously impair its ability to ward off infection, increasing risk significantly. Smoking constricts blood vessels and robs healing tissues of needed oxygen and nutrients, also increasing infection risk, especially to the distal extremities.

Several drugs detract from the body's ability to fight infection. Persons on immunosuppressant medications such as prednisone or cortisone (corticosteroids) are also at increased risk for serious infection. Colchicine, a drug used to treat gout, and nonsteroidal anti-inflammatory drugs (NSAIDs) such as ibuprofen also reduce the body's inflammation response. Neoplastic agents such as methotrexate, which are used to combat rapidly reproducing cells in cancer patients (as well as for other conditions), also disrupt cell regeneration at an injury site.

The wound type strongly affects the likelihood of a wound infection. A puncture wound traps contamination deep within tissue where there is a perfect environment for bacterial growth. Avulsion tears away blood vessels and supporting structures, robbing the damaged tissue of its blood supply, a critical factor in preventing or reducing infection. Crush injuries and other wounds that produce large areas of injured or dead (devitalized) tissue provide an excellent environment for bacterial growth and are at great risk for wound infection.

In a similar fashion, wound location influences infection risk. Well-vascularized areas such as the face and scalp are very resistant to infection. Distal extremities, the feet in particular, are at greater risk.

Clean objects, such as uncontaminated sheet metal or a clean knife, usually leave only small amounts of bacteria in a wound and, consequently, do not often cause infections. However, objects contaminated with organic matter and bacteria, such as a nail on a barnyard floor, a knife used to clean raw meat, or a piece of wood, pose much greater risks of infection. The infection risk associated with bites caused by mammals, and carnivores in particular, is very great. Bites by humans, cats, and dogs are among the most common and most serious types of bites.[2]

The type of treatment provided for a wound affects the risk of infection. Use of sterile dressings and clean examination gloves minimizes wound contamination during prehospital treatment. Gloves protect not only the rescuer but also the patient from contaminants on the rescuer's hands. Wound irrigation with sterile saline using a pressurized stream device has been shown to reduce bacterial loads and reduce infection rates. Closing wounds (with sutures or staples, for example) increases infection risks as compared to leaving wounds open. However, the risks associated with wound closure are frequently accepted in order to achieve the best possible cosmetic outcome and more rapid healing.

In most cases, routine use of antibiotics with wounds does not help reduce infection rates and, in fact, may increase the likelihood of infection with antibiotic-resistant microorganisms. Antibiotics may be helpful if given within the first hour or so after deep major wounds, such as those from gunshots or stabbings, puncture wounds to the feet, and wounds where retention of a foreign body is suspected.

Infection Management

Despite the potential problems previously noted, the mainstay in treatment for infections is the use of chemical antibacterial agents, also known as antibiotics. Antibiotics for the treatment of gram-positive infections include the antistaphylococcal penicillins and cephalosporins. Erythromycin (and similar agents) can be used in patients allergic to penicillin. The pharmacological approach against *Pseudomonas* often requires the use of two drugs, while *Pasteurella* usually can be treated with penicillin.

On occasion, a wound forms a collection of pus called an abscess and requires a minor incision and drainage to correct. Surgical removal of this material helps the body return to normal more quickly.

Gangrene **Gangrene** is tissue decomposition by bacteria resulting from loss of blood supply, crush injury, or infection. It is one of the rarest and most feared wound complications. Gangrene is a deep-space infection usually caused by the anaerobic bacterium *Clostridium perfringens*. These bacteria characteristically produce a gas deep within a wound, causing subcutaneous emphysema and a foul smell whenever the gas escapes. Once they have become established, the bacteria are particularly prolific and can rapidly involve an entire extremity. Left unchecked, gangrene frequently leads to sepsis and death. In the days before antibiotics, amputation was frequently necessary to stop the spread of the disease. Modern treatment with a combination of antibiotics, surgery, and hyperbaric oxygenation effectively arrests most cases of gangrene if caught early in their course.

Tetanus Another highly feared but, fortunately, rare complication of wound infections is **tetanus**, or lockjaw. Tetanus is caused by the bacterium *Clostridium tetani* and, like its cousin

Clostridium perfringens, it is anaerobic. Tetanus presents with few signs or symptoms at the local wound site, but the bacteria produce a potent toxin that causes widespread, painful, involuntary muscle contractions. Early observers noted mandibular trismus, or jaw-clenching ("lockjaw"). There is an antidote for the tetanus toxin, but it only neutralizes circulating toxin molecules, not those already bound to the motor endplates. Thus, treatment is slow and recovery prolonged.

Fortunately, tetanus is preventable through immunization. Widespread immunization has reduced incidence to a very few cases. The standard immunization is a series of three shots in childhood, with boosters every ten years thereafter. It is common practice in emergency departments to provide boosters to wound patients if they have not been immunized in the past five years. Immigrants from Third World countries often have never completed a tetanus vaccine series. In these cases, it is prudent to administer tetanus immune globulin (TIG) in addition to the tetanus vaccine to prevent development of the disease while the body gears up to make new antibodies.

Other Wound Complications

Several circumstances or conditions can interfere with normal wound healing processes. These conditions include impaired hemostasis, rebleeding, and delayed healing.

Impaired Hemostasis

Several medications can interfere with hemostasis and the clotting process. Aspirin and clopidogrel (Plavix) are powerful inhibitors of platelet aggregation, and are used clinically to help prevent clot formation in the coronary and cerebral arteries of patients at risk for myocardial infarction or stroke. Thus, a side effect of aspirin or clopidogrel use is a prolongation of clotting time, an important consideration in a patient who has sustained significant trauma or is undergoing major surgery. Likewise, anticoagulants, such as Coumadin (warfarin) and heparin, and fibrinolytics, such as TPA and streptokinase, interfere with or break down the protein fibers that form clots and are used to prevent or destroy obstructions at critical locations. Additionally, abnormalities in proteins involved in the fibrin formation cascade may result in delayed clotting, as is the case in hemophiliacs.

Rebleeding

Despite treatment that provides adequate initial bleeding control, rebleeding is possible from any wound. Movement of underlying structures, such as muscles or bones, or of the bandage or dressing material may dislodge clots and reinstitute hemorrhage.

Also, hemorrhage that appears to have been stopped may actually be bleeding into an oversized dressing until it saturates the dressing and pushes through it. Monitor your dressings and bandages frequently to ensure that blood loss is not continuing.

Partially healed wounds are also at risk for rebleeding. Postoperative wounds in particular can rebleed with life-threatening results. Because patients are discharged from hospitals more quickly today than in the past and return home sooner after surgery, be wary of this potential complication.

Delayed Healing

In some patients, the wound repair process may be delayed or even arrested, resulting in incomplete wound healing. Persons at greatest risk for this complication are diabetics, the elderly, the chronically ill, and the malnourished. Nutrition must be adequate for wound healing to occur. Patients with multiple injuries often require significantly more calories during the healing phase than normal. Seriously or chronically infected wounds and wounds in locations with limited blood flow (distal extremities) are also at risk for incomplete healing. Incompletely healed wounds remain tender and are easily reinjured. A pale yellow or blood-tinged serous fluid may drain from them. Out-of-hospital treatment of incompletely healed wounds includes frequent changes of sterile, nonadherent dressings, and protection of the wound.

Compartment Syndrome

Compartment syndrome is a complication most commonly associated with closed injuries to the extremities, most commonly a fracture or crushing type injury. In the extremities, major muscle groups are contained in compartments formed by strong and inelastic fascia (Figure 14 ●). Normally, pressure within the fascial compartment is near zero. In compartment syndrome swelling within the compartment or constriction of the compartment from outside forces (as with a circumferential pressure dressing) causes the intracompartmental pressure to rise. If it rises above 30 mmHg it begins to restrict capillary blood flow to muscle tissue and nerves (traveling into and through the compartment). This results in ischemic damage that becomes irreversible after about 10 hours. The muscle mass may die and its contribution to limb function may be lost (Figure 15 ●). Frequently, the resulting scar tissue shortens the length of the muscle strand, thus further reducing the usefulness of the limb after compartment syndrome. All extremities may experience compartment syndrome, but the lower extremities, especially the calves, are at greatest risk because of their bulk and fascial anatomy.

Compartment syndrome most commonly affects the extremities. The most common location is the leg (anterior, lateral, deep posterior, and superficial posterior compartments). It can also affect the thigh (quadriceps compartment) and buttocks (gluteal compartment). In the upper extremity, it may occur in the hand (interosseus compartment), forearm (dorsal and volar compartments), and arm (deltoid and biceps compartments). Most occurrences of compartment syndrome are associated with fracture (about two-thirds) with auto collisions and sports injuries the most common cause. The leg's anterior compartment is the most common location of compartment syndrome.

Abnormal Scar Formation

During the healing process, scar tissue sometimes develops abnormally. A keloid is excessive scar tissue that extends beyond the boundaries of a wound. It develops most commonly in darkly pigmented individuals and develops on the sternum, lower abdomen, upper extremities, and ears. Another healing abnormality is hypertrophic scar formation. This is an excessive

Compartments of the Leg

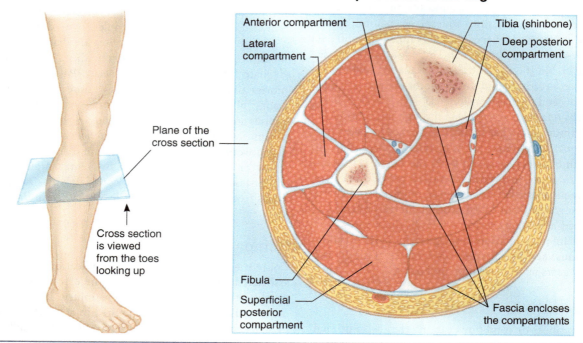

● **Figure 14**   Musculoskeletal compartments segregated by fasciae.

Compartment Syndrome in the Anterior Compartment

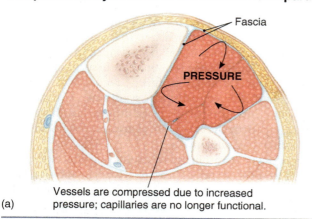

(a)

Fasciotomy Procedure

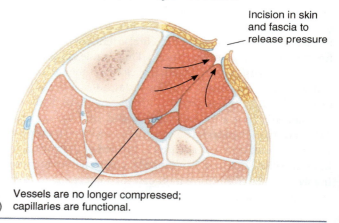

(b)

● **Figure 15**   (a) Compartment syndrome. (b) Compartment syndrome relieved by fasciotomy.

accumulation of scar tissue, usually within the injury border, that is often associated with dynamic skin tension lines, like those at flexion joints.

Pressure Injuries

A special type of soft-tissue injury is the pressure injury, which is caused by prolonged compression of the skin and tissues beneath. This may occur in the chronically ill (bed-ridden) patient, the patient who falls and remains unconscious for hours (due to alcohol intoxication, stroke, or drug overdose), or the patient who is entrapped with no crushing mechanism. The patient's weight against the ground or other surface compresses

tissue and induces hypoxic injury. The injury is similar to a crush injury, although the mechanism is more passive and more likely to go unnoticed. Pressure injury may also occur when a long spine board, PASG, air splint, or rigid splint remains on a patient for an extended period of time.

Crush Injury

Crush injury involves a trauma pattern in which body tissues are subjected to severe compressive forces. A crush injury can be relatively minor—for example, one that involves only a finger or part of an extremity—or it can be massive—one that affects much or all of the body. The mechanisms of injury can be varied. A packing machine might compress a worker's finger or extremity; a collapsed jack might trap a mechanic's leg under a car wheel; the seat and steering column might compress a driver's chest between them in an auto crash; or debris from a building collapse or trench cave-in might bury a construction worker.

A crush injury disrupts the body's tissues—muscles, blood vessels, bone, and, in some cases, internal organs. With such injuries, the skin may remain intact and the limb may appear normal in shape, or the skin may be severely cut and bruised and the extremity mangled and deformed. In both cases, however, the damage within is extensive. The injury often results in a large area of destruction with limited effective circulation, thus creating an excellent growth medium for bacteria. Hemorrhage with crush injuries may be difficult to control for several reasons: The actual source of the bleeding may be hard to identify, or several large vessels may be damaged. Also, the general condition of the limb may not support effective application of direct pressure. The resulting tissue hypoxia and acidosis may result in muscle rigor, with muscles that may feel very hard and "wood-like" on palpation.

Associated Injury

When patients have been subjected to mechanisms that cause crush injuries, those mechanisms or others associated with them often result in additional injuries. For example, patients who have received crush injuries in building collapses or when entrapped by machinery may suffer additional fractures and open or closed soft-tissue injuries. Falling debris can cause direct injury, both blunt and penetrating. Dust and smoke can cause respiratory and eye injuries. Also, entrapment for any length of time leads to dehydration and hypothermia. You should consider all these possibilities when assessing and providing emergency care to victims of crush injury.

Crush Syndrome

Crush syndrome occurs when body parts are entrapped for 4 hours or longer. Shorter periods of entrapment may result in direct body part damage, but they usually do not cause the broad, systemic complications of crush syndrome. The crushed skeletal muscle tissue undergoes necrosis and cellular changes with resultant release of metabolic by-products. This degenerative process, called traumatic rhabdomyolysis (skeletal muscle disintegration), releases many toxins. Chief among these by-products of cellular destruction are myoglobin (a muscle protein), phosphate and potassium (from cellular death), and lactic acid (from anaerobic metabolism). These by-products accumulate in the crushed body part but, because of the entrapment and the resulting minimal circulation through the injured tissue, do not reach the systemic circulation. Once the limb or victim is extricated and the pressure is released, however, the accumulated by-products and toxins flood the central circulation.

High levels of myoglobin can lodge in the kidney's filtering tubules, especially with patients who are in hypovolemic (shock) states. This can lead to renal failure, a leading cause of delayed death in crush syndrome. More immediate problems include hypovolemia and shock from the flow of sodium,

chloride, and water into the damaged tissue. Increased blood potassium (hyperkalemia) can reduce the cardiac muscle's response to electrical stimuli, induce cardiac arrhythmias, and lead to sudden death. Rising phosphate levels (hyperphosphatemia) can lead to abnormal calcifications in the vasculature and nervous system, compounding problems for the patient. As oxygenated circulation returns to the cells, the aerobic process by which uric acid is produced can operate again, thus increasing cellular acidity and injury.

Injection Injury

A unique type of soft-tissue injury is the injection injury. A bursting high-pressure line, most commonly a hydraulic line, may inject fluid through a patient's skin and into the subcutaneous tissues. If the pressure is strong enough, the fluid may push between tissue layers and travel along the limb (Figure 16 ●). The fluid thus injected—for example, a petroleum-based hydraulic fluid—may then chemically damage the surrounding tissue. The body's repair mechanisms are unprepared to remove the great quantities of injected material, and the resulting damage is severe. A limb may be lost due to the direct physical damage from the injection process, from the chemical damage done

---

PATHO PEARLS

High-Pressure Tool Injuries

Although infrequently encountered, high-pressure tools can cause very serious soft-tissue injuries. High-pressure tools are commonly used in repair shops and often contain fluid or grease (hydraulic fluid or grease guns) or simply air. The most common cause of the injury is accidentally discharging the device with the tip in proximity to the skin. This causes a small superficial skin wound. However, tissues below the wound can sustain serious injury from the grease or fluid, the pressure, or a combination of the two. These wounds often cause serious infections and loss of function if not surgically explored and adequately treated. If the injury involves the hand (as is common), the pressure may inject materials into the forearm and even as far as the arm or shoulder. The grease or other foreign substance tends to follow the fascial planes of the hand and forearm and can become embedded within the muscle sheaths. The injury generally presents with a small open wound with some contamination, but its nature is generally far worse than the wound's physical signs and symptoms suggest.

Contaminants introduced deep into the wound exist in an environment with limited air and circulation (anaerobic state). However, the area is warm and moist, providing any bacteria introduced into the wound an ideal environment to proliferate. Hydraulic fluid and grease are toxic to the internal tissues and cause cell injury and death. Because of the depth and extent of contamination, surgical debridement is extremely difficult and may, itself, cause significant and extensive tissue injury. Whenever a patient presents with this type of injury, recognize the likelihood of extensive limb involvement and seek the services of the trauma center.

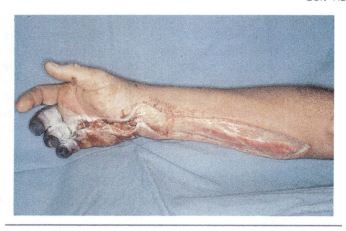

● **Figure 16** An injection injury resulting from the pressurized injection of grease. *(Photo courtesy of Scott & White Healthcare)*

by the injected material, or from infection that develops after the injection. High-pressure, paint-spraying devices are of particular danger because they are designed to provide an open spray that places exposed body parts at constant risk, in contrast to rare exposure resulting from leaks that are the cause of injuries from other pressurized tools. Depending on the type of paint in use, local and systemic toxicity can be substantial.

DRESSING AND BANDAGE MATERIALS

Several types of dressings and bandages are effective in prehospital care. A dressing is material placed directly on the wound to control bleeding and maintain wound cleanliness.[3] A bandage is material used to hold a dressing in place and to apply direct pressure to control hemorrhage. Dressings and bandages have various designs and are used for a variety of purposes in emergency care.

Dressings

Sterile/Nonsterile Dressings

Sterile dressings are cotton or other fiber pads that have been specially prepared to be without microorganisms. They are usually packaged individually and remain sterile for as long as the package is intact. Once the packaging is opened, sterile dressings become contaminated by airborne dust and particles that harbor bacteria and other microorganisms. Sterile dressings are designed to be used in direct contact with wounds.

Nonsterile dressings are clean—that is, free of gross contamination—but are not free of microscopic contamination and microorganisms. Nonsterile dressings are not intended to be applied directly to a wound, but rather to be placed over a sterile dressing to add bulk or absorptive power.

Occlusive/Nonocclusive Dressings

Some dressings, such as sterilized plastic wrap and petroleum-impregnated gauze, are designed to prevent the movement of fluid and air through them. These dressings are called occlusive and are helpful in preventing air aspiration into chest wounds

(open pneumothorax) and open neck wounds (air emboli into the jugular vein). Most dressing material is nonocclusive.

Adherent/Nonadherent Dressings

Adherent dressings are untreated cotton or other fiber pads that will stick to drying blood and fluid that has leaked from open wounds. Adherent dressings have the advantage of promoting clot formation and thus reducing hemorrhage, but their removal from wounds can be quite painful. Removal or disturbance of an adherent dressing is also likely to break the clot and cause rebleeding. Nonadherent dressings are specially treated with chemicals such as polymers to prevent the wound fluids and clotting materials from adhering to the dressing. Nonadherent dressings are preferred for most uncomplicated wounds.

Absorbent/Nonabsorbent Dressings

Absorbent dressings readily soak up blood and other fluids, much as a sponge soaks up water. This property is helpful in many bleeding situations. Nonabsorbent dressings absorb little or no fluid and are used when a barrier to leaking is desired. The clear membrane dressings frequently placed over intravenous puncture sites are good examples of nonabsorbent dressings. Most other dressings used in prehospital care are absorbent dressings.

Wet/Dry Dressings

Wet dressings are sometimes applied to special types of wounds such as burns. They are also used in the hospital to effect healing in some complicated postoperative wounds. Sterile normal saline is the usual fluid used to wet dressings. Wet dressings provide a medium for the movement of infectious material into wounds, however, and are not commonly used in prehospital care, except with injuries such as abdominal eviscerations or burns involving only a limited body surface area. Dry dressings are the type most often employed for wounds in prehospital care.

Hemostatic Dressings

A new development in wound care is the topical hemostatic agents (Figure 17 ●). These products, approved by the FDA, can be applied directly to a bleeding wound and will help to slow or stop the bleeding. There are several products on the market. These include the following:

● *Celox*™ is a granular powder placed immediately on a bleeding wound to control or stop bleeding. The principal ingredient is chitosan, a polysaccharide that is derived from the shells of crustaceans (e.g., shrimp, crabs). When chitosan becomes moistened with blood, it becomes extremely adherent and stops bleeding. Chitosan has antibacterial properties and is hypoallergenic. Celox has a shelf life of three years.

● *HemCon* bandages are dressings impregnated with chitosan. They are supplied in 2″ × 2″, 2″ × 4″, and 4″ × 4″ dressings. They have been widely used in battlefield care.

● *QuickClot*® is a hemostatic agent that is made from zeolite. Zeolite is a proprietary substance derived from volcanic rock. It is supplied in 3.5-ounce packets that can be poured directly on the wound. QuickClot quickly absorbs water, thus concentrating the blood and promoting clot formation. The shelf life is three years.

- *TraumaDEX™* is a starch-based powder derived from plants. It is supplied in a bellows and applied directly to the wound. The hemostatic effects are derived from the absorption of the water from blood, which promotes clot formation.

Bandages

Self-Adherent Roller Bandages

The most common and convenient bandage material is the soft, self-adherent, roller bandage (Kling or Kerlix). It has limited stretch and resists unraveling as it is rolled over itself. It conforms well to body contours and is quick and easy to use. This bandage is most appropriate for injuries located where it can be wrapped circumferentially. It comes in rolls from 1 to 6 inches wide.

Gauze Bandages

Like soft, self-adherent bandages, gauze bandages are a convenient material for securing dressings. They do not stretch, however, and thus do not conform as well to body contours as the self-adherent material, but they are otherwise functional for bandaging. Since gauze bandages do not stretch, they

CONTENT REVIEW

► Types of Bandaging and Dressing Materials

Dressings

- Sterile/nonsterile
- Occlusive/nonocclusive
- Adherent/nonadherent
- Absorbent/nonabsorbent
- Wet/dry
- Hemostatic

Bandages

- Self-adherent roller
- Gauze
- Adhesive
- Elastic
- Triangular

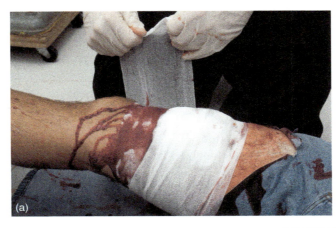

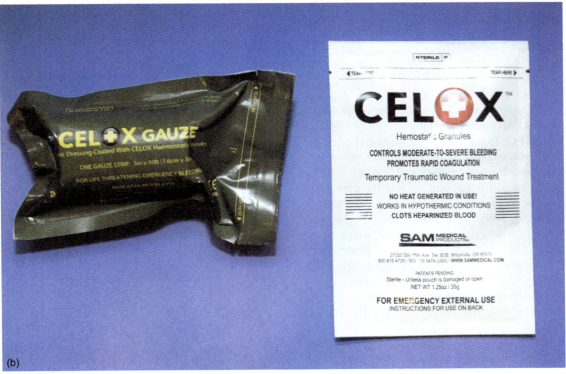

● **Figure 17**   (a) A hemostatic dressing applied to a large wound. (b) Hemostatic agents are available as dressings or granules. *(Photo b: Dr. Bryan E. Bledsoe)*

may increase the pressure associated with tissue swelling at injury sites. Gauze usually comes in rolls from 1/2 to 2 inches wide.

Adhesive Bandages

An adhesive bandage (or adhesive tape) is a strong plastic, paper, or fabric material with adhesive applied to one side. It can effectively secure a small dressing to a location where circumferential wrapping is impractical. When used circumferentially, an adhesive bandage does not allow for any swelling and permits pressure to accumulate in tissues beneath it. Adhesive bandages usually come in widths that range from 1/4 to 3 inches.

Elastic (or Ace) Bandages

Elastic bandages stretch easily and conform to body contours. Elastic bandages provide stability and support for minor musculoskeletal injuries, but they are not commonly used in prehospital care. When you do use these bandages, however, remember that it is very easy to apply too much pressure with them. Each consecutive wrap applied will contain and add to pressure on the wound site. Swelling associated with the wound may increase the pressure until blood flow through and out of the affected limb is reduced or stopped.

Triangular Bandages

Triangular bandages, or cravats, are large triangles of cotton or linen fabric. They are strong, nonelastic bandages commonly used to make slings and swathes and, in some cases, to affix splints. They can also be used to hold dressings in place, but they do not conform as well to body contours as soft, self-adherent bandages and do not maintain pressure or immobilize wound dressings very well.

ASSESSMENT OF SOFT-TISSUE INJURIES

Careful observation of the skin is an essential element of trauma assessment, as any trauma must pass through the skin to cause any deeper injury. Not only is the skin the first body organ to experience the effects of trauma, but it is the first and often the only organ to display them. Therefore, assessment of the skin and its injury must be deliberate, careful, and complete. While the processes that cause soft-tissue injuries and the manifestations of those injuries vary, prehospital assessment is a simple, well-structured process. Follow the assessment process carefully and completely to ensure that you establish the nature and extent of each injury. Doing so enables you to assign soft-tissue injuries, and other injuries associated with them, the appropriate priorities for care.

Assessment of patients with soft-tissue wounds follows the same general progression as the assessment of other trauma patients. First, size up the scene, ruling out potential hazards; identify the mechanism of injury; identify any environmental conditions that will affect extrication, assessment, patient packaging, patient care, and transport; determine the need for additional medical and rescue resources; and integrate with scene oversight (incident command). Next, perform a quick primary assessment

and identify and care for any immediately life-threatening injuries. For the patient with a mechanism of injury or signs and symptoms that suggest serious trauma, you will perform a rapid trauma assessment and use trauma triage criteria to determine the need for rapid transport. For a patient with no significant mechanism of injury and no indication from the primary assessment of a serious injury or life threat, perform a focused trauma assessment and gather vital signs and patient history at the scene. Perform a detailed physical exam only if conditions warrant and time permits. Provide serial reassessments to track your patient's response to his injuries and your care.

Scene Size-Up

During the scene size-up, look for evidence that will help you determine the mechanism of injury and anticipate the likely injuries and their severity. While soft-tissue injuries are not usually life threatening, they can suggest other, serious life threats. Remember: No trauma mechanism can impact the human body without first traveling through the skin. Identify where injury is likely and be prepared to carefully examine the skin for evidence that suggests internal injury. Consider mechanisms of injury that could cause entrapment and either crush injury or crush syndrome.

Be alert because any mechanisms that injured your patient may still be present and pose threats to you and other rescuers. Rule out or eliminate any hazards to yourself or fellow care providers before entering the scene (Figure 18 ●).

Because trauma that penetrates the skin is likely to expose you to the hazards of contact with a patient's body fluids, don

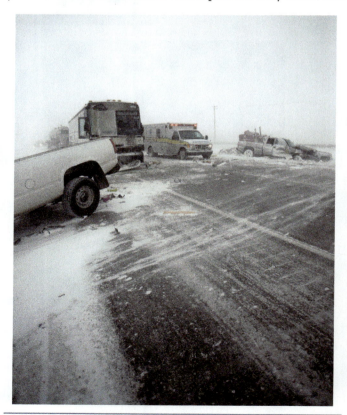

● **Figure 18** During the scene size-up, rule out hazards, don gloves, and analyze the mechanism of injury. (© *Kevin Link*)

clean gloves and observe other Standard Precautions as you approach the patient. Recognize that arterial bleeding and hemorrhage associated with the airway can cause blood to splatter at the scene. If you suspect these injuries, don splash protection for your eyes, mucous membranes, and skin.

Primary Assessment

Begin your primary assessment by forming a general patient impression and establishing manual cervical in-line immobilization—if you suspect significant head or spine injury. Determine the patient's level of consciousness and assess the airway, breathing, and circulation. Assess perfusion by noting skin color, temperature, and condition and by assessing capillary refill.

During this assessment, pay particular attention to the location and types of visible wounds to gain further understanding of the mechanism of injury and whether it produced blunt or penetrating trauma. If responsive, the patient may be able to give you critical information about how the wound occurred. If the patient is unable to speak, first responders or bystanders may be able to provide this information. Correct any immediate threats to the patient's life as you discover them. And, prioritize them for care and transport.

Secondary Assessment

Use the information you have gathered through the primary assessment to determine how to proceed in the secondary assessment process. Patients with serious trauma, suggested by a significant mechanism of injury or the findings of the primary assessment, will receive a rapid trauma assessment. All other patients will receive a focused trauma assessment.

Significant Mechanism of Injury—Rapid Trauma Assessment

In the rapid trauma assessment, you will perform a swift evaluation of the patient's head, neck, chest, abdomen, pelvis, extremities, and posterior body. Examine these areas for signs of internal or life-endangering injuries. Quickly investigate any discolorations, deformities, temperature variations, abnormal muscle tone, or open wounds.

Ensure any wounds you discover, or injuries suggested beneath them, do not involve or endanger the airway or breathing or contribute significantly to blood loss. Focus your immediate care during the rapid trauma assessment on continuing to support the patient's airway and breathing and then on controlling severe blood loss.

Inspect and palpate areas where the mechanism of injury suggests serious injuries may exist. Again, look for discoloration, temperature variation, abnormal muscle tone, and deformity suggestive of trauma (Figure 19 ●). If the mechanism of injury suggests open wounds, sweep body areas hidden from sight with gloved hands; this will rule out the possibility of unseen blood loss and pooling. Control moderate to severe hemorrhage immediately. Hemorrhage control need not be definitive, but should stop continuing significant blood loss. Once more serious injuries are cared for, you can return and dress and bandage wounds more carefully.

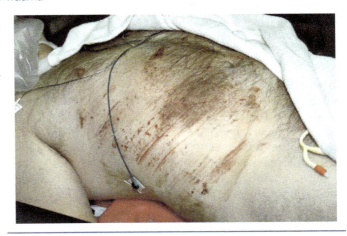

● **Figure 19** Often the only signs of serious internal injury are external soft-tissue injuries. (© *Edward T. Dickinson, MD*)

Survey all bleeding wounds to determine the type of hemorrhage—arterial, venous, or capillary. Attempt to approximate the relative rate of blood lost since the time of the incident.

Carry out your exam using the methods described in "Assessment Techniques" later in this chapter. Apply a cervical spinal immobilization collar once you have completed the rapid assessment of the head and neck. Continue to provide manual immobilization, however, until the patient is fully immobilized to a backboard, rigid orthopedic stretcher, or vacuum mattress.

When the rapid trauma assessment is complete, obtain a set of baseline vital signs, Glasgow Coma Scale score, and a patient history. Be sure to maintain manual in-line immobilization while the signs and history are being gathered. If you have enough personnel, the vital signs, Glasgow Coma Scale score, and history may be obtained simultaneously as the rapid trauma assessment is performed.

When obtaining the history, be sure to question the patient about medications, especially those that may have some direct relevance to soft-tissue injuries. For example, the patient's tetanus history is important with any trauma that breaks the skin. Determine if the patient has had a tetanus booster and how long ago it was given. Note that a patient's routine use of aspirin, clopidogrel, or blood thinners—for example, heparin or warfarin for stroke or MI risk—may impact the body's ability to halt even minimal hemorrhage. Ask about anti-inflammatory medication use, such as prednisone, because those medications reduce the inflammatory response and slow the normal healing process. Question the patient about any preexisting diseases. Note that certain diseases, especially AIDS and hemophilia, increase the risks of infection and the problems of hemorrhage control.

At the conclusion of the rapid trauma assessment, confirm the decision either to transport the patient immediately with further care provided en route to the hospital or to remain at the scene and complete treatment of non-life-threatening injuries. Consider the rate and volume of any blood loss and any uncontrollable bleeding in this decision.

If your patient's condition merits care at the scene, prioritize the soft-tissue wounds you have identified to establish an order of care to follow. The few moments taken to sort out injuries and to plan the management process save valuable time in the field. They also ensure that you provide early care for injuries with the highest priority.

No Significant Mechanism of Injury— Focused Trauma Assessment

When a patient has a soft-tissue injury but neither a significant mechanism of injury nor an indication of a serious problem from the primary assessment—for example, a cut finger or a knee abrasion from a fall—the sequence of assessment steps is different than for a patient with a significant injury mechanism. Begin this phase of the assessment with a focused trauma assessment, which is an exam directed at the injury site—the finger or the knee in the examples previously noted. A full head-to-toe rapid trauma assessment is not necessary in most such cases.

Direct the focused trauma assessment at the chief complaint and any area of injury suggested by the mechanism of injury. Use the examination techniques of inquiry, inspection, and palpation (described in the following sections) to evaluate the injury and the surrounding area. In the case of a wound to an extremity, be sure to check the distal extremity for pulses, capillary refill, color, and temperature. Then, obtain a set of baseline vital signs and a history from the patient. If any of your findings suggest the patient has more serious injuries, perform a rapid trauma assessment and consider rapid transport.

Depending on the nature of the injury, you may decide to provide transport or to refer/release the patient. If you are treating an isolated injury such as a cut finger, your system's protocols may prescribe whether you may release/refer the patient or transport the patient. Increasingly, EMS systems are employing release/referral protocols to improve system efficiency. If you do transport, provide ongoing assessment.

Detailed Physical Exam

Once the rapid or focused trauma assessment has been completed, vital signs and history have been gathered, and necessary emergency care steps have been taken, you may perform a detailed physical exam. Like the rapid trauma assessment, this head-to-toe evaluation of the skin (and the rest of the body) involves the techniques of inquiry, observation, and palpation. The detailed exam should follow a planned and comprehensive process, ideally progressing from head to toe although the order is not critical. The main purpose of the detailed assessment is to pick up any additional information regarding the patient's condition and to search for any unsuspected or subtle injuries. Manage any additional injuries you discover during the examination. The detailed physical exam is usually performed during transport or on scene if transport has been delayed. Never delay transport to perform it, and only perform it if the patient's condition permits.

Assessment Techniques

The assessment techniques that follow can be used during both the rapid trauma assessment and the detailed physical exam.

Inquiry

Question the patient about the mechanism of injury, any pain, pain on touch or movement, and any loss of function or unusual sensation specific to an area. Additionally, attempt to determine the exact nature of the pain or sensory or motor loss by using elements of the OPQRST mnemonic . Question the patient about signs and symptoms before touching an area.

Inspection

Continue the exam by carefully observing a particular body region. Identify any discolorations, deformities, or open wounds in those regions.

Determine if any discoloration is local, distal, or systemic, reflecting local injury, circulation compromise, or systemic complications such as shock. Contusions, blood vessel injuries, dislocations, and fractures may cause local discoloration, including erythema or ecchymosis. Distal discoloration may present as a pale, cyanotic, or ashen-colored limb distal to the point of circulation loss. You may also notice systemic discoloration, such as pale, ashen, or grayish skin in all limbs, suggestive of hypovolemia and shock.

Examine any deformities you find to determine their cause. Is the deformity due to a developing hematoma, to the normal swelling associated with the inflammatory process, or to underlying injuries?

Inspect any wounds you discover in detail. Study the wound to determine its depth and evaluate its potential for damage to underlying muscles, nerves, blood vessels, organs, or bones. If possible, identify the object that caused the wound and determine the amount of force transmitted by it to the body's interior. Ascertain if there are any foreign bodies, contamination, or impaled objects in the wound. Finally, identify the nature and location of any hemorrhage.

Observe each wound carefully so you can describe it to the attending physician after you dress and bandage the injury. This information will help the emergency department staff prioritize the patient's injuries. Careful observation will also aid you in preparation of your prehospital care report. Adequate lighting is crucial for evaluating wounds. If necessary, defer this portion of the detailed physical exam until better lighting is available, as in the back of the ambulance.

If a patient's limb or digit has been amputated, have other rescuers conduct a brief but thorough search for the amputated part. If the part cannot be located immediately or remains entrapped, do not delay transport. Instead, leave someone at the scene to continue the search. Ensure that once the body part is retrieved, it is properly handled, packaged, and brought to the same hospital as the patient.

Palpation

In addition to questioning the patient and inspecting the body regions, you should palpate the body's entire surface. Be alert for any deformity, asymmetry, temperature variation, unexpected mass, or localized loss of skin or muscle tone. Gently palpate all apparent closed wounds for evidence of tenderness, swelling, crepitus, and subcutaneous emphysema. Avoid palpating the interior of open wounds, which may introduce contamination and disturb the clotting process. Ascertain the presence or absence of distal pulses and capillary refill time with any extremity injury. Also, check motor and sensory function distal to any extremity wound and compare findings with those from the opposite limb.

Reassessment

During transport, provide periodic reassessments, reexamining the patient's mental status, airway, breathing, and circulation; gathering additional sets of vital signs; and evaluating the sites of the patient's injuries. Also inspect any interventions you have performed. Provide a reassessment at least every 5 minutes with unstable patients and every 15 minutes with stable patients. If you note any change in the patient's condition, modify your priorities for transport and care accordingly.

MANAGEMENT OF SOFT-TISSUE INJURIES

Once you complete your patient assessment, take steps to manage the soft-tissue injury, either in the field or en route to the hospital. Control of blood loss, prevention of shock, and decontamination of affected areas take priority. The following sections describe some of the most important of these care steps.

Unless you note extensive bleeding, wound management by dressing and bandaging is a late priority in the care of trauma patients. Dress and bandage wounds whose bleeding does not represent a life threat only after you stabilize your patient by caring for higher priority injuries.

Objectives of Wound Dressing and Bandaging

The dressing and bandaging of a wound has three basic objectives. These are to control all hemorrhaging, to keep the wound as clean as possible, and to immobilize the wound. The appearance of the final dressing and bandage is not as critical as the achievement of these three objectives.

Hemorrhage Control

The primary method of controlling hemorrhage associated with soft-tissue injury—and the most effective one—is direct pressure. In cases of serious hemorrhage flowing from a wound with some force, place a small dressing directly over the site of the bleeding and apply pressure directly to it with a finger. If this does not immediately halt the hemorrhage, consider the use of a tourniquet. When the bleeding is the more commonly encountered slow-to-moderate type, use a dressing that has been sized to cover and pad the wound. Then simply wrap the dressing with a soft, self-adherent bandage using moderate pressure to hold the dressing in place and halt the blood loss. Monitor the wound frequently to ensure bleeding has stopped.

Occasionally, bleeding from a soft-tissue injury can be difficult to control. If the bleeding continues despite the use of direct pressure, reassess the wound to be sure you are applying direct pressure to the bleeding site. If your dressing and bandage do not, then reapply direct digital pressure to the precise bleeding point. Often, hemorrhage continues because the bandaging technique distributes pressure over the entire wound site rather than focusing it directly on the bleeding source. The force driving hemorrhage is no greater than the patient's systolic blood pressure, and properly applied digital pressure can exceed this to compress the vessel and halt any blood loss.

In certain circumstances, direct pressure may not control hemorrhage. Crush injuries, amputations, and some penetrating trauma are situations in which normal bleeding control measures may be ineffective. With these traumatic injuries, several blood vessels are jaggedly torn, confounding the body's normal hemorrhage control mechanisms and making it difficult to pinpoint the bleeding source. Even if the source of bleeding can be found, applying firm direct pressure to it may be difficult. In such cases, apply a tourniquet immediately, usually above either the knee or the elbow. A tourniquet applied for the leg or forearm may not be able to control blood flow through arteries that travel between the two bones of a distal extremity. If properly applied, the tourniquet will stop the flow of life-threatening hemorrhage; however, its use has serious associated risks.[4] Keep the following precautions in mind whenever you consider using a tourniquet.

1. If the pressure applied is insufficient, the tourniquet may halt venous return while permitting continued arterial blood flow into the extremity, increasing the rate and volume of blood loss.

2. When the tourniquet is applied properly, the entire limb distal to the device is without circulation. Hypoxia, ischemia, and necrosis may permanently damage the tissue distal to the tourniquet.

3. A tourniquet should be tightened only enough to halt the blood flow. Overtightening may result in crush injury to the body part directly beneath the tourniquet.

4. When circulation is restored, the blood flows and pools in the extremity, adding to any hypovolemia. In addition, any blood that returns to the central circulation is highly hypoxic, acidic, and toxic. This blood can cause shock, lethal arrhythmias, renal failure, and death. The return of circulation may also restart hemorrhage and introduce emboli into the central circulation.

Use a tourniquet when you cannot otherwise control severe bleeding quickly. Place it just proximal to the wound site, but stay well above the elbow or knee joints (Figure 20 ●). Apply the tourniquet in a way that will not injure the tissue

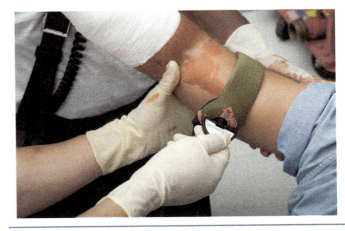

● **Figure 20**   Application of a commercial tourniquet.

143

beneath. For example, do not use very narrow material, like rope or wire, for a tourniquet; applying great pressure to a limb with such material may cause serious injury in the compressed tissue. Instead, select a 2-inch or wider band for compression.

Commercial tourniquets now available are very effective in hemorrhage control, easy to apply, and their design reduces any chance of associated injury. If a commercial tourniquet is not at hand, a readily available tourniquet is the sphygmomanometer (regular for the upper extremity and thigh for the lower). It is wide, simple to apply, rapid to inflate, and easy to monitor. Inflate it to a pressure 20 to 30 mmHg above the patient's systolic blood pressure and beyond the pressure at which the patient's hemorrhage ceases. Once applied—because sphygmomanometers tend to leak air—it is essential to record the initial pressure within the cuff and monitor it frequently to ensure the pressure does not diminish.

Once you apply a tourniquet, leave it in place until the patient arrives at the emergency department. Monitor the tourniquet during transport to ensure that it does not lose pressure, and watch for signs of renewed bleeding. If bleeding starts again, increase the tourniquet pressure. Alert the hospital staff to your use of the tourniquet during transport as well as on arrival. Make sure the receiving physician is aware that a tourniquet has been applied.

In general, a tourniquet is released only when the patient arrives at a facility with blood transfusion and surgical capability.[4] Do not release a tourniquet in the field except under exceptional circumstances and then only during consultation with medical direction. Be prepared to provide vigorous fluid resuscitation, ECG monitoring, arrhythmia treatment, and rapid transport if a tourniquet release is attempted.

Cleanliness

Once you halt severe bleeding, keep the wound as clean as possible. Under field conditions, sterility is impossible but any contamination makes healing more difficult. With very small open wounds, like an IV start or a small laceration, you may consider the application of an antibacterial ointment to help with infection control. However, the effectiveness of such ointments on larger wounds is limited, and ointments are not generally applied to these wounds.

Under normal conditions, you need not cleanse the wound. If a wound is grossly contaminated and there is a longer transport time, consider irrigating it with normal saline solution. A 1,000-mL bag of saline, connected to a macrodrip administration set and pressurized by squeezing the bag under your arm, may allow rapid and gentle wound cleansing. Try to move any contamination from the center of the wound outward. You may also carefully remove larger particles—glass, gravel, debris, and so forth—if you can do this swiftly and without inducing further injury.

Apply a bandage to make the dressing appear as neat as time and the conditions under which you are working will allow. Often, this is as easy as covering the entire dressing with wraps of soft, self-adherent roller bandage. The neat appearance calms and reassures the patient, while the bandaging reduces contamination and the chances of post-trauma infection.

Immobilization

The final objective of bandaging is immobilization. Stability of the wound site helps the natural clotting mechanisms operate and reduces patient discomfort. This is especially true of wounds in or near a joint where motion is most likely to cause the wound to gape, dislodge clots, and bleed more profusely.

Maintaining gentle pressure with the bandage may reduce pain and local swelling as well. Immobilize the limb with bandaging material to the patient's body or to a rigid surface such as a padded board or ladder splint. When immobilizing a limb, do not use elastic bandaging material or apply the bandage too tightly. The edema that develops rapidly with an injury puts increasing pressure on underlying tissue. This pressure may quickly reduce or halt circulation. (See more about controlling pain and edema in the next section.)

Frequently monitor any limb that you bandage circumferentially to ensure that the distal pulse and capillary refill remain adequate and that the distal extremity maintains good color and does not swell. If you cannot locate the distal pulse, monitor capillary refill, skin color, and temperature. If signs or symptoms suggest that the distal circulation is compromised, elevate the extremity, if possible, and consider loosening or reapplying the bandage.

Pain and Edema Control

Treat painful soft-tissue injuries or those likely to cause large debilitating edema with the application of cold packs and moderate-pressure bandages. Cold reduces inflammatory response and local edema. It also dulls the pain associated with soft-tissue trauma. Use a commercial cold pack or ice in a plastic bag wrapped in a dry towel and apply it to the wound. Do not use a cold pack directly against the skin as it cools beyond any therapeutic value. Direct application of a cold pack may also cause tissue freezing, especially in areas with reduced circulation. A mnemonic used by sports medicine (regarding blunt muscle injury)—RICE—stands for Rest, Ice, Compression, and Elevation. Mild compression reduces the edema associated with injury while elevation enhances venous return and also reduced edema.

Gentle pressure over the wound area may also help reduce pain and wound edema.[3] In cases where the patient reports severe pain, consider use of morphine sulfate, fentanyl, or other analgesics for patient comfort. Avoid aspirin or NSAIDs (e.g., ibuprofen [Motrin, Advil], naproxen [Aleve]) as they may reduce clotting.

Anatomic Considerations for Bandaging

Each area of the body has specific anatomic characteristics. Your application of bandages and dressings should take these characteristics into account to provide effective prehospital wound care.

Scalp

The scalp has a rich supply of vessels that can bleed heavily when injured. It's commonly said that head wounds rarely account for shock, but scalp hemorrhage can be severe and difficult to control and can lead to the loss of moderate to large volumes of blood.

In scalp hemorrhage uncomplicated by skull fracture, direct pressure against the skull is effective in the control of bleeding. To hold a dressing in place and maintain pressure, wrap a bandage around the head, capturing the occiput or brow or, in some cases, passing the bandage under the chin (while still allowing for jaw movement and mouth opening).

If a head wound is complicated by fracture, be very careful in your application of pressure. Apply gentle digital pressure around the wound and attempt to locate the small scalp arteries that feed it to use as pressure points. Then simply hold a dressing on the wound without much pressure.

Face

Facial wounds are frequently gruesome and bleed heavily. Gentle direct pressure to these wounds can effectively control hemorrhage. You can maintain this pressure by wrapping a bandage around the head. Be careful to ensure a clear airway and use your bandaging to splint any facial instability.

Remember, blood is a gastric irritant and swallowed blood may induce emesis. Be ready to provide suctioning in patients with oral or nasal hemorrhage because unexpected emesis may compromise the airway.

Ear or Mastoid

Wounds to the ear region can be easily bandaged by wrapping the head circumferentially. Use open gauze to collect, not stop, any bleeding or fluids flowing from the ear canal. These materials may contain cerebrospinal fluid, and halting their flow may add to any increasing intracranial pressure.

Neck

Minor neck wounds may be taped to hold dressings in place. If bleeding is moderate to severe, however, direct manual pressure may be necessary because the amount of pressure applied by circumferential wrapping may compromise both the airway and circulation to and from the head. If the wound is to the side of the neck, consider wrapping bandage material around the side of the neck and through the opposite axilla to hold the dressing in place. In cases of large wounds or moderate to severe bleeding, also consider using an occlusive dressing to prevent aspiration of air into a jugular vein. In any neck wound, careful monitoring of the airway is required as continued bleeding, tissue swelling, or hematoma formation may all obstruct the airway.

Shoulder

The shoulder is an easy area to bandage as soft, self-adherent roller bandages readily conform to body contours. Use the axilla, arm, and neck as points of fixation, but be careful not to put pressure on the anterior neck and trachea.

Trunk

For minor trunk wounds, adhesive tape may be sufficient to hold dressings in place. With larger wounds, bandaging can be more difficult because you must wrap the patient's body

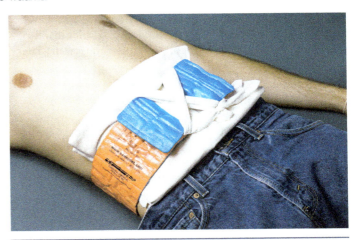

● **Figure 21** Using a formable SAM splint as an anchor may help in circumferential bandaging of a wound to the trunk.

circumferentially to apply direct pressure to a wound. Be aware that applying a circumferential bandage to the thorax may impede the normal chest wall excursion during breathing. Monitor the respiratory rate and depth and the pulse oximeter in such cases. Applying a bandage circumferentially may also require moving the patient and risk causing or worsening an injury. Consider instead using a formable splint that is negotiated beneath the patient's torso and molded to the patient's torso to serve as an anchor for bandaging (Figure 21 ●).

Groin and Hip

The groin and the hip are easy places to affix a dressing. Bandage by following the contours of the upper thighs and waist, similar to the technique of bandaging a shoulder. Be careful here, though. Any patient movement is likely to affect bandage tightness and the amount of pressure over the dressing. With these injuries, therefore, bandage after the patient is in the final position for transport.

Elbow and Knee

Joints, especially the elbow and knee, are difficult to bandage. Bandage using circumferential wraps and then splint the area to ensure that the bandage does not loosen with movement. If possible, place the joint in a position halfway between flexion and extension. This position, called the position of function, relaxes the muscles controlling the joint and the skin tension lines, and is most comfortable for the patient during long transports or periods of immobilization.

Hand and Finger

Hand and finger injuries are easy to bandage by simple circumferential wrapping. Again, consider placing the hand or digit in the position of function, halfway between flexion and extension. Accomplish this by placing a large, bulky dressing in the palm of the patient's hand and then wrapping around it. You may use a malleable finger splint to obtain the position of function and then wrap circumferentially to splint the finger.

If possible, before bandaging, carefully remove any jewelry from the wrist and fingers, as swelling may restrict distal circulation and also make it difficult to remove the jewelry later.

Ankle and Foot

Ankle and foot wounds are also easy to bandage by wrapping circumferentially and by using the natural body contours. If strong direct pressure is needed to maintain hemorrhage control, start your wrapping from the toes and work proximally. This ensures that the bandaging pressure does not form a venous tourniquet and compromise circulation to this very distal injury.

Complications of Bandaging

Bandaging can lead to some complications, although such occurrences are infrequent. If a bandage—particularly a circumferential bandage—is too tight, the area beneath it may continue to swell, increasing pressure in the wound area. This can lead to decreased blood flow and ischemia distal to the bandage. Pressure can build to such an extreme that the bandage acts like a tourniquet. Pain, pallor, tingling, a loss of pulses, and prolonged capillary refill time are typical signs of developing pressure and ischemia. Avoid this complication by making bandages snug but not too tight. A useful technique is to wrap a bandage only so tight that one finger can still be easily slipped beneath it.

Bandages and dressings left on too long can become soaked with blood and body fluids and then serve as incubators for infection. This problem usually takes at least two to three days to develop and is not a common concern in most prehospital settings.

The size of the dressing is an important consideration in bandaging. An unnecessarily large and bulky dressing can prevent proper inspection of a wound and hide contamination and continued serious bleeding. Too small a dressing can become lost in a wound and become, in effect, a foreign body. This is most frequently a problem with large, gaping wounds and deep wounds that penetrate the thoracic or abdominal body cavities. When dressing a wound, choose a dressing just larger than the wound yet not so small as to become lost in it.

Care of Specific Wounds

Some circumstances—amputations, impaled objects, and crush syndrome cases—deserve special attention during the patient management process. These injuries can challenge even the seasoned paramedic to provide the most appropriate care.

Amputations

Amputations may bleed either heavily or minimally. Attempt to control hemorrhage with direct pressure by applying a large, bulky dressing to the wound. If this fails to control hemorrhage, consider using a tourniquet just above the point of severance, above the elbow or knee joint if appropriate. If there is a crushing wound associated with the limb loss, apply the tourniquet just above the crushed area. Do not delay patient transport while locating or extricating the amputated body part. Transport the patient immediately, and then have other personnel transport the part once it is located or released from entrapment.

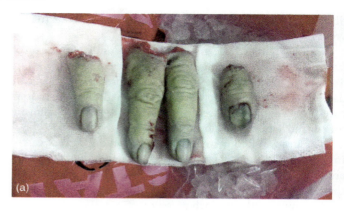

(a)

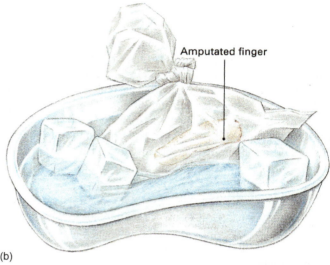

Amputated finger

(b)

● **Figure 22**   (a) Amputated parts should be cooled without direct contact between ice and the amputated part. (b) For transport, put the amputated part in a dry, sealed bag and place it in cool water that contains a few ice cubes. (*Photo a: © Dr. John P. Brosious*)

Current recommendations for managing separated body parts include moist cooling (Figure 22a ●) and rapid transport. For transport, place the amputated part in a plastic bag with the part wrapped in gauze moistened with lactated Ringer's solution or normal saline, and immerse the bag in cold water (Figure 22b ●). The water may have a few ice cubes in it, but avoid direct contact between the ice and the amputated part. Even if the amputated part cannot be totally reattached, skin from it may be used to cover the limb end (Figure 23 ●).

Impaled Objects

When possible, immobilize all impaled objects in place. You may position bulky dressings around the object to stabilize it, and tape over the dressings to hold them in place. Try to make patient movement to the ambulance and transport to the emergency department as smooth and non-jarring as possible. Remember that any movement of an impaled object is likely to cause continued internal bleeding and additional tissue damage.

If the impaled object is too large to transport or is affixed to something that cannot be moved, such as a reinforcing rod set in concrete, consider cutting it. Use appropriate techniques

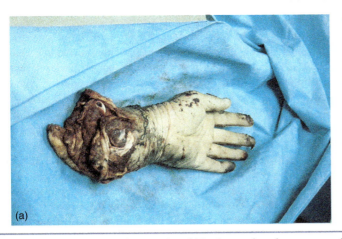
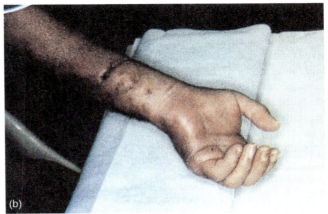

● **Figure 23** Amputated parts should be located and transported with the patient to the hospital for possible replantation. (a) An amputated hand. (b) A successfully replanted hand. *(Both: Dr. Bryan E. Bledsoe)*

and tools depending on the circumstances of the impalement. A hand or power saw, an acetylene torch, or bolt cutters might be employed. Whatever tools and techniques are used, be sure to take steps to limit the heat, vibration, or jolting transmitted to the patient. Provide the best possible support for both the object and the patient during the cutting procedure.

There are some special circumstances in which you *should* remove an impaled object. For example, you may remove an object impaled in the cheek if removal is necessary to maintain a patent airway. In this case, be prepared to apply direct pressure to the wound both from inside the cheek (intraorally) and externally.

Another object that would require removal is one impaled in the central chest of a patient who needs CPR. In such a circumstance, the risk associated with not performing resuscitation outweighs the risk of removing the object. Be aware, however, that a trauma patient who needs CPR has a very poor prognosis.

Another complication associated with an impaled object occurs when a patient is impaled on an object that cannot be cut or moved. In such a case, contact medical direction for advice and guidance. If the object is impaled in a limb, bleeding may be controllable. If it has entered the head, neck, chest, or abdomen, it may not be.

Crush Syndrome

The key to successful prehospital management of a crush syndrome patient is anticipation of the problem and prevention of its effects. Since, by definition, all crush syndrome patients are victims of prolonged entrapment, cases can be identified before extrication is complete. The focus of prehospital crush injury care is on rapid transport, adequate fluid resuscitation, diuresis, and—possibly—systemic alkalinization.

The prehospital approach to crush syndrome is similar to that with other trauma patients. Ensuring scene safety is particularly important in these cases. Crush syndrome victims are often buried in heavy rubble or other large debris, and access may be difficult. You may need to request the assistance of specialized personnel and their equipment—urban search and rescue

teams, or trench, heavy, or confined space rescue teams. Never place yourself or other rescuers in unreasonable danger when providing care or attempting a rescue.

Once the scene is safe and you can reach the patient, conduct a primary assessment. Remove debris from around the head, neck, and thorax to minimize airway obstruction and restriction of ventilation. Control any reachable and obvious bleeding. Perform as much of the primary and rapid trauma assessment as possible, keeping in mind that portions of the patient's body will be inaccessible as a result of the entrapment. The dark, dusty, and cramped conditions of many confined space rescues may force you to improvise. Be alert for signs and symptoms of associated injuries such as dust inhalation, dehydration, and hypothermia.

Remember that the greater the body area compressed and the longer the time of entrapment, the greater the risk of crush syndrome. Initially, a trapped patient will complain only of entrapment symptoms: pain, lack of motor function, tingling, or loss of sensation in the affected limb. The patient may also experience flaccid paralysis and sensory loss in the limb unrelated to the normal distribution of peripheral nerve control and sensation.

As long as the body part is still trapped and the metabolic by-products of the crush injury are confined to the entrapped part, the patient will not experience the full effects of crush syndrome. With extrication, however, toxic by-products are released into the circulation, and the patient may rapidly develop shock and die. If the patient survives the initial release of the by-products, he remains at great risk of developing renal failure with serious morbidity or delayed death. Note, too, that a crush injury may also induce compartment syndrome (explained later), especially with prolonged entrapment.

Once you have ensured the patient's ABCs (airway, breathing, circulation), turn your attention to obtaining IV access. Intravenous fluids and selected medications are important in treating crush syndrome. Initiate a large-bore IV if possible. Because of the entrapment, it may be necessary to consider alternative IV sites such as the external jugular vein, sternal or humoral (IO), or the veins of a lower extremity. Avoid any site distal to a crush injury.

When you encounter crush syndrome, it is unlikely that your protocols will address it. Contact the trauma center for medical direction and communicate, on-line, with the emergency physician. Expect to provide frequent vital sign and patient updates, and be prepared to administer large fluid volumes and, possibly, alkalizing agents.

Alkalinization of the blood and urine is a consideration for preventing and treating crush syndrome. In combination with fluid resuscitation, alkalinization can correct acidosis, help prevent renal failure, and help correct hyperkalemia. Administer sodium bicarbonate 1 mEq/kg initially, followed by 0.25 mEq/kg/hr thereafter.

Diuretics may help keep the kidneys well perfused and more resistant to failure during crush syndrome. Mannitol, an osmotic diuretic, is the drug of choice because it draws interstitial fluid into the vascular space and eliminates it as mannitol is excreted by the kidneys. Furosemide, a loop diuretic, inhibits the reabsorption of both sodium and chloride. Its use is not advisable in hypovolemic states because it may add to the electrolyte imbalance and volume loss.

Consider applying a tourniquet before the entrapping pressure is released if you have been unable to medicate the patient and provide fluid resuscitation. The tourniquet will sequester the toxins and prevent reperfusion injury. Tourniquet use, however, will continue crush injury development and worsen its effects.

In cases where the entrapping object may not be moved for many hours or days, medical direction may consider field amputation. This operation will likely be performed by a physician responding to the scene but, in dire circumstances, may be performed by a paramedic under on-line direction of an emergency physician.

Cardiac (ECG) monitoring is important with all crush syndrome patients. Arrhythmias may develop at any time but are most likely to occur immediately following the release of pressure on extrication. This is because both potassium and lactate are released with the pressure release and travel with the blood to the heart. Sudden cardiac arrest should be treated in the usual fashion with defibrillation and cardiac drugs as appropriate. Consider 500 mg calcium chloride IV push (in addition to the sodium bicarbonate) to counteract life-threatening arrhythmias induced by hyperkalemia. Watch for the tenting, or peaking, of the T-wave, a prolonged P-R interval, and S-T segment depression. Severely elevated blood levels of potassium may induce a widening of the QRS complex that quickly leads to refractory ventricular fibrillation. Be sure to flush the IV line between infusions or to use different lines because calcium chloride and sodium bicarbonate precipitate.

Once the patient is freed from entrapment, be prepared to treat rapidly progressing shock. Continue the normal saline infusions at 30 mL/kg/hr and provide additional boluses of sodium bicarbonate as needed. Rapidly transport the patient to an appropriate hospital (usually a trauma center) for all cases of suspected crush syndrome.

Prehospital care of the crushed limb or body parts requires no special techniques. Cover open wounds and splint fractures, keeping in mind that progressive swelling will necessitate reassessment, with monitoring of distal circulation and the tightness of bandages, straps, and splints. Handle all crushed limbs gently because ischemic tissue is prone to injury.

Care at the hospital for crush injury is aggressive and may use techniques such as debridement and hyperbaric oxygenation. During hyperbaric oxygenation, the patient is placed in a chamber with artificially high concentrations of oxygen under several atmospheres of pressure. This drives oxygen into poorly oxygenated tissue to help with the destruction of anaerobic bacteria and to increase tissue oxygenation for repair and regeneration, ultimately reducing tissue necrosis and edema. Hyperbaric oxygenation is most effective when provided early in the course of care.

Hospital care for crush injuries also includes administration of several medications as well as hemodialysis to help salvage the kidneys from the ravages of myoglobin and other toxic agents. Allopurinol, a xanthine oxidase inhibitor, interferes with the production of uric acid, a by-product of skeletal muscle destruction, and may help reperfusion of both the kidneys and the skeletal muscles. It is most effective if administered immediately before release of the compression. Amiloride hydrochloride is a potassium-sparing diuretic that inhibits the sodium/calcium exchange. Mannitol, tetanus toxoid (if needed), and prophylactic antibiotics may also be administered in the hospital to treat crush syndrome.

Compartment Syndrome

The most prominent symptom of compartment syndrome is severe pain, often out of proportion to the physical findings. Other signs are often subtle or absent, or they may be overshadowed by the original injury such as a fracture or contusion. Some people suggest using the six Ps—pain, pallor, paralysis, paresthesia, pressure (feeling of tension within the extremity), and pulses (diminished or absent distally)—plus a seventh P sometimes cited, poikilothermia (referring to a limb that is cool to the touch). However, many of these signs are not dependable or they appear very late in the course of the injury.

Motor and sensory functions are usually normal with compartment syndrome, as are distal pulses. Even capillary refill shows little or no change. It is important to note that compartment syndrome rarely occurs within the first 4 hours after an acute injury. It is more likely to appear 6 to 8 hours (or as much as a day or more) after the initial injury. Recognition of compartment syndrome can be challenging and requires a healthy suspicion for the problem.

The first step in prehospital treatment for compartment syndrome is care of the underlying injury. Splint and immobilize all suspected fractures, and use traction as appropriate for femur fractures. Apply cold packs to severe contusions. Elevation of the affected extremity is the single most effective prehospital treatment for compartment syndrome. This reduces edema, increases venous return, lowers compartment pressure, and helps prevent ischemia. In the hospital, compartment syndrome is diagnosed by inserting a hollow needle into the affected compartment to directly obtain a pressure reading. Severe cases are treated surgically, through a procedure called a fasciotomy that incises the restrictive fascia.

Special Anatomic Sites

Several anatomic sites provide challenges to the care of soft-tissue injuries. These include the face and neck, the thorax, and the abdomen.

Face and Neck

Soft-tissue injuries to the face and neck present potential challenges owing to the anatomic relationships of the airway and great vessels. Injuries to the face may result in blood and tissue debris in the airway, posing risks of airway obstruction, asphyxia, and aspiration. Pooled secretions and tissue edema may add to airway problems. Trauma to the face or neck may also distort the anatomic structures of the upper airway, leading to airway compromise, and complicating attempts at endotracheal intubation (Figure 24 ●).

Emergency treatment of face and neck injuries can be challenging and may tax your skills. First, gain control of the airway. Open the airway using manual maneuvers. If you suspect the possibility of spinal injury, use the jaw-thrust maneuver in conjunction with in-line manual immobilization. Aggressively suction blood, saliva, and debris from the pharynx to maintain the airway, but limit the depth of suction catheter insertion to that which is necessary to maintain the airway, in order to avoid stimulating the gag reflex. Insert an oro- or nasopharyngeal airway as needed.

Direct visualization of the endotracheal tube passing through the cords is the gold standard for securing the airway, but achieving it is fraught with complications in cases of face and neck trauma. Secretions and blood may prevent adequate visualization even with aggressive suctioning. Airway edema can distort the anatomy beyond recognition, and even prevent passage of the ET tube. Extraglottic airways, such as the newer LMAs and King Airways, may be very effective when injury to the airway is noted. In all cases, meticulous and absolute confirmation of tube placement is mandatory to avoid fatal hypoxia. Continuous waveform capnography is essential to ensure initial and ongoing proper endotracheal tube placement.

In desperate circumstances, needle cricothyrotomy may be lifesaving. Avoid placing the needle through neck hematomas to avoid life-threatening bleeding.

Once you have secured the airway, focus your attention on any serious facial or neck bleeding. Direct pressure is usually successful for bleeding control, but be certain to avoid compressing or occluding the airway. A tourniquet should not be used because of the risks of cerebral ischemia and strangulation. In a similar fashion, as noted earlier, circumferential neck bandaging carries the same risk and should be meticulously monitored if used. Open neck wounds also carry the danger of air aspiration and emboli. Cover any open neck wound with an occlusive dressing, which should then be held or bandaged firmly in place. Because of the neck's anatomy, you may have to maintain digital pressure throughout the course of prehospital care to ensure effective bleeding control.

Thorax

Superficial soft-tissue injury to the thorax may suggest more serious intrathoracic injuries. The pleural space extends superiorly to the supraclavicular fossa and inferiorly to include the entire rib cage both anteriorly and posteriorly. Trauma to this area is likely to injure both the pleura and lungs. Small "lacerations" may actually be deep, penetrating stab or gunshot wounds with resultant hemothorax, pneumothorax, pericardial tamponade, penetrating heart trauma, or injury to the great vessels, esophagus, bronchi, or diaphragm. A seemingly minor "rib bruise" may be the only visible sign of serious lung or cardiac contusions beneath.

Perform a thorough physical examination to detect any signs of internal bleeding, pulmonary edema, arrhythmias, or shock. However, never explore a thoracic wound beyond the skin edges. Probing deeper can convert a minor wound to a pneumothorax or a bleeding disaster. Consider all thoracic wounds to be potentially life threatening until evidence proves otherwise.

Dress all open thoracic wounds with sterile dressings in the usual fashion. As noted earlier, if a circumferential bandage is applied to the thorax, be aware of the risk of impeding the normal chest wall excursion during breathing. Monitor the respiratory rate and depth and the pulse oximeter in such cases. Be alert for the presence of air bubbling, subcutaneous emphysema, crepitus, or other hints of open pneumothorax.

Be extremely cautious about making an airtight seal on any thoracic wound, because doing so can rapidly convert a simple pneumothorax to a tension pneumothorax and death. Instead, use an occlusive dressing sealed on three sides and be prepared to assist ventilations. Watch the occlusive dressing so that it does not seal with blood against the chest wall and convert a simple pneumothorax into a tension pneumothorax. If indicated by deteriorating vital signs, completely unseal an occlusive dressing (even one that was prepared with an opening and sealed

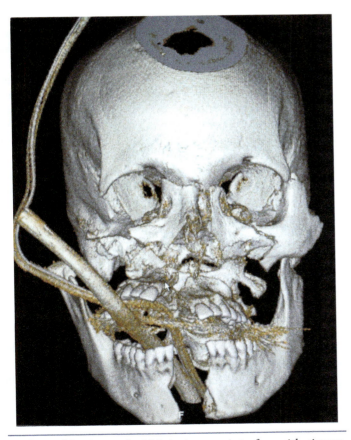

● **Figure 24** Severe facial injuries may interfere with airway control and distort landmarks used for intubation. *(© Dr. Bryan E. Bledsoe)*

on only three sides) to ensure the dressing is not contributing to the development of tension pneumothorax. Auscultate the chest and monitor vital signs frequently.

Abdomen

The peritoneal cavity extends approximately from the symphysis pubis inferiorly to the diaphragm superiorly. Since the diaphragm rises and falls with respiration, so too does the border between the abdominal and thoracic cavities. You cannot know the diaphragm's exact position at the time the injury occurred, so suspect associated injuries to both abdominal and thoracic organs if the soft-tissue injury involves the region between the rib margin and the fifth rib anteriorly, the seventh rib laterally, and the ninth rib posteriorly.

Some abdominal organs are located posterior to the peritoneum and are called retroperitoneal. These include the kidneys, ureters, adrenal glands, most of the pancreas, and the abdominal aorta and inferior vena cava. The retroperitoneal space does not restrict the blood loss as well as the peritoneal space and has a reduced pain response to free blood in this space.

Blunt or penetrating trauma to the abdomen can injure both hollow and solid organs, penetrate or rupture the diaphragm, and cause serious internal bleeding. Anteriorly and just underlying the rib margin are the liver on the right and the spleen on the left. Posteriorly, the kidneys (not true abdominal organs since they lie retroperitoneally) are located in the costovertebral angle region. Hollow organs—the bowel, stomach, and urinary bladder—may rupture. In addition to bleeding copiously, these organs may release their contents and inflame the peritoneum.

Consider any soft-tissue wound in the abdominal region as potentially damaging to the underlying organs. Signs and symptoms of internal damage can be subtle, particularly early on. Eviscerations and other massive injuries are obvious, but other internal injuries that are just as serious may not be apparent. Prehospital treatment is primarily supportive and includes ensuring adequate oxygenation, preventing shock, dressing open wounds, and rapid transport. Be aware that bulky abdominal dressings, especially if they are secured with circumferential bandages, may restrict movement of the abdominal contents during the excursion of the diaphragm. This in turn may compromise breathing. Monitor the rate and depth of breathing and the pulse oximeter in such cases.

Wounds Requiring Transport

Transport any patient with a wound that involves a structure beneath the integument for emergency department evaluation. This includes wounds involving, or possibly involving, nerves, blood vessels, ligaments, tendons, or muscles. Also transport any patient with a significantly contaminated wound, a wound involving an impaled object, or a wound that was received in a particularly unclean environment. Also, transport any patient with a wound with likely cosmetic implications, such as facial wounds or large gaping wounds.

Soft-Tissue Treatment and Refer/Release

In some EMS systems, paramedics are permitted to treat and release patients with minor and superficial soft-tissue injuries or treat and refer them to their personal physicians. This generally occurs under on-line medical direction or according to strict protocols.

In such circumstances, you must evaluate and dress the wound. Then explain to the patient the steps to follow for continuing care of the injury. Tell the patient of the need to change the dressing and to monitor the injury site for further hemorrhage or developing infection. Provide the patient with simple written instructions (approved and/or published by medical direction) explaining wound care, monitoring, protection, dressing change, cleansing, and the signs of problems such as infection or hemorrhage.

Instruct the patient to contact a physician if certain signs and symptoms appear and describe those signs and symptoms thoroughly. Ensure that the patient has the means to obtain physician or health care provider follow-up and again stress the circumstances in which such follow-up care should be sought. During any referral or release, if the patient's tetanus immunization history is unclear or it has been longer than five years since the last immunization, instruct the patient to obtain a tetanus booster as soon as possible (generally within 72 hours).

Document all refer/release incidents carefully in the prehospital care report. The report should include a description of the nature and extent of the wound and of the care provided for it. Note in the report all instructions and materials provided to the patient and any medical direction you received.

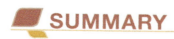

SUMMARY

Soft-tissue injury may compromise the skin—the envelope that protects and contains the human body. Any trauma must penetrate the skin before it can harm the interior organs and threaten life. Any damage to the skin may interfere with its ability to contain water and blood and to prevent damaging agents from entering. For these reasons, the assessment and care of soft-tissue injuries are important parts of prehospital care.

Assess wounds carefully since they may provide the only overt signs of serious internal injury. Realize that discoloration and swelling take time to develop and may not be as apparent in the field as when you present the patient at the emergency department. Look carefully for the early signs of wounds, and use the mechanism of injury to locate potential trauma sites. When caring for soft-tissue injuries, keep in

CHAPTER REVIEW

mind the basic goals: controlling hemorrhage, keeping the wound as clean as possible, and immobilizing the injury site. While soft-tissue injuries are not often assigned a high priority in prehospital care, they do account for a large number of patient injuries and are significant to the overall assessment and care of trauma victims.

YOU MAKE THE CALL

You arrive at the scene of a "foot injury" to find a young child lying on the lawn and surrounded by his parents. As you begin to question his father about what happened, he explains, "My son stepped on a board with a nail in it." After donning gloves, you carefully remove the boy's shoe to discover an almost invisible penetration to the sole of the foot. The child is now resting quietly, without much pain.

1. What type of wound is this and what significance does it have for infection?

2. What elements of history and specifically vaccinations will be important in assessing this patient?

3. What direction would you give this patient if his parents do not wish to have him transported to the local emergency department?

See Suggested Responses at the back of this chapter.

REVIEW QUESTIONS

1. How does the integumentary system prevent pathogens from attacking the body?
a. The skin provides a pathway out of the body for pathogens.
b. Leukocytes in the skin attack pathogens.
c. Antibodies in the skin attack and destroy pathogens.
d. The skin provides a protective barrier against pathogens.

2. Of the open wounds presenting to emergency departments, up to _____ percent will eventually become infected, resulting in significant morbidity.
a. 8
b. 6.5
c. 10
d. 15

3. Glands within the dermis that secrete sweat are called _____.
a. mast cells
b. sebaceous glands
c. sudoriferous glands
d. lymphocyte glands

4. When an artery is ruptured but the skin is not broken, blood can separate the tissues and pool in a pocket. This pocket of blood is known as a(n) _____.
a. contusion
b. abrasion
c. hematoma
d. crush injury

5. _____ are typically the most minor of injuries that violate the protective envelope of the skin.
a. Incisions
b. Avulsions
c. Abrasions
d. Lacerations

6. Specialized white blood cells capable of engulfing bacteria are _____.
a. granulocytes
b. macrophages
c. phagocytes
d. all of the above

7. The anaerobic bacterium *Clostridium perfringens* causes a deep space infection called _____.
a. gangrene
b. tetanus
c. collagen
d. lockjaw

8. You have been called to a scene where a patient has caught one of his hands between two pieces of machinery. As the hand is removed from the machinery, there is no visible injury. You should expect the internal injuries to be _____.
a. extensive
b. unimportant
c. life threatening
d. minimally significant

9. Which type of dressing is designed to be placed over a wound as a barrier to leaking?
a. adherent
b. nonabsorbent
c. absorbent
d. nonadherent

10. As you begin to bandage a soft-tissue injury, you should continue to check distal pulses to ensure proper tissue perfusion. This is primarily because the bandage may fit properly at first but later become too tight and reduce circulation as a result of the _____.
a. shrinking of the bandage
b. development of shock
c. toxins entering central circulation
d. swelling of the damaged tissue

11. When bandaging the foot and ankle to create pressure and maintain hemorrhage control, wrap in a _____.
   a. distal-to-proximal fashion to avoid forming a venous tourniquet
   b. proximal-to-distal fashion to avoid forming a venous tourniquet
   c. proximal-to-distal fashion to help maintain gentle traction
   d. distal-to-proximal fashion to help maintain gentle traction

12. When a soft-tissue injury occurs, a process to stop bleeding starts almost immediately; the vessels constrict, platelets clot, and the blood coagulates. This process is called _____.
   a. inflammation
   b. hemostasis
   c. epithelialization
   d. neovascularization

See Answers to Review Questions at the back of this chapter.

REFERENCES

1. Lieurance, R., J. B. Benjamin, and W. D. Rappaport. "Blood Loss and Transfusion in Patients with Isolated Femur Fractures." *J Orthop Trauma* 6(2) (1992): 175–179.

2. Horswell, B. B. and C. J. Chahine. "Dog Bites of the Face, Head, and Neck in Children." *W V Med J* 107(6) (Nov–Dec 2011): 24–27.

3. Jones, A. P., K. Allison, H. Wright, and K. Porter. "Use of Prehospital Dressings in Soft Tissue Trauma: Is There Any Conformity or Plan?" *Emerg Med J* 26(7) (Jul 2009): 532–534.

4. Kragh, J. F., Jr, et al. "Survival with Emergency Tourniquet Use to Stop Bleeding in Major Limb Trauma." *Ann Surg* 249(1) (Jan 2009): 1–7.

FURTHER READING

Bates, Barbara, and Peter G. Szilagyi. *A Guide to Physical Examination and History Taking.* 9th ed. Philadelphia: J. B. Lippincott, 2007.

Bledsoe, B. E., and D. Clayden. *Prehospital Emergency Pharmacology.* 7th ed. Upper Saddle River, NJ: Pearson/Prentice Hall, 2011.

Bledsoe, B. E., B. J. Colbert, and J. E. Ankney. *Essentials of A & P for Emergency Care.* Upper Saddle River, NJ: Pearson/Prentice Hall, 2010.

Martini, Frederic. *Fundamentals of Anatomy and Physiology.* 7th ed. San Francisco: Benjamin Cummings, 2011.

Rosen, P., and R. Barkin, eds. *Emergency Medicine: Concepts and Clinical Practice.* 7th ed. St. Louis: Mosby, 2009.

Tintinalli, J. E., ed. *Emergency Medicine: A Comprehensive Study Guide.* 7th ed. New York: McGraw-Hill, 2011.

Trott, A. T. *Wounds and Lacerations: Emergency Care and Closure.* 3rd ed. St. Louis, Mosby 2005.

SUGGESTED RESPONSES TO "YOU MAKE THE CALL"

The following are suggested responses to the "You Make the Call" scenarios presented in this chapter. Each represents an acceptable response to the scenario but should not be interpreted as the only correct response.

1. What type of wound is this and what significance does it have for infection?

This is a puncture wound that is vulnerable to a variety of infections. The most concerning complication would be tetanus.

2. What elements of history and specifically vaccinations will be important in assessing this patient?

Are the child's vaccinations up to date and when was his last tetanus shot?

3. What direction would you give this patient if his parents do not wish to have him transported to the local emergency department?

Depending on whether or not the patient has an updated tetanus, advise the patient to be seen by his doctor for a tetanus shot or simply watch for signs of infection, including increased pain, redness, and swelling around the injury site. Especially watch for signs of tetanus, including muscle stiffening, especially in the muscles of the face and jaw.

ANSWERS TO REVIEW QUESTIONS

1. d
2. b
3. c
4. c
5. c
6. d

7. a
8. a
9. b
10. d
11. a
12. b

 ## GLOSSARY

abrasion   scraping or abrading away of the superficial layers of the skin; an open soft-tissue injury.

amputation   severance, removal, or detachment, either partial or complete, of a body part.

avulsion   forceful tearing away or separation of body tissue; an avulsion may be partial or complete.

chemotactic factors   chemicals released by white blood cells that attract more white blood cells to an area of inflammation.

collagen   tough, strong protein that makes up most of the body's connective tissue.

compartment syndrome   muscle ischemia that is caused by rising pressures within an anatomic fascial space.

contusion   closed wound in which the skin is unbroken, although damage has occurred to the tissue immediately beneath.

crush injury   mechanism of injury in which tissue is locally compressed by high-pressure forces.

crush syndrome   systemic disorder of severe metabolic disturbances resulting from the crush of a limb or other body part.

degloving injury   avulsion in which the mechanism of injury tears the skin off the underlying muscle, tissue, blood vessels, and bone.

dermis   true skin, also called the corium; it is the layer of tissue producing the epidermis and housing the structures, blood vessels, and nerves normally associated with the skin.

ecchymosis   blue-black discoloration of the skin due to leakage of blood into the tissues.

epidermis   outermost layer of the skin composed of dead or dying cells.

epithelialization   early stage of wound healing in which epithelial cells migrate over the surface of the wound.

erythema   general reddening of the skin due to dilation of the superficial capillaries.

fascia   a fibrous membrane that covers, supports, and separates muscles and may also unite the skin with underlying tissue.

fibroblasts   specialized cells that form collagen.

gangrene   deep-space infection usually caused by the anaerobic bacterium *Clostridium perfringens*.

granulocytes   white blood cells charged with the primary purpose of neutralizing foreign bacteria.

hematoma   collection of blood beneath the skin or trapped within a body compartment.

hemostasis   the body's three-step response to local hemorrhage, comprising a vascular phase that reduces blood flow, a platelet phase in which aggregating platelets form a weak clot, and a coagulation phase that results in the formation of fibrin, creating a strong clot.

hyperemia   increased blood flow into and through injured or infected tissue, responsible for the reddish skin color, or erythema, associated with inflammation.

impaled object   foreign body embedded in a wound.

incision   very smooth or surgical laceration, frequently caused by a knife, scalpel, razor blade, or piece of glass.

inflammation   complex process of local cellular and biochemical changes as a consequence of injury or infection; an early stage of healing.

integumentary system   skin, consisting of the epidermis, dermis, and subcutaneous layers.

keloid   a formation resulting from overproduction of scar tissue.

laceration   an open wound, normally a tear with jagged borders.

lumen   opening, or space, within a needle, artery, vein, or other hollow vessel.

lymphangitis   inflammation of the lymph channels, usually as a result of a distal infection.

lymphocyte   white blood cell that specializes in humoral immunity and antibody formation.

macrophage   immune system cell that has the ability to recognize and ingest foreign pathogens.

necrosis   tissue death, usually from ischemia.

neovascularization   new growth of capillaries in response to healing.

phagocytosis   process in which a cell surrounds and absorbs a bacterium or other particle.

puncture   specific soft-tissue injury involving a deep, narrow wound to the skin and underlying organs that carries an increased danger of infection.

remodeling   stage in the wound-healing process in which collagen is broken down and relaid in an orderly fashion.

rhabdomyolysis   acute pathological process that involves the destruction of skeletal muscle.

sebaceous glands   glands within the dermis secreting sebum.

sebum   fatty secretion of the sebaceous gland that helps keep the skin pliable and waterproof.

serous fluid   a cellular component of blood, similar to plasma.

skeletal muscle   contractile tissue organized in large bundles that provides locomotion and movement for the body.

subcutaneous tissue   body layer beneath the dermis.

sudoriferous glands   glands within the dermis that secrete sweat.

tendons   long, thin, very strong collagen tissues that connect muscles to bones.

tension lines   natural patterns in the surface of the skin revealing tensions within.

tetanus   a rare wound infection caused by the bacterium *Clostridium tetani*. Also called *lockjaw*.

Orthopedic Trauma

Robert S. Porter, MA, EMT-P

STANDARD
Trauma (Orthopedic Trauma)

COMPETENCY
Integrates assessment findings with principles of epidemiology and pathophysiology to formulate a field impression to implement a comprehensive treatment/disposition plan for an acutely injured patient.

OBJECTIVES

Terminal Performance Objective
After reading this chapter you should be able to assess and manage patients with orthopedic injuries.

Enabling Objectives
To accomplish the terminal performance objective, you should be able to:

1. Define key terms introduced in this chapter.
2. Describe considerations in preventing orthopedic injuries.
3. Describe the anatomy and physiology of the musculoskeletal system.
4. Discuss the effects of aging on the musculoskeletal system.
5. Describe the pathophysiology of the following injury types:
   a. muscular
   b. joint
   c. bone
6. Describe special considerations in pediatric, geriatric, and sports-related orthopedic injuries.
7. Discuss the impact of inflammatory and degenerative conditions on the musculoskeletal system.
8. Given a variety of scenarios, demonstrate the assessment of musculoskeletal injuries.
9. Adhere to the general principles of musculoskeletal injury management.
10. Given a variety of musculoskeletal injury scenarios, select and apply an appropriate splinting device.
11. Describe special considerations in the management of fractures, joint injuries, and injuries of muscle and connective tissue.
12. Describe the special considerations in management of the following fractures:
    a. pelvis
    b. femur
    c. tibia/fibula
    d. clavicle
    e. humerus
    f. radius/ulna

13. Describe the special considerations in management of the following joint injuries:
    a. hip
    b. knee
    c. ankle
    d. foot
    e. shoulder
    f. elbow
    g. wrist/hand
    h. fingers/toes

14. Discuss considerations in pain management in the care of musculoskeletal injuries.

15. Describe considerations for patients with musculoskeletal injuries who refuse treatment or transport.

KEY TERMS

abduction	femur	osteocyte
acetabulum	fibula	osteoporosis
adduction	gout	pelvis
amphiarthroses	greenstick fracture	perforating canals
appendicular skeleton	hairline fracture	periosteum
arthritis	haversian canals	phalanges
articular surface	humerus	pubis
axial skeleton	iliac crest	radius
bursa	ilium	red bone marrow
bursitis	impacted fracture	reduction
calcaneus	innominate bone	rheumatoid arthritis
callus	insertion	scapula
cancellous	ischial tuberosity	septic arthritis
carpal bones	ischium	sesamoid bone
cartilage	joint	spasm
circumduction	joint capsule	spiral fracture
clavicle	ligaments	sprain
closed fracture	malleolus	strain
comminuted fracture	medullary canal	subluxation
cramping	metacarpal	synarthroses
devascularization	metaphysis	synovial fluid
diaphysis	metatarsal	synovial joint
diarthroses	oblique fracture	tendonitis
dislocation	olecranon	tendons
epiphyseal fracture	open fracture	tibia
epiphyseal plate	opposition	tone
epiphysis	origin	transverse fracture
fascicle	osteoarthritis	ulna
fatigue	osteoblast	yellow bone marrow
fatigue fracture	osteoclast	

CASE STUDY

The dispatch center sends Rescue 201 and its assigned paramedics, Mark and Steffany, to an adult care center for a patient who has fallen down a flight of stairs. On arrival, paramedics find the patient lying on the ground. The resident director explains that Mary Herman, a 91-year-old female resident, tripped and fell down three or four steps while walking out of the building on the way to the cafeteria. There are no scene safety issues, and after donning gloves Mark and Steffany begin the primary assessment. Mrs. Herman seems fully oriented and alert and complains of moderate pain to her right thigh and lower back. She denies any neck pain or spinal symptoms, though her mechanism of injury, age, and distracting injury suggest the need for spinal precautions. The remainder of the primary assessment reveals no significant findings, and Mrs. Herman is classified as a stable (S) patient.

The physical exam, patient history, and chief complaint investigation of the focused trauma assessment concentrate on Mrs. Herman's isolated injury. Mrs. Herman denies dizziness, nausea, or any other symptoms either now or prior to the fall. She denies striking her head or other injury symptoms. Both the patient and nursing staff report that Mrs. Herman has had few medical problems. She has no known allergies, and her medications include a daily vitamin and an aspirin. The focused physical exam evaluates the right lower extremity and finds pain and tenderness to the right thigh, crepitus, the foot externally rotated, and instability to the hip joint. Steffany performs a quick pulse, motor, and sensory check, revealing an easily palpable posterior tibial pulse, brisk capillary refill (in less than 2 seconds), good foot strength with extension and flexion, and the ability to discern touch. The same tests on the opposing extremity provide equal results.

Vital sign evaluation reveals a blood pressure of 120/90, a strong and regular pulse of 90, and respirations of normal depth at a rate of 22 per minute. Mark, the senior paramedic, applies manual spinal immobilization. The pulse oximeter shows a saturation of 97 percent, so Mark and Steffany withhold oxygen, and the ECG shows a regular sinus rhythm at 90.

Next, Mark and Steffany move Mrs. Herman to a spine board via an orthopedic stretcher. They place a folded blanket between her legs, maintain her head slightly off the board, pad under the body spaces, and, gently but firmly, strap her to the spine board. They apply a cervical immobilization device and secure the CID and Mrs. Herman's head to the spine board. Once they have loaded the patient into the ambulance, they start an intravenous line, hang a normal saline drip, and set it to run at a to-keep-open rate. The paramedics transport her uneventfully to the emergency department. There, X-rays confirm a hip fracture. Because of her age, Mrs. Herman will spend several days in the hospital and then several months in rehabilitation.

INTRODUCTION TO MUSCULOSKELETAL TRAUMA

In trauma, the incidence of musculoskeletal injury is second only to that of soft-tissue injuries. Musculoskeletal injury usually results from application of significant direct or transmitted blunt kinetic forces. Skeletal or muscular injuries may also occasionally result from penetrating mechanisms of injury. Millions of Americans sustain musculoskeletal injuries each year from a variety of sources including sports injuries, motor vehicle crashes, falls, and acts of violence. These incidents can cause a variety of injuries to the body's bones, cartilage, ligaments, muscles, or tendons.

While injuries to the upper extremities can be painful and sometimes debilitating, they rarely threaten life. Lower extremity injuries, however, are generally associated with a greater magnitude of force and greater secondary blood loss and, thus, more often constitute threats to life or limb. In addition, the same forces responsible for a musculoskeletal injury may damage the spine, internal organs, nerves, and blood vessels, causing serious problems throughout the body. In fact, most patients (up to 80 percent) who suffer multisystem trauma experience significant musculoskeletal injuries.

PREVENTION STRATEGIES

Stopping injury before it occurs—injury prevention—is the optimal way of dealing with musculoskeletal injuries. Strategies for preventing musculoskeletal injuries include application of modern vehicle and highway designs and safe driving practices, including the use of restraint systems. Auto crashes are the greatest single cause of musculoskeletal injuries, and improved vehicle safety has done much to reduce the incidence and severity of such injuries. Workplace safety standards developed by the National Institutes of Safety and Health (NIOSH) and enforced by the Occupational Safety and Health Administration (OSHA) have done much to reduce on-the-job injuries. These standards include criteria for

CONTENT REVIEW

► Functions of the Skeleton

- Gives the body structural form
- Protects vital organs
- Allows for efficient movement
- Stores salts and other materials for metabolism
- Produces red blood cells

proper footwear, scaffolding, fall-protection devices, and the like.

Sports injuries account for a significant number of traumas, which most commonly affect the musculature, joints, and long bones. While protective gear, improved equipment design, and better athlete conditioning can reduce the number of these injuries, the very nature of contact sports means that they remain a significant cause of injury. Household accidents and falls also account for many musculoskeletal injuries, and use of good safety practices—for example, proper footwear, well-designed railings, appropriate stepladder use—can reduce injury incidence at home.

In musculoskeletal injuries, severe forces are directed to the structures of the body. These forces threaten homeostasis by disrupting the tissues responsible for moving the body and by injuring tissues and body systems beyond the muscles and skeleton. To respond properly to musculoskeletal emergencies, you must maintain and build on the knowledge and skills of the EMT. In addition to those fundamentals, you need a deeper understanding of musculoskeletal system structures and functions, a fuller knowledge of the injury progression process, and a complete grasp of assessment and care procedures for these injuries.

MUSCULOSKELETAL ANATOMY AND PHYSIOLOGY

The musculoskeletal system is a complex arrangement of levers and fulcrums powered by biochemical motors that provide motion and support for the body. It has two distinct subsystems, the skeleton and the muscles. The skeleton is the human body's superstructure, while muscles supply the power of motion to this superstructure, organs, and other body components. These subsystems also produce body heat, store essential salts and energy sources, and create blood cells for transporting oxygen and combating disease.

The musculoskeletal system is covered by fascia, over which the skin and subcutaneous tissue lie. These elements protect the skeleton and muscles, as well as other body systems, from trauma, fluid loss, infection, and fluctuations in body temperature. Skin also provides some cushioning for skeletal components, as on the soles of the feet during walking.

Skeletal Tissue and Structure

As the body's living framework, the skeleton has a structure and design that permits it to perform a variety of functions and to repair itself as needed, within limits. The skeleton is a complex, living system of cells, salt deposits, protein fibers, and other specialized elements. It serves five important purposes:

- It gives the body its structural form.
- It protects vital organs.

- It allows for efficient movement despite gravity.
- It stores many salts and other materials needed for metabolism.
- It produces red blood cells used to transport oxygen.

Although the skeleton is not often thought of as alive, it is exactly that. Its cells live within a matrix of protein fibers and salt deposits. These living cells constantly change the structure and dynamics of the human frame. In fact, 20 percent of the total bone mass (salts, protein fiber, and bone cells) is replaced each year by the remodeling process.

Bone Structure

Typical bone structure consists of numerous aligned cylinders of bone. Minute blood vessels travel lengthwise along the bone through small tubes, called haversian canals. These blood vessels are surrounded by salt layers deposited in collagen fibers. Bone cells called osteocytes are trapped within this matrix and maintain collagen and calcium, phosphate, carbonate, and other salt crystals. Other bone cells, osteoblasts and osteoclasts, build or dissolve these salt deposits and protein fibers as necessary. Osteoblasts lay down new bone in areas of stress during growth and during the bone repair cycle. Osteoclasts dissolve bone structures that are not carrying pressures of articulation and support, or when the body requires more salts for electrolyte balance. These three types of bone cells maintain a dynamic and efficient structure for supporting and moving the body.

A continuous blood supply brings oxygen and nutrients to bone tissue and removes carbon dioxide and waste products from them. Blood vessels enter and exit the bone shaft through perforating canals and distribute blood to both bone tissue and structures located within the medullary canal of the shaft and bone ends. As with any other body tissue, if the blood supply is reduced, or ceases, bone tissue becomes ischemic and will eventually die. Bone does not show degeneration evidence for quite some time, and certainly not during prehospital emergency care. However, long-term effects of devascularization may result in loss of bony integrity and failure of the bone to support weight or forces.

Long bones, such as those of the forearm (humerus) and thigh (femur), best demonstrate the organization of bone tissue into structural body elements (Figure 1 ●). The major areas and tissues of the long bones include the diaphysis, epiphysis, metaphysis, medullary canal, periosteum, and articular cartilage.

The Diaphysis

The diaphysis is the central portion or shaft of the long bone. It consists of a very dense and relatively thin layer of compact bone. Because of its tubular structure, the diaphysis efficiently supports weight, yet is relatively light. While bone shaft design enables it to carry weight well, lateral forces may cause the shaft to break rather easily.

The Epiphysis

Long bone structure changes at the bone ends. The bone's diameter increases dramatically, and the underlying thin, hard, compact bone of the shaft changes to a network of skeletal fibers and strands. This network spreads the stresses and pressures of

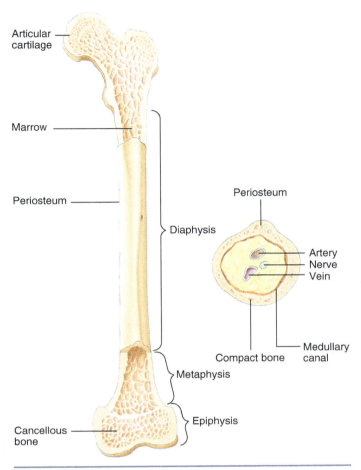

● **Figure 1**   The internal anatomy of a long bone.

weight bearing over a larger surface. This widened, articular bone end is called the **epiphysis**. Tissue within the epiphysis in cross section resembles a rigid bony sponge and is called spongy or **cancellous** bone. Covering this network of fibers is a very thin layer of compact bone supporting the surface that meets and moves against another bone, the **articular surface**.

The Metaphysis

The **metaphysis** is an intermediate region between the epiphysis and diaphysis. It is where the diaphysis's hollow tube of compact bone makes the transition to the bone-fiber honeycomb of the epiphysis's cancellous bone. In this region is the **epiphyseal plate**, or *growth plate*. During childhood, cartilage is generated here and the plate widens. Osteoblasts from the end of the diaphysis deposit salts within the cartilage's collagen matrix to create new bone tissue. This results in lengthening of the infant's and then the child's bone. During this growth period, the epiphyseal plate is also weaker than the rest of the bone and associated joints and is thus a frequent site of fractures in pediatric patients. If damaged, injury may lead to growth discrepancies between the injured and uninjured extremities or to malunion of the fracture.

The Medullary Canal

The chamber formed within the hollow diaphysis and the cancellous bone of the epiphysis is called the **medullary canal**.

The central medullary canal is filled with **yellow bone marrow** that stores fat in a semiliquid form. The fat is a readily available energy source the body can use quickly and easily. **Red bone marrow** fills the cancellous bone chambers of the larger long bones, pelvis, and sternum. It is responsible for manufacturing erythrocytes and other blood cells.

CONTENT REVIEW

▶ Types of Joints

• Synarthroses—immovable
• Amphiarthroses—very limited movement
• Diarthroses (synovial joints)—relatively free movement
  • Monaxial
  • Biaxial
  • Triaxial

The Periosteum

A tough fibrous membrane called the **periosteum** covers the exterior of the diaphysis. With extensive vasculature and innervation, it transmits pain sensation when bones fracture and then initiates the bone repair cycle. Blood vessels and nerves penetrate both the periosteum and compact bone by traveling through small perforating canals. Tendons intermingle with collagen fibers of the periosteum and with collagen fibers of the bony matrix to form strong attachments.

Cartilage

A layer of connective tissue called **cartilage** is a continuous collagen extension of the underlying bone and covers a portion of the epiphyseal surface. It is a smooth, strong, and flexible material that functions as the actual surface of articulation between bones. Cartilage is very slippery and somewhat compressible. It permits relatively friction-free joint movement and absorbs some of the shock associated with activity, such as walking.

Bone Classification

Bones are classified according to their general shape. Those previously described are considered long bones and include the humerus, radius, ulna, tibia, fibula, metacarpals (hand), metatarsals (foot), and phalanges (fingers and toes). The bones of the wrists and ankles, the carpals and tarsals, are short bones. Bones of the cranium, sternum, ribs, shoulder, and pelvis are classified as flat. Irregularly shaped bones include those of the vertebral column and facial bones. Another special type of bone is the **sesamoid bone**, a bone that grows within tendinous tissue; one example is the kneecap, also called the patella.

Joint Structure

Bones move at, and are held together by, a relatively sophisticated structure called a **joint**. There are three basic types of joints, which are classified by the amount of movement they permit.

Synarthroses are immovable joints, such as the sutures of the skull or the juncture between the jaw and teeth (which is called a gomphosis). **Amphiarthroses** are joints that allow some very limited movement. Examples include the joints between vertebrae and between the sacrum and ilium of the pelvis. **Diarthroses**, or **synovial joints**, permit relatively free movement. Such joints include the elbow, knee, shoulder, and hip.

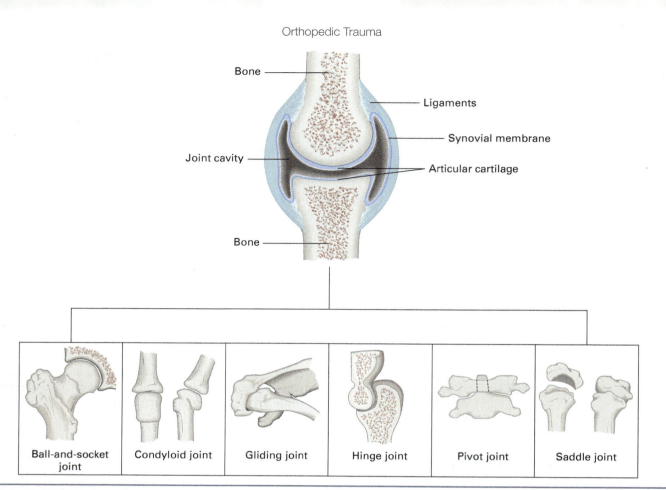

● **Figure 2** Types of synovial joints.

Diarthroses are divided into three joint categories based on movements they allow (Figure 2 ●). These are:

● *Monaxial joints* Hinge joints permit bending in a single plane. Examples include the knees, elbows, and fingers.

   Pivot joints are characterized by articulation between the atlas (the first cervical vertebra) and the axis of the spine. They allow the head to rotate through about 180 degrees of motion.

● *Biaxial joints* Condyloid, or gliding, joints provide movement in two directions. They are located at the joints of carpal bones in the wrist and between the clavicle and sternum.

   Ellipsoidal joints provide a sliding motion in two planes, as between the wrist and the metacarpals.

   Saddle joints allow for movement in two planes at right angles to each other. Examples are the joints at the bases of the thumbs.

● *Triaxial joints* Ball-and-socket joints permit full motion in a cone of about 180 degrees and allow a limb to rotate. Examples include the hip and shoulder.

These joints permit various types of motion. Flexion/extension is a bending motion that reduces/increases the angle between articulating elements. **Adduction/abduction** is the movement of a body part toward/away from the midline. Rotation refers to a turning along the axis of a bone or joint. **Circumduction** refers to movement through an arc of a circle.

Ligaments

Ligaments are connective tissue bands that hold bones together at joints (Figure 3 ●). They stretch and permit joint motion while holding bone ends firmly in position. Ligament ends attach to the joint ends of each of the associated bones.

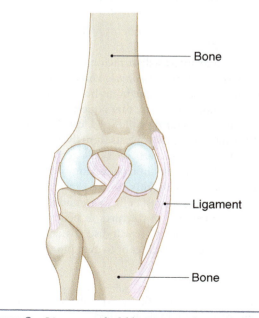

● **Figure 3** Ligaments hold bones together at a joint.

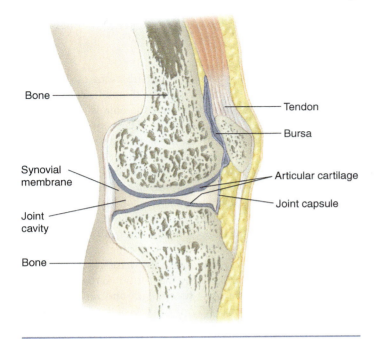

● Figure 4   Structure of a joint.

Ligaments surround the articular region and cross it at many oblique angles. This arrangement ensures that the joint is held together firmly but flexibly enough to permit movement through a designed range of motion.

Joint Capsule

Ligaments surrounding a joint form what is known as a synovial capsule or **joint capsule** (Figure 4 ●). This chamber holds a small amount of fluid to lubricate articular surfaces. This oily, viscous substance, known as **synovial fluid**, assists joint motion by reducing friction. Its lubrication reduces friction to about one-fifth that of two pieces of ice sliding together. Small sacs filled with synovial fluid, known as **bursae**, are also located between tendons and ligaments or cartilage in the elbows, knees, and other joints to reduce friction and absorb shock. Synovial fluid flows into and out of articular cartilage as the joint undergoes compression, relaxation, and movement. Cartilage acts like a sponge, pushing out fluid as it is compressed and drawing in fluid when it is relaxed. This synovial fluid movement circulates oxygen, nutrients, and waste products to and from joint cartilage.

The joint capsule is a very delicate and sterile environment. If it is opened to the environment and infectious agents during trauma (an open wound), those agents may induce damage that will hinder the joint's future function. Cartilage within the joint also does not have the ability to repair itself. If seriously injured during joint trauma, that injury may require surgical intervention and repair. Anticipate that any open wound in the vicinity of a joint involves the joint capsule and ensure it is evaluated in the emergency department.

Skeletal Organization

A human skeleton is made up of approximately 206 bones (Figure 5 ●). These bones form two major divisions, the axial and appendicular skeletons.

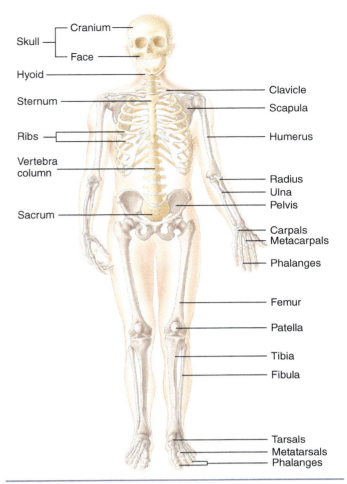

● Figure 5   The human skeleton.

The **axial skeleton** consists of the bones of the head, thorax, and spine. These bones form the axis of the body, protect central nervous system elements, and make up the thoracic cage, which is the dynamic housing for respiration.

The **appendicular skeleton** consists of the upper and lower extremity bones, including both the shoulder girdle and pelvis and excluding the sacrum. These bones provide extremity structure and permit the major articulations of the body. Extremity long bones are similar in design and structure. Both upper and lower extremities are affixed to the axial skeleton and articulate with joints supported by several bones. Each of these extremities has a single long bone proximally and paired bones distally. The terminal member, the hand or foot, is made up of numerous bones with differing purposes, yet parallel designs.

Upper Extremities

Each upper extremity (Figure 6 ●) consists of a shoulder girdle, arm, forearm, and hand. The shoulder is composed of the clavicle and scapula, which sit high on the posterior and lateral thoracic cage. The **scapula** is a triangular bone buried within musculature of the upper back. It is basically a flat plate, called the body, with three major irregular outgrowths. The coracoid and acromion processes are protuberances for muscular attachments. The

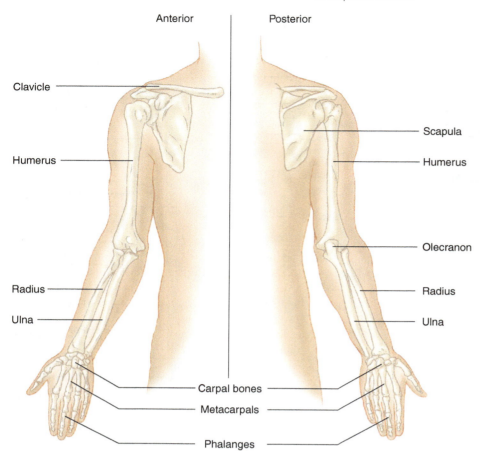

Anterior

Posterior

Clavicle

Humerus

Radius

Ulna

Scapula

Humerus

Olecranon

Radius

Ulna

Carpal bones

Metacarpals

Phalanges

The **radius** and **ulna** form the forearm. The radius is on the thumb (lateral) side of the forearm while the ulna is on the little finger (medial) side. They move in conjunction with the humerus and with each other. This biaxial articulation allows the distal forearm to rotate palm up (supination) or palm down (pronation). This articulation simultaneously permits folding of the elbow. The ulna's proximal end forms the bump of the elbow, known as the **olecranon**.

The radius and ulna articulate with **carpal bones** of the wrist. There are eight carpal bones that form two rows and give the wrist its strength and mobility. The proximal row consists of the scaphoid, lunate, triangular, and pisiform bones. The distal row consists of the trapezium, trapezoid, capitate, and hamate bones. The distal carpal bones, in turn, articulate with the long, thin **metacarpals** of the palm. The carpal bones, with their saddle, gliding, and ellipsoidal joints, provide the wrist with a high degree of flexibility.

Metacarpals articulate with the **phalanges** of the fingers. Each of the four fingers consists of three phalanges—the proximal, middle, and distal. The thumb has only two—the proximal and distal. The combination of these hinge, saddle, and ellipsoidal joints in the metacarpals and phalanges allows fine motion and motor control of the hand and fingers.

glenoid process provides the glenoid fossa, a shallow socket that accepts the head of the humerus. The scapula moves freely over the posterior thorax, providing some of the shoulder's large range of motion. The muscular upper back effectively protects the scapula from fracture in all but the most direct and severe trauma.

The **clavicle** articulates with the acromion of the scapula and the manubrium of the sternum. It is not as well protected as the scapula and is, in fact, the most commonly fractured bone of the human body. It holds the scapula and shoulder joint at a fixed distance from the sternum. The clavicle permits the shoulder to move up and down (shrug) while somewhat restricting anterior and posterior motion. The shoulder joint is one of the most mobile in the body. It permits humerus rotation through about 60 degrees and permits circumduction of the limb through 180 degrees.

The **humerus** is the single bone of the proximal upper extremity (the region properly referred to as the arm). Its rounded or surgical head articulates with the scapula's glenoid fossa, proximally. The head is connected to the humeral shaft by the anatomic neck, which also acts as the terminal end of the articular capsule. Two protuberances, the greater and lesser tuberosities, provide places of attachment for tendons and form the superior portion of the humerus. They, and the anatomic neck and surgical head, are connected to the humerus shaft by the surgical neck, a frequent location of fracture. Distally, the humerus shaft widens into lateral and medial condyles and articulates with the radius and ulna at the elbow.

Lower Extremities

Each lower extremity (Figure 7 ●) is similar in structure to the upper extremities and is made up of the pelvis, thigh, leg, and foot. The **pelvis** is a strong skeletal structure where the lower extremities attach to the body. It consists of two symmetrical structures, called **innominate bones**, and posterior to and joining them, the sacrum. Each innominate is constructed from one large flat bone, the **ilium**, and two irregular bones, the **ischium** and **pubis**, all fused together. Joined anteriorly at the symphysis pubis, the innominates with the sacrum form the pelvic ring. This rigid ring is very strong and provides the basis for support and movement of the lower extremities as well as forming the bony base of the abdomen. Structural pelvic landmarks include the **iliac crests**, lateral bony ridges that hold the belt, and **ischial tuberosities**, bony knobs on which we sit. The pubic bone forms the bony structure at the base of the inguinal area and is divided centrally by the symphysis pubis, the anterior joint between the two innominates. The juncture of the three components of the innominate bones forms the **acetabulum**, a hollow depression in the lateral pelvis. The acetabulum is the socket and actual articular surface for the femoral head.

The **femur** is the largest and strongest bone in the body. During the normal stress of walking, it often withstands pressures

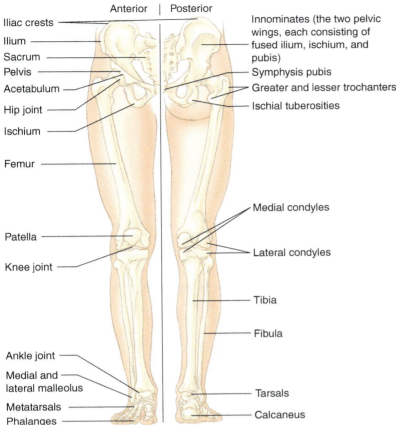

Anterior | Posterior

Iliac crests
Ilium
Sacrum
Pelvis
Acetabulum
Hip joint
Ischium
Femur
Patella
Knee joint
Ankle joint
Medial and lateral malleolus
Metatarsals
Phalanges

Innominates (the two pelvic wings, each consisting of fused ilium, ischium, and pubis)
Symphysis pubis
Greater and lesser trochanters
Ischial tuberosities
Medial condyles
Lateral condyles
Tibia
Fibula
Tarsals
Calcaneus

● **Figure 7**   The lower extremities.

of supporting the entire body over all these bones. The metatarsals articulate with the phalanges of the foot in a configuration parallel to that of the bones of the wrist and hand. The great toe has two phalanges (one proximal and one distal), while the other four toes each have three (proximal, middle, and distal).

Bone Aging

The bones, like all other body tissues, evolve during fetal development and after birth. Bone initially forms in the embryo as loose cartilaginous tissue. Before birth, the skeletal structure is predominantly cartilage, with very little ossified bone evident. This is one reason that infants are highly flexible yet unable to support themselves. Ossified bone begins to appear along the long bone shafts and then extends to the epiphyseal plates. It also develops within the epiphyses and grows outward to form the articular surfaces. Over time, bone formation becomes complete to the epiphyseal plate, and the epiphysis is fully formed. The epiphyseal plate continues to generate cartilage, with the shaft and epiphyses growing from it. As the young adult reaches full height and the end of skeletal growth, epiphyseal plates narrow, become bony, and cease to produce cartilage.

Associated with bone development and aging is the transition from flexible, cartilaginous bone to firm, strong, and fully ossified bone. Bones of the young child remain flexible and do not reach maximum strength until early adulthood. While each bone matures at a different time, almost all maturation is complete by 18 to 20 years of age.

Around the age of 40, the body begins to lose its ability to maintain bone structure. It is unable to rebuild the collagen matrix, and salt crystal deposition is reduced from what it was in earlier years (osteopenia). Effects of these changes appear very slowly. They include a very gradual diminution of bone strength, an increase in bone brittleness, a progressive loss of body height, and some curvature of the spine. Bone fracture incidence also increases, especially at the high-stress points of the lumbar spine and the femur's surgical neck. Osteoporosis is bone mass loss to the point that strength and function are diminished. This increases fracture incidence in the older patient, may lead to poor healing, and may increase likelihood of refracture.

Age-related changes in the skeletal system also affect other body systems. For example, cartilage of the costochondral joints and costal bones (the ribs) becomes less flexible, which leads to shallower, more energy-consuming respirations. Also, intervertebral discs lose water content and become less flexible, more prone to herniation, and narrower, thus shortening and stiffening the trunk.

Muscular Tissue and Structure

More than 600 muscle groups make up the muscular system (Figure 8a ● and 8b ●). As you might expect, a large number of EMS calls involve injuries to this extensive system. Injuries to it may result from excessive forces indirectly expressed to the

of up to 1,200 pounds per square inch along its diaphysis.[1] Like the humerus, the femur is not a straight long bone. At its proximal end, where the head meets the acetabulum, the femur makes an almost 50-degree turn. The femoral head is supported by the surgical neck, a narrow shaft at almost a right angle to the uppermost aspect of the widened femoral shaft. This configuration permits the wide range of motion found in the joint and accounts for the femur's great strength. The greater and lesser trochanters, located at the widening of the femur at its upper end, form attachment points for tendons. The long femoral shaft spreads out for articulation as it meets with the tibia and forms a lateral and medial condyle. The patella, or kneecap, is a free-floating bone (sesamoid) within the quadriceps tendon and is located just proximal to the actual knee joint.

The **tibia** is the only distal bone to articulate with the femur. It pairs with the **fibula**, a smaller and much more delicate bone, just distal to the knee joint. Because of this arrangement, the tibia bears most of the weight supported by the lower extremity. The fibula's primary function is to add control to foot placement and motion during walking. The tibia and fibula are held together by a fibrous interosseous membrane, and they articulate, one against the other, to allow the foot to move through about 45 degrees of rotation.

Both the tibia and fibula join the talus and calcaneus to form the ankle. The tibia forms the medial **malleolus** (inner protuberance of the ankle), while the fibula forms the lateral malleolus. The **calcaneus** is the largest foot bone and forms the heel. The talus articulates with the calcaneus and the tarsals. The tarsals, in turn, articulate with the **metatarsals**, all forming the arch of the foot. There are actually two arches in the foot, one longitudinal and one transverse. This arrangement distributes stresses

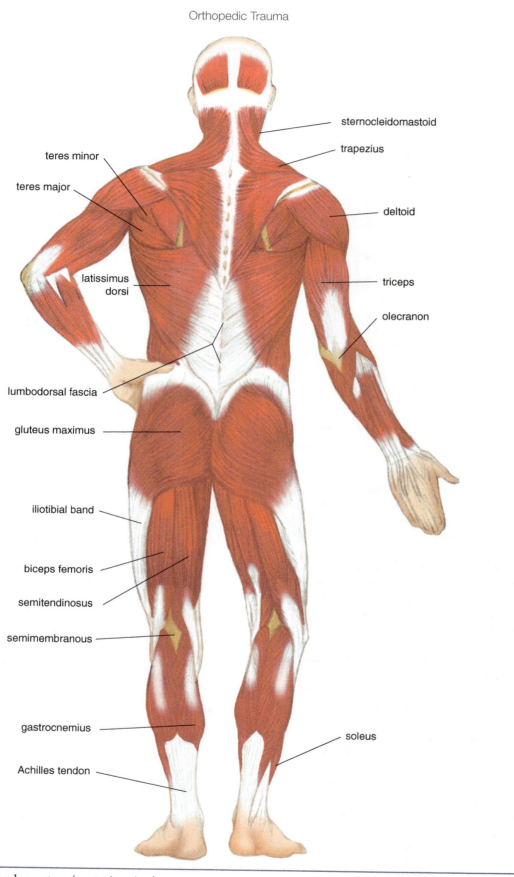

sternocleidomastoid

trapezius

deltoid

triceps

olecranon

teres minor

teres major

latissimus
dorsi

lumbodorsal fascia

gluteus maximus

iliotibial band

biceps femoris

semitendinosus

semimembranous

gastrocnemius

soleus

Achilles tendon

● **Figure 8a**   The muscular system (posterior view).

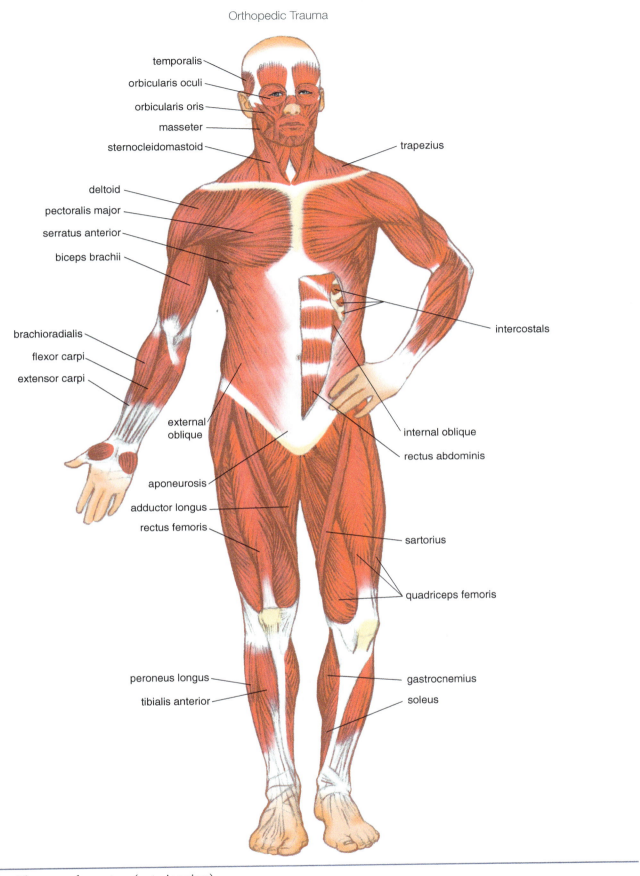

temporalis

orbicularis oculi

orbicularis oris

masseter

sternocleidomastoid

trapezius

deltoid

pectoralis major

serratus anterior

biceps brachii

intercostals

brachioradialis

flexor carpi

extensor carpi

external
oblique

internal oblique

rectus abdominis

aponeurosis

adductor longus

rectus femoris

sartorius

quadriceps femoris

peroneus longus

tibialis anterior

gastrocnemius

soleus

● **Figure 8b**   The muscular system (anterior view).

muscles and their attachments or from direct trauma, either blunt or penetrating.

There are three muscle tissue types within the body—cardiac, smooth, and skeletal (Figure 9 ●). Of these, the most specialized is cardiac muscle, which makes up the myocardium. It contracts rhythmically on its own (automaticity), emitting an electrical impulse in the process (excitability), and passing that impulse along to other cells of the myocardium (conductivity). In this way, the heart provides its lifelong rhythmic contraction and pumping. Cardiac muscle can also be classified according to its structure, which combines characteristics of both skeletal and smooth muscle and is thus called smooth-striated muscle.

The second muscle type is smooth, or involuntary, muscle. It is not under conscious control but functions at the direction of the autonomic nervous system. Smooth muscle is found in arterial and venous blood vessels, bronchioles, bowel, and many other organs. Smooth muscle contracts to reduce (or relaxes to expand) the lumen (diameter) of the vasculature, airways, or digestive tract. Smooth muscles have the ability to contract over a wide lateral distance, enabling them to accommodate great changes in length, such as those that occur during bladder filling and evacuation and arteriole contraction and dilation.

The final type of muscle tissue is skeletal (also called striated or voluntary). We have conscious control over these muscles, which are associated with mobility of the extremities and the body in general. Skeletal muscles are controlled by the somatic nervous system. Skeletal muscles are the largest muscular system component, accounting for 40 to 50 percent of the body's total weight. They are the type of muscle most commonly traumatized.

Skeletal muscles lie directly beneath a protective layer of skin and subcutaneous fat. Because of their hunger for oxygen during activity, they have a more than ample supply of blood vessels. Individual muscle cells layer together to form a muscle fiber, many fibers layer together to form a muscle **fascicle**, and fascicles layer together to form a muscle body, such as the triceps. A muscle body has the strength of about 50 pounds of lift for each square inch of cross-sectional area.

Skeletal muscles attach to bones at a minimum of two locations. These attachment points are called origin and insertion, depending on how the bones move with contraction. An attachment point that remains stationary as the muscle contracts is the **origin**, while an attachment point to the moving bone is the **insertion**.

Muscles usually pair, one on each side of a joint. This configuration is essential because muscles can actively contract, not lengthen. One muscle moves an extremity in one direction by contraction, while an opposing (and relaxed) muscle stretches. The opposing muscle can then in turn contract, stretching the first muscle and moving the extremity in the opposite direction. This arrangement, called **opposition**, permits limb straightening (extension) and then bending (flexion).

With several muscles attached to a joint with different origins and insertions, the body enjoys a wide variety of motions. In the shoulder, for example, the humerus can travel through several types and ranges of motion. These include moving the extremity away from the body (abduction) and toward the body (adduction), turning the humerus (rotation) through about 60 degrees, and circling the entire extremity (circumduction) through a 180-degree arc.

Tendons are specialized bands of connective tissue that accomplish attachment of muscle to bone at the insertion and, in some cases, at the origin (Figure 10 ●). These very fibrous

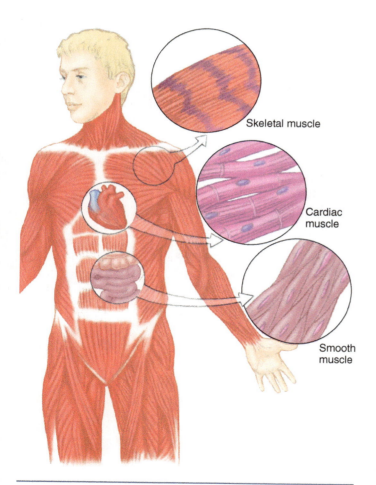

Skeletal muscle

Cardiac muscle

Smooth muscle

● **Figure 9**   Three types of muscle tissue.

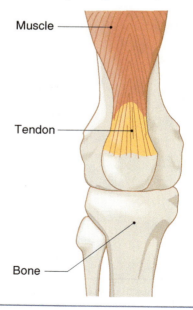

Muscle

Tendon

Bone

● **Figure 10**   Tendons are the bands of tissue that connect muscle to bone.

ribbons of collagen are extremely strong and do not stretch. They originate at muscle ends at what is called the musculoskeletal junction, which is the transition from muscle to tendon. They are so strong that in some instances they will break an area of bone loose rather than tear. The Achilles tendon demonstrates the strength of this particular tissue. It can be felt as the band posterior to the malleoli of the ankle. This tendon is the muscle-controlled cord that allows a person to lift the entire body weight when standing on the toes.

The forearm demonstrates the sophistication of the muscle-tendon relationship. As muscles controlling finger flexion contract, you can feel them tensing in the dorsal forearm. You can also visualize and palpate tendon movement in the distal forearm and wrist as the fingers flex and extend. It is easy to appreciate damage a deep transverse laceration can cause to underlying connective tissues and their control of distal skeletal structures. Tendons are often classified by the action they perform when the muscle associated with them contracts—for example, flexor or extensor, abductor or adductor, and so forth.

Muscle tissue is responsible not only for body movement but also for heat energy production. A chemical reaction between oxygen and simple sugars produces the energy of motion. Heat, water, and carbon dioxide are by-products of this reaction. More than half the energy created by muscle motion is heat that helps maintain body temperature. The body then excretes water and salts in urine or sweat, expels carbon dioxide through respiration, and dissipates excess heat through the skin via radiation, convection, or evaporation. The body must constantly meet muscle tissue requirements for oxygen and nutrients and eliminate waste products of those tissues, including heat.

Muscles are found in a condition of slight contraction called tone. Even while the body is at rest, the central nervous system sends some limited impulses to muscle bodies causing a few fibers to contract. These impulses give the muscles firmness and ensure that they are ready to contract when a need arises. Muscle tone may be very significant in a well-conditioned athlete or absent (flaccid muscle tone) in someone with peripheral motor nerve disruption. Muscle strength is graded from 0 to 5 (Table 1).

TABLE 1 | Muscle Strength Scale

Score	Description
5	Active movement against full resistance with no fatigue
4	Active movement against some resistance and gravity
3	Active movement against gravity
2	Active movement with gravity eliminated
1	Barely palpable muscle contraction with no movement
0	No visible or palpable muscle contraction

MUSCULOSKELETAL PATHOPHYSIOLOGY

The orthopedic injury process is a complicated one, resulting in much more damage than just disruption of an inert structural body element. Bone is alive and requires a continuous supply of oxygenated circulation. Bone lies deep within muscle tissue, and major nerves and blood vessels parallel it as they travel to the distal extremity. At points of articulation, there is a complex arrangement of ligaments, cartilage, and synovial fluid that holds joints together while permitting a wide range of movement. Finally, muscles attach and direct skeletal movement through collections of fibers, fasciculi, and muscle bodies connected to the skeletal system by tendons. This complex arrangement of connective, skeletal, vascular, nervous, and muscular tissue is endangered whenever significant kinetic forces are applied to the extremities. If forces are severe enough, they are likely to cause muscular, joint, or skeletal injury.

Muscular Injury

Muscular injuries may result from direct blunt or penetrating trauma, overexertion, or problems with oxygen supply during exertion. These injuries include contusion, compartment syndrome, penetrating injury, fatigue, cramp, spasm, and strain. Muscular problems usually do not contribute significantly to hypovolemia and shock, with the exceptions of severe contusions with large associated hematomas and penetrating injuries with extensive hemorrhage.

Contusion

Severe trauma frequently crushes muscles between a blunt force and skeletal structures beneath. This damages both muscle cells and blood vessels that supply them. Small blood vessels rupture, leaking blood into interstitial spaces and causing pain, erythema, and then ecchymosis. Blood in interstitial spaces and muscle cell damage set off the body's inflammatory response. Capillary beds engorge with blood, and fluid shifts to the interstitial space, leading to tissue edema. Injury may also cause blood to pool beneath or within tissue layers in a hematoma. In more massive body muscles, like those of the thigh, buttocks, calf, or arm, large blood volumes may accumulate, contributing significantly to hypovolemia. A large hematoma or significant muscular edema will increase the injured limb's diameter, especially as compared to the opposing uninjured limb. For the most part, however, signs of muscle injury and accumulating blood remain hidden beneath the skin or manifest well after prehospital emergency assessment and care.

Compartment Syndrome

The muscular configuration of the extremities, and especially of the leg and forearm, are prone to a specific injury called compartment syndrome. Muscle bodies of these regions are contained in strong inelastic fascial envelopes. When injury damages soft tissue within the compartment, localized swelling results. Contained by fascia, this swelling increases pressure within the compartment, reducing capillary blood flow to muscle and nerve tissues.

CONTENT REVIEW

▶ Types of Muscular Injuries

• Contusion
• Compartment syndrome
• Penetrating injury
• Muscle fatigue
• Muscle cramp
• Muscle spasm
• Muscle strain

Reduced capillary flow causes release of histamine, which increases capillary permeability and worsens swelling and pressure. As pressure builds, blood flow to tissues all but stops. However, pressure necessary to halt capillary blood flow is much less than that needed to stop arterial blood flow to the distal extremity. The patient still has a distal pulse, capillary refill, and venous return from the distal limb. The leg is the most common location associated with this syndrome though it has also been reported with arm, thigh, and hand injuries.

A patient with compartment syndrome most commonly complains of a deep and burning pain that appears out of proportion to the apparent injury. Pain is not reduced by positioning. An increase in pain when you (not your patient) move the extremity and stretch the muscles involved is a related finding (this is called passive stretching). The patient may also report pain when he flexes the affected extremity. Distal pulses and capillary refill may be normal, though the patient may report increased distal sensitivity or numbness that results from nerve compression and injury.[2,3]

Penetrating Injury

Deep lacerations may penetrate skin and subcutaneous tissues, thus affecting the muscle masses and tendons below. Massive wounds involving a large percentage of a muscle body or those injuring or severing a tendon may reduce the distal limb's strength or render muscular control ineffective. When a tendon or muscle is cut, opposing muscle contraction moves the limb while the injured muscle/tendon is unable to return it toward the neutral position. Such injuries call for surgical intervention to identify and rejoin the damaged tendon or muscle body. These wounds may also introduce infectious agents, damage muscle tissue, and affect the muscle's blood supply. The resulting infection, ischemia, or a combination of the two may result in further tissue injury and poor healing.

Fatigue

Muscle **fatigue** occurs as muscles reach their performance limit. Exercise draws down muscle oxygen and energy reserves and results in metabolic by-product accumulation. Cell environment becomes hypoxic, acidic, toxic, and energy deprived. Fewer and fewer muscle fibers are able to contract. Muscle mass strength diminishes, and further exertion becomes painful. Until adequate circulation restores oxygen and muscle cells can replenish energy sources, muscle fibers and the muscle body remain weakened.

Muscle Cramp

Cramping is not really an injury, but a painful muscle tissue spasm. Muscle pain results when exercise consumes available oxygen and energy sources and the circulatory system fails to remove metabolic waste products. Pain begins during or immediately after vigorous exercise or after the limb has been left in an unusual position for a period of time (obstructing circulatory flow). Cramping usually presents with a continuous muscle contraction (spasm).

Changing the limb's position or massaging it may help return the circulation and reduce the pain. Once rest and adequate circulation restore metabolic balance, muscle cramp pain usually subsides. Muscle cramp pain can also be caused by electrolyte imbalances such as hypocalcemia and lactic acid accumulation.

Muscle Spasm

In muscle **spasm**, the affected muscle goes into an intermittent (clonic) or continuous (tonic) contraction. Spasm may be firm enough to feel like deformity associated with a fracture and can confound assessment. As with muscle cramp, muscle spasm usually subsides uneventfully with rest.

Strain

A **strain** occurs when muscle fibers are overstretched by forces that exceed the fiber's strength. Muscle fibers then stretch and tear, causing pain that increases with any further muscle use. Injury may occur with extreme muscle stress, as during heavy lifting or sprinting, or at times of fatigue, when only a limited number of muscle fibers are in contraction. With a strain, fibers are damaged without significant internal bleeding, edema, or discoloration. The injury site is generally painful to palpation, and patients normally report pain that limits affected muscle use.

Joint Injury

Joint injuries include sprain, subluxation, and dislocation. The following sections detail pathologies behind each of these injuries.

Sprain

A **sprain** is a tearing of a joint capsule's connective tissues, specifically a ligament or ligaments. Injury causes acute pain at its site, followed shortly by inflammation and swelling. Ecchymotic discoloration occurs over time, but not usually during prehospital care. Tearing of ligaments weakens the joint. Continued joint use when the tear is significant may lead to its complete failure. Minor tears may actually heal faster if modestly loaded, as in ambulation, as tolerated. Sprains are classified, or graded, according to their severity, using the following criteria:

● *Grade I.* Minor and incomplete tear. The ligament is painful, and swelling is usually minimal. The joint remains stable.

● *Grade II.* Significant but incomplete tear. Swelling and pain range from moderate to severe. The joint is intact but unstable.

● *Grade III.* Complete ligament tear. Due to severe pain and spasm, the grade III sprain may present as a fracture. The joint is unstable.

Subluxation

Subluxation is a partial bone end displacement from its position within a joint capsule. It occurs as a joint separates under stress, stretching the ligaments. Subluxation differs from a sprain in that it more significantly reduces a joint's integrity. The injured joint is painful and swells quickly, its range of motion is limited, and the joint is unstable. Hyperflexion, hyperextension, lateral rotation beyond the normal range of motion, or application of extreme axial force are common causes of subluxations.

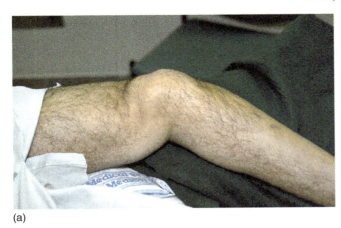

(a)

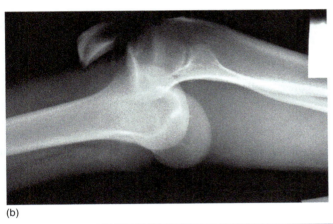

(b)

● **Figure 11**   Knee dislocation. (a) Presentation of a knee dislocation. (b) X-ray of the dislocation. *(Both: © Edward T. Dickinson, MD)*

Dislocation

A **dislocation** is a complete displacement of bone ends from their normal joint position (sometimes referred to as a luxation) (Figure 11 ●). The joint then fixes in an abnormal position with noticeable deformity. The site is painful, swollen, and immobile. This injury carries with it the danger of entrapping, compressing, or tearing blood vessels and nerves. Dislocation occurs when a joint moves beyond its normal range of motion with great force. By its nature, a dislocation has serious associated ligament damage and may involve joint capsule and articular cartilage injury.

Bone Injury

Fracture is an involved process that ultimately disrupts bone continuity. A bone fractures when extreme axial forces or significant lateral forces exceed the bone's tensile strength.

A fracture may be caused by direct injury—for example, an auto bumper impacts a patient's femur or a high-powered rifle bullet slams into a patient's thigh and, then, femur. A fracture cause may also be indirect. This might occur when a bike rider is thrown over the handlebars and braces the fall with an outstretched upper extremity. In this case, impact energy is transmitted from the hand to the wrist, to the forearm, to the arm, to the shoulder, to the clavicle. Transmitted force fractures the clavicle and may cause internal injury to blood vessels and the upper reaches of the lung. For this reason, always analyze mechanism of injury carefully, recognizing that kinetic forces may be transmitted and cause injury far from the impact point. Remember, 80 percent of multisystem trauma cases have associated serious musculoskeletal injury.

CONTENT REVIEW

► Types of Joint Injury

• Sprain
• Subluxation
• Dislocation

As kinetic energy is transmitted to a bone and the bone fractures, collagen, osteocytes, salt crystals, blood vessels, nerves, and medullary canal of the bone, as well as its periosteum and endosteum (the inner lining of the medullary canal), are disrupted. If broken bone ends displace, they may further injure surrounding muscles, tendons, ligaments, nerves, veins, and arteries. The result is a serious insult to limb structure.

Vascular damage may restrict distal blood flow to the limb, increasing capillary refill time, diminishing pulse strength and limb temperature, and causing discoloration and paresthesia (a "pins-and-needles" sensation). Nerve injury may result in distal paresthesia, anesthesia (loss of sensation), paresis (weakness), and paralysis (loss of muscle control). Muscle or tendon damage may interfere with a victim's ability to move the limb. If muscle tissue is badly damaged and swells where fasciae firmly contain it, compartment syndrome may develop.

If the bone does not seriously displace and the forces causing fracture do not penetrate, surrounding skin remains intact and the resulting injury is termed a **closed fracture**. If sharp bone ends displaced by forces causing fracture or other subsequent limb motion lacerate through the muscle, subcutaneous tissue, and skin, the result is termed an **open fracture** (Figure 12 ●). An open fracture may also occur when an object such as a bullet travels through a limb and fractures a bone. Open fractures carry risk for infection within disrupted soft, bone, and medullary tissues. Such an infection may seriously reduce a bone's ability to heal. Where bones are located very close to the skin, as with the tibia (the shin), an open fracture can occur with relatively minimal bone displacement. Note that any break in the skin overlying, or in close association to, a fracture is considered open.

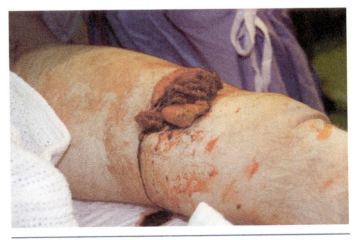

● **Figure 12**   An open fracture. *(© Edward T. Dickinson, MD)*

Surprisingly, some fractures may be relatively stable (Figure 13 ●). When a bone suffers a small crack that doesn't disrupt its total structure, the injury is termed a **hairline fracture**. This injury type weakens the bone and is painful, but the bone remains in position, retaining some of its strength. Another relatively stable bone injury is the **impacted fracture**. With a compression mechanism of injury, a bone may impact on itself resulting in a compressed but aligned bone. As in a hairline fracture, an impacted fracture remains in position and retains some of its original strength. The danger with both hairline and impacted fractures is that further stress and movement may fracture the remaining bone and displace the bone ends, increasing both the injury's severity and its healing time.

There are several fracture types whose physical characteristics can be revealed only by X-rays. For example, the **transverse fracture** is a complete break in a bone that runs straight across it at about a 90-degree angle. This is usually a high-energy injury pattern caused by a bending force. A fracture that runs at an angle across the bone is considered an **oblique fracture**. A fracture in which the bone has splintered into several smaller fragments is a **comminuted fracture**; this type of fracture is often associated with crushing injuries or high-velocity bullet impact. It generally represents a significant energy exchange and is often associated with extensive soft-tissue damage. Fractures involving a twisting motion may result in a curved break around the bone shaft known as a **spiral fracture**. Spiral fractures can occur when a child's arm is pulled and rotated by an adult or when an adult's limb is pulled into machinery like an auger.

Fatigue fracture is associated with prolonged or repeated stress. The bone generally weakens and fractures from repetitive application of modest forces, and not through a single great kinetic force. Most stress fractures occur in the lower extremities in association with vigorous aerobic training such as walking and running. An example is the metatarsal fatigue fracture, also known as a march fracture.

A very infrequent but serious fracture complication is fat embolism. Bone disruption may damage adjacent blood vessels and the medullary canal. Injury may then release fat, stored in a semi-liquid form, into the wound site where it enters the venous system, becomes emboli, and travels to the heart. The heart distributes the emboli to the pulmonary circulation where it lodges (pulmonary emboli). Fat embolism is usually associated with severe or crush injuries or post-injury manipulation of larger long bone fractures, especially the femur.

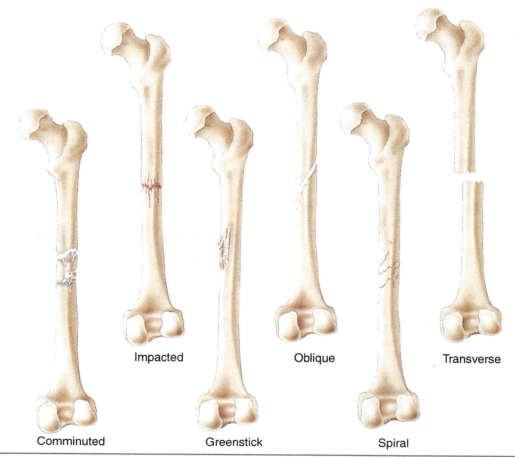

Impacted   Oblique   Transverse

Comminuted   Greenstick   Spiral

● **Figure 13**   Types of fractures.

Pediatric Considerations

Physiologically, bones of infants, young children, and, to a degree, older children contain a greater percentage of cartilage than those of adults and are still growing from the epiphyseal plate. Pediatric patients thus often sustain different types of fractures than do adults.

The flexible nature of pediatric bones is responsible for a **greenstick fracture**, a type of partial fracture. Like a severely bent green twig, the greenstick fracture disrupts only one side of the long bone. It remains angulated and resisting alignment due to the disrupted periosteum and bone tissue on the fracture side and the intact periosteum and bone tissue on the uninjured side. During the bone repair process, the injured side experiences more rapid growth than the uninjured side. This results in increasing angulation as the bone heals. Surgeons sometimes complete a greenstick fracture by breaking the bone fully, thereby ensuring proper healing. Another incomplete fracture in pediatric patients is the buckle or torus fracture. The fracture is a buckling of the bone on one side due to increased cartilage and flexibility of the child's bone. Buckle fractures heal very well.

A child's bone grows at the epiphyseal plate, which forms a weak spot in the long bone. In pediatric trauma, this is a common site of long bone disruption called an **epiphyseal fracture**. If the growth plate is disrupted, disruption may lead to a reduction or halt in bone growth, a condition most commonly involving the proximal tibia.

Fracture repair and remodeling are aggressive in children. Increased pediatric metabolism and normal bone tissue replacement generally ensure that a fracture site will stabilize more quickly than in an adult. In pediatric patients, the aggressive bone remodeling process (where bone is laid down along lines of stress and dissolved in areas of reduced stress) ensures a rapid return to normal bone shape when circulation to the site is good and injured bones are relatively aligned.

Pediatric joint fractures are classified according to the Salter-Harris Pediatric Scheme (Figure 14 ●). While definitive diagnosis is performed by X-ray and other diagnostic techniques not available in the ambulance, a short discussion of the scheme may help in understanding the various types of growth plate (epiphyseal) fractures. The fractures are classified according to

involvement of the growth plate, the adjacent bone, and joint. A type I fracture traverses the growth plate without affecting either the bone above or the joint tissue below. A type II fracture involves both the growth plate and the bone of the limb (diaphysis). A type III fracture involves the growth plate and the joint structure below (epiphysis). A type IV fracture involves the bone above, crosses through the growth plate, and involves the joint structure below. Finally, a type V fracture is generally a crushing type of injury involving the entire joint area. In general, the greater the Salter-Harris fracture, the longer and more difficult the healing.

Geriatric Considerations

The aging process causes several changes to the musculoskeletal system. A gradual, progressive decrease in bone mass and collagen structure begins at about the age of 40 and results in bones that are less flexible, more brittle, and more easily fractured. The bones also heal more slowly. Aging adults also lose some muscle strength and coordination, increasing the likelihood of skeletal injury. Lumbar spine and femoral neck fractures occur because of stress, often without a history of significant trauma.

Another age-related and more significant problem secondary to poor bone remodeling is called **osteoporosis**. Osteoporosis is an accelerated bone tissue degeneration due to bone mineral loss, principally calcium. It typically affects women more than men and becomes most serious after menopause. The condition leads to increases in bone structure degeneration, spinal curvature, and incidences of fractures. A less significant and more common bone density condition is osteopenia. This is a natural condition where bone deterioration with age (generally after 40 years) reduces the bone mass and strength.

Pathological Fractures

Pathological fractures result from disease pathologies that affect bone development or maintenance. Such problems may be caused by tumors (cancer) of the bone, periosteum, or articular

CONTENT REVIEW

► Types of Fractures

- Closed
- Open
- Hairline
- Impacted
- Transverse
- Oblique
- Comminuted
- Spiral
- Fatigue
- Greenstick
- Epiphyseal

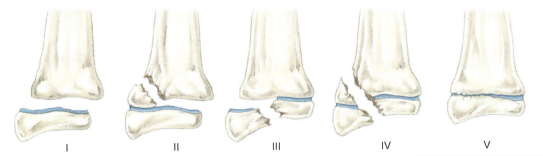

● **Figure 14** The Salter-Harris system of classifying growth-plate injuries. The likelihood of a permanent growth-plate deformity increases as the classification number increases.

cartilage or by diseases that release agents that increase osteoclast activity and osteoporosis. Other diseases and infections can have the same impact on bone tissue and result in fracture, especially in older patients. Radiation treatment may also kill bone cells, resulting in localized bone degeneration, weakened bones, and fractures. These fractures are not likely to heal well, if they heal at all. Be suspicious of pathological fractures in patients with a past medical history (PMH) of cancer, or in low-energy mechanisms that cause fractures in young, otherwise healthy, or non-osteoporotic elderly patients.

General Considerations with Musculoskeletal Injuries

The potential effects of trauma can be better anticipated when skeletal structure and musculature are examined together. It is important to note that long bones are smallest through the diaphysis and largest at the epiphyseal area, or joint. However, the external extremity diameter is greatest surrounding the mid-shaft due to skeletal muscle placement. This anatomic relationship is significant when looking at the potential for nervous and vascular injury.

Since there is limited soft tissue surrounding joints, joint fractures, dislocations, and—to a lesser degree—subluxations and sprains may cause severe problems beyond direct skeletal injury. Any swelling, deformity, or displacement may compromise nerve and vascular supply to the distal extremity. Fractures near a joint are more likely to compress or sever blood vessels or nerves. With shaft fractures, neurovascular injury is less likely, although fracture site manipulation or gross deformity may still endanger blood vessels and nerves running along the bone.

Areas around joints are further endangered because blood vessels supplying the epiphysis enter the long bone through the diaphysis. If a fracture close to the epiphysis displaces the bone ends, it may compromise this blood supply with devastating results. Distal bone tissue may die without adequate circulation, destroying the joint and its function.

Once injury occurs, extremity stability is reduced. Any additional movement can increase pain, damage soft tissues, and injure nerves and blood vessels. Even slight manipulation can cause internal trauma. For example, a fractured femur has bone ends that are about the size of a broken broom handle. If, during extrication, splinting, and patient transport, these bone ends move about within soft tissue, resulting damage may be much more severe than that which initially occurred with fracture. Injury site manipulation may also increase the likelihood of introducing bone fragments or fat emboli into the venous system, causing pulmonary embolism.

Another complication associated with long bone fracture is muscle spasm induced by pain. In a long bone fracture, pain causes surrounding muscles to contract. This contraction forces broken bone ends to override the fracture site. The result, in the case of the femur, is two broom-handle-sized bones driven into the thigh muscles, causing a cycle of more pain, more spasm, and more damage.

Bone Repair Cycle

The bone repair cycle is a complex process that normally results in almost complete healing. When trauma fractures a bone, the periosteum, local blood vessels, soft tissues, and endosteum tear. Blood fills the injured site and congeals, establishing a clot consisting of red blood cells and collagen called a fracture hematoma. This hematoma halts further hemorrhage and forms a relatively weak fracture site immobilization. Special cartilage-forming cells migrate into this hematoma from the broken bone ends and begin to strengthen the site. As cartilage grows together it forms a more rigorous mass to stabilize the site. This elemental skeletal stabilization is called the **callus**. The bone-developing cells, osteoblasts, migrate into the callus and begin to lay down calcium within protein fibers. This forms spongy bone and a stronger stabilization of the fracture site. The callus becomes rigid and is significantly larger than the bone it is splinting. Eventually (in about four months) the callus will approximate the original strength of the bone it is splinting.

With time, bone remodeling occurs. Osteoblasts lay down calcium along stress lines in the bone while osteoclasts remove calcium from areas with limited stress. The result is gradual bone shaping (remodeling) that will eventually resemble the original bone. If a patient is young when a fracture occurs and the bone ends are well aligned, there may be little evidence that an injury ever occurred.

If bone ends are misaligned or if the fracture site experiences stress, infection, or movement before it has a chance to heal properly, it may never return to normal and may leave the person with some disability. Conditions such as smoking, infection, diabetes or poor health, and NSAIDs and immunosuppressive drug use may impair the healing process. In some cases, preexisting conditions may disrupt the bone-healing process to a degree that two broken bone ends do not rejoin (nonunion).

Inflammatory and Degenerative Conditions

Patients suffering from inflammatory and degenerative conditions may complain of joint pain, tenderness, and fatigue. These patients may also have difficulty walking and moving, may require additional assistance with their normal daily activities, and may be prone to musculoskeletal injuries. Common inflammatory diseases of the musculoskeletal system include bursitis, tendonitis, and arthritis.

Bursitis

Bursitis is an acute or chronic inflammation of the bursae, the small synovial sacs that reduce friction and cushion ligaments and tendons from trauma. Bursitis may result from repeated trauma, gout, infection, and, in some cases, unknown etiologies. A patient with bursitis experiences localized pain, swelling, and tenderness at or near a joint. Commonly affected locations include the olecranon (elbow), the area just above the patella (prepatellar bursa), and the shoulder.

Tendonitis

Tendonitis is characterized by inflammation of a tendon and its protective sheath and has a presentation similar to that of bursitis. Repeated trauma to a particular muscle group is a common cause of the condition, which usually affects the major tendons of the upper and lower extremity.

Arthritis

Arthritis is literally joint inflammation, frequently caused by damage to or destruction of the joint's cartilage. Four of the most common types of arthritis are osteoarthritis, septic arthritis, rheumatoid arthritis, and gout (more formally known as gouty arthritis).

Osteoarthritis, which is also known as degenerative joint disease, is the most common connective tissue disorder. It is characterized by a general degeneration, or "wear-and-tear," of articular cartilage that results in irregular bony overgrowths. Signs and symptoms include pain, stiffness, and diminished movement in the joints. Joint enlargement may be visible, especially in the fingers. Predisposing factors for osteoarthritis include trauma, obesity, and aging.

Septic arthritis is caused by joint capsule infection. An agent may be introduced through an open wound, by blood-borne pathogens, or may be introduced from adjacent infection. Common agents include *staphylococcus* and *streptococcus* species, and *Neisseria gonorrhoeae*. A patient will present with fever and a warm, swollen joint.

Rheumatoid arthritis is a chronic, systemic, progressive, and debilitating disease resulting in deterioration of peripheral joint connective tissue. It is characterized by synovial joint inflammation, which causes immobility, pain, increased pain on movement, and fatigue. The disease occurs two to three times more frequently in women than in men. In extreme cases, flexion contractures may develop due to muscle spasms induced by inflammation.

Gout is a joint and connective tissue inflammation produced by an accumulation of uric acid crystals. It occurs most frequently in males who often have high concentrations of uric acid in the blood. Uric acid is a metabolism end-product that is not easily dissolved. Signs and symptoms of gout include peripheral joint pain, swelling, and possible deformity. Pseudogout is a gout-like disease caused by the deposition of a crystalline substance similar to uric acid.

Lyme disease, a tick-introduced infectious agent (*Borrelia burgdorferi*), may produce joint inflammation. The infection usually also causes small red lesions and symptoms such as fever, fatigue, headache, and muscle and joint pain. Untreated, the disease commonly leads to arthritis. Interestingly, the arthritis is not septic; that is, the joint contains no infectious agent. Instead, the Borrelia agent stimulates the production of inflammatory agents that affect the joint. Several viruses also cause arthritis in this fashion.

MUSCULOSKELETAL INJURY ASSESSMENT

With musculoskeletal trauma patients, fractures, dislocations, or muscular injuries infrequently threaten life or seriously contribute to shock's development. In most circumstances, a patient with an isolated fracture, dislocation, or trauma to muscular or connective tissue will receive a focused trauma assessment and management at the scene.

However, serious musculoskeletal injury is common in patients who present with other serious injuries. As noted earlier, energy is often transmitted from the impact point along the skeletal system to internal organs. Thus, when you discover a skeletal injury, always look for indications of trauma force severity and the possibility that those forces caused internal injuries.

As with any trauma patient, assessment progresses through scene size-up, primary assessment, either rapid or focused trauma assessment, detailed physical examination when appropriate, and serial reassessments. You will usually focus your attention on musculoskeletal injuries during the rapid or focused trauma assessment and then as part of a detailed physical exam.

Scene Size-Up

Remember to ensure scene safety and don appropriate personal protective equipment (Standard Precautions) before approaching any scene. Gloves are mandatory when dealing with open musculoskeletal wounds, but those wounds, by themselves, do not usually suggest a need for protective eyewear, mask, or gown. (The only exception would be severe arterial hemorrhage.) Since musculoskeletal injuries result from trauma, analyze the mechanism of injury to anticipate the nature and severity of those injuries. Enhance your mechanism of injury analysis by talking with the patient, family members, and bystanders to identify what happened and how. Identify any impact environmental considerations might have on assessment, care, and transport and integrate with any incident command. Lastly, ensure you have all the resources you need to secure the scene, access the patient, and extricate him, if necessary.

Primary Assessment

It is imperative that trauma patient assessment begin with an evaluation of the patient's mental status and ABCs. During this primary assessment, you must also identify any potential for spinal injury and a need for spinal precautions. Remember, any serious musculoskeletal injury suggests kinetic energy forces sufficient to cause spinal injury, so always take spinal precautions with such an injury. Remember too that a serious fracture is a distracting injury and may mask symptoms of spinal injury. Proceed with the primary assessment and ensure that any life-threatening injuries are addressed before moving on with the secondary assessment. Never let a gruesome musculoskeletal injury distract you from first identifying and caring for life-threatening injuries.

Patients with musculoskeletal injuries are classified into four categories:

- Patients with life- and limb-threatening injuries
- Patients with life-threatening injuries and minor musculoskeletal injuries
- Patients with non-life-threatening injuries but serious limb-threatening musculoskeletal injuries
- Patients with non-life-threatening injuries and only isolated minor musculoskeletal injuries

Perform a rapid trauma assessment for those patients with possible life- or limb-threatening injuries. A patient without life threat but with serious musculoskeletal injury may receive a rapid trauma assessment or a focused trauma assessment, depending

CONTENT REVIEW

► Classification of Patients with Musculoskeletal Injuries

- Life- and limb-threatening injuries
- Life-threatening injuries, minor musculoskeletal injuries
- Non-life-threatening injuries, serious limb-threatening injuries
- Non-life-threatening injuries, isolated minor musculoskeletal injuries

on mechanism of injury and information you discover during your primary assessment. Provide patients presenting with isolated and simple musculoskeletal injuries with a focused trauma assessment, though you must remain watchful for any sign or symptom of more serious injury and a need for both a rapid trauma assessment and rapid patient transport to a trauma center.

Secondary Assessment

Secondary assessment includes either a rapid trauma assessment or a focused trauma assessment.

Rapid Trauma Assessment

Rapid trauma assessment is performed on any patient with any sign, symptom, or mechanism of injury that suggests serious injury. While musculoskeletal injuries do not often cause life-threatening hemorrhage, remember that 80 percent of patients with serious multisystem trauma have associated musculoskeletal injury. When you have evidence of serious musculoskeletal injury, maintain a high index of suspicion for serious internal injury.

Perform a rapid trauma assessment in a carefully ordered way, progressing through an evaluation of the head, neck, chest, and abdomen, and arriving at the pelvis. Pay particular attention to possible pelvic fracture, because such an injury may account for hemorrhage of more than 2 liters. If no other signs of pelvic fracture exist, check pelvic ring stability by directing firm pressure downward, then inward on the iliac crests, and then directing gentle downward pressure on the symphysis pubis. Suspect pelvic fracture if pressure reveals any instability or crepitus, or elicits a painful response from the patient. Crepitus is a grating sensation felt as bone ends rub against one another. If you feel crepitus once, presume that bone injury exists and do not attempt to re-create the sensation, as it represents continued damage to the fractured bone ends and surrounding tissue. It is also quite painful. Consider the patient a possible candidate for rapid transport with fluid resuscitation initiated en route.

In assessing the thighs, look for signs of tissue swelling and femur fracture. Each femur fracture may account for as much as 1,500 mL of blood loss. Evidence of this loss may be hidden within tissue and thigh muscle, so compare one thigh to the other to evaluate swelling. If you find evidence of either pelvic or bilateral femur fracture, consider a pelvic sling or binder and spine board immobilization or pneumatic anti-shock garment (PASG), and inflate all compartments to a pressure that immobilizes the pelvis and the lower extremities. Monitor for signs that the patient is compensating for blood loss, and consider both rapid transport and fluid resuscitation.

While extremity fractures and muscular injuries may not by themselves produce shock, they may significantly contribute to hypovolemia. Consider the effects of these injuries in your

decision on whether to provide rapid transport or on-scene care. Further, fractures and dislocations may entrap or damage blood vessels or nerves, thus seriously threatening the future use of a limb. Quickly survey each limb and check the distal pulses, capillary refill, temperature, muscle tone, and, if the patient is conscious, sensation and motor function.

Complete the rapid trauma assessment by gathering a patient history and a baseline set of vital signs and Glasgow coma score (simultaneously with physical assessment). If the rapid trauma assessment reveals a serious threat to life or limb, rapidly transport the patient to the nearest appropriate facility.

Focused Assessment

The focused trauma assessment directs your attention to injuries found or suggested during primary assessment, by mechanism of injury or by patient signs and symptoms. This assessment is performed for patients without life-threatening injuries and directs both assessment and care to isolated injuries.

Begin a focused trauma assessment by observing and inquiring carefully for signs and symptoms of fracture, dislocation, or other musculoskeletal injury in each limb with suspected injury (Figure 15 ●). Expose and visualize the entire limb by removing any restrictive jewelry and clothing or cutting it away carefully. In

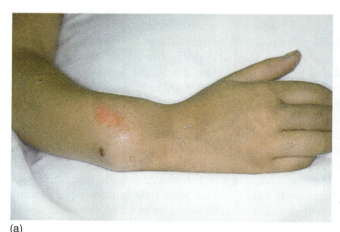

(a)

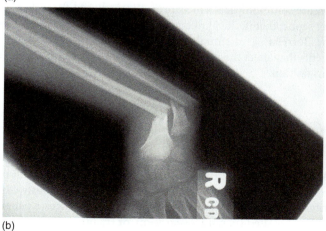

(b)

● **Figure 15** Presentation of a forearm fracture. (a) A fracture will often present with deformity. (b) An X-ray of the fracture. (*Both: © Charles Stewart, MD, MPH*)

doing so, avoid any potential injury site manipulation. Inspect the injury site carefully by looking at the medial, lateral, anterior, and posterior surfaces to locate any deformities (angulation or swelling), discolorations (unlikely in the first minutes after the incident), and indications of soft-tissue wounds that suggest injury beneath. Any unusual limb placement, asymmetry, or inequality in limb length (when compared to the opposing limb) should also arouse suspicion of musculoskeletal injury. Remember that tendon separation may cause the muscle to contract away from the injury and create a muscle mass near one end of the long bone. Consider that any open wounds communicate with an associated fracture or dislocation. Observe for any contamination or sign of the bone protruding. Question the patient about pain, pain with attempted movement, pain on touch, discomfort, or unusual feeling or sensation. Also inquire about weakness, paralysis, paresthesia, or anesthesia. It may be helpful to think of the "six Ps" as a way to remember key elements when evaluating an extremity:[4]

- **Pain.** The patient may report this on palpation (tenderness) or movement.
- **Pallor.** The patient's skin may be pale or flushed, and capillary refill may be delayed.
- **Paralysis.** The patient may have inability to, or difficulty in, moving an extremity.
- **Paresthesia.** The patient may report numbness or tingling in the affected extremity.
- **Pressure.** The patient reports a feeling of tension within the extremity.
- **Pulses.** These may be diminished or absent in the distal extremity.

An additional "P" sometimes cited is poikilothermia, referring to a limb that is cool to the touch.

If you do not identify a specific injury, palpate the extremity for instability, deformity (swelling or angulation), crepitus, unusual motion (joint-like motion where a joint shouldn't exist), muscle tone (normal, flaccid, or spasming), or any regions of unusual warmth or coolness. Palpate the entire anterior and posterior surfaces, then lateral and medial surfaces. Your assessment must be gentle, yet complete. Record any abnormal signs. When assessing the feet, carefully evaluate the distal circulation. Assess pulses for presence and relative strength, and then compare bilaterally. Test the skin for humidity and warmth. Suspect circulatory compromise if capillary refill time is prolonged compared to the uninjured limb. Observe the skin for discoloration, noting any erythema, ecchymosis, or any abnormal hue (pale, ashen, or cyanotic). Approximate the level at which any deficit begins, and note any relation to possible extremity injury.

In a conscious and responsive patient, evaluate sensation and muscle strength distal to the injury (Figure 16 ●). Check tactile (touch) response by touching or stroking the bottom of the foot with the blunt end of a bandage scissors or other similar instrument. Ask the patient to describe the feeling. If the limb appears uninjured, ask the patient to push down with the balls of both feet (plantar flexion) against your hands. Then ask the patient to pull upward with the top of both feet (dorsiflexion), again against your hands. If you feel any unilateral or bilateral weakness or

the patient reports any pain, document any findings on the prehospital care report and look for a cause. Check abnormal sensation and the patient's ability to wiggle the toes or fingers. If the limb appears uninjured, ask the patient to move each joint through its normal range of motion and note any patient symptoms or restrictions to normal movement.

Assess for potential upper extremity injury in a manner similar to your lower extremity assessment. Expose, observe, question about, and then palpate the limb as previously described. Determine tactile response by using the back of the patient's hand. Test muscular strength by having the patient squeeze two of your fingers. Compare strength and sensation bilaterally, identify any deficit, and attempt to locate a cause. Evaluate an upper extremity and ensure it is uninjured before you use it for blood pressure determination.

When extremity assessment suggests injury, treat the limb as though a fracture or dislocation exists. The only definitive way to rule out these injuries is by X-ray evaluation. Also note that splinting protects strains, sprains, and subluxations as well as fractures and dislocations from further injury. Treating a soft-tissue or muscular injury as a fracture or dislocation produces nothing more harmful than providing slight patient discomfort. Failure to immobilize an injury properly, however, may lead to additional soft, skeletal, connective, vascular, or nervous tissue damage and possibly cause permanent harm.

If possible, find the exact injury site and determine if it involves a joint area or a long bone shaft. Form a clear visual image of the injury site in your mind so you can describe it in the patient care report and to the receiving physician. Remember that a splinting device (e.g., a padded board splint for a wrist fracture) may hide the site from view, leaving the attending physician unable to determine what exists beneath it. A good wound description may

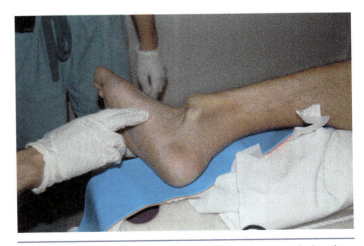

● **Figure 16**   Evaluate sensation and muscle strength distal to the injury. (© Edward T. Dickinson, MD)

CONTENT REVIEW

► Early Indicators of Compartment Syndrome

- Feelings of tension within limb
- Loss of distal sensation (especially in webs of fingers and toes)
- Complaints of pain
- Condition more severe than mechanism of injury would indicate
- Pain on passive extension of extremity
- Pulse deficit (late sign)

delay the need to remove a splint to view an injury.

One important complication of musculoskeletal injury to an extremity is compartment syndrome. This condition results from bleeding into, or edema within, a muscle mass surrounded by fasciae that do not stretch. Pressure buildup within fascia then compresses capillaries and nerves, leading to a reduction in local circulation. This, in turn, leads to local tissue ischemia and then necrosis, with some distal sensation loss. A pulse deficit or delayed capillary refill may be late findings in compartment syndrome as building pressure within fascia may not restrict arterial blood flow early in the syndrome. Suspect compartment syndrome in any patient who has any paresthesia, especially in the webs between medial toes or fingers; who has an extremity injury with a firm mass or increased skin tension at the injury site; who has pain out of proportion to the injury nature; or who has pain that increases when you move the limb (passive stretching). Also suspect compartment syndrome in any unconscious patient with a swollen limb. Compartment syndrome most often occurs in the forearm or leg. Compartment syndrome takes a long time to develop and may not be recognizable in the prehospital setting. It may be seen in patients well after an emergency department visit for musculoskeletal injuries, in patients with casts in place, and with snake bite envenomations.

During the physical exam, question the patient about injury symptoms. Ensure that your verbal investigation is detailed and complete. Determine the nature and location of pain, tenderness, or dysfunction. The patient's event description regarding a fracture or dislocation may also be helpful. The patient may state that he felt the bone "snap" or joint "pop out." Determine if the bone snapped, thus causing a fall, or whether a fall caused the fracture. Evaluate for the amount of pain (0 to 10 scale) and discomfort the patient is experiencing with injury. For example, an elderly patient may present with a fractured hip and limited pain, a presentation usually related to a degenerative disease and secondary fracture. These findings may suggest that you adopt a less aggressive approach to care for this patient, focusing on patient comfort rather than on traction splinting and shock care. Also identify pertinent patient allergies, medications, past medical history, last oral intake, and events leading up to the incident.

Compare any assessment findings to your index of suspicion for injury developed during scene size-up. If you have found less significant injury than you suspected, consider reevaluating the patient to ensure that no injury has been overlooked. If you find a more significant injury, suspect other severe injuries have occurred elsewhere and expand your focused exam.

As you conclude the focused trauma assessment, identify all injuries found, prioritize them, and establish an order of care for them. Identify the extent to which each injury may contribute to

hemorrhage and shock. Then prioritize the patient for transport. Taking these few moments to sort out what is wrong with the patient and to plan care steps increases your patient care efficiency, reduces on-scene time, and ensures the patient receives proper care at the right time.

Detailed Physical Exam

After you have ruled out or addressed potential threats to patient life or limb, attended to any serious problems, and assessed any suspected injuries, you may perform a detailed physical exam. You will most likely perform a detailed physical exam on a patient who is unconscious or has a lowered level of consciousness. The exam may be performed at the scene or, more likely, while en route to the hospital. A detailed physical exam is a search for signs and symptoms of further injury not suggested by the mechanism of injury analysis, by patient complaints, or by assessment to this point. It is performed as a head-to-toe evaluation, looking specifically where you have not looked before and with enough intensity to identify any subtle indications of injury. Be alert for signs and symptoms of internal or external injury or hemorrhage. Use the same assessment techniques for evaluating musculoskeletal injuries during a detailed physical exam that you employed during the rapid trauma assessment and focused history and physical exam.

Record the results of your assessment carefully. It may be helpful to use the mnemonic "NO LARD" to help remember the critical elements of fracture assessment: Name (of the bone involved), Open (versus closed injury), Location (distal, mid-shaft, or proximal), Angulation (the approximate angle of the distal segment), Rotation (either internal or external), and Displacement (shortened or lengthened in inches or centimeters.).

Reassessment

Reassessment focuses on serial measurement of patient vital signs, level of consciousness, and signs and symptoms of major trauma affecting the patient. For patients with musculoskeletal injuries, monitor distal sensation, motor function, capillary refill, and pulses frequently. Remember to ask the patient about how the musculoskeletal injury feels, watching for any change in response. As time passes and the "fight-or-flight" response effects wear off, a patient may display more significant and specific injury symptoms. A patient may also begin to complain of other injuries, major and moderate pain or discomfort masked earlier by the chief complaint or complaints. If this occurs, provide a focused trauma assessment for the area of complaint and modify your patient priorities as additional injuries are found and evaluated.

Sports Injury Considerations

Many musculoskeletal injuries you attend to as a paramedic are associated with sports activities. Activities such as football, basketball, soccer, hockey, baseball, in-line skating, skiing, snowboarding, bicycling, wrestling, hiking, and rock climbing often lead to participant injury. When you are called to a sports injury scene, assess the mechanism of injury and determine whether there was a major kinetic force involved, a hyperextension or flexion injury (or other injury mechanism involving moving a limb beyond its normal range of motion), or a fatigue-type injury. Athletic injuries often affect major body joints like the shoulder, elbow, wrist, knee, and ankle. Injuries in these areas are especially troubling for patients because serious ligament damage might preclude future sports participation and limit limb usefulness. It is imperative that any potentially significant sports injury be attended to by an emergency physician. Competitive natures of players, teammates, coaches, and athletic trainers may lead them to downplay injuries in order to keep an injured athlete in competition. Allowing an injured athlete to keep playing, however, places additional stress on the injury and may result in further, and more debilitating and/or permanent, damage.

A specific and serious musculoskeletal injury associated with sports is the sprain, especially of the knee. A sprain affects joint ligaments and is graded from minor (first degree) to complete rupture (third degree). Third-degree sprains destabilize the joint, require long-term healing, and may result in continuing or recurring joint instability. Sprains should be considered as serious orthopedic injuries. The most commonly sprained ligament of the knee is the anterior cruciate ligament. It prevents anterior displacement of the tibia on the femur and is frequently injured with hyperextension or twisting motions of the knee. A patient will likely report that the knee "gave out" during strenuous activity or impact. The injury will likely present with pain, swelling, and inability to support weight.

Strains can be equally significant as injuries. They are graded, with the third-degree strain resulting in a tear of the muscle mass or tendon or with complete tendon detachment from the bone. Third-degree injury to major tendons (Achilles, quadriceps, or patellar tendons) will result in complete limb instability and may require surgical repair. The shoulder is a complicated and extremely mobile joint and a common location of strain injury. The humerus is held in position with a grouping of four muscles that are collectively known as the rotator cuff. These muscles hold the joint together and provide much of the strength associated with shoulder motion. Their tear or rupture leaves the shoulder joint painful and unstable.

Care for orthopedic sports injury calls for affected limb immobilization and suspicion of potential spine injury. Keep in mind that limb injury may account for serious pain (a distracting injury) and make the patient an unreliable reporter of spinal symptoms.

MUSCULOSKELETAL INJURY MANAGEMENT

Musculoskeletal injury management is not normally a high priority in trauma patient care. It usually does not occur until after you have completed primary assessment; stabilized airway, breathing, and circulation; and finished rapid trauma assessment, if needed. While care focus for a serious trauma patient is for life threats, provide some protection for serious musculoskeletal injuries by moving the patient as a unit (with axial alignment) and by packaging the patient for transport using a long spine board. These techniques help you reduce risks of aggravating musculoskeletal injuries, increasing hemorrhage, and worsening shock. However, do not let a gruesome musculoskeletal injury distract you from trauma patient management priorities.

Pelvic and, to a lesser degree, femur fractures can significantly contribute to hypovolemia and shock. These injuries deserve a high priority in patient care. Other musculoskeletal injuries that merit a priority for care include those that threaten a limb, such as injuries with loss of distal circulation or sensation (most commonly joint injuries), and those that cause compartment syndrome (most likely crushing leg or forearm injuries). You may prioritize other injuries by relative size of the bone fractured or body area involved and by energy that was required to cause injury. Prioritize patient musculoskeletal injuries for care and then proceed with splinting and transport.[5]

General Principles of Musculoskeletal Injury Management

Objectives of musculoskeletal injury care are to reduce any further injury during patient care and transport and to reduce patient discomfort. Accomplish these goals by protecting open wounds and soft tissues, positioning the extremity properly, immobilizing the injured extremity, and monitoring neurovascular function in the distal limb (Figure 16). In some cases, care involves manipulating the injury to reestablish distal circulation and sensation or simply to restore normal anatomic position for the patient expecting prolonged extrication or transport. In most cases, care for musculoskeletal injuries involves application of a splinting device.[5]

As you begin to care for a patient with musculoskeletal injuries, talk to him and explain what you are doing, why, and what impact it will have on him. Alignment and splinting will likely first cause an increase in pain followed by a significant reduction in it. By telling a patient of this in advance, you increase his confidence in both your intent to help and your ability to provide care.

Protecting Open Wounds

If there is any open wound in proximity to the fracture or dislocation, consider the fracture or dislocation to be an open one. Carefully observe the wound and note any signs of muscle, tendon, ligament, or vascular injury and be prepared to describe it in your report and at the emergency department. Cover the wound with a sterile dressing held in place with bandaging or a splint. Frequently, attempts to align a limb, application of traction, or the splinting process itself will draw protruding bones back into the wound. This is an expected consequence of proper care but must be brought to the attention of the attending emergency physician.

CONTENT REVIEW

► Basics of Musculoskeletal Injury Care

- Protecting open wounds
- Proper positioning
- Immobilizing the injury
- Monitoring of neurovascular function

With high-energy mechanisms, the wounding energy may fracture (or even destroy) the bone and/or joint, thus amputating (partially or completely) the limb. The resulting amputated part should be placed in a clean, dry plastic bag, and kept cool with ice or an ice pack. Do not allow any portion of the amputated part to freeze.

Positioning the Limb

Proper limb positioning is essential to ensure patient comfort, to reduce chances of further limb injury, and to encourage venous drainage. Proper positioning is different with fractures and dislocations, although splinting with a limb in a normal anatomic position, the position of function, is beneficial for both.

Limb alignment is appropriate for any midshaft fracture of the femur, tibia/fibula, humerus, or radius/ulna. Alignment can be maintained by using an air splint, padded rigid splint, PASG, vacuum, or traction splint. Proper fracture alignment enhances circulation and reduces potential for further injury to surrounding tissue. It is also very difficult to immobilize a limb with a fracture in an unaligned, angulated position because fracture segments are short and buried in soft tissue. Perform any limb alignment with great care so as not to damage tissue surrounding the fracture site. During limb alignment, the proximal limb should remain in position while you bring the distal limb to alignment using gentle axial traction. Stop the process when you detect any resistance to movement or when the patient reports any significant increase in pain or discomfort.

Generally, you should not attempt alignment of dislocations or fractures within 3 inches of a joint. Only manipulate these injury sites when distal circulation is compromised. Then, try to move the joint while another care provider palpates the distal pulse. If the pulse is restored, if you meet significant resistance to movement, or if the patient complains of greatly increasing pain, stop the manipulation and splint the injured limb as it is. Be sure to transport the patient quickly, because circulation loss can endanger future limb usefulness.

If you suspect a limb will remain dislocated for an extended period, as during lengthy transports or prolonged patient entrapments, consider reducing the dislocation. Apply a firm and progressive traction to the limb, which draws the dislocated ends away from each other and moves the joint toward normal positioning. When (and if) the bone ends "pop" back into position, ensure there is a distal pulse and immobilize the limb in the position of function.

Proper positioning of injured limbs is important for maintaining distal circulation and sensation and increasing patient comfort. Deformities and extremes of flexion or extension put pressure on soft tissues and may compress nerves and blood vessels. These positions also fatigue surrounding muscles and increase pain associated with injury. By placing uninjured joints halfway between flexion and extension in what is called the position of function, you place the least stress on joint ligaments and muscles and tendons surrounding the injury. Place the limb in the position of function whenever possible (Figure 17 ●). Note, however, that some injuries and some splinting devices commonly used for musculoskeletal injuries may preclude this positioning.

When practical, elevate an injured limb. This assists venous drainage and reduces edema associated with musculoskeletal injury.

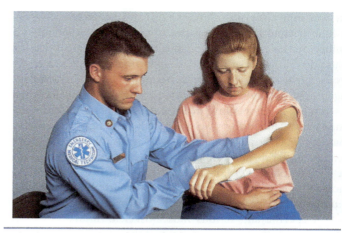

● **Figure 17**   Gently position the limb in the position of function, unless your attempts meet with resistance or a significant increase in pain or the injury is within 3 inches of a joint.

Immobilizing the Injury

The aim of immobilizing musculoskeletal injuries is to prevent further injury caused by post-injury movement of a strain, sprain, subluxation, dislocation, or fracture. Immobilization restricts fractured bone ends from further lacerating soft tissues, blood vessels, and nerves and from dislodging any clot development and internal hemorrhage control. In dislocations, immobilization prevents movement of dislodged bone ends at a joint where they may entrap or compress nerves and blood vessels and place further stress on ligaments, muscles, or tendons already injured by the injury mechanism. Immobilization of strains, sprains, and subluxations also reduces stress on ligaments, muscles, and tendons and protects the injury from further trauma. Immobilization of orthopedic injury is also an effective technique to reduce injury pain, especially that likely with limb movement during further care and patient transport. Orthopedic immobilization is usually accomplished using a splinting device.

Since most long bones are buried deep within an extremity's musculature, it is very difficult to immobilize them directly. Hence, we immobilize the joint above and joint below the injury, regardless of whether the injury occurs at a joint or mid-shaft of a long bone. This ensures that no motion is transmitted through the injury site as might occur, for example, with the rotation (supination/pronation) of the radius against the ulna at the elbow when the wrist turns.

Securing a splint to immobilize a limb often involves wrapping a limb circumferentially. Wrap any bandage associated with a splinting device from a distal point to a proximal one. This ensures that bandaging pressure moves any blood into the systemic circulation and does not trap it in the distal limb. This wrapping method assists venous drainage and the healing process. Apply firm pressure when wrapping, but be sure you can easily push a finger beneath the wrapping.

Checking Neurovascular Function

It is imperative that you identify circulation, motor function, and sensation status distal to the injury site before, during, and after splinting of all musculoskeletal injuries. A neurovascular check before splinting identifies a baseline condition and establishes whether or not an initial injury disrupts circulation. A neurovascular check during splinting ensures that inadvertent limb movement or circumferential pressure does not compromise distal circulation. The check after splinting identifies any restriction caused by progressive swelling of the injured area against the splinting device. Clearly identify and document these evaluations whenever you apply a splint.

To perform neurovascular evaluation, first palpate for a pulse and ensure it is equal in strength to that of the opposing limb. If the pulse cannot be located or is weak, check capillary refill and skin temperature, color, and general skin condition. Again compare your findings to the opposing limb. Ask the patient to describe the sensation when you rub or pinch the bottom of the foot or back of the hand and ask him to move the fingers or toes. Patient response establishes your baseline circulation, sensory, and motor findings. Reevaluate pulse, motor function, and sensation frequently during the remaining care and transport. If a care provider is holding the limb while you apply the splint, have him or her monitor pulse and skin color and temperature. That care provider then immediately recognizes any compromise in circulation.

A pulse oximeter can be used to monitor distal pulse during the splint process. Affix a probe to a free finger or toe and ensure a good reading. Then monitor the oximeter, watching for any change, especially if readings becoming erratic or the device becomes unable to obtain a reading at all. This suggests a compromise in distal circulation (loss of pulsing necessary to obtain a reading) and a need to reassess distal pulse, skin temperature, and capillary refill.

Local Cooling and Gentle Compression

As a general care principle for orthopedic injuries, supply local cooling and gentle pressure to the injury site. Limb structure injuries often result in local tissue inflammation and edema. This results in pain and swelling with a potential to increase pressure in tissues surrounding the limb (and especially surrounding joints). This swelling may reduce circulation to, and through, the injury site. Immediate local cooling reduces local pain, inflammation, and swelling. Provide local cooling with the application of cold packs wrapped in a towel. Be careful not to apply cold packs or ice directly to skin or a wound as it may cause further injury. Gentle pressure applied by firm bandaging to apply a splint may also assist in reducing swelling and pain. However, be sure the pressure does not affect distal circulation. Frequently monitor distal circulation, motor function, and sensation to ensure they remain adequate.

Splinting Devices

An essential part of managing any musculoskeletal system injury is the use of devices to immobilize a limb and permit patient transport without causing further injury. These devices, called splints, are designed to help reduce or eliminate movement of an injured extremity. Splints come in several forms that can assist in immobilizing common fractures and dislocations associated with musculoskeletal trauma. They include rigid, formable, vacuum, soft, traction, and other splints.

Rigid Splints

Rigid splints, as the name implies, are firm supports for an injured limb. They can be constructed of plastic, metal, synthetic products, wood, or cardboard. Such devices very effectively immobilize injury sites but require adequate padding to lessen patient discomfort. This padding may be built into the splint or may simply be a bulky dressing affixed to the splint with soft bandaging. Several types of commercially available rigid splints are used in prehospital care. They are usually flat and rigid devices and are about 3 inches wide and from 16 to 48 inches long. Cardboard splints are enjoying great popularity as they store flat, are folded to create a firm splinting surface, are disposable, and are relatively inexpensive (Figure 18 ●). A special form of rigid splint is the preformed splint. It is usually a stamped metal or preformed plastic or fiberglass device shaped to limb contours. These splints are usually available for ankles, forearms, and hands.

An aligned injured limb is immobilized to or within the splint using tape, cravats, or bandaging material to circumferentially wrap the limb. If the limb remains angulated, it may be held in position by cross-wrapping between the limb and splint at two locations.

Formable Splints

Another rigid splint type is the formable, or malleable, splint. It is made up of material that you can easily shape to match limb angulation. You then affix the formed splint to the limb with circumferential bandaging. Formable splints include both the ladder splint, which is a matrix of soft metal wires soldered together, and the metal sheet splint, which is made up of thin aluminum or another easily shaped metal. The SAM (Structural Aluminum Malleable) splint is an example of a sheet splint covered with padding and easily formed to a limb's shape.

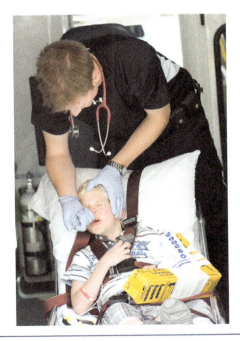

● **Figure 18** Cardboard splints are enjoying great popularity. (The medic in this photo is administering intranasal fentanyl for pain to the patient with the splinted arm.) (© *Kevin Link*)

Vacuum Splints

Vacuum splints sized for almost all long-bone fractures are available. The device is an airtight fabric bag filled with small plastic particles. The splint is negotiated around an injured limb, conformed to limb shape, and secured around it. As air is withdrawn from the device and small particles lock in position, a firmly fixed shape around the limb is created (Figure 19 ●). The splint firmly and comfortably secures a limb in position, although there is a small amount of shrinkage with air evacuation.

Soft Splints

Soft splints use padding or gentle air pressure to immobilize an injured limb. Soft splint varieties include air splints, the pelvic sling or binder, and pillow splints.

Though less frequently used than in the past, some systems continue to use the air splint. Air splints provide immobilization as air pressure fills the splint and compresses a limb. Since the splint is a formed cylinder, and may include shaping for the foot, it immobilizes the limb in an aligned position. Air splints should not be used with long bone injuries at or above the knee or elbow because they cannot prevent movement of hip or shoulder joints and are thus unable to immobilize the proximal limb joints. Air splints apply a pressure that may be helpful in controlling both external and internal hemorrhage. While these devices may limit distal extremity assessment, they do permit observation because they are transparent.

Monitor air splints carefully with any changes in temperature or atmospheric pressure. Increases in ambient heat or decreases in pressure, as during an ascent in a helicopter, increase splint pressure. Conversely, decreases in temperature or a descent in a helicopter decrease splint pressure. Constantly monitor air splint pressure to ensure they do not rise or fall during your care. You can easily do this by depressing the splint with your thumb and comparing the pressure you use and the indentation with earlier experiences.

Pelvic slings or binders are either commercially made devices or improvised fabric sheets that encompass the pelvis. They are tightened to contain, compress, and immobilize the pelvis. They are used for unstable pelvic ring fractures.

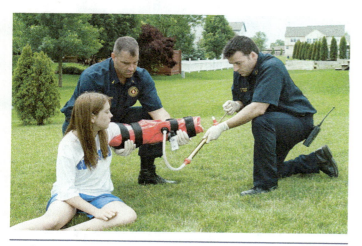

● **Figure 19** Suction the air out of a vacuum splint until the device is rigid. Reassess pulse, motor function, and sensation in the extremity after application.

Pillow splints are comfortable and effective for ankle and foot injuries. The foot is simply placed on a pillow while the outer pillow cover fabric is drawn around the foot and pillow. The outer fabric is pinned together or wrapped circumferentially with bandage material (Kling, Kerlix, or cravats) placed tightly around the injury site. This device applies gentle and uniform pressure to effectively immobilize the distal extremity. Using a bulky blanket or two to cradle the ankle and wrapping the blankets firmly may also provide effective immobilization.

Traction Splints

Traction splints were developed during World War I and used extensively during World War II. These splints dramatically reduced both mortality and limb loss from femur fractures caused by projectile wounds, blast injuries, and other battlefield traumas. Today, however, isolated mid-shaft femur fractures are relatively infrequent, as is the need for traction splinting.

The traction splint is a frame that applies a pull (traction) to an injured extremity and against the trunk. Traction application

---

PATHO PEARLS

The Traction Splint: Past, Present, and Future

The traction splint has been a mainstay of prehospital emergency care ever since J. D. (Deke) Farrington penned the pamphlet entitled "Death in a Ditch" and began what is today's modern EMS system. The traction splint was developed in the late 1800s and its worth was proven during the trench warfare of World War I. The old half-ring splint evolved into the "Hare" and then the "Sager"-style splints we find on almost every ambulance today. And, surely everyone who has been in EMS more than a decade can remember instances when its application turned a patient writhing in pain into someone with only limited discomfort. However, does the traction splint deserve to be a standard of care in the modern EMS system?

The traction splint is limited in its application to isolated femur fractures. In fractures of the hip or those in the vicinity of the knee, traction risks nervous or vascular complications, and the splint is likewise contraindicated in pelvic fractures or any serious skeletal injury to the distal extremity. It may also be contraindicated in multisystem trauma due to the time required for application and the likelihood of contraindicating injuries.[6] Recent research suggests that the incidence of injury requiring the traction splint is about five times in 10,000 prehospital patients. The study further identifies that 40 percent of patients with indications for the traction splint never had it applied, and an equal number of patients (two) had it applied when contraindications existed.

As we examine past, current, and future prehospital care skills, we must evaluate the traction splints' incidence of use and weigh their benefit against equipment costs and the training time necessary to ensure their proper use. As paramedic practitioners, we are aware that we may need to lay aside some mainstays of current prehospital practice as we strive to do the most good for the greatest number of patients.

is necessary when splinting a fractured femur, which is surrounded by very heavy musculature. Frequently, fracture pain initiates muscle spasm that causes bone ends to override each other, further aggravating the original injury and increasing pain and muscle spasm. Traction splinting sometimes lessens patient pain and may help relax any muscle spasm.

There are basically two styles of traction splint, the bipolar frame device and the unipolar device. The bipolar traction splint has a half ring that fits up and against the ischial tuberosity of the pelvis. A distal ratchet connects to a foot harness and pulls traction from the foot and against the pelvis. The frame lifts and supports the limb and a foot stand holds the injured limb and splint off the ground. This construction helps prevent limb motion during patient movement, while elevation supplied by the stand enhances venous drainage. A variation of the bipolar frame device is the Reel Splint (Figure 20 ●). It has the design features of the bipolar frame traction splint with the added feature that the frame can be bent at the knee. It can accommodate knee dislocations and may provide more comfortable limb positioning for femur fractures.

The unipolar (Sager) traction splint uses a single lengthening shaft to pull a foot harness against pressure applied to the pubic bone. The unipolar splint does not elevate or stabilize the extremity, so you must observe greater care whenever you move the patient.

Other Splinting Aids

Cravats or Velcro straps can augment the effectiveness of rigid splints. You can secure the lower extremities, one to the other, to help the patient control musculoskeletal injury sites or you can use a sling and swathe to help immobilize a splinted upper extremity to the chest. Humerus fractures are difficult to immobilize because the shoulder is such a large and mobile body region. A sling around the neck and across the wrist may hold the elbow at a fixed angle, while a swathe secures the limb against the chest to limit further shoulder motion (cuff and collar sling and swath). By holding a thumb in the fold of the elbow, the patient can easily reduce any limb motion and complement the splinting process.

In patients with serious multisystem trauma, other injuries preclude splinting individual fractures and dislocations. In such cases, you may splint limbs to the body with cravats or bandage material and immobilize the patient to a long spine board. Simply strap the body and limbs to the board and transport the patient as a unit. While this is not definitive splinting, it will provide reasonable protection for musculoskeletal injuries. If time and patient priorities permit, provide a more definitive splint while transporting the patient.

Fracture Care

A fracture occurring near a joint (generally within 3 inches) carries a high probability of blood vessel, nerve, and joint capsule involvement. To protect against further complicating this injury, treat any musculoskeletal injury in the proximity of a joint as a joint injury. This necessitates carefully immobilizing the limb in the position found unless there is a significant circulatory or nervous deficit.

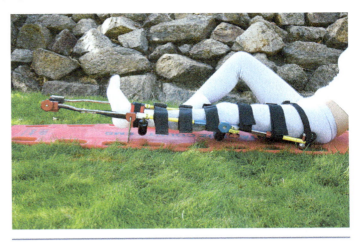

● **Figure 20a**   The Reel Splint has features of the bipolar frame traction splint. (© *Reel Research and Development*)

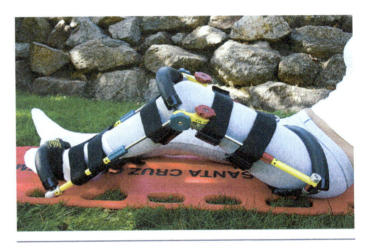

● **Figure 20b**   The Reel Splint can be bent at the knee. (© *Reel Research and Development*)

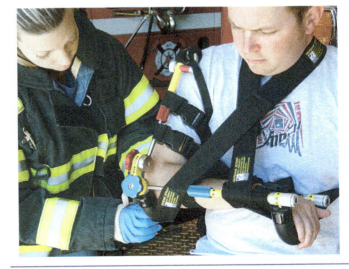

● **Figure 20c**   A pediatric-size Reel Splint can be used to splint an adult arm. (© *Reel Research and Development*)

Begin fracture care by ensuring distal pulses, sensation, and motor function. Then align the limb for splinting. Quickly recheck distal circulation and motor and sensory function. If you identify any neurovascular deficit, attempt to correct it by gentle repositioning, even if a limb is relatively aligned. If the limb is angulated, proceed with realignment. Remember that most splinting devices are designed to immobilize aligned limbs and that alignment provides the best chance for ensuring good neurovascular function.

To move an injured limb from an angulated position into alignment, use gentle distal traction applied manually. Also consider aligning a limb if a bone end is close to the skin and in danger of converting a closed fracture into an open one. Have an assisting EMT immobilize the proximal limb in the position found. Grasp the distal limb firmly and apply traction along and in the direction of the proximal limb's axis, gently moving it from angulated to an aligned position. Should you feel any resistance to movement or notice a great increase in patient discomfort, stop alignment and splint the limb as it lies. Once you complete alignment, recheck distal neurovascular function. If it is adequate, proceed with splinting. If function is inadequate, move the limb around slightly while another care provider monitors for a pulse. If one attempt at gentle manipulation does not reestablish a pulse, splint and transport the patient quickly.

Proceed with splinting by selecting an appropriate device and secure the limb to it in a way that ensures you immobilize both the fracture site and adjacent joints. Have a care provider who is holding the limb apply a gentle traction to stabilize the limb (and monitor the distal pulse) during splinting. If you apply your splint properly, the device may maintain this traction and provide greater limb stabilization and greater patient comfort. Secure the limb to the body (upper extremity) or to the opposite limb (lower extremity) to protect it and to give the patient some control over the limb.

Joint Care

Joint care, too, begins with assessment for distal neurovascular function. Immobilize the joint in the position found if you find adequate circulation, sensation, and motor function. Use a ladder, vacuum, or other malleable splint, shaped to the limb's angle, or cross-wrap with a padded rigid splint to immobilize the joint in place. Ensure that your splinting immobilizes the injured joint and both the joint above and the joint below the injury. If not, secure the limb firmly to the body to immobilize these joints.

If circulation or motor or sensory function is lost below the joint injury, consider moving the limb to reestablish it. Have another care provider stabilize the proximal limb in position while you monitor the circulation and sensation and gently move the limb. If you can reestablish neurovascular function quickly, splint the limb in the new position. If not, splint and provide quick transport.

With some joint injuries, you may attempt to return the displaced bone ends to their normal anatomic position. This process is called **reduction** and has both benefits and hazards. An early return to normal position reduces stress on the ligaments and basic joint structure and facilitates better distal circulation and sensation. However, the process has a risk of trapping blood vessels or nerves as bone ends return to their normal anatomic position. Attempt dislocation reduction only when you are sure the injury *is* a dislocation, when you expect the patient's arrival at the emergency department to be delayed (prolonged extrication or long transport time), or when there is a significant neurovascular deficit. Do not attempt a reduction if the dislocation is associated with other serious patient injuries. Consult your protocols and medical direction to identify criteria for attempting dislocation reduction used in your system.

When performing a joint reduction, you attempt to protect the articular surface while directing the bones back to their normal anatomic position. Begin the process by providing the patient with analgesic therapy to reduce pain associated with the injury and the reduction itself. Then have an assisting care provider hold the proximal extremity in position and provide counter-traction during the reduction. You apply increasing traction to pull the bone surfaces apart, reducing pressure between non-articular surfaces. Slowly increase traction and direct the displaced limb toward its normal anatomic position. Successful relocation is indicated when you feel the joint "pop" back into position, the patient experiences a lessening of pain, and the joint becomes mobile within at least a few minutes of the procedure. Carefully evaluate distal circulation, sensation, and motor function after reduction. If the procedure does not meet with success within a few minutes, splint the limb as it is and provide rapid patient transport. If reduction is successful, splint the limb in the position of function and transport.

Muscular and Connective Tissue Care

Injuries to musculoskeletal system soft tissues deserve special care. While such injuries are not usually life threatening, they can be very painful and, in some cases, threaten limbs. For example, compartment syndrome can restrict capillary blood flow, venous blood return, and nerve function at and beyond the site of the injury. If such an injury is not discovered and remedied, it may produce severe disability. Deep contusions and especially large hematomas can also contribute to blood loss and hypovolemia. Once you care for life threats, fractures, joint injuries, and other limb threats, give injuries to muscular and connective tissues your attention.

To manage muscle, tendon, and ligament injuries, immobilize the region surrounding them. Doing so reduces associated internal hemorrhage and pain. Provide gentle circumferential bandaging (loose enough to let you slide a finger underneath) to further reduce hemorrhage, edema, and pain, but be sure to monitor distal circulation and loosen the bandage further if there are any signs of neurovascular deficit. Local cooling reduces both edema and patient discomfort. Be careful to wrap any cold or ice pack in a dressing or towel to prevent too drastic a cooling and consequent injury. You may apply heat to the wound after 48 hours to enhance both circulation and healing. If possible, place the limb in the position of function and elevate the extremity to ensure good venous return, limit swelling, and reduce patient discomfort. Monitor distal neurovascular function to ensure your actions do not compromise circulation, sensation, or motor function.

Care for Specific Fractures

Pelvis

Pelvic fractures involve either the iliac crest or pelvic ring. While iliac crest fractures may reflect serious trauma, they do not represent the patient life-threat suggested by ring fractures. Iliac crest fractures are often isolated and stable injuries that you can care for by simple patient immobilization. The pelvis may also suffer isolated fractures at the symphysis pubis or sacroiliac joint. Pelvic ring fracture due to a high-energy trauma event, and especially if it is associated with hypotension, carries a high mortality rate and is considered a critical/high-priority injury.

The pelvis is a very large, strong and important skeletal structure. It supports the abdomen, thorax, upper extremities, neck, and head. It protects the genitalia, urinary bladder, terminal end of the alimentary canal, and the major blood vessels serving the lower extremities. It also serves as the articulation point with the lower extremities and lumbar spine. In addition, the pelvis is actively involved in blood cell production, has a rich blood supply of bridging vessels supplying its interior, and its interior surface is adjacent to major blood vessels that perfuse the lower extremities.

Pelvic fractures can be divided into four types of fracture. Type I fractures involve fractures not involving the pelvic ring and include avulsion fractures and those of the pubis, sacrum, coccyx, ischium, or iliac wing. Type II fractures involve a single break in the pelvic ring, maintain pelvic stability, and include unilateral ring fractures and symphysis pubis and sacroiliac fractures. Type III fractures involve high energy and multiple ring fractures (and likely hypovolemia). Type IV fractures involve the acetabulum.

A specific type of pelvic fracture is the open-book fracture. It is caused by an anterior-posterior compression mechanism that disrupts the sacroiliac joint and separates the symphysis pubis. This injury increases the volume of the pelvic space and may permit severe, difficult-to-control hemorrhage.

The pelvic ring shape gives it great strength, but when this ring breaks, the injury often results in fractures at two sites. Kinetic forces necessary to fracture the pelvic ring are significant and are likely to produce fractures and internal injuries elsewhere. Veins in this area are without valves, have limited musculature, and may experience retrograde blood flow when they are torn. Injury to the pelvic ring, therefore, can result in heavy hemorrhage that is likely to empty into the pelvic and retroperitoneal spaces. This loss can easily exceed 2 liters. Such injury may also result in circulation impairment to one or both lower extremities. Pelvic fractures may also be associated with hip dislocations and injuries to the bladder, female reproductive organs, urethra, prostate in the male, and alimentary canal (anus and rectum).

Pelvic injury care objectives include stabilizing the fractured pelvis, supporting the patient hemodynamically, and providing rapid transport to a trauma center. Because of the severe blood loss potential and difficulty in immobilizing a broken pelvic ring, application of the PASG or a pelvic sling or binder is sometimes recommended for pelvic fractures (Figure 21a ●). The pelvic sling or binder is a wide band, either commercially available (Figure 21b ●) or made from a sheet. To make a pelvic sling, fold a sheet to about 10 inches wide and gently negotiate

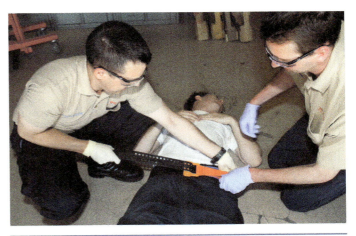

● **Figure 21a**   The SAM pelvic wrap. (© Dr. Bryan E. Bledsoe)

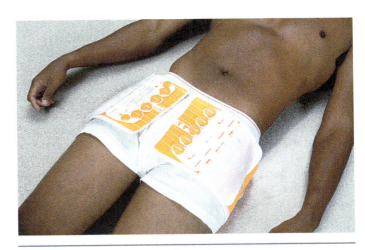

● **Figure 21b**   A T-POD pelvic splint system.

it under a patient, or move the patient to the spine board with the device in place. The band should engage the pelvis with the band's upper border just below the iliac crests. Secure the commercial device or sheet firmly to immobilize the pelvis with firm but not excessive pressure. Place a folded blanket between a patient's lower extremities and tie them together. If necessary for comfort, place a pillow under a patient's knees.[7]

If the patient is hypotensive, start a large-bore IV, and hang one 1,000-mL bag of normal saline. Set up using trauma tubing, and administer fluid boluses as needed to maintain a systolic blood pressure of at least 80 mmHg. Monitor for a palpable pulse and any changes in level of consciousness. Always consider a pelvic fracture patient to be a candidate for rapid transport.

Femur

Femur fractures may be traumatic, resulting from very strong and violent forces, or atraumatic, resulting from degenerative diseases. Patients with disease-induced fractures usually are of advancing age and present with a history of a degenerative disease, a clouded or limited trauma history, and only moderate discomfort. The patient often displays some limb shortening, external rotation, and limited deformity. Care for such patients by immobilizing them as found and then providing gentle transport. Generally, you can provide effective splinting by placing the patient on a long spine board and padding with pillows and blankets for patient comfort. Traction splint use is not essential because pain is not inducing spasms that cause broken bone ends to override.

A patient who has suffered a traumatic femur fracture usually experiences extreme discomfort, and is often writhing in pain. In such patients, providing distal traction immobilizes both bone ends, relieves muscle spasms, and reduces associated pain. Traction splinting is the best avenue for care of the hemodynamically stable patient with an isolated femur fracture. However, the traction splint is not indicated if the patient has concurrent serious pelvic, knee, tibia, or foot injuries.

Proximal fractures (surgical neck and intertrochanteric fractures) are frequently caused by hip injuries, transmitted forces, or the degenerative effects of aging. These proximal femur fractures, which are commonly referred to as hip fractures, do not benefit from traction splinting, and a traction splint should not be used. In contrast, mid-shaft fractures often result from high-energy, lateral traumas and are associated with significant blood loss. Injuries to the distal femur (condylar and epicondylar fractures) can be extensive and are likely to involve blood vessels, nerves, and connective tissue. The energy necessary to fracture the femur may be sufficient to dislocate the hip and cause serious internal injuries elsewhere. Mid-shaft femur fractures without associated hip or pelvis injuries gain the most benefit from traction splinting.[8]

You may find it difficult to differentiate between proximal femur fractures (hip fractures) and anterior hip dislocations. Generally, a femur fracture presents with the foot externally rotated (turned outward) and the injured limb shortened when compared to the uninjured limb. This difference may be slight and may be unnoticeable if the patient's legs are not straight and parallel. An anterior dislocation presents similarly to the femur fracture, but with the femoral head protruding into the inguinal region. In either case, treat as a dislocation. Traction splints should not be used in either case or if a joint injury (hip or knee) is suspected.

If you suspect an isolated mid-shaft femur fracture, align the limb, determine the circulation and sensory and motor function status, and apply the traction splint or possibly the PASG. (If you use manual traction to align the femur, maintain it until the splint is applied and continues that traction.) Adjust splint length to the uninjured extremity, position the device against the pelvis, and secure it in position with the inguinal strap. With a bipolar splint, apply the ankle hitch, provide gentle traction, and elevate the distal limb to place the splint's ring against the ischial tuberosity. With a unipolar splint, position the T-shaped support against the pubic bone and simply apply the ankle hitch. Ensure that the hitch and splint hold the foot and limb in an anatomic position as you apply firm traction. Position and secure the limb to the splint with straps, then gently move the patient and splint to a long spine board. Firmly secure the patient and limb for transport.

Guide your traction application by your patient's response. Ask the patient how the limb feels as you initiate and increase the traction. Stop the traction application when the limb is immobilized and patient discomfort eases. Remember, as traction prevents bone end overriding, injury pain should decrease. This reduces muscle spasm strength and lets the limb return toward its initial length. This, in turn, reduces traction provided by the splint, which means that bone ends are no longer well immobilized. Check traction frequently to ensure that it does not lessen during your care. If the patient reports increasing pain, consider increasing traction gradually until some reduction in pain is noted.

When other patient injuries or the need for rapid transport preclude using a traction splint, consider placing the patient on a long spine board for immobilization and transport. Use long, padded rigid splints, one medial and one lateral, to quickly splint the injured limb, and then tie that limb to the uninjured one. Use an orthopedic stretcher or another device or movement technique to transfer the patient to a long spine board and secure the patient firmly on it.[8]

Tibia/Fibula

Fractures of leg bones, the tibia and fibula, can occur separately or together. The tibia is the most commonly fractured leg bone and may be broken by direct force, crushing injury, or twisting forces. Tibial fracture is likely to cause an open wound. Fibular fractures are often associated with damage to the knee or ankle. If the tibia is fractured and the fibula is intact, the extremity may not angulate, but it is not able to bear weight. If only the fibula is broken, the limb may be relatively stable. Injuries to either bone may result in compartment syndrome. Direct trauma suffered during an auto crash or athletic impact frequently causes these tibia and fibula injuries.

Align the injured limb; assess circulation, sensation, and motor function; and then immobilize the limb with gentle traction. A full-leg air splint (one that accommodates the foot and knee), vacuum, or lateral or medial padded rigid splint provide effective immobilization (Figure 22 ●). You may also use a cardboard splint as long as it accommodates the full limb and is rigid enough to maintain immobilization. After you splint an injured limb, secure it to the uninjured leg. This affords some protection against uncontrolled movement and may reassure a patient that they still have some control over the extremity.

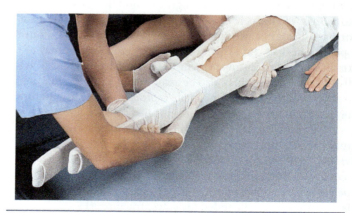

● **Figure 22** Placement of long padded board splints laterally and medially can effectively splint tibia/fibula fractures.

Clavicle

The clavicle is the most frequently fractured bone in the human body. Fractures to it usually result from transmitted forces directed along the upper extremity that cause relatively minor skeletal injury. The clavicle, however, is located adjacent to both the upper reaches of the lung and the vasculature serving the upper extremity and head. Hence, a clavicle injury may cause serious internal injury, especially if very powerful injury mechanisms are involved. The clavicular fracture patient often presents with pain and a shoulder shifted forward with palpable deformity along the clavicle. Accomplish splinting by immobilizing the affected limb in a sling and swathe against the chest. Monitor the patient carefully for any internal hemorrhage signs or respiratory compromise.

The clavicle may also dislocate with severe forces. A dislocation at the sternum (sternoclavicular) joint can be immobilized with a figure-of-eight dressing, gently pulling the shoulders back. A dislocation at the shoulder (acromioclavicular) is best immobilized with a sling and swath.

Humerus

A fractured humerus is very difficult to immobilize at its proximal end. The proximal humerus is buried within arm and shoulder muscles, and the shoulder joint is very mobile atop the thoracic cage. The axillary artery runs through the medial aspect of the shoulder joint (the axilla), making it difficult to apply any mechanical traction to the limb without compromising circulation. Hence, the most effective techniques for splinting this fracture are to apply a sling and swathe to immobilize the bent limb against the chest or to secure the extended and splinted limb against the body.

The preferred technique to secure a fractured humerus is to use a "cuff and collar" sling and swath. Apply a short, padded rigid splint to the arm's lateral surface to distribute any pressure of the swathing and better immobilize the arm. Sling the forearm with a cravat, catching just the wrist region and not the elbow. This permits some gravitational traction in the seated patient and prevents inadvertent pressure application by the sling, which could flex the limb. Then use several cravats to gently swathe the arm and forearm to the chest. If the patient is conscious, have him place the thumb of the uninjured extremity in the elbow's fold to help control the injured limb's motion. This gives your patient control over the limb, decreases limb movement, and increases patient comfort.

You may also immobilize a limb by using a long, padded rigid splint affixed to the extended limb. Place the splint along the medial aspect of the upper extremity and ensure that it does not apply pressure to the axilla. Such pressure disrupts axillary artery blood flow to the limb and is uncomfortable for the patient. Secure the splint firmly to the limb, wrapping from the distal end toward the proximal end. Then secure the splint to the supine patient's body, and move the patient and splint to a long spine board.

Radius/Ulna

The forearm may fracture anywhere along its length and fracture may involve the radius, ulna, or both. Most commonly, fracture occurs at the distal end of the radius, just above its articular surface, and displaces the bone end in a volar (toward the palm) direction. This is known as Colles' fracture, and it presents with the wrist turned up at an unusual angle. Another term for this injury is "silver fork deformity" because it is contoured like a fork and the distal limb often becomes ashen. As with most joint fractures, a major concern is for distal circulation and innervation. If you find a neurovascular injury, use only slight adjustments to restore nervous or circulatory function because movement in this area is likely to cause further neurovascular injury.

Splint forearm fractures with a short, padded rigid splint affixed to the forearm and hand. Secure the hand in the position of function by placing a large dressing material wad in the palm to maintain a position like that of holding a large ball. Place a rigid splint along the medial forearm surface and wrap circumferentially from fingers to elbow. Leave at least one digit exposed to permit checking for capillary refill and skin color. Bend the elbow across the chest and use a sling and swathe to hold the limb in position. This provides relative elevation and improves venous drainage in both seated and supine patients.

An air splint or long, padded rigid splint, tied firmly to the body's side, may also adequately immobilize forearm fractures (Figure 23 ●). When using these devices, remember to place the hand in the position of function to increase patient comfort.

Care for Specific Joint Injuries

Hip

The hip may dislocate in two directions, anteriorly and posteriorly. Anterior dislocation presents with the foot turned outward and the femur's head palpable in the inguinal area (Figure 24 ●). Posterior dislocation is most common and presents with the knee flexed and foot rotated internally. The femur's displaced head is buried in the buttocks muscle and may impinge on the sciatic nerve. Sciatic nerve injury may result in the inability to flex the knee and in reduced sensation in the foot and posterior and lateral leg.

Immobilize a patient with either dislocation on a long spine board using pillows and blankets as padding to maintain patient position and provide comfort. If distal circulation, sensation, or

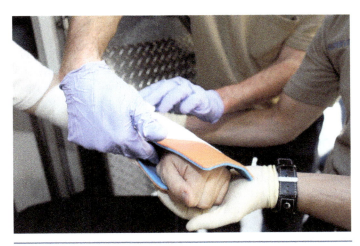

Figure 23 A "sugar tong" flexible (SAM) splint can effectively splint a forearm fracture. (© Dr. Bryan E. Bledsoe)

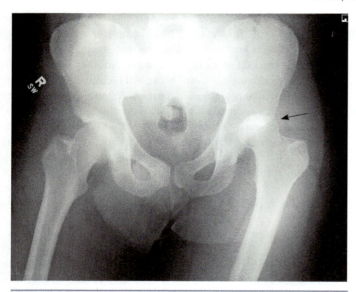

● **Figure 24** An anterior hip dislocation (patient's left, readers right). *(© Dr. Bryan E. Bledsoe)*

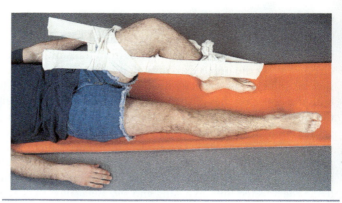

● **Figure 25** Angulated knee dislocations can be immobilized with two padded rigid splints.

motor function is severely compromised, consider one attempt at posterior dislocation reduction. (Consult local protocols and medical direction to identify criteria for reduction attempts.) However, do not attempt reduction if there are other serious injuries, like a pelvic fracture, associated with the hip dislocation. Anterior dislocations in general cannot be managed by reduction in the prehospital setting.

For reduction of a posterior hip dislocation, have a care provider hold the pelvis firmly against a long spine board or other firm surface by placing downward pressure on the iliac crests. Flex both the patient's hip and knee at 90 degrees and apply a firm, slowly increasing traction along the femur's axis. Gently rotate the femur externally (outward). It takes some time for the thigh muscles to relax, but when they do the femur head will "pop" back into position. If you feel this "pop" or if the patient reports a sudden pain relief and is able to easily extend the leg, reduction has likely been successful. Immobilize the patient in a comfortable position, either in flexion (not to exceed 90 degrees) or fully supine with the hip and leg in full extension. Reevaluate sensation, motor function, and circulation. If the femur head does not move into the acetabulum after a few minutes of your attempted reduction, immobilize the patient as found and consider rapid transport. Because of the strength of the hip joint, posterior and anterior hip dislocation reductions often take several strong providers and possible patient sedation. Again, consult your protocols and medical direction before beginning this procedure.

Knee

Knee injuries may include fractures of the femur, tibia, or both; patellar dislocations; or frank dislocations of the knee. The knee joint is held together by four major ligaments: the anterior and posterior cruciate and medial and lateral collateral ligaments. Because the knee is such a large joint and bears such a great amount of weight, the ligaments may be injured by compression, twisting, torsion (when the body is twisted against a firmly planted foot), or hyperextension. These injuries can be serious

and may threaten a patient's future ability to walk. Another concern with knee injury is possible injury to the major blood vessel traversing the area, the popliteal artery. This artery is less mobile than blood vessels in other joints, which leaves it more subject to injury and resulting distal vascular compromise.

Immobilize knee joint fractures and patellar dislocations in the position found unless distal circulation, sensation, or motor function is disrupted. If the limb is flexed, splint it with two medium rigid splints, placing one medially and one laterally (Figure 25 ●). Cross-wrap the splint and limb with bandage material to secure the limb in position. You may also use ladder or malleable splints, conformed to the limb's angle and placed anteriorly and posteriorly, or form and evacuate a vacuum splint to immobilize the knee. If the limb is extended, simply apply two padded rigid splints or a full-leg air splint.

Patellar dislocations are more common than frank knee dislocations and usually leave the knee in a flexed position with lateral patella displacement. The injured knee appears significantly deformed, though patellar dislocation has a lower incidence of vascular injury than does knee dislocation.

Anterior knee dislocations produce an extended limb contour that lifts at the knee (moving from proximal to distal) while posterior dislocations produce a limb that drops at the knee. (Ensure that the injury is not a patellar dislocation.) If there is neurovascular compromise, have another care provider immobilize the femur firmly in position. You then grasp the calf muscle, just above the ankle, and apply firm and progressive traction, first along the axis of the tibia and then pulling the limb toward alignment with the femur. With posterior dislocations, a third care provider may provide moderate downward pressure on the distal femur and upward pressure on the proximal tibia to facilitate reduction. As with most dislocations, success is measured by feeling the bone end "pop" back into place, hearing the patient report a dramatic reduction in pain, and noting freer limb movement at the knee joint. Once you reduce a knee dislocation, immobilize the joint in the position of function and transport the patient. If you cannot reduce a dislocation within a few minutes with distal traction, immobilize the extremity in the position found and transport quickly. Perform a knee dislocation reduction even if the patient has good distal circulation and nervous function when the time to definitive care will exceed 2 hours.

Ankle

Ankle injuries often produce a distal lower limb that is grossly deformed, either due to malleolar fracture, dislocation, or both. Sprains are also injuries of concern, although the limb remains in anatomic position. Splint sprains or nondisplaced fractures with an air splint (shaped to accommodate the foot) or with long rigid splints positioned on either side of the leg and ankle, padded liberally, and wrapped firmly. You may also use a pillow splint, especially if there is any ankle deformity (Figure 26 ●). Apply local cooling to ease the pain and reduce swelling.

Ankle dislocation may occur in any of three directions: anteriorly, posteriorly, or laterally. Anterior dislocation presents with a dorsiflexed (upward pointing) foot that appears shortened. Posterior dislocation appears to lengthen a plantar flexed (downward-pointing) foot. Lateral dislocation is most common and presents with a foot turned outward with respect to the ankle. If distal neurovascular compromise indicates a need for reduction, have a care provider grasp the calf, hold it in position, and pull against the traction you apply. You then grasp the heel with one hand and the metatarsal arch with the other. Pull a distal traction to disengage bone ends and protect articular cartilage during relocation. For anterior dislocations, move the foot posteriorly with respect to the ankle; with lateral dislocations, rotate the foot medially; with posterior dislocations, pull the heel toward you and the foot toward you, then away. The joint should return to a normal position with a "pop," a reduction in patient pain, and an increase in the mobility of the joint. Apply local cooling and immobilize the limb. If the procedure does not result in joint reduction within a few minutes, splint the joint as found and provide rapid transport.

Foot

Injuries to the foot include dislocations and fractures to calcanei (heel bones), metatarsals, and phalanges. Injuries to calcanei generally result from falls and can cause significant pain and swelling and are sometimes associated with lumbar vertebral fractures. Injuries to metatarsals and phalanges can result from penetrating or blunt trauma or typical "stubbing" of a toe. Fatigue fractures of metatarsal bones, or "march fractures," are relatively common. These injuries are reasonably stable, even though the extremity cannot bear weight. When foot or ankle injury is suspected, anticipate both bilateral foot injuries and lumbar spinal injury.

Immobilize foot injuries in much the same way you do with ankle injuries. Use pillow, vacuum, ladder, or air splints (with foot accommodation). If possible, leave some portion of the foot accessible so you can monitor distal capillary refill or, at least, skin temperature and color.

Shoulder

Shoulder fractures most commonly involve the proximal humerus, lateral scapula, and distal clavicle. Dislocations can include anterior, posterior, and inferior displacement of the humoral head. Anterior dislocations displace the humoral head forward, resulting in a shoulder that appears "hollow" or "squared-off," with a patient holding the arm close to the chest and forward of the mid-axillary line. Posterior dislocations rotate the arm internally, and a patient presents with the elbow and forearm held away from the chest. Inferior dislocations displace the humoral head downward, with the result that a patient's arm is often locked above the head.

You should immobilize shoulder injuries, like all joint injuries, as found, unless pulse, sensation, or motor function distal to the injury is absent. Immobilize anterior and posterior dislocations with a sling and swathe and, if needed, place a pillow under the arm and forearm. Immobilization of any inferior dislocation (with the upper extremity fixed above the head) will call for ingenuity on your part in splinting. In such cases, immobilize the extended arm in the position found. Using cravats, tie a long, padded splint to the torso, shoulder girdle, arm, and forearm to immobilize the upper extremity above the head. Gently move the patient to a long spine board and secure both splint and patient to the spine board.

Reduce anterior and posterior shoulder dislocations by placing a strap across the patient's chest, under the affected shoulder (through the axilla) and across the back. Have a care provider prepared to pull countertraction across the chest and superiorly using the strap. You, meanwhile, should flex the patient's elbow, drawing the arm somewhat away from the body (abduction) and pull firm traction along the axis of the humerus. Some slight internal and external humerus rotation may facilitate reduction. For reduction of inferior dislocations, have one care provider hold the thorax while you flex the elbow. Gradually apply firm traction along the axis of the humerus and gently rotate the arm externally. If the joint does not relocate in a few minutes, immobilize it as it lies and transport the patient. If reduction is successful, immobilize the upper extremity in the normal anatomic position with a sling and swathe.

Elbow

Elbow injuries display a high incidence of nervous and vascular involvement, especially in children. As in the knee, blood vessels running through the elbow region are held firmly in place. The probability is good, therefore, that any fracture or dislocation will involve the brachial artery and medial, ulnar, and radial nerves. Assess distal neurovascular function and, if you detect a deficit, move the joint very carefully and minimally to restore distal circulation. Then splint the elbow with a single padded rigid splint,

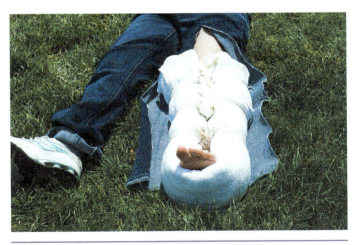

● **Figure 26** A pillow splint is made with readily available soft material such as a pillow, or a blanket.

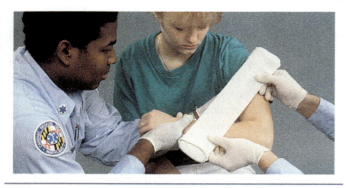

● **Figure 27** Use a padded board splint to immobilize angulated fractures or dislocations of the elbow.

providing cross-strapping as necessary, or use a ladder splint bent to conform to the limb's angle (Figure 27 ●). Keeping the wrist slightly elevated above the elbow, secure the limb to the chest using a sling and swathe. This position increases venous return and reduces swelling and pain associated with injury.

Wrist/Hand

Hand and wrist fractures are commonly associated with direct trauma. They present with very noticeable deformity and significant pain reported by the patient. These fractures are of serious concern to the patient. Since the hand and wrist bones are small, any fracture is close to a joint. Exercise caution as you care for these injuries because of possible vascular and neural involvement.

You can effectively immobilize musculoskeletal injuries of the forearm, wrist, hand, or fingers with a padded rigid, vacuum, or air splint. Place a roll of bandaging, a wad of dressing material, or some similar object in the patient's hand to maintain position of function. Then secure the extremity to a padded board with circumferential wrapping or inflate the air splint. Be sure to leave some portion of the distal extremity accessible so that you can monitor perfusion adequacy and sensation. Place the wrist above the elbow to assist venous return and reduce distal swelling.

Hand and wrist injuries are very common, particularly among athletes and children. A particular type of wrist fracture is Colles' fracture in which the wrist has a "silver fork" appearance (explained earlier). Fortunately, such injuries are seldom serious and can be managed in the prehospital setting quite easily.

Finger or Toe

Forces may displace phalanges from their joints, resulting in deformity and pain. Dislocation usually occurs between phalanges or between the proximal phalanx and metacarpal with the distal bone displaced either anteriorly or posteriorly. (Amputations are multisystem injuries that severely damage the musculoskeletal system.

Splint finger fractures using tongue blades or small, malleable splints shaped to the injured finger positioning. The finger may also be taped to adjoining fingers (buddy taping) to limit additional motion. The hand is then placed in the position of function and further immobilized.

Finger dislocations usually involve the proximal joint (and sometimes the distal joint) with the digit commonly displacing

posteriorly. If reduction is indicated, grasp the distal finger and apply a firm distal traction. Then direct the digit toward the normal anatomic position by moving its proximal end. You should feel the finger "pop" into place, and the digit should resume its normal alignment when compared to an uninjured finger on the other hand. Splint the finger with a slight bend (10 to 15 degrees) and immobilize the hand in the position of function.

Toe fractures and dislocations are generally treated in a fashion similar to finger injuries. Because of their small size and low likelihood of long-term problems, toe injuries are a low-priority problem and should be addressed after all other significant injuries are assessed and treated. In most cases, buddy taping and a loose-fitting shoe is an adequate splint for most toe fractures and dislocations of the toes.

Soft and Connective Tissue Injuries

Tendon, ligament, and muscle injuries are rarely, if ever, life threatening. Massive muscular contusions and hematomas can, however, contribute to hypovolemia, while ligament and tendon injuries can endanger future limb function. Be careful about permitting the patient to put further stress on a limb, especially with higher grades of sprains. Weakened ligaments may fail completely, resulting in complete joint instability or dislocation. Treat tendon, ligament, and muscle injuries as you would dislocations and immobilize adjacent joints. Monitor distal neurovascular function because tissue swelling and resulting pressure within circumferential wrapping of a splint may compress blood vessels and nerves. Care for muscular injuries with immobilization, gentle compression with snug (but not overly tight) dressings, and local cooling to suppress edema and pain using cold packs or ice wrapped in dressing material or a towel. Be watchful for compartment syndrome signs, especially in the calf and forearm.

Open wounds involving muscles, tendons, and ligaments can be severe and debilitating. Carefully evaluate such wounds for connective tissue involvement. Be especially watchful with deep open injuries close to joints. With such wounds, tendon and ligament disruption is likely and may adversely affect future use of the joint, muscles controlling the joint, or muscles controlling joint movement proximal or distal to the injury. Carefully evaluate for circulation, sensation, and motor function below these injuries.

Injury to a muscle or tendon may limit its ability to either extend or flex the limb. The opposing muscle moves the limb, while injured muscle cannot return it to a normal position. With limb injuries, note any unusual limb position, especially if the patient is unable to return the limb to a neutral position. At any sign of pain or dysfunction, splint the limb.

Medications

Medications are frequently administered to patients with musculoskeletal injury to relieve pain and to premedicate before relocation of a dislocation. Medications used include diazepam, morphine, and fentanyl.

Sedatives/Analgesics

Diazepam Diazepam (Valium) is a benzodiazepine with both anti-anxiety and skeletal muscle relaxant qualities. Although it does not have any pain-relieving properties, diazepam does reduce patient perception and memory of pain. It is used with musculoskeletal injuries and to premedicate patients before painful procedures such as cardioversion and dislocation reduction. It is administered in a slow IV bolus of 5 to 15 mg, not to exceed 5 mg/minute, into a large vein. Diazepam is rather fast acting, with IV effects occurring almost immediately and reaching peak effectiveness in 15 minutes. Its duration of effectiveness is from 15 to 60 minutes. Do not mix diazepam with any other drugs, and flush the IV line before and after administration. Administer diazepam as close to the IV catheter as possible, and do not inject it into a plastic IV bag. Diazepam is readily absorbed by plastic, which quickly reduces its concentration.

Diazepam is usually supplied in single-use vials or preloaded syringes containing 2 mL of a 5 mg/mL solution (10 mg). Administer 5 to 15 mg IV and repeat in 10 to 15 minutes if necessary.

Diazepam's effects may be reversed by flumazenil administration. Usually, 2 mL of a 0.1 mg/mL solution is given IV (over 15 seconds) with a second dose repeated, as needed, at 60 seconds.

Morphine Morphine sulfate (Duramorph, Astramorph) is an opium alkaloid used to relieve pain (narcotic analgesic), to sedate, and to reduce anxiety. It is used with musculoskeletal injuries for its ability to reduce pain perception. Morphine may increase vascular (container) volume and reduce cardiac preload by increasing venous capacitance and may thus decrease blood pressure in the hypovolemic patient. It should not be administered to a patient with hypovolemia or hypotension. Its major side effects are respiratory depression and possible nausea and vomiting. A mild, red, itchy rash often accompanies the administration of morphine and is caused by the release of histamine. It should not be confused with an allergic reaction, but if it is severe, the histamine reaction can be treated with diphenhydramine (Benadryl) orally or intravenously.

Morphine is available in 10-mL single-use vials or Tubex units of a 1 mg/mL solution or as 1 mL of a 10 mg/mL solution vial for dilution with 9 mL normal saline. Administer a 2-mg bolus slowly IV, repeating as necessary every few minutes to effect.

Naloxone hydrochloride (Narcan) is a narcotic antagonist that can quickly reverse narcotic effects (morphine, fentanyl, and nalbuphine) and should be available anytime you use any of these drugs. Naloxone is administered as an IV bolus of 0.4 to 2 mg, repeated every 2 to 3 minutes until effective. Naloxone is a shorter-acting drug than morphine, so repeat doses may be necessary.

Fentanyl Fentanyl is an opiate narcotic, chemically unrelated to morphine, that provides immediate and effective pain control. Fentanyl's onset of action is more rapid than morphine's and it is considerably more potent, thus requiring lower doses. Fentanyl does not cause hypotension to the same degree as does morphine, which makes it an ideal agent for trauma.

Fentanyl is supplied in various doses. The typical starting dose is 25 to 50 mcg IV. Repeat doses of 25 mcg IV can be provided as needed. As with all opiates, continuously monitor the patient's vital signs. Fentanyl may also be administered intranasally (1–2 mcg/kg). This can be very useful when an IV line has not yet been established or in pediatric patients when the pain of an IV start may be a consideration.[9,10]

Other Musculoskeletal Injury Considerations

Other areas for special consideration with musculoskeletal injuries include pediatric injuries, athletic injuries, patient refusals and referrals, and the psychological support for the patient with musculoskeletal injury.

Pediatric Musculoskeletal Injury

Children are at higher risk than adults for musculoskeletal injuries due to their activity levels and incompletely developed coordination. Special injuries affecting them include greenstick fractures and epiphyseal fractures.

The incomplete nature of the greenstick fracture produces a stable but angulated limb in the young child. The injured limb is painful and will not bear weight. In these cases, do not attempt to realign the limb and understand that the orthopedic specialist will probably complete the fracture to permit proper healing.

Epiphyseal fractures disrupt a child's bone's growth plate and endanger future bone growth. This injury is likely with fractures within a few inches of the joint because the epiphyseal plate is a point of skeletal weakness. Treat these fractures as you would for an adult, but recognize that they are potentially limb-threatening injuries.

Assess for possible abuse during evaluation of a pediatric patient with musculoskeletal injuries. Look for injuries not consistent with the described mechanism of injury or multiple injuries in different stages of healing. Report any suspicions as appropriate under state law and your protocols.

Athletic Musculoskeletal Injuries

Athletes, especially those involved in contact sports like football, soccer, basketball, and wrestling, have a higher incidence of musculoskeletal injuries than the general public. Injuries to joints, often serious knee and ankle sprains, are common reasons for calls to EMS. Such injuries are especially important because they occur in individuals who are at least moderately well conditioned and result from significant kinetic force application. When you are called to an injured athlete's side, be especially sensitive to the potential for residual disability caused by these injuries and be predisposed to transport instead of permitting the patient to remain at the scene.

Knowing athletic trainers in your area may help your on-scene operations run more smoothly and efficiently. In many cases, athletic trainers work under local physician supervision much as you work under medical direction. It is important for trainers to understand that, once you are called to the scene, an injured athlete becomes an EMS system patient and will be treated under system medical direction and protocols. Also, as a system representative, you are likely to assume responsibility for decisions about patient care and transport. Ensuring that trainers understand these circumstances may eliminate confrontations over injured athlete care.

Athletic trainers use the acronym RICE to identify the recommended treatment for sprains, strains, and other soft-tissue injuries. RICE stands for *R*est the extremity, *I*ce for the first 48 hours, *C*ompression with an elastic bandage, and *E*levation for venous drainage. This is consistent with standard emergency care for sprains and strains. (Note, however, that the application of the elastic bandage in this case is to strengthen a limb for further activity and is not recommended for prehospital care.)

► RICE Procedure for Strains, Sprains, and Soft-Tissue Injuries

- *R*est the extremity
- *I*ce for the first 48 hours
- *C*ompress with elastic bandage
- *E*levate extremity

Patient Refusals and Referral

In some situations, you may encounter a patient suffering from an isolated sprain or strain with no significant mechanism of injury and no other injury signs, symptoms, or complaints. This patient may refuse your assistance or be a candidate for on-scene treatment and referral for follow-up medical care. Evaluate the need for immobilization and X-rays and determine if the patient should seek immediate care in an emergency department or see a personal physician. Any referral to a personal physician or patient refusal must be done in conjunction with medical direction and follow local protocols.

Psychological Support for the Musculoskeletal Injury Patient

Regardless of the specific type of injury sustained, patients need psychological as well as physiologic support. Too often, we concentrate all efforts on a patient's injuries, forgetting the emotional impact that an incident and emergency care measures employed have on a patient. Keep in mind that patients are not frequently exposed to injuries. They do not know what effects injuries will have on their lives or what to expect from medical care in the prehospital, emergency department, or in-hospital settings. Remember that you can have a significant impact on a patient's emotional response to trauma. Displaying a concerned attitude and a professional demeanor and communicating frequently and compassionately with patients will go far to calm and reassure them. Simple attention paid to a patient may make his experience with prehospital emergency medical service one that is remembered positively.

CHAPTER REVIEW

SUMMARY

Injuries to the bones, ligaments, tendons, and muscles of the extremities rarely threaten your patient's life. Major exceptions to this statement are pelvic and serious or bilateral femur fractures, in which associated hemorrhage can contribute significantly to hypovolemia and shock. In addition, serious musculoskeletal trauma suggests the possibility of other, life-threatening trauma and, in fact, occurs in about 80 percent of cases of major multisystem trauma. The presence of serious musculoskeletal trauma should increase your index of suspicion for other serious internal injuries.

Care for isolated musculoskeletal trauma is usually delayed until the primary assessment and patient life threats are stabilized. Musculoskeletal care goals are to protect any open wounds, position affected limbs properly, immobilize the injury area, and carefully monitor distal extremities to ensure neurovascular function.

Pelvic and bilateral femur fractures are immobilized through PASG or pelvic sling and long spine board application. The PASG provides splinting for the pelvis and upper portion of the lower extremities and helps control internal blood loss. The pelvic sling immobilizes the unstable pelvis. Manage other fractures by aligning the extremity with gentle traction and immobilizing it by splinting. In cases where you discover a loss of distal neurovascular function, move the extremity slightly to restore neurovascular function and then splint.

Joint injuries carry a greater risk of damage to distal circulation, sensation, and motor function. Splint these injuries as you find them unless there is distal neurovascular compromise. If that is the case, employ gentle manipulation to restore circulation, motor function, or sensation. If gentle manipulation is unsuccessful and transport is to be delayed, attempt dislocation reduction for the hip, knee, ankle, shoulder, or finger as permitted by local protocol.

Care for injuries to connective and muscular tissues by immobilizing the area of injury in the position of function. Evaluate distal extremities for pulse, capillary refill, color, temperature, sensation, and motor function before, during, and after any immobilization or movement of a limb and provide frequent monitoring thereafter. Consider local cooling, gentle wrapping (most probably associated with splinting), and possibly medication to reduce musculoskeletal injury pain.

YOU MAKE THE CALL

You and your partner are called to 1616 Hampton Avenue for a patient who has tripped in the yard and injured his ankle. Dispatch reports that the patient is a 16-year-old male who is conscious, alert, and breathing; there is no bleeding present. Bystanders are on the scene performing first aid.

On arrival at the scene, you find the patient, Hank Tomlin, leaning against a tree in the front yard of his mother's home. As you interview Hank and bystanders, you discover that he is complaining of pain, swelling, and deformity to his right ankle. Hank tells you that he was running after his dog when his foot twisted in the grass and he fell to the ground. You suspect that the patient has probably dislocated or fractured his ankle.

While your partner continues to obtain a patient history and vital signs, you assess the site of the injury. A third off-duty paramedic is also on the scene to assist.

1. When assessing the injury site, what signs of fracture will you be evaluating?

2. What are the three main factors to consider when evaluating distal neurovascular status?

3. What steps should you take if you determine the patient is suffering from distal neurovascular impairment and choose to realign the injury?

4. How many attempts are permitted when realigning an injury?

5. How would you splint this injury once realignment has taken place?

See Suggested Responses at the back of this chapter.

REVIEW QUESTIONS

1. The skeleton gives the body its structural form and it also _____.
   a. protects the vital organs
   b. allows for efficient movement despite the forces of gravity
   c. stores salts and other materials needed for metabolism
   d. all of the above

2. Bones are classified according to their _____.
   a. size
   b. shape
   c. weight
   d. diameter

3. Minute blood vessels, surrounded by layers of salts deposited in collagen fibers, travel lengthwise along the bone through small tubes known as _____.
   a. osteocytic pores
   b. osteoblastic pores
   c. perforating canals
   d. haversian canals

4. There are approximately 206 bones in the human body. Many are arranged in a contiguous fashion into jointed systems. The connective tissue(s) holding these bones together at a joint is/are _____.
   a. tendons
   b. cartilage
   c. bursal tissue
   d. ligaments

5. Biaxial joints allow movement in two planes. An example from this category of joints would be the _____.
   a. knee
   b. shoulder
   c. thumb bases
   d. fingers

6. Age-related changes in the skeletal system begin to occur as early as 40 years of age. These changes include _____.
   a. calcium retention
   b. progression in body height
   c. loss of ability to maintain bone structure
   d. an increase in flexibility of costochondral joints

7. Skeletal muscles provide the ability for voluntary movement associated with the mobility of the body and its extremities. These muscles are controlled by the _____ nervous system.
   a. somatic
   b. autonomic
   c. sympathetic
   d. musculoskeletal

8. More than half of the energy created by muscle motion is _____.
   a. heat energy
   b. chemical energy
   c. electrical energy
   d. mechanical energy

9. Joints can move beyond their normal range of motion with a sufficiently large applied force. This movement causes a complete displacement of bone ends from their normal position and is known as a(n) _____, and is characterized by _____.
   a. oblique fracture; pain, edema, and possibly bleeding
   b. dislocation; pain, edema, and immobility
   c. grade III sprain; severe pain and spasm without joint instability
   d. subluxation; pain, rapid edema, and an unlimited range of motion

10. Red marrow is found within the cancellous bone chambers of the long bones, sternum, and pelvis. The function of the marrow in these sites is _____.
    a. destruction and recycling of old and fragile blood cells
    b. manufacturing of erythrocytes and other blood cells
    c. storage of essential salts and minerals for bone aggregation
    d. storage of a readily available source of energy generation

11. A grade _____ sprain may present as a fracture.
    a. I
    b. II
    c. III
    d. IV

12. A small crack in a bone that does not disrupt its total structure is called a(n) _____ fracture.
 a. open
 c. impacted
 b. closed
 d. hairline

13. A common disintegration of the articular joints often associated with the aging process describes degenerative joint disease. Another disorder, characterized by inflammation of the synovial joints and causing immobility, pain, and fatigue, is known as _____.
 a. osteoarthritis
 b. costrochondritis
 c. inflammatory gout
 d. rheumatoid arthritis

14. A femur fracture may account for as much as _____ mL of blood loss.
 a. 1,000
 c. 2,000
 b. 1,500
 d. 2,500

15. Your patient has been involved in a motor vehicle collision. You suspect concurrent femur and pelvic fractures. Treatment of this patient would best be provided by _____.
 a. traction device, long board, transport to trauma center
 b. long board, one IV line, transport to emergency department
 c. traction device, PASG, transport to trauma center
 d. padded rigid splints, long board, transport to trauma center

See Answers to Review Questions at the back of this chapter.

REFERENCES

1. American Medical Association. *The Wonderful Human Machine* (1979).

2. Badhe, S., et al. "The 'Silent' Compartment Syndrome." *Injury* 40(2) (Feb 2009): 220–222.

3. Flynn, J. M., et al. "Acute Traumatic Compartment Syndrome of the Leg in Children: Diagnosis and Outcome." *J Bone Joint Surg Am* 93(10) (May 18, 2011): 937–941.

4. Oprel, P. P., et al. "The Acute Compartment Syndrome of the Lower Leg: A Difficult Diagnosis?" *Open Orthop J* 4 (2010): 115–119.

5. Melamed, E., et al. "Prehospital Care of Orthopedic Injuries." *Prehosp Disaster Med* 22(1) (Jan–Feb 2007): 22–25.

6. Wood, S. P., M. Varhas, and S. K. Wedel. "Femur Fracture Immobilization with Traction Splints in Multisystem Trauma Patients." *Prehosp Emerg Care* 7(2) (Apr–Jun 2003): 241–243.

7. Tan, E. C., S. F. van Stigt, and A. B. van Vugt. "Effect of a New Pelvic Stabilizer (T-POD®) on Reduction of Pelvic Volume and Haemodynamic Stability in Unstable Pelvic Fractures." *Injury* 41(12) (Dec 2010): 1239–1243.

8. Abarbanell, N. R. "Prehospital Midthigh Trauma and Traction Splint Use: Recommendations for Treatment Protocols." *Amer J Emerg Med* 19(2) (Mar 2001): 137–140.

9. Garrick, J. F., S. Kidane, J. E. Pointer, W. Sugiyama, C. Van Luen, and R. Clark. "Analysis of the Paramedic Administration of Fentanyl." *J Opiod Manag* 7(3) (May–June 2011): 229–234.

10. Kanowitz, A., T. M. Dunn, E. M. Kanowitz, et al. "Safety and Effectiveness of Fentanyl Administration for Prehospital Pain Management." *PreHospital Emergency Care* 10(1) (2006).

FURTHER READING

American College of Surgeons, Committee on Trauma. *Advanced Trauma Life Support Course: Student Manual.* 8th ed. Chicago: American College of Surgeons, 2008.

Bates, Barbara, and Peter G. Szilagyi. *A Guide to Physical Examination and History Taking.* 9th ed. Philadelphia: J. B. Lippincott, 2007.

Bledsoe, B. E., and D. Clayden. *Prehospital Emergency Pharmacology.* 7th ed. Upper Saddle River, NJ: Pearson/Prentice Hall, 2011.

Bledsoe, B. E., B. J. Colbert, and J. E. Ankney. *Essentials of A & P for Emergency Care.* Upper Saddle River, NJ: Pearson/Prentice Hall, 2010.

Campbell, John E. *International Trauma Life Support for Emergency Care Providers.* 7th ed. Upper Saddle River, NJ: Pearson/Prentice Hall, 2012.

Martini, Frederic. *Fundamentals of Anatomy and Physiology.* 7th ed. San Francisco: Benjamin Cummings, 2011.

Rosen, P., and R. Barkin, eds. *Emergency Medicine: Concepts and Clinical Practice.* 7th ed. St. Louis: Mosby, 2009.

Tintinalli, J. E., ed. *Emergency Medicine: A Comprehensive Study Guide.* 7th ed. New York: McGraw-Hill, 2011.

SUGGESTED RESPONSES TO "YOU MAKE THE CALL"

The following are suggested responses to the "You Make the Call" scenarios presented in this chapter. Each represents an acceptable response to the scenario but should not be interpreted as the only correct response.

1. *When assessing the injury site, what signs of fracture will you be evaluating?*

   You are looking for instability, deformity such as swelling or angulation, crepitus, unusual motion, abnormal muscle tone, and regions of unusual warmth or coolness. Consider the "six Ps"—pain, pallor, paralysis, paresthesia, pressure, and pulses.

2. *What are the three main factors to consider when evaluating distal neurovascular status?*

   Circulation, motor function, and sensation.

3. *What steps should you take if you determine the patient is suffering from distal neurovascular impairment and choose to realign the injury?*

   Have your partner immobilize the proximal limb in the position found. Grasp the distal limb firmly and apply traction along the axis.

If you feel resistance to movement or great increase in patient discomfort, stop and splint the limb as it lies. Once you complete alignment, recheck distal neurovascular function. If function is inadequate, move the limb around. If one attempt at gentle manipulation does not reestablish a pulse, splint and transport the patient quickly.

4. *How many attempts are permitted when realigning an injury?*

   This should only be attempted once.

5. *How would you splint this injury once realignment has taken place?*

   Splinting the injury in a "position of function" or natural position is the best method for splinting and maintaining distal function. A manufactured splint will accomplish this. Another very effective method for splinting an ankle is with a pillow.

ANSWERS TO REVIEW QUESTIONS

1. d
2. b
3. d
4. d
5. c
6. c
7. a
8. a
9. b
10. b
11. c
12. d
13. d
14. b
15. d

GLOSSARY

abduction   movement of a body part away from the midline.

acetabulum   hollow depression in the lateral pelvis that forms the articular surface for the femoral head.

adduction   movement of a body part toward the midline.

amphiarthroses   joints that permit a limited amount of independent motion.

appendicular skeleton   bones of the extremities, shoulder girdle, and pelvis (excepting the sacrum).

arthritis   inflammation of a joint.

articular surface   surface of a bone that moves against another bone.

axial skeleton   bones of the head, thorax, and spine.

bursa   sac containing synovial fluid that cushions adjacent structures.

bursitis   acute or chronic inflammation of the small synovial sacs.

calcaneus   the largest bone of the foot; the heel.

callus   thickened area that forms at the site of a fracture as part of the repair process.

cancellous   having a lattice-work structure, as in the spongy tissue of a bone.

carpal bones   bones of the wrist.

cartilage   connective tissue providing the articular surfaces of the skeletal system.

circumduction   movement at a synovial joint where the distal end of a bone describes a circle but the shaft does not rotate.

clavicle   bone that holds the scapula and shoulder joint at a fixed distance from the sternum and permits the shoulder to move up and down (shrug).

closed fracture   a broken bone in which the bone ends or the forces that caused it do not penetrate the skin.

comminuted fracture   fracture in which a bone is broken into several pieces.

cramping   muscle pain resulting from overactivity, lack of oxygen, and accumulation of waste products.

devascularization   loss of blood vessels from a body part.

diaphysis   hollow shaft found in long bones.

diarthroses   synovial joints.

dislocation   complete displacement of a bone end from its position in a joint capsule.

epiphyseal fracture   disruption in the epiphyseal plate of a child's bone.

epiphyseal plate   area of the metaphysis where cartilage is generated during bone growth in childhood. Also called the growth plate.

epiphysis   end of a long bone, including the epiphyseal, or growth plate, and supporting structures underlying the joint.

fascicle   small bundle of muscle fibers.

fatigue   condition in which a muscle's ability to respond to stimulation is lost or reduced through overactivity.

fatigue fracture   break in a bone associated with prolonged or repeated stress.

femur   large bone of the proximal lower extremity.

fibula   the small bone of the lower leg.

gout   inflammation of joints and connective tissue due to buildup of uric acid crystals.

greenstick fracture   partial fracture of a child's bone.

hairline fracture   small crack in a bone that does not disrupt its total structure.

haversian canals   small perforations of the long bones through which the blood vessels and nerves travel through the bone itself.

humerus   the single bone of the proximal upper extremity.

iliac crest   lateral bony ridge that is a landmark of the pelvis.

ilium   large, flat innominate bone.

impacted fracture   break in a bone in which the bone is compressed on itself.

innominate bone   one of the structures of the pelvis.

insertion   attachment of a muscle to a bone that moves when the muscle contracts.

ischial tuberosity   one of the bony knobs of the posterior pelvis.

ischium   irregular innominate bone.

joint   area where adjacent bones articulate.

joint capsule   chamber formed by ligaments surrounding a joint that holds a small amount of synovial fluid to lubricate articular surfaces.

ligaments   bands of connective tissue that connect bone to bone and hold joints together.

malleolus   the protuberance of the ankle.

medullary canal   cavity within a bone that contains the marrow.

metacarpal   one of the bones of the palm.

metaphysis   growth zone of a bone, active during the development stages of youth. It is located between the epiphysis and the diaphysis.

metatarsal   one of the bones forming the arch of the foot.

oblique fracture   break in a bone running across it at an angle other than 90 degrees.

olecranon   proximal end of the ulna.

open fracture   a broken bone in which the bone ends or the forces that caused it penetrate the surrounding skin.

opposition   pairing of muscles that permits extension and flexion of limbs.

origin   attachment of a muscle to a bone that does not move (or experiences the least movement) when the muscle contracts.

osteoarthritis   inflammation of a joint resulting from wearing of the articular cartilage.

osteoblast   cell that helps in the creation of new bone during growth and bone repair.

osteoclast   bone cell that absorbs and removes excess bone.

osteocyte   bone-forming cell found in the bone matrix that helps maintain the bone.

osteoporosis   weakening of bone tissue due to loss of essential minerals, especially calcium.

pelvis   skeletal structure where the lower extremities attach to the body.

perforating canals   structures through which blood vessels enter and exit the bone shaft.

periosteum   the tough exterior covering of a bone.

phalanges   bones of the fingers and toes.

pubis   irregular innominate bone.

radius   bone on the thumb side of the forearm.

red bone marrow   tissue within the internal cavity of a bone responsible for the manufacture of erythrocytes and other blood cells.

reduction   returning of displaced bone ends to their proper anatomic orientation.

rheumatoid arthritis   chronic disease that causes deterioration of peripheral joint connective tissue.

scapula   triangular bone buried within the musculature of the upper back.

septic arthritis   joint capsule infection from an agent introduced through an open wound, bloodborne pathogens, or an adjacent infection, causing fever and a warm, swollen joint.

sesamoid bone   bone that forms in a tendon.

spasm   intermittent or continuous contraction of a muscle.

spiral fracture   a curving break in a bone as may be caused by rotational forces.

sprain   tearing of a joint capsule's connective tissues.

strain   injury resulting from overstretching of muscle fibers.

subluxation   partial displacement of a bone end from its position in a joint capsule.

synarthroses   joints that do not permit movement.

synovial fluid   substance that lubricates synovial joints.

synovial joint   type of joint that permits the greatest degree of independent motion.

tendonitis   inflammation of a tendon and/or its protective sheath.

tibia   the larger bone of the lower leg that articulates with the femur.

tone   state of slight contraction of muscles that gives them firmness and keeps them ready to contract.

transverse fracture   a break that runs across a bone perpendicular to the bone's orientation.

ulna   bone on the little finger side of the forearm.

yellow bone marrow   tissue that stores fat in semiliquid form within the internal cavities of a bone.

Abdominal Trauma

Robert S. Porter, MA, EMT-P

STANDARD
Trauma (Abdominal and Genitourinary Trauma)

COMPETENCY
Integrates assessment findings with principles of epidemiology and pathophysiology to formulate a field impression to implement a comprehensive treatment/disposition plan for an acutely injured patient.

OBJECTIVES

Terminal Performance Objective
After reading this chapter you should be able to assess and manage patients with abdominal trauma.

Enabling Objectives
To accomplish the terminal performance objective, you should be able to:

1. Define key terms introduced in this chapter.
2. Describe the anatomy and physiology of the abdominal cavity and its contents.
3. Describe changes in anatomy and physiology associated with pregnancy.
4. Discuss the pathophysiology of blunt and penetrating mechanisms of abdominal trauma.
5. Describe the pathophysiology of the following types of abdominal injuries:
   a. abdominal wall
   b. hollow organ
   c. solid organ
   d. vascular structure
   e. mesentery and bowel injury
   f. peritoneal injury
   g. pelvic fracture
   h. injury in pregnancy
   i. abdominal injuries in pediatric patients
6. Given a variety of scenarios, demonstrate assessment of patients with abdominal injuries.
7. Given a variety of scenarios, develop a management plan for patients with abdominal injuries.

KEY TERMS

abruptio placentae
chyme
digestive tract
evisceration
guarding
hematemesis

hematochezia
hematuria
mesentery
pelvic space
peristalsis
peritoneal space

peritoneum
peritonitis
rebound tenderness
retroperitoneal space
supine hypotensive
 syndrome

From Chapter 9 of *Paramedic Care: Principles & Practice, Volume 5,* Fourth Edition. Bryan Bledsoe, Robert Porter, and Richard Cherry. Copyright © 2013 by Pearson Education, Inc. All rights reserved.

Janice and her paramedic partner Doug respond to a "shots fired" call in the early hours of Saturday morning. They arrive at an apartment complex, noting that there are several police vehicles on scene. Officers tell the paramedics that the wife is in custody and are directed by an officer to a hallway where a middle-aged male sits propped against a wall. The man holds what appears to be a blood-soaked towel against his abdomen.

Janice introduces herself as a paramedic and begins the patient's primary assessment. The victim, Marty, is a 43-year-old who was shot by his wife during a domestic dispute. He reports "she shot me once with my 9-mm handgun" at close range. Janice coaxes Marty to lift the towel and observes a small entrance wound to the left upper quadrant, above and to the left of the navel. The wound is oozing just a small amount of blood. Inspection of Marty's back and flank reveals no exit wound. Doug assesses vital signs and obtains a blood pressure of 110/86, a strong and regular pulse at a rate of 90, and respirations of 22. Marty's ECG traces a sinus rhythm with no abnormalities, and his oxygen saturation is 99 percent. He is alert and oriented to time, place, and person. He describes his abdominal pain as sharp at the entrance wound, although the area surrounding the wound feels "burning" in nature.

Janice does not administer oxygen because of the high saturation reading. She and Doug prepare to move Marty quickly to the waiting stretcher and then to the ambulance.

As Janice prepares Marty for the ride to the hospital, Doug informs her that the nearest trauma center has just received several seriously injured patients from an auto crash, and Janice and Doug are directed to a more distant Level II trauma center.

En route, Janice initiates an IV line with a large-bore catheter, trauma tubing, and a 1,000-mL bag of normal saline solution, running at a to-keep-open rate. During transport Janice questions Marty about his symptoms and some thirst. Janice's reassessment reveals a blood pressure of 112/94, a strong pulse at 86, and respirations that are now somewhat shallow at 24. Oxygen saturation remains at 99 percent and the ECG still displays a normal sinus rhythm. Blood is no longer draining from the entrance wound, and further examination does not reveal an exit wound. Janice auscultates the chest and abdomen and, though road sounds limit auscultation clarity, she hears only clear breath sounds in the chest and no bowel sounds.

Janice completes a final set of vital signs as they arrive at the emergency department. Marty's pulse is 88, blood pressure is 112/96, and respirations are 22 and somewhat shallow. Janice quickly reports her assessment findings and care to the trauma team. In the emergency department Marty is crossmatched for blood and prepared for exploratory laparotomy in the operating room. During her next trip to the trauma center the staff informs Janice that Marty's surgery was successful. They found the stomach to be perforated, the spleen to be torn, and over 400 mL of blood was in the abdomen. Marty did well during surgery and is on his way to a quick recovery.

INTRODUCTION TO ABDOMINAL TRAUMA

The abdominal cavity is one of the body's largest cavities, contains many organs essential to life, and is not well protected by skeletal structures as are most other body cavities. Blunt and penetrating trauma may damage these vital organs, and large blood volumes can be lost in the cavity. However, injuries to the abdomen do not always present as dramatically as they do elsewhere because of the few skeletal structures. Transmitted injury signs—deformity, swelling, and discoloration—take time to develop and are not often seen in the prehospital setting. These considerations make anticipation of abdominal injuries and careful abdominal assessment critical for patients with trauma to this region.

Abdominal injury severity and death associated with blunt trauma have also decreased thanks to improvements in highway design and vehicle structure and to greater seat belt use and air bag deployment. However, overall mortality and morbidity from penetrating trauma is on the rise due to the increasing violence in our society, most specifically in the growing use and increasing power of handguns. Penetrating trauma is approaching trauma associated with auto crashes as the number one trauma killer. Nowhere is this more apparent than with abdominal injuries.[1]

Prevention of abdominal injuries, as with most other types of trauma, is the best way to reduce mortality and morbidity. As noted, highway and vehicle design improvements and employing safe practices at home and in the workplace play important roles in reducing both abdominal injury incidence and seriousness.

There remains room for further improvements in safety practices, however. For example, many people still do not use seat belts. Failure to use the seat belt increases abdominal injury incidence secondary to impact with the steering wheel, dash, or other auto interior surfaces and of impact after ejection. (Side impact air bags have the potential to reduce the incidence of pelvic fracture and internal abdominal injuries frequently associated with this mechanism of injury.)

One area of special concern is proper lap belt application. If the belt rides too high on the abdomen, deceleration may direct forces both to abdominal cavity contents and the lumbar spine. Severe compression may result in serious associated abdominal injury. Proper placement, in which the belt rests on the iliac crests, transmits severe deceleration forces to the pelvis and body's skeletal structure, thus sparing abdominal contents and the spine from injury. Proper positioning of seat belts is especially important with children. Too low a belt placement may impinge on the femurs and, with severe impact, fracture them near the pelvis.

ABDOMINAL ANATOMY AND PHYSIOLOGY

The abdominal cavity is bound by the diaphragm, superiorly; pelvis, inferiorly; vertebral column, posterior and inferior ribs, and back muscles (psoas and paraspinal muscles), posteriorly; flank muscles, laterally; and abdominal muscles, anteriorly (Figure 1 ●). The cavity is divided into three spaces: the **peritoneal space** (containing those organs or portions of organs covered by the abdominal [peritoneal] lining); the **retroperitoneal space** (containing those organs posterior to the peritoneal lining); and the **pelvic space** (containing organs within the pelvis). Anatomic landmarks of this area include the centrally located umbilicus (the navel), xiphoid process (tip of the sternum) at the upper and central abdominal border, bony pelvic ridges (the iliac crests) inferiorly and laterally, and pubic prominence inferiorly.

The abdomen is divided into four subregions by vertical and horizontal lines intersecting at the umbilicus and forming the right and left upper and lower quadrants. The right upper quadrant contains the gallbladder, right kidney, most of the liver, some small bowel, a portion of the ascending and transverse colon, and a small portion of the pancreas. The left upper quadrant contains the stomach, spleen, left kidney, most of the pancreas, and portions of the liver, small bowel, and transverse and descending colon. The right lower quadrant contains the appendix, and portions of the urinary bladder, small bowel, ascending colon, rectum, and female genitalia. The left lower quadrant contains the sigmoid colon and portions of the urinary bladder, small bowel, descending colon, rectum, and female genitalia.

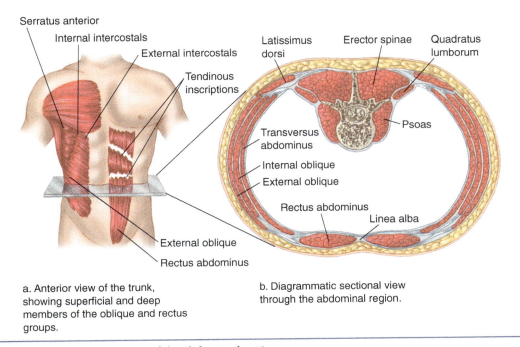

a. Anterior view of the trunk, showing superficial and deep members of the oblique and rectus groups.

b. Diagrammatic sectional view through the abdominal region.

● **Figure 1**   Muscles protecting the organs of the abdominal cavity.

Major structures within the abdomen include the digestive tract, accessory organs of digestion, structures and organs of the urinary system, spleen, and, in the female, genitals. The digestive tract (also called the alimentary canal) is the muscular tube that physically and chemically breaks down and absorbs fluids and nutrients from the food we eat. The accessory digestive organs include the liver, gallbladder, and pancreas. These organs prepare and store digestive enzymes and perform other important body functions. The spleen is a component of the immune system, while the paired kidneys and ureters, urinary bladder, and urethra make up the urinary system. In the female, the ovaries, fallopian tubes, uterus, and vagina also occupy some of the abdominal cavity.

Digestive Tract

The **digestive tract** is a 25-foot-long hollow muscular tube responsible for churning material to be digested, for excreting digestive juices to be mixed with it, and for absorbing nutrients and then water (Figure 2 ●). Abdominal components of the digestive tract consist of the stomach, small bowel (duodenum, jejunum, and ileum), large bowel (or colon), rectum, and anus. These structures fill the anterior and lateral aspects of the abdominal cavity, except for the area occupied by the liver.

The esophagus enters the abdomen through the hiatus of the diaphragm (just posterior to the xiphoid process) and then conveys its contents into the stomach. The stomach is a J-shaped muscular container that mixes ingested material with hydrochloric acid and enzymes (both produced in the gastric wall) into a thick fluid called **chyme**. Acid released by the stomach increases gastric acidity (pH) to between 1.5 and 2.0. This is a very acidic fluid that would damage the stomach and initial small bowel lining if not for the continuous production of protective mucus. The stomach is highly variable in size, depending on the amount of material it contains. It can distend to hold as much as 1.5 liters of food after a large meal.

Chyme is released in small boluses into the beginning of the small bowel, the duodenum. The duodenum is approximately 1 foot in length and is where the digesting material is mixed with bile from the liver (stored in the gallbladder) and pancreatic digestive juices. These agents raise the pH of the chyme (returning it toward neutral), begin the breakdown of fats, and help release the nutrients chyme contains.

Digesting food is propelled along the small and large bowel by waves of contraction called **peristalsis**. Digestive tract muscles constrict the bowel's lumen behind a mass of food, then progressively constrict the lumen in the direction of desired movement. The resulting rhythmic constriction moves digesting material through the tract. As chyme enters the next two segments of the small bowel (the jejunum and the ileum), the mixing decreases and nutrients, released by the physical and chemical digestion processes, are absorbed, directed to the liver for detoxification, and then released into the circulatory system.

As the food continues its travel through the digestive tract, it arrives at the large bowel. Here masses of bacteria assist in releasing vitamins and water from the digesting food, which are readily absorbed. Water serves to hydrate the body while digestive juices are reabsorbed and reprocessed to rejoin the digestive process upstream. The large bowel ascends superiorly along the right side of the abdomen (ascending colon), traverses the abdomen just below the liver and stomach (transverse colon), then descends along the left lateral abdomen (descending colon). It aligns with the rectum through the S-shaped sigmoid colon where waste products of the digestive process (feces) await excretion (defecation) through the terminal valve, the anus.

Accessory Organs

The liver is a vascular structure responsible for detoxifying blood, providing bile, removing damaged or aged erythrocytes, and storing glycogen and other important agents for body metabolism. The liver also assists in osmotic fluid regulation and produces proteins used in the clotting process. Finally, the liver detoxifies materials absorbed by the digestive system and either stores or releases nutrients to ensure metabolic needs are met. It is located in the right upper quadrant, just below the diaphragm, and extends into the medial portion of the left upper quadrant. It is the largest abdominal organ, accounting for 2.5 percent of total body weight. It receives about 25 percent of cardiac output and holds the greatest blood reserve of any body organ. The lower portion of its mass can occasionally be palpated just below the margin of the rib cage. It is suspended in its location by several ligaments, including the ligamentum teres, and connects to the omentum inferiorly. The liver is a solid organ but is rather delicate in nature. It is contained within a fibrous capsule (visceral peritoneum) that serves to retard hemorrhage and helps hold the liver together if injured by blunt trauma. When injured, the liver will regenerate to some degree but will not function as efficiently as before the injury.

The gallbladder is a small hollow organ located behind and beneath the liver. It receives bile (a by-product of red blood cell reprocessing) from the liver and stores it until it is needed during fatty food digestion. It then constricts and sends bile through the bile duct and into the duodenum. Bile helps emulsify (breaking apart and suspending) ingested fats that would otherwise remain as indigestible clumps during the digestive process.

Another accessory digestive organ is the pancreas. It is responsible for production of glucagon and insulin, hormones responsible for blood glucose regulation and glucose transport across cell membranes. The pancreas also produces very powerful digestive enzymes that help return chyme pH toward normal and break down proteins. These enzymes pass through the pancreatic duct, which joins the bile duct just before entering the duodenum. Like the liver, the pancreas is a solid, though delicate, organ, encapsulated in a serous membrane. It is located in the medial and lower portion of the left upper quadrant and extends into the medial right upper quadrant. The duodenum wraps around the right pancreatic border. If the pancreas is damaged, pancreatic enzymes may become active and begin to "self-digest" pancreatic tissue. If these enzymes are released into the retroperitoneal space, they will also damage surrounding tissue.

The Digestive System

ORGANS OF THE DIGESTIVE SYSTEM

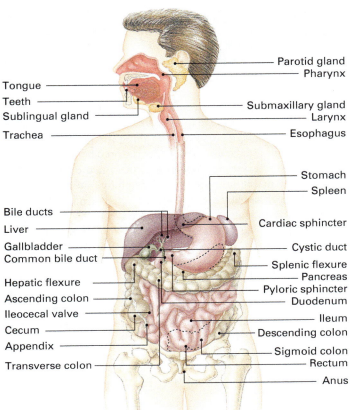

Parotid gland
Pharynx
Tongue
Teeth
Submaxillary gland
Sublingual gland
Larynx
Trachea
Esophagus
Stomach
Spleen
Bile ducts
Liver
Cardiac sphincter
Gallbladder
Cystic duct
Common bile duct
Splenic flexure
Pancreas
Hepatic flexure
Pyloric sphincter
Ascending colon
Duodenum
Ileocecal valve
Ileum
Cecum
Descending colon
Appendix
Sigmoid colon
Rectum
Transverse colon
Anus

LIVER, STOMACH, AND PANCREAS

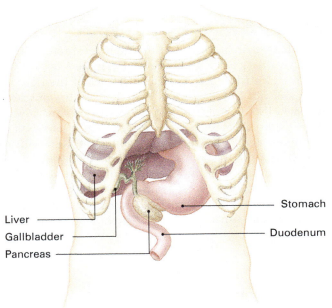

Stomach
Duodenum
Liver
Gallbladder
Pancreas

LARGE INTESTINE

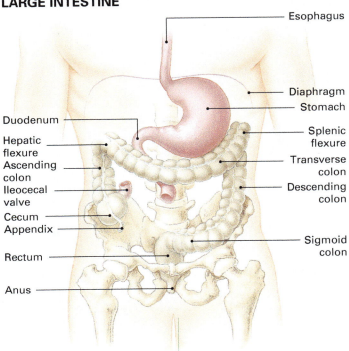

Esophagus
Diaphragm
Stomach
Duodenum
Hepatic flexure
Splenic flexure
Ascending colon
Transverse colon
Ileocecal valve
Descending colon
Cecum
Appendix
Rectum
Sigmoid colon
Anus

SMALL INTESTINE

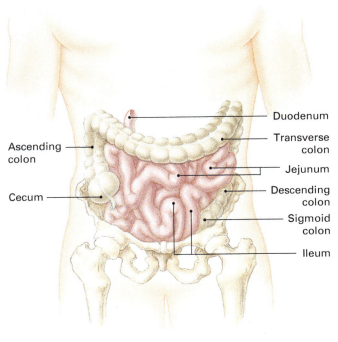

Duodenum
Ascending colon
Transverse colon
Jejunum
Cecum
Descending colon
Sigmoid colon
Ileum

● **Figure 2**   The digestive tract and accessory organs.

Spleen

The spleen is not an accessory digestive organ but rather a part of the immune system. It is a very vascular organ about the size of the palm of the hand and is located behind the stomach and lateral to the kidney in the left upper quadrant. The spleen performs some immunologic functions and also stores a large blood volume. Although the spleen is well protected in its location by the rib cage, spine, and flank and back muscles, it can be injured during blunt trauma, especially with impacts affecting the left flank.

Urinary System

The urinary system consists of the kidneys (or renal glands), ureters, urinary bladder, and urethra (Figure 3 ●). The kidneys are located in the posterior portions of the right and left upper quadrants and are protected by the muscles of the back, the thoracic and lumbar spine, and the muscles of the flanks. The kidneys have direct connections with the abdominal aorta and receive an abundant blood supply. They collect the waste products found in the bloodstream and concentrate them in a watery fluid called urine. They exert significant regulatory control over the salt/water (osmotic) balance of the body by retaining or releasing water or sodium and other body salts. The kidneys also play an important role in controlling body pH and monitoring and maintaining blood pressure.

Just above and attached to the kidneys are the adrenal glands. These structures are a part of the endocrine system and are responsible for production and release of the sympathetic hormones epinephrine and norepinephrine. Adrenal injury can have a profound effect on autonomic system control. However, since there are two kidneys and also two adrenal glands, it is unlikely that both would be seriously injured at the same time.

The kidneys each connect to a small tube, called a ureter, which transports urine to the urinary bladder. The bladder is a hollow muscular organ located along the pelvic floor and just posterior to the pubic bone. Urine is stored here until it is convenient or necessary to void. After urination, the bladder contains about 10 mL of fluid. However, when fully distended it may contain more than 500 mL. Urine is excreted through the urethra, a small tube slightly more than 1 inch (25 to 30 mm) long in the female and 7 to 8 inches (18 to 20 cm) long in the male.

Genitalia

Female sexual organs are located internally within the peritoneum and lower abdominal cavity (Figure 4 ●). These organs consist of ovaries, fallopian tubes, uterus, and vagina.

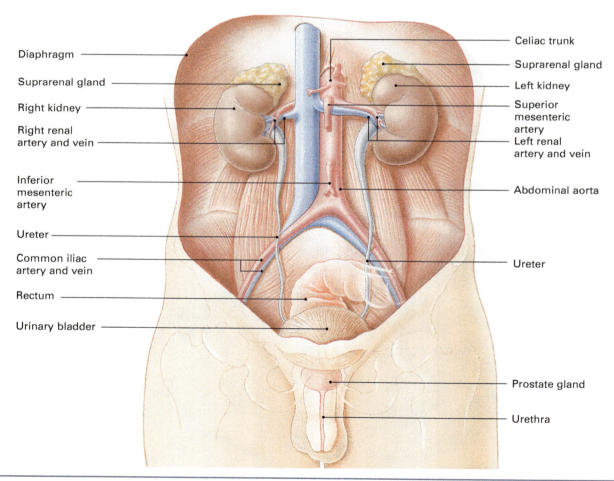

Diaphragm

Suprarenal gland

Right kidney

Right renal artery and vein

Inferior mesenteric artery

Ureter

Common iliac artery and vein

Rectum

Urinary bladder

Celiac trunk

Suprarenal gland

Left kidney

Superior mesenteric artery

Left renal artery and vein

Abdominal aorta

Ureter

Prostate gland

Urethra

● **Figure 3**   Major elements of the urinary system.

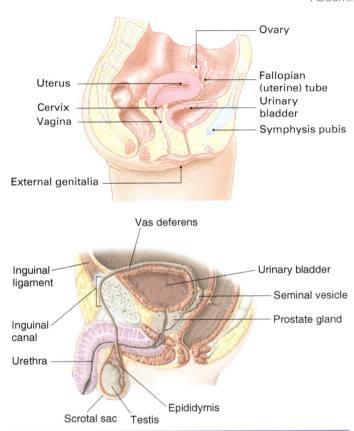

● **Figure 4**   The female and male reproductive systems.

travels to the uterus. The uterus is a pear-shaped muscular organ located within the central pelvis. In the nonpregnant state it is about 3 inches long and 2 inches in diameter at its largest point. A fertilized egg will attach itself to the inner surface of the uterus or the uterine surface will be sloughed if fertilization does not occur. The inferior portion of the uterus is the cervix, a muscular valve that contains a developing fetus until time for delivery. The cervix opens to the vaginal canal, the female organ of copulation and the canal for fetal passage during delivery. The vagina opens at the pelvic base, just behind the pubic bone. The vagina, uterus, and fallopian tubes represent an open passage to the abdominal cavity's interior.

Male sexual organs are external to the abdomen, just anterior to the pubic bone. They include the testes, the sac that contains them (called the scrotum), and the penis. The testes generate sperm, which then move through a small, convoluted tube, the epididymis, to the prostate. At sexual climax, the sperm is mixed with seminal fluid, propelled through the prostate and the urethra, and expelled. The penis is a highly vascular cylindrical structure composed of special tissue surrounding the urethra. Cells of this tissue engorge with blood during sexual excitement and stiffen the penis.

Pregnant Uterus

Dynamics of pregnancy greatly affect female abdominal cavity anatomy (Figure 5 ●). The uterus and its contents grow rapidly from conception until delivery and are well protected during the first trimester (three months) of pregnancy. During the second trimester (12 to 24 weeks), progressive uterine enlargement displaces most abdominal contents upward as the growing uterus rises out of the pelvis and its upper border extends above the umbilicus. By 32 weeks and until the pregnancy ends, the uterus fills the abdominal cavity to the level of the

Ovaries are almond-shaped solid organs that store, mature, and then release an unfertilized egg approximately every 28 days. The egg is released into the abdominal cavity and directed to the adjacent fallopian tube, through which it then

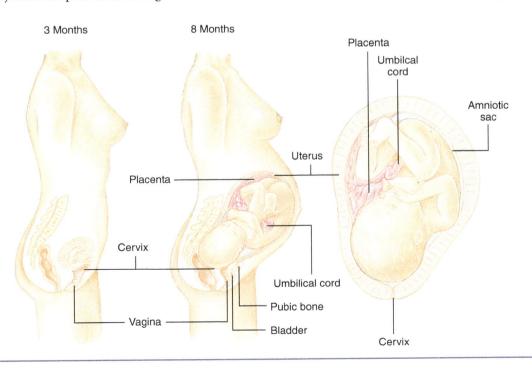

● **Figure 5**   The pregnant uterus.

lower rib margin. This enlarging abdominal mass also increases intraabdominal pressure and displaces the diaphragm upward. This displacement reduces lung capacity at the same time that the physiologic changes of pregnancy require an increase in tidal volume.

Pregnancy also affects maternal physiology by raising circulatory volume by about 45 percent. By the third trimester, pregnancy raises the cardiac rate by about 15 beats per minute and cardiac output by up to 40 percent. The increase in vascular volume is accompanied by a less significant increase in erythrocytes. The result is a relative anemia that becomes an important consideration with aggressive fluid resuscitation for the mother in shock. In the last trimester of pregnancy, the uterus is significant in both size and weight and may compress the vena cava, reducing venous return to the heart (cardiac preload) and inducing a temporary hypotension in the supine patient (supine hypotensive syndrome) that is easily corrected with repositioning. Finally, the developing fetus means there are now two

lives to protect when the mother suffers any trauma, especially involving the abdomen.

Vasculature

Abdominal contents are supplied with blood via the abdominal aorta, which travels along and to the left of the spinal column. It sends forth many branches to discrete organs and the bowel (Figure 6 ●). The abdominal aorta bifurcates at the upper sacral level into two large iliac arteries. These eventually become the femoral arteries as they traverse and then exit the pelvis. The attachment of these arteries to the pelvic structure is quite firm and may result in their tearing if the pelvis is fractured and displaced. The inferior vena cava is located along the spinal column and collects venous blood from the lower extremities and the abdomen, relatively parallel to the arterial system, returning it to the heart. The abdomen also houses a special circulatory system, the portal system. This venous subsystem

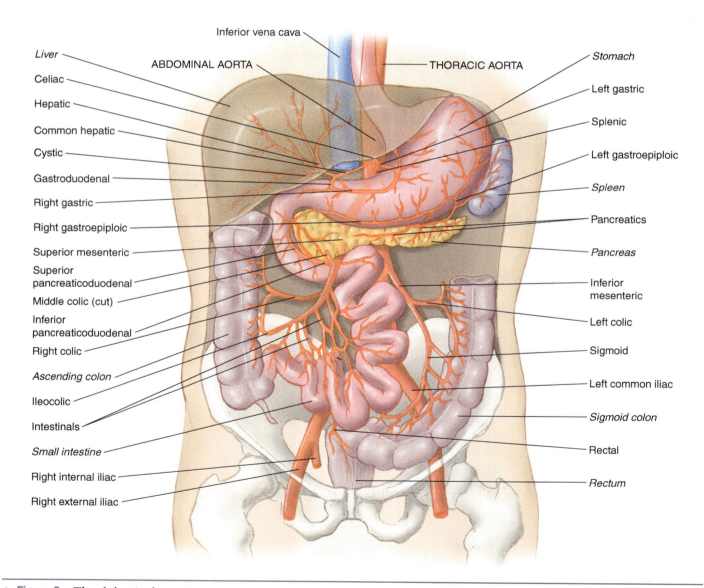

● **Figure 6** The abdominal arteries.

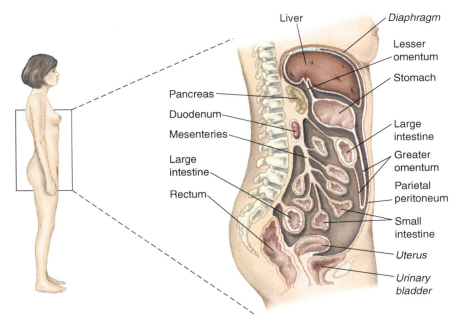

Liver
Diaphragm
Lesser omentum
Stomach
Pancreas
Duodenum
Large intestine
Mesenteries
Greater omentum
Large intestine
Parietal peritoneum
Rectum
Small intestine
Uterus
Urinary bladder

● **Figure 7**   Reflections of the peritoneum.

The abdominal cavity is a dynamic place. The diaphragm moves up and down, displacing abdominal contents with each breath. With deep expiration, the central diaphragm moves as far upward as the fourth intercostal space, anteriorly (the nipple line), and the seventh intercostal space (the inferior tips of the scapulae), posteriorly. (The diaphragm's edge attaches to the rib cage's border.) During forced and maximal inspiration, the diaphragm moves as much as 3 inches (9 cm) inferiorly. This movement displaces abdominal contents up and down with each breath. Additionally, the volume of substance within the hollow organs varies—an empty (10 mL) versus a distended (500 mL) bladder or a full (1.5 L) versus an empty stomach. The digestive tract is also suspended from the posterior abdominal cavity and is permitted some movement as it digests food. This dynamic movement becomes an important consideration when anticipating blunt or penetrating abdominal injury.

PATHOPHYSIOLOGY OF ABDOMINAL TRAUMA

Mechanism of Injury

Unlike other major body containers (skull, spine, and thorax), the abdomen is bound by muscles rather than skeletal structures. This results in a greater trauma energy transmission to internal organs and structures. Concurrently, overt physical energy transmission signs are limited.

Penetrating Trauma

Penetrating trauma imparts its energy directly to tissues touched by the offending object (Figure 8 ●) or, as with high-velocity

collects venous blood and fluids and nutrients absorbed by the bowel and transports them to the liver. The liver detoxifies the fluid, stores excess nutrients, adds nutrients when they are deficient, and then sends the blood/nutrient/fluid mixture into the inferior vena cava, just below the heart. There it mixes with venous blood and is circulated through the heart and then to the rest of the body.

Peritoneum

Many abdominal organs are covered by a serous membrane called the **peritoneum** (Figure 7 ●). This tissue resembles the lung's pleura and functions in a similar manner. The parietal peritoneum covers most of the interior surface of the anterior and lateral abdominal cavity, while the visceral peritoneum covers individual organs. A small amount of fluid is found between peritoneal layers and permits free bowel movement during digestion. The digestive tract is restrained and prevented from tangling by a structure called the **mesentery**. The mesentery is a double peritoneal fold containing blood vessels, lymphatic vessels, nerves, and fatty tissue. It suspends the bowel from the posterior abdominal wall. An additional fold of mesentery, called the omentum, also covers, insulates, and protects the anterior abdominal cavity. The omentum thickness varies with the size and percentage of body fat. It may be several inches thick in an obese patient or very narrow in a thin and muscular patient. Some abdominal structures are covered by peritoneum, excepting the kidneys, spleen, duodenum, pancreas, urinary bladder, the posterior portions of the ascending and descending colon, and the rectum. Most major vascular structures within the abdomen are also retroperitoneal. An organ's relation to the peritoneum becomes important in trauma because peritoneal irritation (peritonitis) caused by free blood in the peritoneal space presents with more apparent signs and symptoms than does hemorrhage or other fluid release into the retroperitoneal space.

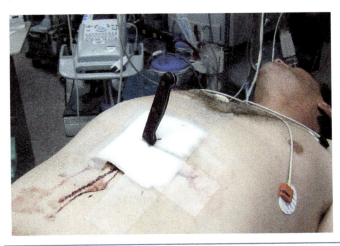

● **Figure 8**   Stab wound to the upper abdomen. (© *Michael Casey, MD*)

projectiles (from handguns, shotguns, and rifles), transmits energy and injury some distance from the projectile pathway. The bullet injury process causes damage as the projectile contacts tissue, sets that tissue and surrounding tissue in motion, then compresses and stretches surrounding tissue. The projectile adds to the damage as it draws debris and contaminants into the wound, potentially causing wound infection or poor healing. Tissue disruption from penetrating trauma may permit uncontrolled hemorrhage, organ damage, spillage of hollow organ contents, and, eventually, abdominal lining (peritoneum) irritation. Gunshot wounds to the abdomen, especially those from rifles, high-powered handguns, and shotguns at close range, impart tremendous energy and tend to cause a mortality and morbidity about ten times greater than that associated with the lower velocity stab wounds.[2] When penetrating trauma induces injury, it affects the liver 40 percent of the time, the small bowel about 25 percent of the time, and the large bowel about 10 percent of the time. Injuries to the spleen, kidneys, and pancreas follow in decreasing order of incidence.

A special type of penetrating trauma is induced by a shotgun blast. A shotgun often delivers numerous round pellets (called shot) through the hollow gun barrel. Shot aerodynamics and the rapid expansion of their distribution (pattern) cause the impact energy to decrease rapidly the farther the projectiles travel from the barrel. Generally, shotgun blasts at short range (under 3 yards) are extremely lethal. Between 3 and 7 yards, projectile penetration is great but often survivable. At distances greater than 7 yards, penetration depth and subsequent injury fall off quickly. These parameters change somewhat with the decreasing gauge size (gun barrel diameter) and the shot size.

Blunt Trauma

Blunt trauma to the abdomen produces the least visible signs of injury and causes trauma through three mechanisms: deceleration, compression, and shear (Figure 9 ●). As the exterior of the abdomen decelerates (or accelerates) during impact, its contents slam into one another in a chain reaction. They are first injured by the force changing their velocity, then by the forces of compression, as they are trapped between the impacting object and the more posterior organs. The entire contents of the cavity may be compressed between the force impacting the anterior abdominal cavity and the spinal column. Shear forces induce damage when one part of an organ is free to move while another part is restricted by trauma forces or by ligamentous or vascular attachments. Blunt trauma is responsible for about 20 to 25 percent of the incidences of splenic injury and 20 to 29 percent of hepatic (liver) injury. The bowel and kidneys are the next most frequently injured abdominal structures in blunt trauma.[3]

Careful mechanism of injury evaluation, including identification of the impact force and direction as it relates to the abdomen, is important to anticipating injuries within the region. Special attention is drawn to the potential for seat belt injury or direct injury as the abdomen impacts the steering wheel in a vehicle crash, impacts with objects or the ground during a fall, or receives striking blows during an assault. Remember that the early presentation of a contusion will likely be a simple reddening (erythema) of the affected area, not the more dramatic discoloration of ecchymosis. Hence it is critically important to analyze the mechanism of injury, identify a high index of suspicion for intraabdominal injury, and carefully investigate the abdomen for signs and symptoms of injury. The abdominal wall, hollow organs, solid organs, vascular structures, mesentery, and peritoneum all respond differently to trauma.

Abdominal Wall Injury

Any injury to the abdominal contents must first disrupt, or be transmitted through, the abdominal wall. Since the skin and muscular lining of the abdomen are more resistant to injury than many of the internal organs, they are likely to be uninjured or minimally injured by blunt trauma forces that cause serious injury within. Even when injured, the skin and underlying muscle may only show erythema during the first hour or so. The more visible discoloration of ecchymosis and any noticeable swelling require several hours to develop. Penetrating wounds may also be difficult to assess properly because musculature and skin tension close the wound opening. Bullet and knife wounds look especially small and may appear much less lethal than they are.

Penetrating abdominal injury may permit abdominal contents to protrude through the opening. This type of injury, called an **evisceration**, occurs most frequently through the anterior abdominal wall and is usually associated with a large and deep laceration (Figure 10 ●). The omentum and/or small bowel are most likely to protrude, though the large bowel may be involved. The evisceration endangers the protruding bowel because of compromised circulation, associated bowel obstruction, and drying of this delicate intraabdominal tissue. However, replacing the protruding abdominal contents risks introducing bacteria into the peritoneal space. If the bowel is torn, there is an additional danger of its contents leaking into the peritoneal space when it is replaced.

Penetrating trauma to the thorax, buttocks, flanks, and back may also enter the abdomen and injure its contents. Abdominal organs extend well into the thorax and move up to the nipple line anteriorly and to the tips of the scapulae posteriorly during deep expiration. Injury to the lower chest may lacerate the

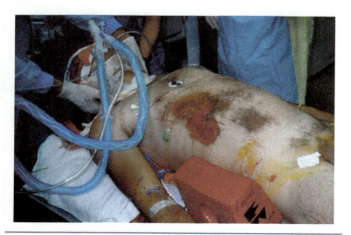

● **Figure 9** Blunt trauma to the upper abdomen. (© *Edward T. Dickinson, MD*)

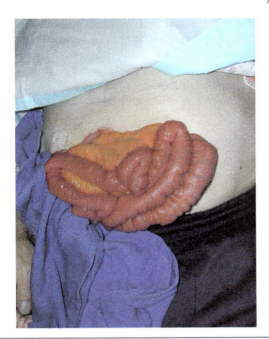

● Figure 10 Abdominal evisceration. *(© Charles Stewart, MD, and Associates)*

diaphragm and injure the stomach, liver, spleen, or gallbladder. Flank, back, and buttock muscles are thick and resist penetrating trauma very well. However, deep wounds in these locations can penetrate into the abdominal cavity and cause injury to adjacent organs. High-powered projectiles, especially those from hunting or military rifles, may have enough energy to deflect when striking bone and enter the abdomen from as far away as a proximal extremity wound.

Tears in the diaphragm may also disrupt the abdominal container. These tears may occur when the patient holds his breath just before an impact or with penetrating injury to the lower thorax or upper abdomen. Not only may such an injury compromise the important role of the diaphragm in respiration, but it may also permit or force abdominal contents (like those of the stomach, liver, or a portion of the small bowel) to enter the thoracic cavity. This reduces thoracic cage volume available during respiration and compromises the blood supply to the herniated organs. Diaphragmatic injury occurs from stab injuries most frequently on the left side because this is where right-handed assailants strike. Gunshot wounds affect both sides equally. Small tears are unlikely to permit abdominal contents to enter the thorax nor are they likely to greatly affect respiration. Large tears are more likely to do both.

Hollow Organ Injury

Hollow organs like the stomach, small bowel, large bowel, rectum, urinary bladder, gallbladder, and pregnant uterus may rupture with compression from blunt forces, especially if the organ is full and distended. They may also tear as penetrating objects disrupt their structure. The small bowel is the most frequently injured hollow abdominal organ during penetrating trauma because it rests anteriorly and just beneath the thin anterior abdominal muscles and omentum.[1] Hollow organ damage results

in hemorrhage and in content spillage into the retroperitoneal, peritoneal, or pelvic spaces. The jejunum, ileum, colon, and rectum contain progressively higher bacterial concentrations, and their rupture and the subsequent leakage into the abdomen will likely induce severe but delayed infection. The other hollow organs are more likely to release contents that cause a chemical irritation of the abdominal lining. The urinary bladder will release urine; the gallbladder, bile; and the stomach and duodenum, chyme; which is acidic and rich in digestive enzymes. Injury to the hollow organs may result in frank blood in the stool (**hematochezia**), blood in emesis (**hematemesis**), and blood in the urine (**hematuria**).

Solid Organ Injury

Solid organs such as the spleen, liver, pancreas, and kidneys are also subject to blunt and penetrating trauma. These organs are especially dense and are not held together as strongly as the more muscular hollow organs. They are prone to contuse, resulting in organ damage and minimal bleeding, or to rupture. If the organ's capsule remains intact, it will limit hemorrhage. However, if the capsule is disrupted by penetrating trauma or torn by the mechanism of blunt trauma, unrestricted hemorrhage may result.

The spleen is especially well protected by the lower ribs, back and flank muscles, and spinal column. It may be injured with severe abdominal compression, blunt left flank trauma, or penetrating injury to its location. The spleen can bleed profusely, resulting in shock. Occasionally, blood loss may accumulate against the diaphragm (especially in the supine patient) and result in referred pain to the left shoulder region (Kehr's sign).

The pancreas is central to the upper abdomen, somewhat less delicate than the spleen, and well protected from blunt trauma by its location deep in the central abdominal cavity. Penetrating trauma may lacerate its structure and permit blood and digestive enzymes to flow into the abdominal cavity. These pancreatic enzymes may actually begin to digest pancreatic and surrounding tissues, leading to severe internal injury. Pancreatic injury does sometimes result from severe blunt trauma to the upper abdomen that compresses the pancreas between the trauma force and the vertebral column. This may occur when a patient impacts a steering wheel or the handlebars of a motorcycle during a crash. Such a patient frequently complains of upper abdominal pain that may radiate to the back.

The kidneys are equally well protected by their location deep in the retroperitoneal cavity. They are somewhat more resistant to injury than the pancreas, have a more substantial serous capsule, and are attached by large renal arteries to the aorta. They are most frequently injured with trauma to the flanks.[4] Renal injury may result in regional (back or flank) pain as well as hematuria.

The liver is the largest single organ within the abdomen. Being a peritoneal organ, it is surrounded by the strong visceral peritoneum, which resists injury and will hold the organ together if injured. The liver is firmer than both the spleen and pancreas and is somewhat protected by the inferior border of the thorax. When trauma forces are directed to this region, however, they are likely to damage the liver, especially if they induce lower rib fracture on the right side. The liver is restrained from forward motion by the ligamentum teres. During severe deceleration, the liver's weight forces it into the ligament, causing shear forces, laceration, and hemorrhage. Liver injury often presents with tenderness along the right lower thoracic border and, as blood accumulates against the diaphragm, pain in the upper right shoulder. The liver is a very vascular organ and may account for serious internal hemorrhage and the need for massive in-hospital fluid resuscitation.

Vascular Structure Injury

Arteries and veins within the abdomen are prone to injury with serious consequences. The abdominal aorta and its major tributaries (gastric, superior and inferior mesenteric, splenic, hepatic, renal, gonadal, and iliac) can be injured by direct blunt or penetrating trauma or may be injured as abdominal organs decelerate and pull on their vascular attachments during an auto crash or similar impact. Penetrating trauma does not frequently involve the very large abdominal vessels, but when the aorta or other major artery is damaged, internal hemorrhage can be severe. The vena cava and its tributaries and the portal system can likewise be injured and may bleed heavily because the limited musculature in the large veins does not close the lumen as well as with arterial vessels. Most vascular injuries are associated with penetrating trauma and carry a mortality rate of between 30 and 60 percent.[3]

Vascular injury in the peritoneal, retroperitoneal, and pelvic spaces can be serious for several reasons. These spaces expand easily, and do not progressively resist continuing hemorrhage that would occur with vascular injury within a muscle mass elsewhere in the body. Without this pressure, both the rate and volume of blood loss do not diminish. These spaces also contain organs that require significant circulation supplied by rather large arterial and venous vessels. The abdomen's dynamic nature and its anatomic size mean that greater blood volumes can accumulate before swelling becomes noticeable. Further, due to vagal stimulation caused by blood in the peritoneal cavity, an increasing heart rate (a common sign of internal hemorrhage and impending shock) may not be present.

Mesentery and Bowel Injury

The mesentery provides the bowel with circulation, innervation, and attachment. Blunt injury occurs as the mesentery stretches during impact. This injury occurs most frequently at points of relative immobility such as the duodenal/jejunal juncture (where the small bowel is affixed by the ligament of Treitz) or where the small bowel joins the large bowel at the ileocecal junction. Injury involving the mesentery may disrupt blood vessels supplying the bowel and eventually cause ischemia, necrosis, and possible rupture. Mesenteric injuries do not usually bleed profusely because peritoneal layers contain the hemorrhage. Deceleration or compression may tear or rupture the full bowel. With penetrating trauma, the omentum is frequently disrupted and the bowel may be torn anywhere along its length, though tears to the small bowel (jejunum and ileum) are the most likely because of its central and anterior location. Even though a tear

may release bowel contents (digesting materials and possibly air) into the peritoneal space, signs and symptoms of such release are often delayed. The duodenum is less frequently injured because of its location deep within the abdomen. Penetrating trauma to the lateral abdomen is likely to injure the large bowel (ascending colon on the right and descending colon on the left).

Peritoneal Injury

The peritoneum is the very delicate and sensitive lining of the anterior abdominal cavity. Its inflammation, called **peritonitis**, can be caused by two major mechanisms, bacterial and chemical irritation. Bacterial peritonitis is an irritation due to infection, which is often caused by bacteria released into the space by a torn bowel or open wound. It takes the bacteria between 12 and 24 hours to grow in sufficient numbers to produce inflammation and hence the condition is usually not apparent during prehospital care. Chemical peritonitis occurs more rapidly than bacterial peritonitis because of the caustic nature of digestive enzymes and acids (from the stomach or duodenum), and, to a lesser degree, urine. These agents quickly irritate the peritoneum and induce the inflammatory response. Blood induces limited peritoneal inflammation, and hence serious hemorrhage into the peritoneal cavity is unlikely, by itself, to cause this condition.

Peritonitis is a progressive process that presents with characteristic signs and symptoms. It usually begins with a slight tenderness at the injury location. Over time, the area of inflammation expands, as does the area of tenderness. Any abdominal jarring, as occurs with percussion or when you quickly release the pressure of deep palpation, causes a twinge of pain (rebound tenderness). **Rebound tenderness** is a sign of great historical importance, but testing for it is painful and offers no information not gained by ordinary palpation. The practice of eliciting rebound tenderness is considered obsolete and is discouraged in modern care. In response to pain induced by movement of the irritated abdominal tissue, the anterior abdominal muscles contract, even in the unconscious patient. This is called **guarding**. When assessing the abdomen, be aware that local muscle injury caused by trauma may result in local or regional abdominal muscle tenderness and spasm that mimics peritonitis. Tenderness or frank pain from the physical injury may coexist with the signs of peritonitis.

Pelvic Injury

A pelvic fracture represents a serious skeletal injury, serious and often life-threatening hemorrhage, and potential injury to organs within the pelvic space. These organs—the ureters, bladder, urethra, female genitalia, prostate, rectum, and anus—can all be injured by severe kinetic forces, crushing mechanisms, or by displaced bone fragments. Pelvic fracture can also cause serious injury to the pregnant uterus.

Trauma and sexual assault may also injure the reproductive structures located internally in the female and externally in the male. Direct trauma to external female genitalia or injury caused by objects inserted into the vagina may tear the soft tissues of this region. Since these tissues are both very sensitive and vascular, the injury may bleed heavily and be very painful. The same is true for the male genitalia, though they are more prone to injury because of their external location.

Injury during Pregnancy

Trauma is the number one killer of pregnant females. Penetrating abdominal trauma alone accounts for as much as 36 percent of overall maternal mortality. Gunshot wounds to the abdomen of the pregnant female also account for fetal mortality rates of between 38 and 67 percent.[5] In blunt trauma, auto collisions are the leading cause of maternal and fetal mortality and morbidity. Proper seat belt placement can significantly reduce injury to the pregnant mother and fetus, while improper placement increases the incidence of both uterine rupture and placental separation from the uterine wall. Unrestrained or improperly restrained mothers in serious auto collisions are three times more likely to suffer fetal mortality.[5]

Physiologic changes associated with pregnancy protect both the mother and her abdominal organs. With the increasing uterine size, most abdominal organs are displaced higher in the abdominal cavity (Figure 11 ●). This generally protects them, unless blunt or penetrating trauma impacts the upper abdomen. If that happens, then the injury may involve numerous organs with increased morbidity and mortality. Direct penetrating injury to the central and lower abdomen of the late pregnancy mother often spares her from serious injury; the resulting injury, however, often damages the uterus and endangers the fetus.

The late-term female is at additional risk of vomiting and possible aspiration. Increasing uterine size increases intraabdominal pressure, while pregnancy hormones relax the cardiac sphincter (the valve that prevents stomach contents reflux). The bladder is displaced superiorly early in pregnancy and then becomes more prone to injury and, when injured, bleeds more heavily.

Increasing uterus and fetal size and weight have several maternal effects that should be considered after trauma. The uterus of a supine patient in late pregnancy may compress the inferior vena cava and reduce venous return to the heart. This may induce hypotension in the uninjured patient and have severe consequences in the hemorrhaging trauma patient. Increased intraabdominal pressure complicated by inferior vena cava compression (by the large and heavy uterus) raise venous pressure in the pelvic region and lower extremities. This pressure engorges the vessels and may increase the venous hemorrhage rate from any pelvic fracture or lower extremity wounds.

The increased maternal vascular volume (up by 45 percent) helps protect the mother from hypovolemia. However, this increase in maternal blood volume does not protect the fetus. (Maternal hypotension will reduce the blood flow to the placenta early in its progression.) In fact, it may take a maternal blood loss of between 30 and 35 percent before changes in maternal blood pressure or heart rate are evident. During this time, reduced placental circulation may endanger the developing fetus. Therefore, it becomes very important to ensure early and aggressive resuscitation of the potentially hypotensive pregnant mother.

In pregnant females, the thick and muscular uterus contains both the developing fetus and amniotic fluid. This container is strong, distributing trauma forces uniformly to the fetus and thereby reducing chances for injury. Significant blunt trauma may cause uterine rupture, and penetrating trauma may

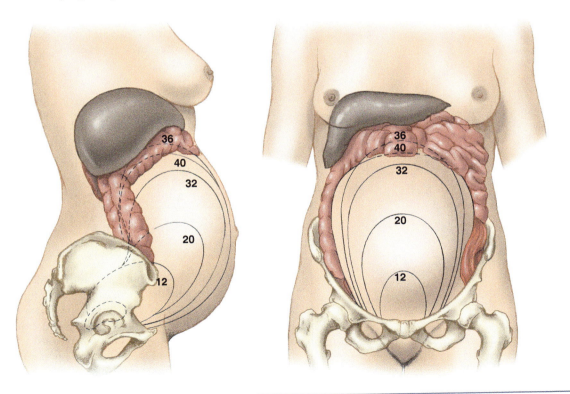

● **Figure 11**   Changing dimensions of the pregnant uterus. Numbers represent weeks of gestation.

perforate or tear it. Here, the dangers of severe maternal hemorrhage and fetal blood supply disruption present life threats to both. The potential release of amniotic fluid into the abdomen is also of great concern. Uterine and fetal injury risk increase with gestation length and are greatest during the third trimester. Frank uterine rupture is a rare complication of trauma, but it does occur with severe blunt impact, pelvic fracture, and—very infrequently—with stab or shotgun wounds.

Blunt trauma to the uterus that causes forceful uterine flexing may result in the placenta detaching from the uterine wall. This is because the placenta is rather inelastic while the uterus is very flexible. This condition, called **abruptio placentae**, presents a life-threatening risk to both mother and fetus because the separation permits both maternal and fetal hemorrhage (Figure 12 ●). Abruptio placentae may present with vaginal bleeding, although hemorrhage is often contained within the uterus. Blunt trauma may also cause premature amniotic sac rupture (breaking of the "membranes" or "bag of waters") and may induce early labor.

Pediatric Abdominal Trauma

Another special patient affected by abdominal injuries is the child. Children have poorly developed abdominal musculature and a reduced anterior/posterior diameter. The rib cage is more cartilaginous and flexible and more likely to transmit injury to the organs beneath. These factors increase the incidence and seriousness of pediatric abdominal injury, especially to the liver, spleen, and kidneys. Children also compensate very well for blood loss and may not show any signs or symptoms until they have lost over half of their blood volume. This is

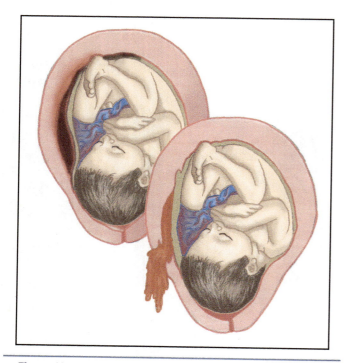

● **Figure 12**   Blunt trauma to the uterus may cause separation of the placenta from the uterine wall (abruptio placentae), shown at left, or even rupture of the uterus, shown at right.

especially important with abdominal injuries, because a large blood volume may be lost into the abdomen with little pain or noticeable distention.

ASSESSMENT OF THE ABDOMINAL TRAUMA PATIENT

Assessment of the abdominal trauma patient is somewhat abbreviated because definitive care for such injury may be surgical intervention. Hence, it is imperative that you quickly assess the patient and, if indications of serious abdominal injury exist, you package and transport him expeditiously. Abdominal injury patient assessment is like that for any trauma patient, with pertinent and significant information gained during the scene size-up, primary assessment, rapid or focused trauma assessment, and serial reassessments.[6]

Scene Size-Up

Ensure that the scene is safe for you, fellow rescuers, bystanders, and the patient. Always use Standard Precautions before moving to the patient's side. Identify the mechanism of injury and begin to develop an index of suspicion and assess any impact the environment might have on assessment, care, and transport. Also determine the number of expected patients, any need for additional EMS, police, fire, and other service resources, and integrate with incident oversight.

For a patient who has sustained abdominal injury, mechanism of injury analysis is a very important scene size-up element. However, forming an index of suspicion for individual abdominal injuries is critical because the signs and symptoms are, for the most part, limited and nonspecific. In fact, more than 30 percent of patients with serious abdominal injury may present with no specific signs or symptoms whatsoever. Additionally, other less life-threatening but more painful injuries may overshadow signs and symptoms of a patient's abdominal injury. Also, those signs and symptoms that are present may become less specific in nature with time and the progressive nature of peritonitis. Lastly, the patient's reporting of his condition may be unreliable due to the effects of alcohol or drug ingestion, head injury, or shock.[7] Because of these factors, a well-developed index of suspicion may direct you to injuries that may otherwise be difficult to identify.

If the patient has suffered blunt trauma, identify the strength and direction of the forces and the location on the body they were delivered. Focus your observation and palpation on that site during the primary and rapid trauma assessments and place your highest suspicion of injury there. Begin to develop a list of possible organs injured (the index of suspicion) and the immediate and delayed effects they will have on the patient's condition. In serious blunt trauma or deep penetrating trauma, expect internal and uncontrolled hemorrhage.

If a patient was involved in an auto crash, identify if seat belts were used and if they were used properly (Figure 13 ●). Remember that improper placement (above the iliac crests) may increase the likelihood of abdominal compression (and lumbar spine) injury. Lack of seat belt use increases the incidence and severity of all types of trauma, including abdominal injury. Examine the vehicle interior for impact signs like deformity of a bent steering wheel, a deflated air bag, or a structural intrusion into the occupant compartment. Air bag deployment is likely to reduce the incidence of abdominal injury, but serious injury may still occur. Frontal impact is most likely to compress the abdomen, injuring the liver and spleen and possibly rupturing distended hollow organs like the stomach and bladder. Right side impact frequently induces liver, kidney, ascending colon, and pelvic injury, while left side impact induces splenic, kidney, descending colon, and pelvic injuries. Pedestrians, and especially children, are likely to sustain lower abdominal injury, especially if the vehicle impacts the patient's midsection. It is important to determine the impact velocity and the distance the patient was thrown. Motorcyclists and, to a lesser degree, bicyclists are likely to sustain abdominal injury as they are propelled forward while the handlebars restrain the pelvis and lower abdomen. In assaults and other isolated impacts, be observant for left flank impact and splenic or renal damage and right-side impact causing renal or hepatic (liver) injury. If impact involves the superior abdomen, suspect liver, stomach, spleen, and pancreatic injury, while impact to the middle or lower abdomen will likely damage the small bowel, kidneys, and bladder.

With a patient who has experienced penetrating trauma, determine the mechanism of injury. If it is a knife, arrow, or impaled object, approximate the probable insertion angle and depth, if possible (Figure 14 ●). Do not move or remove an impaled object.

With gunshot wounds, quickly determine what you can about the mechanism of injury: whether the weapon was a handgun, shotgun, or rifle; the gun's caliber; the distance from the gun to the victim; the number of shots fired; and, if possible, the angle from which the gun was fired. Expose the patient and carefully examine for wounds, including possible exit wounds. Attempt to estimate blood lost at the scene and communicate this, with the other information previously listed, to the emergency department physician. However, always keep in mind that your chief goal is

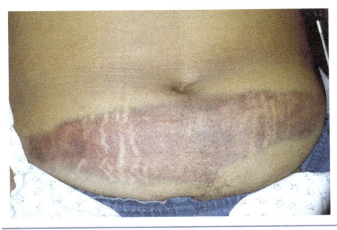

● **Figure 13**   Use the mechanism of injury to identify where signs of injury might be found—for example, contusions resulting from compression by a seat belt. (© *Charles Stewart, MD, FACEP*)

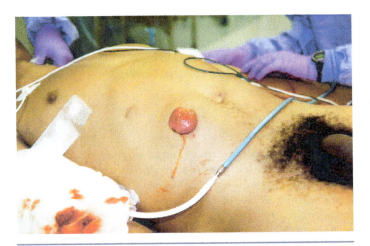

● **Figure 14**   Analyze the mechanism of a penetrating trauma in an attempt to determine the probable angle and depth of the wound. (© *Edward T. Dickinson, MD*)

to assess quickly and transport expeditiously the victim of any gunshot wound.

With either significant blunt or any penetrating trauma to the abdomen, suspect serious and continuing internal hemorrhage. Be especially watchful of the patient during your assessment and initiate shock care at the first signs and symptoms of hypoperfusion. These signs and symptoms include diminishing level of consciousness or orientation, increasing anxiety or restlessness, thirst, increasing pulse rate, decreasing pulse pressure, and increasing capillary refill time.

Information you gather at the scene is invaluable to the attending emergency department physician. That information, however, will be unavailable unless you document it carefully and report it on your arrival at the hospital. Doing this is essential to ensuring that patients receive the best care in both the prehospital and in-hospital settings.

Primary Assessment

As you begin the primary assessment, carefully note your patient's level of consciousness and orientation as well as any indication that he may be affected by alcohol, drugs, head injury, or shock. These agents and conditions reduce your patient's reliability in reporting signs and symptoms of abdominal trauma. Any decrease in the level of orientation or consciousness should alert you to the need to maintain a higher index of suspicion for abdominal injury and to perform more careful primary and rapid trauma assessments. The patient may also complain of dizziness or light-headedness when moving from a supine to a seated or standing position. (Do not ask the patient to move; however, he may have moved on his own before your arrival.) Any of these signs and symptoms should lead you to suspect hypovolemia, possibly from an abdominal injury. Use your initial evaluation as a baseline against which to trend any changes in the patient's consciousness or orientation level.

As you evaluate airway, breathing, and circulation, be observant for any associated signs and symptoms of hypovolemia, especially if they occur early in your care or are out of proportion with the obvious or expected injuries. Note any rapid shallow respirations, diminished pulse pressure, rapid pulse rate, slow capillary refill time, or thirst. Limited chest movement may be due to peritonitis or blood irritating the diaphragm. Shallow respirations may be due to abdominal contents in the thorax from a ruptured diaphragm. Be prepared to protect the airway because abdominal trauma patients are likely to vomit.

Secondary/Rapid Trauma Assessment

Perform the usual full rapid trauma assessment, but if you have developed a high index of suspicion for abdominal injury, pay particular attention to that region. Carefully examine the abdomen for evidence of injury as suggested by the mechanism of injury or by signs or symptoms observed during the primary assessment. When you suspect that a patient has received blunt trauma, look carefully over the entire abdominal surface for the slight reddening of erythema or minor abrasions associated with superficial soft-tissue injury. Remember that any trauma must pass through the abdomen's surface before it can do

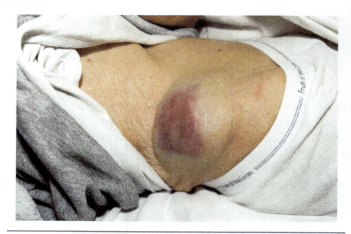

● **Figure 15** Examine the abdomen and flanks for signs of injury. *(© Dr. Bryan E. Bledsoe)*

damage within. Note the patient's positioning as it may suggest abdominal injury. Often the patient with abdominal pain will be in the fetal position to relax the abdominal muscles. He may also be very quiet and non-complaining.

Quickly examine the anterior abdominal surface and then flanks (Figure 15 ●). Then carefully and gently log roll the patient to examine the back, looking for any signs of injury, erythema, ecchymosis, contusions, or open wounds, including eviscerations and impaled objects Discoloration of the flank region is called Grey-Turner's sign, while discoloration around the umbilicus is called Cullen's sign. They result from accumulating blood and take time to develop. If you note a frank black and blue discoloration of an abdominal region, suspect an earlier injury or pathology.

Also look at the abdomen's general shape and any signs of distention. Visualize the inguinal area for injury or hemorrhage signs. Jeans or trousers may contain hemorrhage without any indication, so they should be cut away or removed to assess this region when injury is possible. Remember that the abdominal cavity can contain a very large volume of blood (on the order of 1.5 liters) before it becomes noticeably distended. In obese patients the blood volume loss may be even greater before distention is visible. Also be aware that signs and symptoms of peritoneal (hemoperitoneum) or retroperitoneal hemorrhage are limited.

Visualize and palpate the pelvis for signs of injury or instability. Apply gentle pressure directed posteriorly, then medially, on the iliac crests, then place pressure downward on the symphysis pubis. If you note any crepitus or instability, suspect pelvic fracture and both injury to lower abdominal organs and severe internal hemorrhage. If you already suspect pelvic injury, do not test or apply any pressure and be very careful during movement to the ambulance and transport to the hospital. Any fracture site manipulation may start, restart, or increase hemorrhage.

Question the patient about pain or discomfort in each quadrant, then palpate the quadrants individually, leaving any quadrant with anticipated injury or patient complaint of pain for last. If you palpate an injured quadrant first, the pain may lead the patient to splint or voluntarily contract the abdominal muscles during any remaining palpation. Feel for any spasm or guarding as you palpate. If you palpate an abdomen that is board hard, expect injury to the pancreas, duodenum, or stomach, especially if the time since the injury has been short. Also be observant for any patient pain with patient movement during assessment or care.

Also note any unusual pulsations in the abdomen. You may visualize some pulsing in the thin, young, healthy, athletic patient, but most patients will not have any visible or palpable pulses in the abdomen. Abnormal pulsation suggests arterial injury. Injuries to the thorax or pelvis also suggest abdominal injury, especially if there are lower rib fractures or the pelvic ring is unstable. Auscultation is not beneficial during abdominal trauma patient assessment. It takes a great deal of time to adequately listen for bowel sounds, and their presence or absence neither confirm nor rule out possible injury.

When evaluating the patient with penetrating trauma to the abdomen, look carefully at the entrance wound and note its appearance, size, and depth. Point-blank discharge of a gun against tissue will introduce barrel exhaust into the open wound created by the bullet. You may notice powder debris and the crackling of subcutaneous emphysema. Look for contamination and any signs of serious blood loss. Then examine the patient for an exit wound. Exit wounds may look more "blown out" in nature and are generally larger and more serious in appearance than entrance wounds. Exit wounds are more likely to reflect the nature and extent of internal injury. Count the number of entry and exit wounds and note whether they are paired or if an inequality suggests that some projectiles did not exit. The wounds from a projectile may be very small and difficult to see, while still carrying the potential to cause lethal injury. (It is not advisable to note entrance and exit wounds on the patient care report as it is often difficult to distinguish between the two and there are legal ramifications to misidentifying wounds. Instead, simply describe the wound location and characteristics without reference to "entrance" or "exit.")

A new assessment technique now becoming available in the prehospital setting is ultrasonography. A device creates high-frequency sound waves (small and rapid pressure waves oscillating millions of times per second) that are transmitted into the abdomen. They reflect off organs, tissues, and fluids differently, based on density, and form a cross-sectional image. The device creates an image much the same way that radar does. This image can be used to identify the location of pooling blood within the abdomen (e.g., retroperitoneal) after abdominal trauma. Reassessments can also identify if the pooled blood volume is increasing or stable in size. While sonography use in prehospital care is still new and evolving, it is important to recognize that to be valuable, the sonographic findings must change patient management in some meaningful way. In blunt abdominal trauma, the presence of fluid in the peritoneal cavity suggests blood and could signal the need for transport to a trauma center. Conversely, in penetrating abdominal trauma (e.g., gunshot wound), transport to a trauma center is always indicated, and sonography is unlikely to change prehospital management. Consequently, sonographic imaging in penetrating abdominal trauma is not a priority.[8,9,10]

Anticipate injuries that occurred as the object or bullet sped into and through the body, but remember that it is not uncommon for a bullet to alter its path. Be suspicious of any projectile wound in the proximal extremities because the projectile may travel along the limb and into the body's interior. Also keep in mind that a bullet wound to the thorax may then deflect and penetrate the abdomen, or vice versa.

While performing the rapid trauma assessment, carefully question the patient about the characteristics of any pain he feels and ask specifically about any abdominal sensations or other symptoms. Serious injury may result while the patient feels limited pain or injury sensation, especially when other more painful injuries elsewhere might be distracting him. Abdominal pain evaluation may, however, be subjective as patients often vary in their response to pain. It may be necessary to watch the patient's response to further assessment or his ease in distraction to accurately gauge the patient's degree of pain. In the male, retroperitoneal pain may be referred to the testicular region. Thirst may be one of the few symptoms of abdominal injury as significant hemorrhage draws down the body's blood volume. Be sure to record any symptoms in the patient's own words and ensure these comments and your findings are documented on the prehospital care report and reported to the attending physician.

When investigating patient history, give special consideration to the last oral intake. The bladder, bowel, and stomach are much more likely to rupture if full and distended. Ask about when the patient last ate or drank and how much he consumed. Relate the intake to the type of impact received, especially blunt trauma to the trunk. Conclude the rapid trauma assessment by gathering a set of baseline vital signs. At the end of the rapid trauma assessment, reevaluate your patient's priority for transport. The potential for an abdominal injury must factor into this determination. Remember that serious internal hemorrhage from blunt or penetrating trauma frequently occurs with few overt signs and symptoms. Any patient with a history of significant blunt trauma or any penetrating trauma to the torso is a candidate for rapid transport to the trauma center. Always err on the side of providing more patient care and early transport rather than underestimating the seriousness of abdominal trauma.

Special Assessment Considerations with Pregnant Patients

If a patient you are treating is pregnant, pay special attention to the abdomen and the possibility of injury. Remember that the maternal blood volume is increased by up to 45 percent in the third trimester, and blood loss can exceed 30 percent before the normal signs and symptoms of hypovolemia reveal themselves. Watch for the earliest signs of shock. Ensure the uterus does not compress the vena cava by placing the noticeably pregnant mother in the left lateral recumbent position. If spinal injury is also suspected, immobilize her firmly to the spine board and, after she is placed on the stretcher, rotate the entire board and patient 15 degrees to the left side. Carefully evaluate maternal vital signs and remember that the fetus is likely to experience distress before the mother shows any signs of hypotension or hypoperfusion.

Abdominal trauma in late pregnancy may cause several specific uterine injuries and requires careful assessment. The normal uterus will be firm and round to palpation. It will be palpable above the iliac crests after the first 12 weeks of pregnancy and progress upward in the abdominal cavity until it

▶ Management of the Abdominal Injury Patient

• Position the patient properly
• Ensure adequate oxygenation and ventilation
• Control external bleeding
• Be prepared for fluid resuscitation
• Stabilize impaled objects

▶ When a serious mechanism of injury is found and the patient does not present with the signs and symptoms of shock, act in anticipation of it.

reaches the costal border at about 32 weeks. Your palpation of the injured uterus may result in tenderness and muscular contractions, which are normal with uterine contusions. These contractions will often be self-limiting; however, any tenderness, pain, or contractions should raise your suspicions of abruptio placentae. The mother may complain of cramping, generally related to palpable uterine contractions and, in some cases, experience vaginal hemorrhage. Abruptio placentae represents a serious fetal and maternal risk and is a true emergency requiring rapid transport.

Uterine palpation that reveals an asymmetrical uterus or permits you to recognize the irregular features of the fetus suggests uterine rupture. This condition may also present with uterine contractions, but the uterine fundus is not palpable and the mass does not harden with the contractions.

If uterine rupture or abruptio placentae are suspected or if you suspect any serious abdominal injury to the pregnant patient, ask for the mother's Rh status and report it to the emergency department. Alert the emergency department well before your arrival if you are transporting a pregnant mother who was injured by trauma. This allows department personnel to prepare for the special monitoring necessary for both the mother and fetus.

Reassessment

Reassessment is an essential part of the continuing care process for abdominal injury patients. During it, you will look for the signs of progressing abdominal injury or continuing hemorrhage. Perform it every 5 minutes in patients with any significant suggestion of abdominal injury. Often the progressive nature of peritonitis leads to greater and greater patient complaints or may make abdominal signs and symptoms more evident as you care for and reduce the pain of other injuries. Ongoing hemorrhage signs are equally progressive and may not clearly present until well into your patient care.

Pay close attention to the signs of hidden hemorrhage during reassessments of the patient with potential abdominal injury. Watch blood pressure, pulse rate, capillary refill time, oxygen saturation, and the patient's appearance and level of consciousness and orientation. A decrease in the difference between the systolic and diastolic blood pressures (the pulse pressure) suggests shock compensation. An increasing pulse rate (especially if the pulse strength is diminishing) and an increasing capillary refill time both suggest hypovolemic compensation. Also observe for the skin becoming cool, clammy, cyanotic, or ashen, and watch for pulse oximetry readings that become more erratic. A change in either the level of consciousness or, more subtly, a lowering of the patient's orientation suggests the brain is being hypoperfused. These findings all indicate the body

is employing increasing levels of shock compensation. If you cannot account for a continuing blood loss elsewhere, suspect internal and continuing abdominal hemorrhage. Subtle changes may be the only apparent signs of gradually worsening shock.

Another sign of continuing blood loss from an abdominal hemorrhage is fluid resuscitation that appears ineffective. Note your patient's response to fluid resuscitation. If it takes significant fluid volumes to maintain a patient's vital signs and all external hemorrhage is controlled, suspect continuing internal hemorrhage.

MANAGEMENT OF THE ABDOMINAL TRAUMA PATIENT

Abdominal injury patient management is supportive, with the major emphasis on bringing the patient to the emergency department as quickly as possible. Prehospital care centers on rapid packaging and transport and fluid resuscitation, as needed. Specific care steps for the abdominal injury patient include proper positioning, general shock care, fluid resuscitation, and care for specific injuries (open wounds and eviscerations).[11]

The patient with any abdominal pain should be positioned for comfort (unless the positioning is contraindicated by likely spinal injury). Flex the patient's knees to relax the abdominal muscles. If injuries permit, place the patient in the left lateral recumbent position to maintain knee flexure, relax abdominal muscles, and facilitate airway clearing of emesis.

Ensure good ventilation and consider early administration of high-concentration oxygen for the abdominal injury patient if the patient's pulse-oximetry values are less than 96 percent. Pain associated with peritonitis or diaphragmatic irritation may reduce respiratory excursion, adding to early shock development in these patients.

Control any moderate or serious external hemorrhage with direct pressure and bandaging. Minor bleeding may be controlled during transport, if at all.

When a serious mechanism of injury is found and the patient does not present with the signs and symptoms of shock, act in anticipation of it. Be prepared to administer fluid boluses if the signs of shock develop and the blood pressure drops below a systolic reading of 80 mmHg. Monitor pulse rate and blood pressure. If the pulse does not slow and the pulse pressure does not stabilize, consider administering an additional fluid bolus. Do not delay transport to initiate any IV access. Start the IV access en route to the hospital, if necessary. Prehospital infusion is usually limited to 3,000 mL of fluid. Titrate your administration rate to maintain a systolic blood pressure of 80 mmHg and ensure that you do not exceed this fluid volume limit during field care and transport.[12]

As you should with all serious trauma patients, communicate frequently with the abdominal injury patient to reduce anxiety and provide emotional support. Also watch for any changes in the patient's description of the pain or injury's character or intensity. Consider pain management, probably with Fentanyl because of its hemodynamic stability. Be wary of patient hypothermia, especially when providing fluid resuscitation. Provide ample

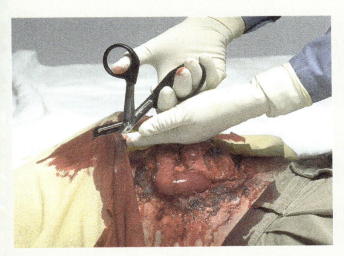

1a ● Remove clothing from around the abdominal wound.

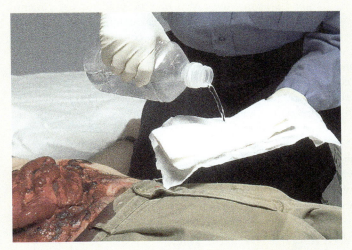

1b ● Cover the wound with a sterile dressing soaked with sterile normal saline.

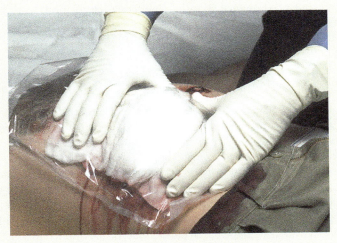

1c ● Cover the moistened dressing with a sterile occlusive dressing to prevent evaporative drying.

blankets, keep the patient compartment warm, take patient complaints of being cold seriously, and warm infusion fluids when possible. Hypothermia is a special consideration with pediatric patients because they have a disproportionately large body surface area to body volume and will rapidly lose heat to the environment.

Cover any exposed (eviscerated) abdominal organs with a dressing moistened with sterile saline (Procedure 1). Be careful to keep the region clean and do not replace any exposed organs. Cover the wet dressing with a sterile occlusive dressing like clear plastic wrap to keep the site as clean as possible and yet retain the moisture. If the transport is lengthy, check the dressing from time to time and remoisten as necessary.

Another wound that deserves special attention is the impaled object. Do all that you can to keep the object from moving and do not remove it. Any motion causes further injury, disrupts clotting mechanisms, and continues hemorrhage. Removal may withdraw the object from a blood vessel, thereby permitting increased internal and uncontrollable hemorrhage. Pad around the object with bulky trauma dressings and wrap around the trunk with soft, self-adherent roller bandaging to secure it firmly. Apply direct pressure around the object if hemorrhage is anything but minor. If the object is too long to accommodate during transport or it is affixed to an immovable object, attempt to cut it. Use a saw, cutter, or torch, but be very careful to ensure that vibration, jarring, and heat are not transmitted to the patient.

Carefully observe and care for penetrating wounds that may traverse both the abdominal and thoracic cavities. If the wound is large and may have penetrated the diaphragm or otherwise entered the thoracic cavity, seal the wound with an occlusive dressing taped on three sides to permit air pressure release that occurs in a tension pneumothorax. Be especially watchful of respiratory excursion and effort.

In some systems, the PASG may be used for the patient with blunt abdominal injury and the early signs of shock. However, it should not be used if there is concurrent penetrating chest trauma. The PASG applies circumferential pressure to the abdominal cavity, thereby raising intraabdominal pressure and reducing the rate of intraabdominal hemorrhage. Its use is generally contraindicated (inflate the leg sections only) in females in late pregnancy, abdominal evisceration patients, or patients with impaled objects. If the patient with an evisceration experiences a blood pressure below 50 mmHg, consider inflating the abdominal section of the garment because the risks associated with injury to the exposed bowel are less than those of profound hypotension. Incrementally inflate the PASG to maintain blood pressure and pulse rate, not to return them to preinjury levels.

Management of the Pregnant Patient

Special care is offered to the pregnant patient because of the anatomic and physiologic changes induced by pregnancy. Place the late-term mother, when possible, in the left lateral recumbent position. If the patient is on a spine board, tilt it to the left 15 degrees to achieve a similar effect. This ensures that the uterus's weight does not compress the vena cava, reduce blood return to the heart, and cause hypotension. It also facilitates airway care. Administer oxygen as needed early in your care; the mother's respiratory reserve volume is diminished because the effort necessary for her to move air is greater due to increased intraabdominal pressure and because the fetus is especially susceptible to hypoxia. If necessary, employ intermittent positive-pressure ventilation early in your care. Also consider aggressive airway care. The pregnant mother is prone to vomiting and aspiration. If she has a significantly reduced level of consciousness, consider rapid sequence intubation.

Maintain a high index of suspicion for internal hemorrhage since the increased blood volume of the third-trimester mother may permit an increased blood loss before signs and symptoms of hypovolemia become evident. The fetus may be at risk early in the blood loss, well before the mother displays any signs. Initiate IV therapy early, but remember that pregnancy induces a relative anemia and that aggressive fluid resuscitation may further dilute the erythrocyte concentrations and lead to ineffective circulation.

CHAPTER REVIEW

SUMMARY

Blunt or penetrating abdominal trauma can result in serious organ damage and life-threatening hemorrhage. Concurrently, injury signs are limited, nonspecific, and do not reflect the seriousness of abdominal pathology. It is thus very important to carefully determine the mechanism of injury and the region of the abdomen it affects. This information must be communicated to the emergency department to ensure its personnel acknowledge the significance of your first-hand knowledge of the mechanism of injury.

Care for significant abdominal injury is provided by rapid transport to the trauma center. Most significant abdominal injury results in serious internal bleeding or organ injury that can neither be cared for nor stabilized in the prehospital setting. Further, the definitive care for the patient with serious abdominal injury is provided via surgery. The patient must be transported to a facility capable of providing immediate surgical intervention when needed. This is a trauma center. Prehospital abdominal injury care is supportive of the airway and breathing, and preventive for shock.

The pregnant patient with abdominal injury deserves special attention because her vascular volume is increased and she will likely not show the signs of shock until the fetus is at risk. Careful observation while preparing for rapid transport to the trauma center is in order. If any of the slightest signs of hypoperfusion are noted, initiate fluid resuscitation.

YOU MAKE THE CALL

You arrive at the scene of a car–pedestrian collision. The victim is a young female about 12 years of age. She is lying on her side, in the fetal position, on the ground. She is conscious and alert, though confused as to where she is and what happened. The patient complains of right shoulder pain, although there is no injury visible in the region. Physical assessment reveals a tender left upper quadrant, just below the margin of the rib cage, with some guarding and no rebound tenderness.

1. Given the signs and symptoms, what is the most likely injury and why?

2. What relation does the right shoulder pain have to the suspected injury?

3. What care will you provide for this patient?

See Suggested Responses at the back of this chapter.

REVIEW QUESTIONS

1. Your patient has a history of trauma to the left flank and complains of pain in that region. Which of the following organs might you suspect to be injured?
   a. liver
   b. heart
   c. spleen
   d. gallbladder

2. All of the following statements regarding bile are correct except _____.
   a. bile is a waste product of the reprocessing of red blood cells
   b. bile is released into the colon in response to fatty foods
   c. bile aids in the digestion of fats
   d. bile is produced by the gallbladder

3. The kidneys serve the body in all of the following ways except _____.
   a. pH regulation
   b. waste product collection
   c. salt/water balance control
   d. fat emulsification

4. Penetrating trauma most frequently involves the _____ and small bowel.
   a. liver
   b. spleen
   c. kidneys
   d. aorta

5. A protrusion of organs from a wound is called an _____.
   a. extravasation
   b. evisceration
   c. ecchymosis
   d. exsanguination

6. One of the functions of the pancreas is _____.
   a. destroying spent RBCs
   b. producing new RBCs
   c. secreting glucagon
   d. manufacturing new WBCs

7. _____ is the number one killer of pregnant females.
   a. Hypertension
   b. Toxemia
   c. Trauma
   d. Sepsis

8. The appendix and portions of the urinary bladder, small bowel, ascending colon, rectum, and female genitalia are located in the _____.
   a. left lower quadrant
   b. right upper quadrant
   c. right lower quadrant
   d. left upper quadrant

9. The spleen is not an accessory organ of digestion but rather a part of the _____ system.
   a. integumentary
   b. respiratory
   c. nervous
   d. immune

10. It is very important to ensure early fluid resuscitation of the potentially hypotensive pregnant mother. This statement is true because it may take a maternal blood loss of between _____ and _____ percent before changes in maternal blood pressure or heart rate are evident.
    a. 10, 15
    b. 20, 25
    c. 30, 35
    d. 40, 45

See Answers to Review Questions at the back of this chapter.

REFERENCES

1. Isenhour, J. and J. Marx. "Abdominal Trauma." *Emergency Medicine: Concepts and Clinical Practice.* 7th ed. St. Louis: Mosby, 2009.

2. Eachempati, S. R., et al. "Factors Associated with Mortality in Patients with Penetrating Abdominal Vascular Injury." *J Surg Res* 108(2) (Dec 2002): 222–228.

3. Hubble, M. and J. Hubble. "Abdominal and Genitourinary Trauma." *Principles of Advanced Trauma Care.* Albany: Delmar, 2002.

4. "Abdominal and Pelvic Trauma." *Advanced Trauma Life Support Course: Student Manual.* 8th ed. Chicago: American College of Surgeons, 2008.

5. Bhatia, K. and H. Cranmer. "Trauma in Pregnancy." *Emergency Medicine: Concepts and Clinical Practice.* 7th ed. St. Louis: Mosby, 2009.

6. Collopy, K. T. and G. Friese. "Abdominal Trauma. A Review of Prehospital Assessment and Management of Blunt and Penetrating Abdominal Trauma." *EMS Mag* 39(3) (Mar 2010): 62–66, 68–69.

7. Mulholland, S. A., et al. "Prehospital Prediction of the Severity of Blunt Anatomic Injury." *J Trauma* 64(3) (Mar 2008): 754–760.

8. Heegaard, W., et al. "Prehospital Ultrasound by Paramedics: Results of Field Trial." *Acad Emerg Med* 17(6) (Jun 2010): 624–630.

9. Hoyer, H. X., et al. "Prehospital Ultrasound in Emergency Medicine: Incidence, Feasibility, Indications and Diagnoses." *Eur J Emerg Med* 17(5) (Oct 2010): 254–259.

10. Snaith, B., M. Hardy, and A. Walker. "Emergency Ultrasound in the Prehospital Setting: The Impact

of Environment on Examination Outcomes." *Emerg Med J* 28(12) (Dec 2011): 1063–1065.

11. Spaite, D. W., et al. "The Impact of Injury Severity and Prehospital Procedures on Scene Time in Victims of Major Trauma." *Ann Emerg Med* 20(12) (Dec 1991): 1299–1305.

12. Yaghoubian, A., R. J. Lewis, B. Putnam, and C. Virgilio. "Reanalysis of Prehospital Intravenous Fluid Administration in Patients with Penetrating Truncal Injury and Field Hypotension." *Am Surg* 73(10) (2007): 1027–1030.

FURTHER READING

American College of Surgeons, Committee on Trauma. *Advanced Trauma Life Support Course: Student Manual.* 8th ed. Chicago: American College of Surgeons, 2008.

Bates, Barbara, and Peter G. Szilagyi. *A Guide to Physical Examination and History Taking.* 9th ed. Philadelphia: J. B. Lippincott, 2007.

Bledsoe, B. E. and D. Clayden. *Prehospital Emergency Pharmacology.* 7th ed. Upper Saddle River, NJ: Pearson/Prentice Hall, 2011.

Bledsoe, B. E., B. J. Colbert, and J. E. Ankney. *Essentials of A & P for Emergency Care.* Upper Saddle River, NJ: Pearson/Prentice Hall, 2010.

Campbell, John E. *International Trauma Life Support for Emergency Care Providers.* 7th ed. Upper Saddle River, NJ: Pearson/Prentice Hall, 2012.

Ivatury, R. R. and G. C. Cayten, eds. *Textbook of Penetrating Trauma.* Media, PA: Williams & Wilkins, 1996.

Martini, Frederic. *Fundamentals of Anatomy and Physiology.* 7th ed. San Francisco: Benjamin Cummings, 2011.

McSwain, N. E. and S. B. Frame, eds. *Prehospital Trauma Life Support.* 6th ed. St. Louis: Mosby, 2010.

Rosen, P. and R. Barkin, eds. *Emergency Medicine: Concepts and Clinical Practice.* 7th ed. St. Louis: Mosby, 2009.

Tintinalli, J. E., ed. *Emergency Medicine: A Comprehensive Study Guide.* 7th ed. New York: McGraw-Hill, 2011.

SUGGESTED RESPONSES TO "YOU MAKE THE CALL"

The following are suggested responses to the "You Make the Call" scenarios presented in this chapter. Each represents an acceptable response to the scenario but should not be interpreted as the only correct response.

1. *Given the signs and symptoms, what is the most likely injury and why?*

Splenic injury is most likely because of the level of the vehicle in relation to her size when she was struck.

2. *What relation does the right shoulder pain have to the suspected injury?*

The right shoulder pain is most likely caused by being thrown to the ground following the injury. Referred pain from the spleen, Kehr's sign, is pain in the left shoulder region.

3. *What care will you provide for this patient?*

You will provide immediate spinal immobilization, oxygen, IV therapy, and rapid transport to the nearest trauma center.

ANSWERS TO REVIEW QUESTIONS

1. c
2. d
3. d
4. a
5. b
6. c
7. c
8. c
9. d
10. c

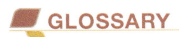

GLOSSARY

abruptio placentae   a condition in which the placenta separates from the uterine wall.

chyme   semifluid mixture of ingested food and digestive secretions found in the stomach and small intestine.

digestive tract   internal passageway that begins at the mouth and ends at the anus.

evisceration   a protrusion of organs from a wound.

guarding   protective tensing of the abdominal muscles by a patient suffering abdominal pain.

hematemesis   vomiting of blood.

hematochezia   passage of stools containing red blood.

hematuria   blood in the urine.

mesentery   double fold of peritoneum that supports the major portion of the small bowel, suspending it from the posterior abdominal wall.

pelvic space   division of the abdominal cavity containing those organs located within the pelvis.

peristalsis   wavelike muscular motion of the esophagus and bowel that moves food through the digestive system.

peritoneal space   division of the abdominal cavity
containing those organs or portions of organs covered by the peritoneum.

peritoneum   fine fibrous tissue surrounding the interior of most of the abdominal cavity and covering most of the small bowel and some of the abdominal organs.

peritonitis   inflammation of the peritoneum caused by chemical or bacterial irritation.

rebound tenderness   pain caused by any abdominal jarring as occurs with percussion or when the pressure of deep palpation is released quickly.

retroperitoneal space   division of the abdominal cavity containing those organs posterior to the peritoneal lining.

supine hypotensive syndrome   inadequate return of venous blood to the heart, reduced cardiac output, and lowered blood pressure resulting from pressure on the inferior vena cava by the fetus and uterus late in pregnancy.

Thoracic Trauma

Robert S. Porter, MA, EMT-P

STANDARD
Trauma (Chest Trauma)

COMPETENCY
Integrates assessment findings with principles of epidemiology and pathophysiology to formulate a field impression to implement a comprehensive treatment/disposition plan for an acutely injured patient.

OBJECTIVES

Terminal Performance Objective
After reading this chapter you should be able to assess and manage patients with thoracic trauma.

Enabling Objectives
To accomplish the terminal performance objective, you should be able to:

1. Define key terms introduced in this chapter.
2. Describe the anatomy and physiology of the thorax and the structures within it.
3. Describe the pathophysiology of blunt and penetrating thoracic trauma.
4. Describe the pathophysiology, assessment, and management of the following types of thoracic injuries:
   a. Chest wall injuries
   b. Pulmonary injuries
   c. Cardiovascular injuries
   d. Injuries to the diaphragm, esophagus, and tracheobronchial tree
   e. Traumatic asphyxia
5. Given a variety of scenarios, demonstrate the assessment and management of patients with thoracic injuries, including specific management of the following:
   a. rib fractures
   b. sternoclavicular dislocation
   c. flail chest
   d. open pneumothorax
   e. tension pneumothorax
   f. hemothorax
   g. blunt cardiac injury
   h. pericardial tamponade
   i. aortic dissection
   j. tracheobronchial injury
   k. traumatic asphyxia

From Chapter 8 of *Paramedic Care: Principles & Practice, Volume 5,* Fourth Edition. Bryan Bledsoe, Robert Porter, and Richard Cherry. Copyright © 2013 by Pearson Education, Inc. All rights reserved.

aneurysm

atelectasis

commotio cordis

electrical alternans

epicardium

flail chest

great vessels

hemopneumothorax

hemoptysis

hemothorax

ligamentum arteriosum

pericardial tamponade

pericardium

pneumothorax

precordium

pulmonary hilum

pulsus alternans

pulsus paradoxus

rhabdomyolysis

tension pneumothorax

tracheobronchial tree

xiphisternal joint

CASE STUDY

Medic 101 responds to a shooting call at a southside tavern. There a man was reportedly shot during a robbery attempt. Victoria and Christian are the responding paramedics. On arrival, they quickly size up the scene and determine it to be safe. Police are on-scene, have an assailant in custody, and have controlled the gathering crowd.

At the patient's side, paramedics find a supine male, just inside the tavern door. The tavern owner reports the man had tried to take cash from the register when he shot him with a .38 caliber handgun at close range. Primary assessment reveals a confused, yet weakly combative patient with pale, ashen skin. He says his name is Conrad and his age is 34. Conrad's speech is not broken by his respirations and he appears conscious, alert, and oriented. His trachea is midline, jugular veins are flat, and he is breathing with only slight distress. Victoria notes minimal bleeding without air leak from four wounds found just below the left clavicle along the midclavicular line, just left of the upper sternum, just right of the lower sternum, and close to the right nipple (and fifth intercostal space) along the midclavicular line. Conrad is slightly tachypneic with symmetrical chest rise and slightly diminished breath sounds on the right. During assessment, his level of consciousness begins to diminish. Radial pulses are not palpable, but weak, thready carotid pulses are present. No exit wounds are noted when Conrad is log rolled to place him on a long backboard to move him from the floor to the stretcher. The carotid pulse suggests a blood pressure between 60 and 80 mmHg. Pulse oximetry reads erratically between 88 and 92 percent.

Conrad is immediately placed on 100 percent oxygen and his color improves somewhat. He is rapidly loaded into the ambulance, where bilateral antecubital large-bore IV lines are initiated and run wide open. Christian administers a 500 mL bolus en route to Southside Hospital. After the bolus, Victoria rechecks the vital signs and notes the pulse remains rapid and weak and blood pressure is 72 by palpation. Conrad now only mumbles to verbal stimuli. Christian alerts medical direction and asks to have a trauma team standing by.

As Victoria addresses potential life threats identified during the primary assessment, she quickly reassesses the chest and notes more labored respirations and that chest rise is no longer symmetrical. The right chest is somewhat hyperexpanded, exhibiting decreased breath sounds in comparison to the left. Conrad appears more ashen, with carotid pulses now absent. His trachea appears somewhat deviated to the left with increasing jugular venous distention. Christian, suspecting tension pneumothorax, asks Victoria to decompress the right chest. Victoria inserts a 3-inch-long 14-gauge IV catheter into the right second intercostal space along the midclavicular line and notes a significant outrush of air. She now observes improvement in Conrad's color and chest rise with less labored breathing. A subsequent reassessment finds that weak, thready carotid pulses have returned as the ambulance arrives at the hospital.

The emergency physician and trauma team take over Conrad's care, initiate a transfusion of packed red blood cells, intubate him, and place bilateral chest tubes for hemopneumothoraces. A trauma X-ray series reveals one bullet in the area of the left scapula, another right of the thoracic spine, one in the right upper abdominal quadrant, and one in the midline upper abdomen. Bedside FAST ultrasound examination reveals blood in the abdomen. Conrad is rapidly transferred to an operating room and an abdominal exploration is performed, revealing a liver laceration and partial abdominal aorta laceration. These injuries are repaired, and Conrad survives.

INTRODUCTION TO THORACIC TRAUMA

The thoracic cavity contains many vital structures, including the heart, great vessels, esophagus, tracheobronchial tree, and lungs. Trauma to any one of these structures could be life threatening. Twenty to twenty-five percent of all trauma deaths are due to thoracic trauma (about 16,000 per year in the United States). The majority of these deaths are related to motor vehicle trauma. Immediate death from thoracic trauma is often due to myocardial or aortic rupture with delayed mortality related to tension pneumothorax, cardiac tamponade, airway rupture, and uncontrolled hemorrhage.[1]

An increase in penetrating trauma associated with violent crime has also been observed in urban areas (Figure 1 ●). Weapons in years past were likely to be of the "Saturday night special" variety: cheap, small-caliber revolvers often producing just single wounds. In recent years, semiautomatic handguns and high-velocity semiautomatic rifles with larger magazine capacities have become more popular, This has increased the incidence of patients receiving multiple chest wounds. With multiple wounds, there is a higher likelihood of vital structure injury and therefore higher mortality.

In this chapter, we will discuss thoracic trauma as a result of penetrating and blunt injuries. These mechanisms are not just simple injury categories but have real clinical significance. Certain injuries are almost exclusively associated with one type

of chest trauma but are unlikely with the other. For example, pericardial tamponade is almost exclusively associated with penetrating thoracic trauma, while cardiac rupture is almost exclusively caused by blunt forces. By considering mechanism of injury, understanding injury pathology, and being aware of a patient's physical injury signs and symptoms, you will be better able to predict, identify, and treat potentially life-threatening thoracic trauma.

THORACIC ANATOMY AND PHYSIOLOGY

The thoracic cage is a chamber that moves air in and out and where oxygen and carbon dioxide exchange to support metabolism. This chamber consists of the thoracic skeleton, diaphragm, and associated musculature. It is also the location of the heart, major blood vessels, trachea, bronchi, lungs, and other important structures essential for body function.

Thoracic Skeleton

The thoracic skeleton forms the thoracic cage and is defined by 12 pairs of C-shaped ribs. These ribs articulate posteriorly with the thoracic spine and then extend in an anterior and inferior direction (Figure 2 ●). The upper seven rib pairs join the sternum at their cartilaginous endpoints. The 8th through 10th ribs

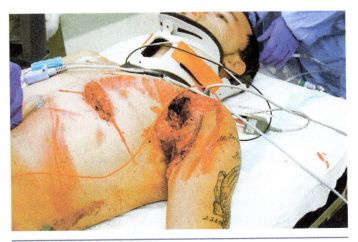

● **Figure 1**   An example of penetrating trauma to the chest. (© *Edward T. Dickinson, MD*)

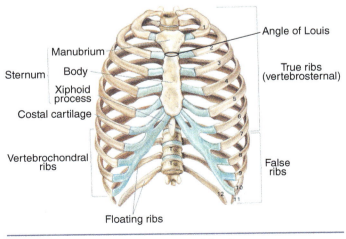

● **Figure 2**   Skeletal components of the thorax.

223

have indirect cartilage connections at their anterior ends where they join the 7th rib at the inferior sternal margin. The 11th and 12th ribs are often termed floating ribs and have no anterior attachment. The sternum completes the anterior bony thorax structure and is made up of three sections: the manubrium, the sternal body, and the xiphoid process. The manubrium is the sternum's superior portion and is the medial endpoint of the clavicle and first rib. The sternal angle (also known as the angle of Louis) is the junction of the manubrium and sternal body and is palpable through the skin as an elevated ridge or prominence. This ridge has clinical significance as it is the attachment site of the second rib and topographical landmark to help identify the second intercostal space. Knowing this location is important, because it helps you locate where to perform needle chest decompression in tension pneumothorax. The xiphoid process, the most inferior portion of the sternum, meets the sternal body just below the costal cartilages of the lower ribs (xiphisternal joint).

The thorax is divided by imaginary vertical lines used to describe positions lateral to the sternum. These lines include the midclavicular line, anterior axillary line, midaxillary line, posterior axillary line, and medial scapular line. When combined with a rib level, these lines serve as landmarks for describing wounds, for locating underlying structures, and for identifying locations to perform procedures. The space just inferior to each rib is called an intercostal space and is given the number of the rib above it. For example, the midsternal line extends from the middle of the sternum inferiorly along the thoracic wall. Its intersection with the second intercostal space is generally used as the site to place a needle to decompress the chest in tension pneumothorax.

The thoracic inlet is the superior thorax opening. It is narrow in comparison to the thoracic diameter and outlet, and is defined by the curvature of the first rib, with its posterior attachment to the first thoracic vertebra and ending anteriorly, at the manubrium. The thoracic outlet is formed posteriorly by the 12th vertebra, laterally by curvature of the 12th rib, and extends anteriorly and superiorly along the costal margin to the xiphisternal joint.

Diaphragm

The diaphragm is a domelike, muscular sheet that separates the abdominal cavity from the thoracic cavity. It is affixed to the rib cage's lower border, while its central and superior margin may extend to the fourth intercostal space anteriorly and sixth intercostal space posteriorly during maximal expiration. This superior positioning may allow penetrating wounds to the mid and lower thorax to penetrate the diaphragm and enter the abdominal cavity. The aorta, esophagus, and inferior vena cava exit the thoracic cavity through separate openings in this structure. The diaphragm is a major respiratory muscle, contracting to displace the thoracic cavity floor downward during inspiration and relaxing and moving upward with expiration.

Associated Musculature

Chest wall muscles found between ribs, called intercostal muscles, along with the diaphragm and sternocleidomastoid muscles are major muscles of respiration. Sternocleidomastoid muscles raise the upper rib and sternum and, with the sternum, raise the anterior attachments of the next nine ribs. Intercostal muscles contract to further elevate ribs and increase the thorax's anterior–posterior dimension. Simultaneously, the diaphragm, which forms the floor of the thorax, contracts and flattens to further increase thoracic cavity volume. As thoracic volume increases, pressure within it falls to less than atmospheric pressure. Air rushes in through the tracheobronchial tree and into alveoli, filling the lungs and alveoli and equalizing this pressure gradient.

As the naturally elastic musculature relaxes and recoils, the diaphragm again intrudes upward into the thoracic cavity, ribs and sternum move inferiorly, and ribs move closer together in an inferior and posterior direction. This decreases thoracic volume and increases intrathoracic pressure. When pressure within the thorax exceeds that of the surrounding atmosphere, air rushes out. Therefore, exhalation in a resting state is largely passive, aided by elastic lung recoil. This changing of volume to move air in and out is called the bellows effect.

Changing volume and arterial pressure within the thoracic cage also assist with moving blood into the systemic circulation and back to the heart. Increasing intrathoracic pressure during exhalation pushes blood away from the heart and thorax, while decreasing intrathoracic pressure during inspiration draws venous blood toward the thorax and heart. Changing intrathoracic pressure affects blood pressure and pulse strength, as well. Normally, systolic blood pressure and pulse strength fall slightly during inspiration and rise again during expiration.

Trachea, Bronchi, and Lungs

Contained within the thoracic cavity are the tracheobronchial tree and lungs. The tracheobronchial tree is a series of progressively narrowing and dividing tubes beginning with the trachea and ending at the alveoli. The trachea is a hollow, cartilage-supported respiratory pathway through which air moves in and out of the thorax and lungs. The trachea enters through the thoracic inlet and divides into right and left mainstem bronchi at the carina, located in the upper central thorax. Right and left mainstem bronchi extend for about 3 centimeters and enter each respective lung at the pulmonary hilum. The pulmonary hilum is also where pulmonary arteries enter and pulmonary veins exit and is the lung's sole fixation point in the thoracic cage. Bronchi then further divide into bronchioles, which ultimately terminate in alveoli. Lungs contain millions of these tiny "grape"-shaped alveoli, which are the basic unit of lung structure and function.

Each lung occupies one side of the thoracic cavity and is divided into lobes. The right lung has three lobes: upper, middle, and lower. The left lung has two lobes: upper and lower. The left upper lobe contains the cardiac notch against which the heart rests. The lower section of the left upper lobe (the lingula) projects around the lateral border of the heart and corresponds to the right lung's middle lobe.

Lungs are covered with a thin, smooth membrane called visceral pleura. It folds over on itself at the pulmonary hilum and then lines the thoracic cavity's interior, where it is called parietal pleura. The potential space that is formed between these dual layers of pleura contains a small amount of serous (pleural) fluid. This fluid lubricates the pleural layers and permits the lungs to move effortlessly against the interior thoracic wall during inspiration and expiration. The dual layers of pleura and pleural fluid also create a seal between the lungs and the thoracic cage that causes the lungs to expand and contract with changing thoracic cavity volume. If air is allowed to enter this potential space freely, the lung collapses, producing a pneumothorax.

Two respiratory centers in the pons also contribute to respiratory control. The apneustic center located in the lower pons acts as a shutoff switch to inspiration. If it becomes nonfunctional, respiratory patterns exhibit prolonged inspiration interrupted by occasional expirations. The pneumotaxic center is located in the upper pons, above the apneustic center, and acts to moderate activity of the apneustic center and provide further fine tuning of respiratory patterns.

Two respiratory reflexes are protective of air passages. The sigh reflex is a deeper than normal inspiration followed by a slower than normal exhalation. It occurs irregularly and occasionally in the normal physiologic state. This reflex recruits and expands alveoli that may become atelectatic (collapsed) with normal quiet respiration. If mechanical ventilation is required after traumatic chest injury, a sigh is often programmed into ventilator settings to prevent atelectasis. The cough reflex is a spasmodic diaphragm contraction to expel foreign material from the bronchi, trachea, and larynx.

Mediastinum

The mediastinum is the central space within the thoracic cavity bounded laterally by the lungs, inferiorly by the diaphragm, and superiorly by the thoracic inlet (Figure 3 ●). The heart is located within and fills most of the mediastinum. The great vessels, trachea, and esophagus as well as the vagus and phrenic nerves enter the mediastinum through the thoracic inlet. The esophagus then courses anterior to the aorta before exiting through the diaphragm at the thoracic outlet (esophageal hiatus or foramen). The vagus nerve, which provides parasympathetic innervation of thoracic and abdominal viscera, traverses the mediastinum—giving branches to the larynx, esophagus, trachea, bronchi, and supraventricular tissues of the heart—then exits the thorax through the esophageal hiatus in the diaphragm. The phrenic nerve traverses the thorax to innervate the diaphragm.

Heart

The heart is a four-chambered muscular pump, divided into right and left chambers by the cardiac septum and into upper and lower chambers by the cardiac valves. The right heart circulates blood to the lungs (pulmonary circulation) and the left heart circulates blood to the rest of the body (systemic circulation). The heart receives a rigorous supply of blood from vessels on its surface, the coronary arteries.

A membranous lining, the pericardium, surrounds the heart. It is similar to the pleura of the lungs. The portion of this lining that covers the heart's outer surface is the epicardium, or visceral pericardium. It then extends to the root of the great vessels before folding back on itself. This folding back forms the parietal pericardium, which is the pericardial sac's outer lining that surrounds the heart. These two layers make up the serous pericardium and, like pleura, also form a potential space, the pericardial space. This space usually contains a small amount (up to 35 to 50 mL) of straw-colored fluid. Pericardial fluid functions as a lubricant between visceral and parietal layers and permits the heart to move easily against the lungs during contractions. External to the serous pericardium is a tough fibrous sac called the fibrous pericardium that, unlike the serous pericardium, resists distention. The fibrous pericardium originates at the base of the great vessels and surrounds the heart and serous pericardium before fusing with the central tendon of the diaphragm. This pericardial structure fixes the heart in the mediastinum and prevents kinking of the great vessels. If the pericardial space rapidly fills with blood, the fibrous pericardium resists passive heart filling during diastole and thereby reduces cardiac output (pericardial tamponade).

Great Vessels

Great vessels are found in the mediastinum and include the aorta, superior and inferior vena cava, pulmonary arteries, and pulmonary veins. Injury to these large vascular structures can lead to

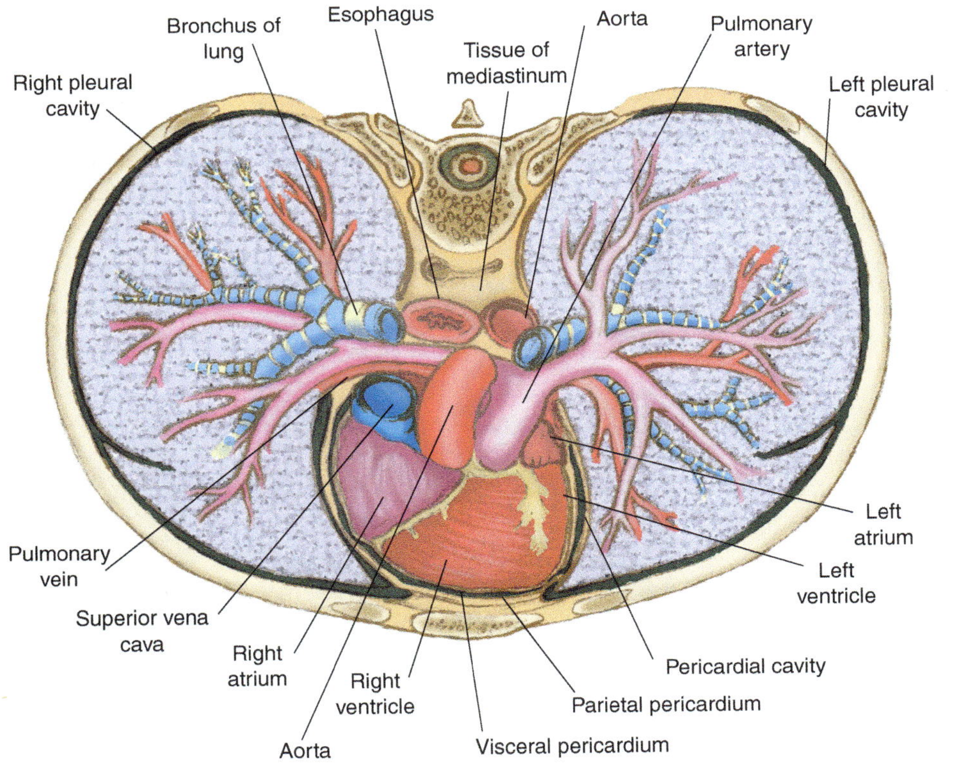

● **Figure 3** Structures of the mediastinum and thorax.

Labels: Bronchus of lung; Esophagus; Tissue of mediastinum; Aorta; Pulmonary artery; Right pleural cavity; Left pleural cavity; Pulmonary vein; Superior vena cava; Right atrium; Right ventricle; Aorta; Visceral pericardium; Parietal pericardium; Pericardial cavity; Left ventricle; Left atrium

rapid blood loss and death if the condition is not quickly recognized and repaired. The aorta, which is fixed at three positions within the thorax, is not only susceptible to penetrating injury, but also to blunt injury by rapid deceleration or shear forces. It is fixed at the annulus where it leaves the heart, at the **ligamentum arteriosum** near the bifurcation of the pulmonary artery, and at the aortic hiatus where it passes through the diaphragm and enters the abdomen.

Other major vessels that branch from great vessels in the upper thorax include subclavian arteries and veins, jugular veins, common carotid arteries, and brachiocephalic artery (which is the first large branch off the aortic arch dividing into the right common carotid and right subclavian arteries). Internal mammary vessels are inferior branches of the subclavians running along the anterior surface of the pleura, posterior to the costochondral (rib-cartilage) junction. They are often harvested for coronary artery bypass grafts. Intercostal arteries are thoracic aorta branches (except for the first two, which arise from branches of the subclavian) that run along lower rib margins along with intercostal nerves. Finally, bronchial arteries (one right and two left) are usually branches of the thoracic aorta that nourish the nonrespiratory (parenchymal) lung tissues.

Esophagus

The esophagus is a smooth muscular tube that enters the thorax through the thoracic inlet with, and just posterior to, the trachea. It continues the length of the mediastinum and exits through the esophageal hiatus of the diaphragm. It is contiguous with the posterior tracheal wall.

PATHOPHYSIOLOGY OF THORACIC TRAUMA

Thoracic trauma is classified into two major categories by mechanism: blunt and penetrating. It is important to examine these injury mechanisms and their effects on thoracic organs.

Blunt Trauma

Blunt thoracic trauma is injury resulting from kinetic energy forces transmitted through tissues. These injuries may be further subdivided by mechanism into blast, crush (compression), and deceleration injuries.

Blast injuries result from an explosive chemical reaction that creates a pressure wave traveling outward from the explosion's epicenter. This pressure wave causes tissue disruption by dramatic compression and then decompression as the wave passes and may be particularly damaging to hollow, air-filled structures. In the thorax, this action may tear blood vessels and disrupt alveolar tissue. These injuries may lead to hemorrhage, pneumothoraces, and air embolism (air entering disrupted pulmonary vasculature and subsequently returning to the central circulation). Other injuries associated with a blast mechanism can include tracheobronchial tree disruption and traumatic diaphragm rupture. When a blast occurs

in a confined space, the pressure wave may be contained and accentuated. The result is an increase in the incidence and severity of associated injuries.

Crush injuries occur when the body is compressed between an object and a hard surface. This leads to direct injury or disruption of the chest wall, diaphragm, heart, or tracheobronchial tree. If a victim remains pinned between two objects, significant restriction in ventilation and venous return may occur, also known as traumatic asphyxia. Crush injuries may also result in impaired organs and soft-tissue perfusion, resulting in organ ischemia and cellular acidosis. Prolonged crush injury may also result in **rhabdomyolysis**, a breakdown of muscle fibers and release of degraded muscle fiber contents into circulation. Some of these contents, in particular myoglobin, can be highly toxic to the kidneys.

Deceleration injuries occur when the body is in motion and impacts a fixed object, such as when the chest impacts against the steering column in a front-end collision (Figure 4 ●). This impact causes a direct blunt chest wall injury while internal thoracic organs continue in motion. Organs and structures then impact with the internal thoracic cavity surface and may be compressed as more posterior structures collide with them. If the organ or structure has points of fixation, as with the aorta at the ligamentum arteriosum, the force of the organ moving against this point of fixation (shear force) can lead to a traumatic disruption. These sudden deceleration and shear forces can cause disruption of the myocardium, great vessels, lungs, trachea, and bronchi. Rapid chest compression, especially against a closed glottis, may also cause alveolar and tracheobronchial rupture and pneumothorax, a phenomenon referred to as "paper bag syndrome."

Age and physiology may alter the effects of the forces causing blunt trauma. The cartilaginous nature of the pediatric thorax spares infants or children from rib fractures but more easily transmits trauma energy to vital organs below. The result is less-significant injury signs, few rib fractures, and a greater incidence of serious internal injury. Geriatric patients respond very differently to blunt chest trauma. They suffer more frequent rib fracture than younger adults because of skeletal calcification and brittleness. Though the greater incidence of rib fracture may somewhat protect the underlying organs,

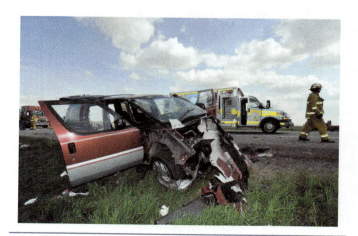

● **Figure 4** Frontal impact auto crashes frequently result in chest trauma. (© *Kevin Link*)

preexisting disease and progressive reduction of respiratory and cardiac reserves result in a greater morbidity and mortality from serious chest trauma.

Penetrating Trauma

Penetrating thoracic trauma induces injury as an object enters the chest. There it causes either direct trauma or secondary injury from transmitted forces related to the cavitational wave of high-velocity projectiles. Penetrating chest trauma can be subdivided into three categories: low-energy, high-energy, and shotgun wounds.

Low-energy wounds are those caused by arrows, knives, handguns, and other relatively slow-moving objects (Figure 5 ●). They cause injury by direct contact or very limited temporary cavity creation. Injury that occurs from this wound type is related to the direct path that missiles or objects take.

High-energy wounds are caused by military and hunting rifles (and some high-powered handguns at close range) that fire missiles at very high velocity. Their velocity gives the projectile very high kinetic energy. As a projectile passes through tissue, it creates a shock wave, tissue movement (including compression and stretching), and a large temporary cavity, a phenomenon known as cavitation. These wounds cause extensive tissue damage perpendicular to the projectile's track. The effect is accentuated by bullet construction that "mushrooms" on striking tissue, thereby increasing their profile (presenting surface) and causing greater cavitation. Tumbling, a bullet rotating along its long axis, also accentuates cavitation but greatly decreases projectile penetration.

Penetrating thoracic trauma is often related to the structures involved. Lung tissue is very resilient when impacted by high-energy projectiles. The "spongy" nature of air-filled alveoli absorbs cavitation energy and reduces the temporary cavity size and injury associated with compression and stretching. The great vessels and the heart (if it is distended with blood) respond much differently. Fluid transmits kinetic energy very well and may result in cardiac or vessel rupture. On the other hand, simple penetration may result with slower moving projectiles or if the heart is struck while in diastole. While a projectile tends to move in a straight line, it is easily deflected by contact with a rib, clavicle, scapula, or the spinal column. Contact with skeletal structures may also fragment a projectile (as well as the skeletal structure it strikes), increasing the energy exchange rate and injury seriousness. Penetrating trauma frequently leads to pneumothorax, which may be bilateral, depending on the missile or knife track. Table 1 lists common injuries associated with penetrating thoracic trauma.

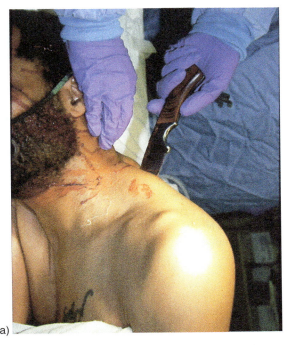

(a)

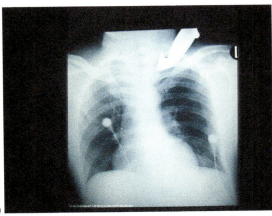

(b)

● **Figure 5** (a) Penetrating (stab) wound to the chest. (b) X-ray shows deep penetration. *(Both: © Edward T. Dickinson, MD)*

TABLE 1 | Injuries Associated with Penetrating Thoracic Trauma
Closed pneumothorax
Open pneumothorax (including sucking chest wound)
Tension pneumothorax
Pneumomediastinum
Hemothorax
Hemopneumothorax
Laceration of vascular structures, including the great vessels
Tracheobronchial tree lacerations
Esophageal lacerations
Penetrating cardiac injuries
Pericardial tamponade
Spinal cord injuries (rare)
Diaphragmatic penetration/laceration/rupture
Intra-abdominal penetration with associated organ injury

CONTENT REVIEW

▶ Signs and Symptoms
of Chest Wall Injuries

- Blunt or penetrating trauma
  to chest
- Erythema
- Ecchymosis
- Dyspnea
- Pain on breathing
- Limited breath sounds
- Hypoventilation
- Crepitus
- Paradoxical motion
  of chest wall

Chest Wall Injuries

Chest wall injuries are by far the most common injuries encountered in blunt chest trauma. As previously discussed, an intact and moving chest wall is necessary to develop pressures essential for air movement into and out of the lungs (the bellows effect). Chest wall injury may disrupt this motion and result in respiratory insufficiency. Closed chest wall injuries include contusions, rib fractures, sternal fractures/dislocations, and flail chest. Open chest wall injuries are almost entirely the result of penetrating trauma and are often associated with deep structure injury in addition to disruption of the changing intrathoracic pressure necessary for respiration.

Chest Wall Contusion

Chest wall contusion is the most common result of blunt thoracic injury. Injury damages soft tissue covering the thoracic cage and causes pain with respiratory effort. Like contusions elsewhere, chest wall contusion may present with erythema initially, then ecchymosis. Discoloration may outline the object causing trauma, may outline the ribs as soft tissue is trapped between the ribs and offending agent, or may outline a combination of both. The most noticeable chest wall contusion symptom is pain, made worse with deep breathing and which may reduce chest expansion. The contusion site will be tender, and you may observe decreased chest wall movement because of the pain.

You may auscultate limited breath sounds because of decreased air movement resulting from limited chest expansion.

Chest wall contusion pain and associated limiting of deep inspiration may lead to hypoventilation. Hypoventilation may not be apparent in a young, otherwise healthy individual and may not pose a significant life threat because of the individual's significant pulmonary reserves. Aged patients, however, often have preexisting medical problems, little pulmonary reserve, and do not tolerate this injury as well. Such patients quickly become hypoxemic (low blood oxygen levels) without proper respiratory support. Pediatric patients have very flexible ribs that resist fracture and easily transmit trauma forces. The result may be chest wall contusion and internal injury without rib fracture.

Rib Fracture

Rib fractures are found in more than 50 percent of serious chest trauma from blunt mechanisms.[2] Rib fractures are likely to occur at the impact point or along the object's border as it impacts the chest (Figure 6 ●). Fractures may also occur at a location remote from the injury site. The thoracic cage is a hollow cylinder with some flex to it. As compressional blunt trauma force deforms the thorax, ribs flex and may fracture at their weakest point, the posterior angle (along the posterior axillary line).

Ribs 4 through 8 are most commonly fractured because they are least protected by other structures and are firmly fixed at both ends (to the spine and sternum). It takes great force to fracture ribs 1 through 3 because the shoulder, scapula, and heavy musculature of the upper chest protect them. Their fracture is sometimes associated with severe intrathoracic injuries (tracheobronchial tree injury, aortic rupture, and other vascular injuries), especially if multiple ribs are involved. Ribs 9 through 12 are less firmly attached to the sternum, relatively mobile, and thus less likely to fracture. However, they more easily transmit trauma energy to internal organs and may permit

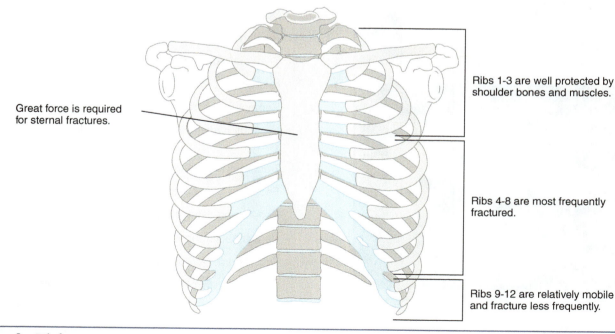

Great force is required for sternal fractures.

Ribs 1-3 are well protected by shoulder bones and muscles.

Ribs 4-8 are most frequently fractured.

Ribs 9-12 are relatively mobile and fracture less frequently.

● **Figure 6** Rib fractures.

more intra-abdominal injury without fracture. Fractures of ribs 9 through 12 are frequently associated with serious trauma and splenic or hepatic injury.

The incidence and significance of rib fracture vary with age. Pediatric patients have very cartilaginous ribs that bend easily. Ribs resist fracture and transmit forces to the thoracic and abdominal structures underneath. Pediatric patients hence have decreased rib fracture incidence and increased underlying injury incidence. Geriatric patients, however, have ribs that are calcified, less flexible, and more easily fractured. Geriatric patients are also more likely to have comorbidity like COPD, which reduces respiratory reserves and compounds the effects of rib injury. If multiple rib fractures are noted in a young adult, they are probably associated with severe trauma and may lead to significant pain, splinting, hypoventilation, and inadequate cough. They also are likely to be associated with significant internal injuries. Mortality associated with rib fractures increases with the number of fractures, extremes of age (the very young or very old), and associated chronic respiratory or cardiac problems, especially in the elderly trauma victim.

Rib fracture is likely to be associated with an overlying chest wall contusion and presents with those signs and symptoms. The fracture site may also demonstrate a grating sensation (crepitus) as bone ends move against each other, either during chest wall movement or during direct palpation. Pain associated with rib fracture is greater than that with chest wall contusion and will more greatly limit respiratory excursion. Deep inspiration pain in patients with rib fractures may also serve to limit the sigh reflex, the body's physiologic response to atelectasis. Pediatric patients may grunt during exhalation if atelectasis is present. Grunting, or partial expiration against a closed glottis, increases positive end expiratory pressure (PEEP) and helps limit atelectasis. This reduced chest wall excursion frequently leads to hypoxia, hypoventilation, and muscle spasms at the fracture site.

Hypoventilation can result in a progressive alveolar collapse (atelectasis). This collapse reduces the lung surface available for gas exchange and contributes to hypoxia. These atelectatic segments also may become filled with blood or tissue fluid from the injury and set the stage for secondary infection such as pneumonia. While pneumonia does not develop in the emergency setting, it causes significant mortality in blunt chest injury patients. Serious internal injuries may also result as jagged rib ends move about and lacerate structures beneath them. Intercostal artery laceration may result in hemothorax, while intercostal nerve damage may result in a focal neurologic deficit (numbness or weakness) of the affected intercostal muscle and associated skin and soft-tissue structures. Lower rib fracture and displacement may injure the liver (right) or spleen (left).

Sternal Fracture and Dislocation

Sternal fractures and dislocations are usually associated with blunt anterior chest trauma. Sternal fracture results only from severe impact, as this chest region is well supported by the ribs and clavicles. The most likely mechanism is a direct blow, a fall against a fixed object, or blunt force of the sternum against the steering wheel or dashboard in a motor vehicle crash. Overall, sternal fracture incidence in serious thoracic trauma patients is around 3 percent. Mortality associated with sternal fracture may be as high as 45 percent, although recent studies suggest the mortality is significantly lower.[3] Almost all sternal fracture mortality is due to underlying blunt cardiac injury, cardiac rupture, pericardial tamponade, and pulmonary contusion. If surrounding ribs or costochondral joints are disrupted, injury may result in a flail chest. Sternal fracture may result in a noticeable deformity and possible crepitus with chest wall movement or palpation.

Dislocation at the sternoclavicular joint is uncommon and also requires significant force. It too may occur with blunt anterior chest trauma or with a lateral compression mechanism, as in side impact collisions or falls with the patient landing on the shoulder. The clavicle may dislocate from the sternum in one of two ways, anteriorly or posteriorly. Anterior dislocation creates a noticeable deformity anterior to the manubrium. Posterior dislocation displaces the clavicle head behind the sternum and leaves a void just lateral to the manubrium (any deformity is more difficult to identify though the shoulder may noticeably displace anteriorly and medially). Posterior clavicular dislocation may compress or lacerate underlying great vessels or compress or injure the trachea and esophagus. Tracheal compression may result in stridor and voice change.

Flail Chest

Flail chest is a chest segment that becomes free to move with respiratory pressure changes. The condition occurs when three or more adjacent ribs fracture in two or more places (Figure 7 ●). It is one of the most serious chest wall injuries because it is often associated with severe underlying pulmonary injury (contusion) and it reduces respiratory volume while increasing respiratory effort. This underlying injury adds to mortality in serious thoracic trauma (between 20 and 40 percent), as does age, head injury, shock, and other associated injuries.[4] The most common injury mechanisms causing

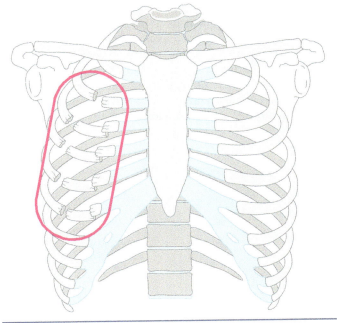

● **Figure 7** Flail chest occurs when three or more adjacent ribs fracture in two or more places.

flail chest are blunt traumas from falls, motor vehicle crashes, industrial injuries, and assaults.

The flail segment is no longer a controlled chest wall component of the bellows system. Increasing intrathoracic pressure associated with expiration moves the flail segment outward while the rest of the chest moves inward. This moves air from uninjured lung alveoli to alveoli under the flail segment. This movement reduces tidal volume, increases respiratory effort associated with ventilation, and moves the mediastinum toward the injury. During inspiration, intrathoracic pressure falls as respiratory muscles move the chest wall outward and the diaphragm drops caudally (tail-ward). Reduced intrathoracic pressure draws the flail segment inward as the adjacent chest wall moves outward. Lung tissue beneath the flail segment moves inward with the inward-moving segment, reducing the air volume moving into the thorax and displacing the mediastinum away from the injury. In summary, the injury produces a chest wall segment that moves in opposition to the chest's normal respiratory effort (paradoxical movement), reduces air volume moved through the airway, and displaces the mediastinum toward and then away from the injury site with each breath (Figure 8 ●). In flail chest, the patient takes more energy to move less air, and respiratory volume is further reduced as rib fracture pain produces chest wall splinting.

It takes tremendous energy to create these six fracture sites (three or more ribs fractured in two or more places) and, accordingly, flail chest is often associated with serious internal injury. In addition, flail segment movement, which is opposite to the rest of the chest wall, damages surrounding tissue. With each breath, bone fracture sites move against one another causing further muscle damage, soft-tissue damage, and pain. Small flail segments may go undetected as associated intercostal muscle spasm naturally splints the segment. With time, however, these muscles suffer further injury and fatigue and the flail segment's paradoxical movement becomes more and more apparent.

Positive-pressure ventilation of a flail chest patient reverses the pressures that cause paradoxical chest wall movement,

restores tidal volume, and reduces pain of chest wall movement. It accomplishes this by pushing the chest wall and flail segment together outward with positive pressure. Passive expiration then causes both the flail segment and the remaining chest to move inward, again, together. However, with underlying injury, positive-pressure ventilation may induce pneumothorax. It must also be noted that positive-pressure ventilation may limit blood return through the vena cava that is normally enhanced by negative intrathoracic pressure that occurs during normal inspiration. Careful monitoring for changes in hemodynamic status is necessary.

Pulmonary Injuries

Pulmonary injuries are injuries to lung tissue or injuries that damage the system that holds the lung to the thoracic cavity interior. They include simple pneumothorax, open pneumothorax, tension pneumothorax, hemothorax, and pulmonary contusion.

Simple Pneumothorax

Simple **pneumothorax** (also known as closed pneumothorax) occurs when lung tissue is disrupted and air leaks into the pleural space (Figure 9 ●). In simple pneumothorax air enters the pleural space from ruptured airways. Some simple pneumothorax cases occur with penetrating trauma; however, air does not enter through the wound but through airway injuries it causes. In pneumothorax, pressure within the thorax does not exceed normal expiratory pressures and there is no mediastinal shift. As more and more air accumulates in the pleural space, the lung collapses. With lung collapse, alveoli collapse (atelectasis) and blood flowing past collapsed alveoli does not exchange oxygen or carbon dioxide. As more and more alveoli collapse, this condition, called ventilation/perfusion mismatch, becomes

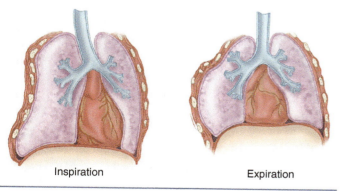

Inspiration   Expiration

● **Figure 8** Paradoxical movement of the chest wall seen in flail chest.

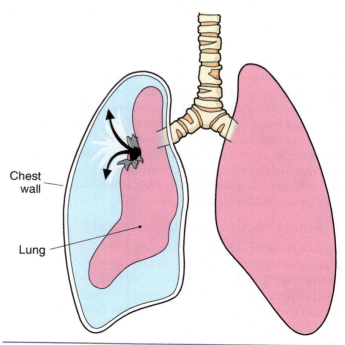

Chest wall

Lung

● **Figure 9** Simple (closed) pneumothorax.

more pronounced and begins to lower blood oxygen levels (hypoxemia) and increases its carbon dioxide content (acidosis). This could become life endangering, especially if there are other associated injuries or shock.

Simple pneumothorax can occur with penetrating and blunt mechanisms. Blunt trauma may cause a pneumothorax when a rib fracture directly punctures the lung. Another mechanism may cause alveolar rupture from a sudden increase in intrathoracic pressure as the chest impacts the steering column with fully expanded lungs and a closed glottis (much like a paper bag filled with air that is compressed suddenly between two hands). Pneumothorax incidence in serious thoracic trauma is between 15 and 50 percent, and its morbidity is related to the degree of atelectasis and ventilation/perfusion mismatch.[1] Penetrating chest trauma is frequently associated with simple pneumothorax, or with an injury that allows air to enter the pleural space through an external wound (open pneumothorax).

A simple pneumothorax reduces respiratory efficiency and may lead to hypoxia. Hypoxia and increases in CO_2 blood levels trigger the medulla to increase respiratory rate (tachypnea) and volume. If the pneumothorax is limited, there may be no apparent signs or symptoms. A larger pneumothorax may cause mild dyspnea, or complete lung collapse may result in severe dyspnea and hypoxia. Simple pneumothorax signs, symptoms, and significance increase with any preexisting disease. Pneumothorax may produce local chest pain with respiration as pleurae become irritated (respirophasic pain). This pathology may cause the chest to hyperinflate and breath sounds to diminish on the affected side (usually in the extremes of the upper and lower lung first). A small pneumothorax involving less than 15 percent of the affected lung may be difficult to detect clinically and requires only supportive measures. Often a small pneumothorax will seal itself and air in the pleural cavity will be reabsorbed. A larger pneumothorax is often clinically apparent and requires more aggressive therapy such as high-concentration oxygen and chest tube placement (in the emergency department).

Open Pneumothorax

Open pneumothorax is most commonly noted in military conflicts when a high-velocity bullet creates a significant chest wall wound (usually an exit wound). Recently use of high-velocity assault weapons has become more common in civilian settings and thus the frequency of these injuries is on the increase. Another open pneumothorax cause is a shotgun blast at close range with an associated large chest wall wound. This chest wall disruption leads to free air passage between the atmosphere and pleural space (Figure 10 ●). Air is drawn into the wound as the chest moves outward and the diaphragm moves downward during inspiration. Internal thoracic pressure drops and air rushes through the wound and into the chest cavity. This air replaces lung tissue, permits lung collapse, and results in a large functional dead space. Inspiratory effort of the contralateral chest draws the mediastinum toward it and away from the injury. This prevents the uninjured lung from fully inflating. On exhalation, the contracting chest wall and rising diaphragm increase internal pressure and force air outward through the wound. This air movement into and out of the chest through the wound causes a "sucking" sound that leads to the wound's common name, "sucking chest wound."

For air movement to occur through a chest wall opening, the opening must be at least two-thirds the tracheal diameter. Remember, trachea size is about that of the patient's little finger. This must be the unimpeded size of the chest opening, not the wound size. The chest wall's thickness and resiliency often closes a wound to air movement unless it is quite large. Such wounds rarely occur with handgun rounds, but may be possible with high-velocity rifle rounds. Then the remaining defect may permit free air movement and create an open pneumothorax.

Open pneumothorax can be recognized by a large open thoracic wound and the characteristic air movement (or sound) it produces. Air passage through the wound and the wound's associated hemorrhage may produce frothy blood around the opening, another open pneumothorax characteristic. A patient is likely to experience increased dyspnea, and possibly hypovolemia from associated hemorrhage. A patient's condition is further compromised because reduced intrathoracic pressures developed during inspiration do not complement venous return as they do with an intact thorax and normal respiratory effort.

Tension Pneumothorax

Tension pneumothorax is an open or simple pneumothorax that generates and maintains a pressure greater than atmospheric pressure within the thorax. It may be caused by a traumatic mechanism of injury or possibly by positive-pressure ventilation of a patient with chest trauma or congenital defect affecting the respiratory tree. Tension pneumothorax may also

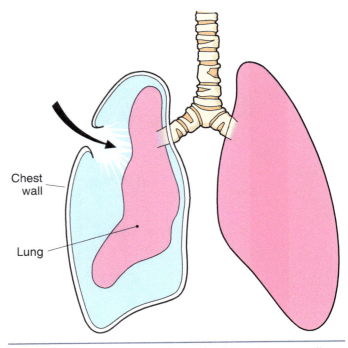

● **Figure 10** Open pneumothorax (sucking chest wound).

Chest wall

Lung

CONTENT REVIEW

► Signs and Symptoms
of Tension Pneumothorax

- Chest trauma
- Severe dyspnea
- Ventilation/perfusion mismatch
- Hypoxemia
- Hyperinflation of affected side of chest
- Hyperresonance of affected side of chest
- Diminished, then absent breath sounds
- Cyanosis
- Diaphoresis
- Altered mental status
- Jugular venous distention
- Hypotension
- Hypovolemia

occur as an open pneumothorax is sealed and an internal injury or defect acts as a valve and permits a pressure buildup.

Tension pneumothorax occurs because the mechanism of injury (either an external wound, or an internal injury) forms a one-way valve. Air flows into the pleural space through the defect during inspiration because the pressure within the pleural space is less than atmospheric pressure. With expiration, increasing pleural pressure closes the defect and does not permit air to escape. With each breath, air volume and pressure within the pleural space increase. Increasing intrapleural pressure collapses the lung on the ipsilateral (same or injury) side, causes intercostal and suprasternal bulging, and begins to exert pressure against the mediastinum. As pressure continues to build, it displaces the mediastinum, compressing the uninjured lung and crimping the vena cava as it enters the thorax through

the diaphragm and/or where it attaches to the heart. This reduces venous return (which reduces cardiac output), results in an increase in venous pressure, causes jugular venous distention (JVD), and narrows pulse pressure. Tracheal shift may occur as mediastinal structures are pushed away from increasing pressure. This is a very late and rare finding and is more commonly seen in young trauma victims as the pediatric mediastinum is more mobile than an adult's. Atelectasis occurs in the ipsilateral side from the initial lung collapse and on the contralateral (uninjured or opposite) side from mediastinal shift and compression of that lung. These mechanisms lead to ventilation/perfusion mismatch, further hypoxemia, and systemic hypoxia.

Tension pneumothorax begins with simple or open pneumothorax (Figure 11 ●). As pleural space pressure begins to rise, dyspnea, ventilation/perfusion mismatch, and hypoxemia develop. The ipsilateral chest becomes hyperinflated and hyperresonant to percussion, and respiratory sounds become very faint, then absent. Increasing pressure may cause intracostal tissues to bulge outward. The contralateral chest becomes somewhat dull to percussion, with progressively fainter respiratory sounds as tension pneumothorax worsens. Severe hypoxia results in cyanosis, diaphoresis, and altered mental status while increased intrathoracic pressure reduces venous return and may cause JVD and hypotension. If the condition is not quickly recognized and promptly treated, it may lead to death. Often the most obvious clinical finding is a pneumothorax and associated hemodynamic compromise.

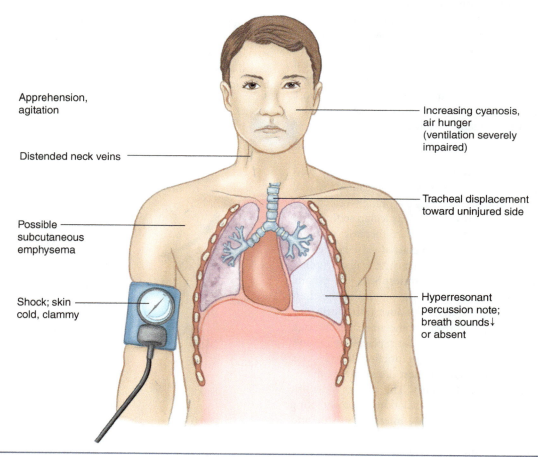

● **Figure 11**   Physical findings of tension pneumothorax.

Tension pneumothorax is a serious, progressive, and immediate life threat. It is corrected by relieving intrapleural pressure by inserting a needle through the chest wall to convert tension pneumothorax to open pneumothorax. As long as the catheter remains open, it will relieve any building pressure, help ensure venous return, and help the patient maintain adequate ventilation.

Hemothorax

Hemothorax is simply an accumulation of blood in the pleural space from internal hemorrhage. It can be very minor and not detectable in the field or, when associated with serious or great vessel injury, may result in rapid patient deterioration. Serious hemorrhage may displace a complete lung and accumulate over 1,500 mL of blood quickly. Hemothorax is most commonly caused by penetrating trauma but may occur when a rib is fractured in blunt trauma.[5] Hemothorax is primarily a blood loss problem as each hemithorax may hold up to 3,000 mL of blood (or half the total blood volume). However, blood lost into the thorax reduces tidal volume and respiratory efficiency in a patient who has already suffered trauma and is likely to move quickly into shock.

Hemothorax is frequently associated with rib fractures and can be associated with either blunt or penetrating mechanisms. It often accompanies pneumothorax (a **hemopneumothorax**) and occurs 25 percent of the time with penetrating trauma. Hemorrhage into the pleural space may occur from a lung laceration (most common) or laceration to the intercostal artery, pulmonary artery, great vessel, or internal mammary artery. Intercostal arteries can bleed at a rate of 50 mL/min. Bleeding into the chest is more rapid than would occur elsewhere because pressure within the chest during inspiration is less than atmospheric pressure. Blood lost into a hemothorax contributes to hypovolemia and displaces lung tissue. If accumulation is significant, it may cause hypovolemia and shock, hypoxemia, respiratory distress, and respiratory failure.

A patient with hemothorax will have either a blunt or penetrating injury like those associated with open or simple pneumothorax. A patient may also display shock signs and symptoms and some respiratory distress (Figure 12 ●). Blood pools in the lower chest in the seated patient or posterior chest in the supine patient. The lungs present with normal percussion and breath sounds except directly over accumulating fluid. There, lung percussion is very dull and breath sounds are muffled and distant, if they can be heard at all.

Pulmonary Contusion

Pulmonary contusion is simply soft-tissue contusion affecting the lung. They are present in 39 percent of patients with respiratory failure from blunt chest trauma and are frequently associated with rib fracture. Pulmonary contusions range in severity from very limited, minor, and unrecognizable injuries, to those that are extensive and quickly life threatening. They result in a mortality rate of about 18 percent for serious chest trauma patients.[3]

There are two specific injury mechanisms that allow energy transfer to pulmonary tissue and result in pulmonary contusions. They are deceleration or the pressure wave associated with either passage of a high-velocity bullet or explosion. Deceleration injury occurs as a moving body strikes a fixed object. A common example of this mechanism is chest impact with the steering wheel during an auto crash. As the chest wall contacts the wheel and stops, the lungs continue forward, compressing and stretching alveolar tissue or shearing it from the relatively fixed tracheobronchial tree. This causes alveolar/capillary membrane disruption leading to microscopic hemorrhage and edema.

The second mechanism, an explosion or bullet's pressure wave passage, dramatically compresses and stretches

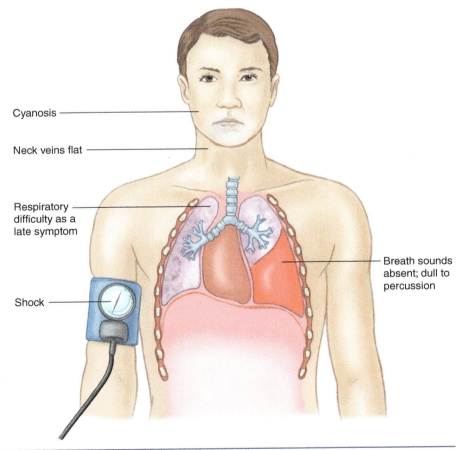

Cyanosis

Neck veins flat

Respiratory difficulty as a late symptom

Shock

Breath sounds absent; dull to percussion

● **Figure 12**   Physical findings of massive hemothorax.

CONTENT REVIEW

▶ Signs and Symptoms of Pulmonary Contusion

- Blunt or penetrating chest trauma
- Increasing dyspnea
- Hypoxia
- Increasing crackles
- Diminishing breath sounds
- Hemoptysis
- Signs and symptoms of shock

lung tissue. Because of the nature of lung tissue (air-filled sacs surrounded by delicate and vascular membranes), pressure passage is partially reflected at the gas/fluid (alveolar/capillary) interface. This leaves small, flame-shaped disruption areas throughout the membrane leading to microhemorrhage and edema (called the Spalding effect). Pulmonary contusion is not generally associated with low-speed chest penetration and lung tissue and structure laceration.

Pulmonary injury magnitude depends on the degree of deformity or stretch, and the velocity at which it occurs. Similar pulmonary contusions may result from different mechanisms. For example, a high-velocity bullet (> 30 m/sec) striking body armor and deforming the chest wall nearly instantaneously by 1 to 2 cm may cause pulmonary contusions similar to a chest impact during an MVA where the chest is deformed 50 percent as it strikes the steering wheel at 15 m/sec (low velocity).[2]

Microhemorrhage into alveolar tissue associated with pulmonary contusion may be extensive and result in up to 1,000 to 1,500 mL of blood loss. This hemorrhage into lung tissue also causes tissue irritation, initiates the inflammation process, and causes fluid to migrate into the interstitial space. Fluid accumulation in the alveolar/capillary membrane (pulmonary edema) progressively increases its dimension and decreases the rate at which gases, and especially oxygen, can diffuse across it. Fluid accumulation also stiffens the membrane, makes the lung less compliant, and increases work necessary to move air in and out of affected tissue.

Thickening alveolar walls reduce respiratory efficiency and result in hypoxemia, while stiffening makes respiration more energy consuming. Edema development also increases pressures necessary to move blood through capillary beds. This increases pulmonary vascular system pressure (pulmonary hypertension) and the right heart's workload. In combination, these effects lead to atelectasis, hypovolemia, ventilation/perfusion mismatch, hypoxemia, hypotension, and, possibly, respiratory failure and shock. Although isolated pulmonary contusions can occur, they are frequently associated with chest wall injury and injuries elsewhere (87 percent of the time).[4]

A patient with pulmonary contusion presents with a mechanism of injury and evidence of blunt or penetrating chest impact. While associated injuries may display immediate signs and symptoms (as in rib fracture pain), pulmonary contusion signs and symptoms take time to develop. A patient will likely complain of increasing dyspnea, demonstrate increasing respiratory effort, and show progressing hypoxia signs. Oxygen saturation may gradually fall as the pathology develops. Careful chest auscultation may reveal increasing crackles and fainter breath sounds. Serious pulmonary contusion may cause **hemoptysis** (coughing up blood) and shock signs and symptoms.

Cardiovascular Injuries

Cardiovascular injuries are the thoracic trauma subset that leads to the most mortality. They include blunt cardiac injury, pericardial tamponade, myocardial aneurysm or rupture, aortic aneurysm or rupture, and other vascular injuries.

Blunt Cardiac Injury

Blunt cardiac injury is a frequent trauma result and may occur in up to 55 percent of all serious chest trauma.[1] It carries a high mortality rate and occurs most commonly with severe blunt anterior chest trauma. Here, the chest is struck by, or strikes, an object. The heart, which is relatively mobile within the chest, impacts the anterior chest wall and then is compressed between the sternum and thoracic spine as the thorax flexes with impact. The resulting contusion will most likely affect the right atrium and ventricle (Figure 13 ●). This results from the heart's position in the chest, rotated somewhat counterclockwise and presenting the right atrial and ventricular surfaces toward the sternum.

Cardiac contusion is similar to any other muscle tissue contusion. Injury disrupts muscle cells and microcirculation, resulting in muscle fiber tearing and damage, hemorrhage, and edema. Injury may reduce cardiac contraction strength and reduce cardiac output. Because of cardiac muscle automaticity and conductivity, contusion may disturb the cardiac electrical system. If injury is serious, it may lead to hematoma, pericardial tamponade (blood in the pericardial sac), and necrosis and may result in cardiac irritability, ectopic (abnormal origin) beats, and conduction system defects such as bundle branch blocks and arrhythmias. If injury is very extensive, it may lead to tissue necrosis (death), decreased ventricular compliance, congestive heart failure, cardiogenic shock, myocardial aneurysm, and acute or delayed myocardial rupture. In contrast to a myocardial infarction from coronary artery disease, cellular damage from blunt cardiac injury heals with less scarring and there is limited injury progression in the absence of associated coronary artery disease.

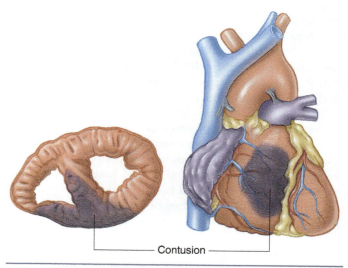

Contusion

● **Figure 13** Blunt cardiac injury most frequently affects the right atrium and ventricle as they collide with the sternum.

A patient experiencing blunt cardiac injury has a significant blunt chest trauma history, most likely affecting the anterior chest. The patient will likely complain of chest or retrosternal pain, very much like that of myocardial infarction, and may have associated chest injuries such as anterior rib or sternal fractures. Cardiac monitoring most frequently reveals sinus tachycardia (though it may be caused by the fight or flight response, pain, hypovolemia, or hypoxia from associated chest injury). Other arrhythmias associated with blunt cardiac injuries are atrial flutter or fibrillation, premature atrial or ventricular contractions, tachyarrhythmia, bradyarrhythmia, bundle branch patterns, T wave inversions, and ST segment elevations. A pericardial friction rub and murmur may be auscultated over the *precordium* but is more likely to occur weeks after injury and is associated with development of inflammatory pericardial effusion.

Commotio Cordis   *Commotio cordis* is a rare event in which ventricular fibrillation is induced by a direct chest blow. Often the impact is seemingly modest, such as being struck in the chest by a baseball. Although commotio cordis is rare, it is the leading cause of sudden death in young athletes. The average age of occurrence is 13 years with a range of 3 months to 50 years. Approximately 15 percent of victims are successfully resuscitated. Survival rates are low because the condition is initially unrecognized or misdiagnosed during the time when CPR or defibrillation should be provided.[6]

Treatment for commotio cordis is the same as for ventricular fibrillation and should include CPR and immediate defibrillation.

Pericardial Tamponade

Pericardial tamponade is a restriction to cardiac filling caused by blood (or other fluid) within the pericardial sac. It occurs in less than 2 percent of all serious chest trauma patients and is almost always related to penetrating injury.[7] Penetrating trauma is the most frequent mechanism and carries a high overall mortality, often resulting in rapid hemorrhage through the myocardial wall and then out the defect in the pericardium.

Pericardial tamponade begins with a tear in a superficial coronary artery or myocardium penetration. Blood seeps into the pericardial space and accumulates (Figure 14 ●). The fibrous pericardium does not stretch and accumulating blood exerts pressure on the heart. Even limited pressure limits cardiac filling, first affecting the right ventricle where filling pressure is the lowest. This restricts atrial, then ventricular filling and venous return to the heart, increases central venous pressure, and

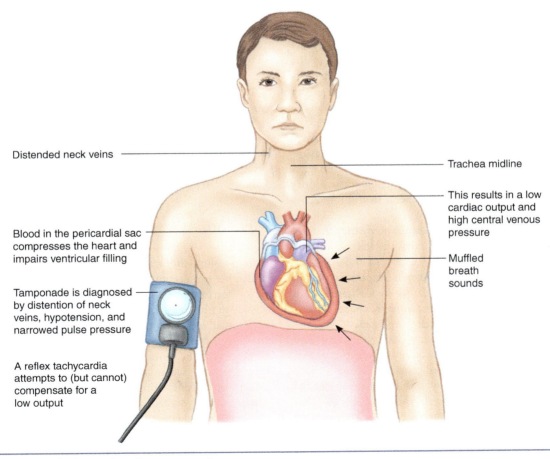

Distended neck veins

Trachea midline

This results in a low cardiac output and high central venous pressure

Blood in the pericardial sac compresses the heart and impairs ventricular filling

Muffled breath sounds

Tamponade is diagnosed by distention of neck veins, hypotension, and narrowed pulse pressure

A reflex tachycardia attempts to (but cannot) compensate for a low output

● **Figure 14**   Physical findings of cardiac tamponade.

► Signs and Symptoms of Pericardial Tamponade

- Dyspnea and possible cyanosis
- Jugular venous distention
- Weak, thready pulse
- Decreasing blood pressure
- Shock
- Narrowing pulse pressure

causes jugular vein distention. Reduced right ventricular output limits outflow to pulmonary arteries and then venous return to the left heart. Tamponade results in a decreasing cardiac output and systemic hypotension. Pressure exerted by blood in the pericardium also restricts blood flow through coronary arteries and to the myocardium. This may result in myocardial ischemia and infarct. It takes about 150 to 300 mL of blood to exert a pressure necessary to induce frank tamponade, while removing as little as 20 mL may provide significant relief. Pericardial tamponade progression depends on the blood flow rate into the pericardium. It may occur very rapidly and result in death before emergency medical services arrival or may gradually progress over hours.

A patient experiencing pericardial tamponade will likely have penetrating trauma to the anterior or posterior chest, though blunt trauma can also cause this problem. While missile and knife blade trajectories are difficult to predict, consider pericardial tamponade with any thoracic or upper abdominal penetrating wound, especially if it is over the precordium (central lower chest). Pericardial tamponade diminishes pulse strength, decreases pulse pressure, and distends jugular veins (JVD). A patient will likely be agitated, tachycardic, diaphoretic, and ashen in appearance. Cyanosis may be noted in the head, neck, and upper extremities. Heart tones may be muffled or distant sounding. Beck's triad (JVD, distant heart tones, and hypotension) is indicative of pericardial tamponade but may not be recognized early in the injury's progression. Another sign of pericardial tamponade is Kussmaul's sign, the decrease or absence of JVD during inspiration. As a patient inspires, reduced intrathoracic pressure increases venous return and decreases the pressure accumulating pericardial fluid exerts on the heart. This then translates to a better venous return and cardiac output during inspiration, and the effect is then seen in jugular veins (Figure 15 ●).

Other findings during pericardial tamponade may include pulsus paradoxus and electrical alternans. **Pulsus paradoxus** is a systolic blood pressure drop of greater than 10 mmHg as the patient inspires during the normal respiratory cycle. (Normally systolic blood pressure drops just slightly with each inspiration.) Pulsus paradoxus results because cardiac output increases with tamponade relief associated with reduced intrathoracic inspiration pressure. As systolic pressure varies with pulsus paradoxus, you may notice an alternation between strong and weak pulses called **pulsus alternans**. **Electrical alternans**, which is only rarely seen in acute pericardial tamponade, is noted on a cardiac rhythm strip as P, QRS, and T amplitude decreases with every other cardiac cycle. In profound pericardial tamponade, the heart displays a rhythm without producing a pulse (PEA).

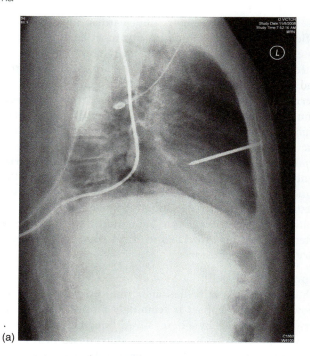

(a)

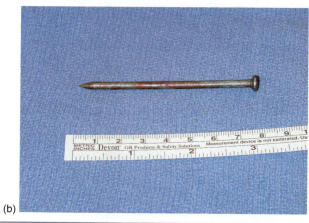

(b)

● **Figure 15**   Penetrating trauma to the heart (nail) (a) as seen on lateral chest X-ray and (b) following surgical removal. *(Both: © Edward T. Dickinson, MD)*

Myocardial Aneurysm or Rupture

Myocardial **aneurysm** or rupture occurs almost exclusively in extreme blunt thoracic trauma, such as automobile collisions. It also has been reported in cases where blunt forces are not extreme; for example as a result of CPR. The condition can affect any of the heart's chambers, the interatrial septum, the interventricular septum, or involve the valves and their supporting structures. Multiple heart chambers or structures are involved 30 percent of the time.[7] Aneurysm and delayed myocardial rupture also occur secondary to necrosis from a myocardial infarction, repaired penetrating injury, or blunt cardiac injury. Necrosis usually develops around two weeks after injury as inflammatory cells degrade injured cells, weakening myocardial tissue and leading to ventricular wall aneurysm and/or subsequent rupture. Rupture can also occur with high-energy projectile injuries.

A patient who experiences myocardial rupture will likely have suffered serious blunt or penetrating trauma to the chest and may have severe rib or sternal fracture. Specific symptoms may depend on the actual pathology. The victim may have pericardial tamponade signs and symptoms if rupture is contained within the pericardial sac. If the pathology affects only ruptured valves, the patient may present with right or left heart failure. If there is a myocardial aneurysm, rupture may be delayed. When it happens, the patient will suddenly present with absent vital signs or signs and symptoms of pericardial tamponade.

Traumatic Dissection or Rupture of the Aorta

Aortic dissection and rupture are extremely life-threatening injuries resulting from either blunt or penetrating trauma. Aortic injury is most commonly caused by blunt trauma, carries an overall mortality of 85 to 95 percent, and is responsible for 15 percent of all thoracic trauma deaths. Dissection and rupture are usually associated with high-speed automobile crashes (most commonly lateral impact) and in some cases with high falls. Unlike myocardial rupture, a significant number, possibly as high as 20 percent, of these victims will survive the initial insult and aneurysm. Some 30 percent of these initial survivors will die in 6 hours if not treated, increasing to about 50 percent at 24 hours, and just under 70 percent by the first week's end. It is the patient subset that survives initial impact and is alive when you arrive that can benefit most by your recognizing the potential injury and then by rapidly extricating, packaging, and transporting him to the trauma center.[7]

The aorta is a large, high-pressure vessel that provides outflow from the left ventricle for distribution to the systemic circulation. It is fixed at three points as it passes through the thoracic cavity and, because of this, experiences shear forces secondary to severe chest deceleration. The fixation points are where the aorta joins the heart (aortic annulus), where it is joined with the ligamentum arteriosum (aortic isthmus), and where it exits the chest (through the diaphragm) (Table 2). Traumatic aortic dissection occurs infrequently to the ascending aorta and most commonly to the descending aorta. With severe deceleration, shear forces separate arterial layers, specifically the interior surface (tunica intima) from the muscle layer (the tunica media).

TABLE 2 | Incidence and Anatomic Location of Traumatic Aortic Rupture

Aortic annulus	9 percent
Aortic isthmus	85 percent
Diaphragm	3 percent
Other	3 percent

This allows blood to enter and, because it is under great pressure, begin to dissect the aortic lining, forming a false lumen. It is likely to rupture if it is not surgically repaired.

A patient with aortic rupture will be severely hypotensive, quickly lose all vital signs, and die unless moved into surgery immediately. Aortic dissection progresses more slowly, though a dissection may rupture at any moment. The patient will probably have a history of a high fall or severe auto impact and deceleration. Lateral impact is an especially high risk factor for aortic aneurysm. The patient may complain of severe tearing chest pain that may radiate to the back. The patient may have a pulse deficit between the left and right upper extremities and/or reduced pulse strength in the lower extremities. Blood pressure may be high (hypertension) because of the stretching of sympathetic nerve fibers present in the aorta near the ligamentum arteriosum, or the pressure may be low because of leakage and hypovolemia. Auscultation may reveal a harsh systolic murmur caused by turbulence as blood exits the heart and passes the disrupted blood vessel wall.

Other Vascular Injuries

Pulmonary arteries and venae cavae are other thoracic vascular structures that can sustain injury during chest trauma. Their injury, and resulting hemorrhage, may cause significant hemothorax, possibly leading to hypotension and respiratory insufficiency. Blood may also flow into the mediastinum and compress the great vessels, esophagus, and heart. Penetrating trauma is a primary cause of injury to pulmonary arteries and venae cavae.

A patient with pulmonary artery or vena cava injury will likely have a penetrating chest or neck wound with a likelihood of central chest involvement. These injuries present with signs and symptoms of hypovolemia and shock and result in hemothorax or hemomediastinum and signs and symptoms associated with those pathologies.

Other Thoracic Injuries
Traumatic Rupture or Perforation of the Diaphragm

Traumatic diaphragm rupture or perforation can occur in both high-energy blunt and penetrating thoracoabdominal trauma. Incidence is estimated from 1 to 6 percent of all patients with multiple trauma. It is more common in patients sustaining blunt trauma from motor vehicle crashes or falls from heights.[3] Penetrating trauma to the lower chest can also cause perforation of the diaphragm. Remember that during expiration the diaphragm may move superiorly to the fourth intercostal space (nipple level) anteriorly and sixth intercostal space posteriorly. Any penetrating injuries at these levels or below may penetrate the diaphragm. Diaphragmatic perforation and herniation occur most frequently on the left side, because assailants are most frequently right handed and the liver's size and solid nature protect the right diaphragm. The liver is also unlikely to herniate through a torn diaphragm unless the injury is sizeable.

If traumatic diaphragmatic rupture occurs, abdominal organs may herniate through the defect into the thoracic cavity.

This herniation may cause bowel strangulation or necrosis, ipsilateral lung restriction, and mediastinal displacement. Mediastinal displacement occurs when displaced abdominal contents place pressure on the lung and mediastinal structures, moving them toward the contralateral side through much the same mechanism as is seen in tension pneumothorax.

Diaphragmatic rupture presents with signs and symptoms similar to tension pneumothorax, including dyspnea, hypoxia, hypotension, and JVD. The patient will have blunt abdominal or penetrating trauma to the lower thorax or upper abdomen. The abdomen may appear hollow, and bowel sounds may be noted in one side of the thorax (most commonly the left). The patient may be hypotensive and hypoxic if the herniation is extensive. The patient may complain of upper abdominal pain, though this symptom is often overshadowed by other injuries. If the diaphragmatic tear is small, there may be no herniation. Even with serious tearing, herniation may not occur or it may be delayed months to years. Without serious herniation, it may be difficult to recognize a diaphragmatic rupture.

Traumatic Esophageal Rupture

Traumatic esophageal rupture is a rare blunt thoracic trauma complication. Esophageal rupture occurs with only about 0.4 percent of penetrating chest trauma.[8] Since the esophagus is centrally located within the chest, its injury usually coincides with other mediastinal injuries. (Esophageal rupture may also result from medical problems such as violent emesis, carcinoma, anatomic distortion, or gastric reflux.) Esophageal rupture carries a 5 to 25 percent mortality, even if quickly recognized, and mortality is much greater if this injury is not diagnosed promptly.[3] Mortality from esophageal rupture is related to material entering the mediastinum as it passes down the esophagus or as emesis passes upward. This results in serious infection or chemical irritation and serious mediastinal structure damage. Air may also enter the mediastinum through an esophageal rupture, especially during positive-pressure ventilation.

Trauma patients with esophageal rupture will likely have deep penetrating trauma to the central chest and may complain of difficult or painful swallowing, respirophasic chest pain, and pain radiating to the midback. Patients may also display subcutaneous emphysema around the lower neck.

Tracheobronchial Injury (Disruption)

Tracheobronchial injury is a relatively infrequent finding in thoracic trauma with an incidence of less than 3 percent in patients with significant chest trauma.[1] It may occur from either blunt or penetrating injury mechanisms and carries a greater than 50 percent mortality rate. Half of tracheobronchial deaths occur at the scene. Disruption can occur anywhere in the tracheobronchial tree but is most likely to occur within 2.5 cm of the carina.[9]

A patient with tracheal or mainstem bronchi disruption is generally in respiratory distress with cyanosis, hemoptysis, and, in some cases, massive subcutaneous emphysema. The patient may also experience pneumothorax and, possibly, tension pneumothorax. Intermittent positive-pressure ventilation drives air into the pleura or mediastinum and makes the condition worse.

Traumatic Asphyxia

Traumatic asphyxia occurs when severe compressive force is applied to the thorax. It leads to a reverse blood flow from the right heart into the superior vena cava and into venous vessels of the upper extremities. (Traumatic asphyxia is not as much a respiratory problem as it is a vascular problem.) Traumatic asphyxia engorges veins and capillaries of the head and neck with desaturated venous blood, turning the skin in this region a deep red, purple, or blue. Blood backflow damages microcirculation in the head and neck, producing petechiae (small hemorrhages under the skin—Figure 16a ●) and subconjunctival hemorrhages (to the whites of the eyes—Figure 16b ●), and stagnating blood above the compression point. Backflow may damage cerebral circulation, resulting in numerous small strokes in the older patient whose venous vessels are not very elastic. If flow restriction continues, toxins and acids accumulate in the blood. These toxins may have a devastating effect when they return to the central circulation with the release of pressure. If thoracic compression continues, it restricts venous return and may prevent or seriously restrict victim respirations. This results in hypotension, hypoxemia, and shock. Death may follow rapidly.

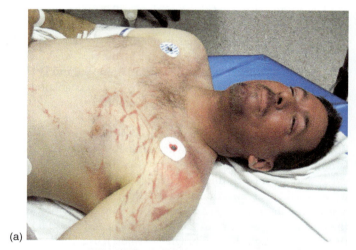

(a)

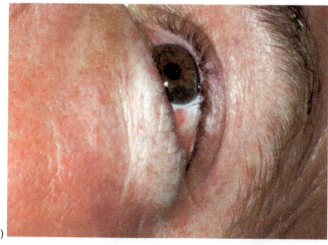

(b)

● **Figure 16** (a) Traumatic asphyxia. (b) Subconjunctival hemorrhage associated with traumatic asphyxia. *(Both: © Dr. Bryan E. Bledsoe)*

Patient extrication may result in rapid injury site hemorrhage with pressure release. Compression release may likewise result in rapid patient deterioration and death from internal hemorrhage.

Traumatic asphyxia patients suffer severe chest compression that is likely to continue until extrication. Compression-induced blood flow restriction and backflow are dramatic and can cause classic head and neck discoloration. The victim's face appears swollen (plethora), eyes bulge, and there are numerous conjunctival hemorrhages. The patient may have severe dyspnea related to the compression and injuries associated with severe chest impact. Once pressure is released, the patient may show signs of hypovolemia, hypotension, and shock as well as signs related to any coexisting respiratory problems.

ASSESSMENT OF THE CHEST INJURY PATIENT

Proper assessment of the chest injury patient is critical to anticipating and detecting injury and providing correct interventions. While chest injury patient assessment follows the standard

PATHO PEARLS

Detecting the Effects of Thoracic Trauma

The thoracic cavity contains three general regions: the pericardial region, the pulmonary region, and the mediastinum. The pericardial region contains the heart and the origin of the great vessels. The pulmonary region contains the lungs, the airways, and the pulmonary vasculature. The mediastinum contains the esophagus, the vagus nerve, the thoracic duct, and other essential structures. Despite these, the thoracic cavity primarily involves respiratory and cardiac functions. Thus, with any thoracic injury, you would expect to see first a variation in respiratory function, cardiac function, or both. With a pneumothorax, you initially will see a subtle increase in respiratory rate and then, as the process progresses, increased respiratory effort and, finally, signs and symptoms of poor oxygenation. If this is allowed to progress untreated, cardiovascular impairment will follow. Cardiovascular impairment can result from incomplete ventricular filling due to increased intrathoracic pressure or from blood loss within the lung parenchyma.

Similarly, a penetrating injury to the heart can lead to cardiovascular collapse. With low-energy wounds, such as knife stab wounds, the pericardial sac may fill with blood, thus preventing adequate ventricular filling (pericardial tamponade). This will be manifest as an initial increase in heart rate, narrowing of the pulse pressure (due to restricted ventricular filling), and distended neck veins. As cardiac efficiency declines, the pulmonary vasculature can become congested, resulting in poor oxygenation. High-energy wounds, such as gunshot wounds, that penetrate the heart are usually mortal wounds—even in the best of EMS systems and trauma centers.

Any time you have a patient with a suspected thoracic injury, first look at the respiratory and circulatory systems for signs of impairment. These findings can help guide you to the nature of your patient's injury.

prehospital assessment process, special considerations regarding chest injury occur during the scene size-up, primary assessment, and especially during the rapid trauma assessment. Reassessment is also critical for tracking injury progression during serious chest trauma.

Scene Size-Up

Chest injury care, like that for any other serious trauma, requires Standard Precautions with gloves as a minimum. Consider a face shield if you will be attending to the airway and a gown for splash protection with serious penetrating thoracic trauma. Ensure a safe scene, including protection from any assailant, if violence is suspected.

Examine the mechanism of injury carefully and determine if the central chest (heart, great vessels, trachea, and esophagus) might be in the pathway of penetrating trauma. In gunshot injuries, determine weapon type, caliber, distance between the gun barrel and victim, and the probable projectile pathway. Determine the direction of blunt trauma impact as it may also have a bearing on which organs sustain injury. Anterior impact may rupture lung tissue and contuse the lung and heart. Lateral impact or landing on one's feet from a great height may tear the aorta as the heart displaces laterally and stresses the aorta's ligamentous attachments.

Primary Assessment

During primary assessment, determine a patient's mental status, potential for spine injury, and the airway, breathing, and circulation status. Intervene as necessary to correct life-threatening conditions. It is during primary assessment that you will first identify signs and symptoms of serious chest trauma. Be especially watchful for any dyspnea; asymmetrical, paradoxical, exaggerated, or limited chest movement; chest hyperinflation; or an abdomen that appears hollow. Notice any general patient skin color reflective of hypoxia such as cyanotic or ashen discoloration. Look for distended jugular veins, costal or suprasternal retractions, and use of accessory muscles of respiration. Also look for any changing neck and facial features caused by air collecting under the skin.

Ensure that ventilation and oxygen saturation levels are adequate. If the patient has an SpO_2 of 96 percent or less, administer supplemental oxygen. Administer any positive-pressure ventilations with care, as thoracic injury may weaken lung tissue and makes the patient prone to pneumothorax or tension pneumothorax. Positive-pressure ventilations may induce these problems. Be suspicious of internal hemorrhage and plan to initiate at least one large-bore intravenous catheter and line or nonrestrictive saline lock in anticipation of hypovolemia, hypotension, and shock. With anterior blunt or penetrating trauma that may involve the heart, attach the ECG electrodes and monitor for arrhythmias. Attach a pulse oximeter and monitor oxygen saturation to evaluate respiration effectiveness. Waveform capnography may also be useful in detecting early or minute changes in ventilation and perfusion. If there is any mechanism suggesting serious chest trauma or any physical signs of either hypoventilation or hypovolemia compensation, perform rapid trauma assessment with a special focus on the chest and prepare for rapid patient transport to the trauma center.[10]

Secondary/Rapid Trauma Assessment

During rapid trauma assessment examine the patient's chest in detail, carefully observing, questioning about, palpating, and auscultating the region.

Observe

Observe the chest for impact evidence. Look for erythema that develops early in the contusion process, especially as it outlines ribs or forms a pattern reflecting contours of the object the chest hit. Look carefully for penetrating trauma and try to determine the entry angle and penetration depth. Also look for exit wounds. Lateral chest injury is likely to involve the lungs, while an energy pathway through the central chest is likely to involve the heart, great vessels, trachea, or esophagus. Injury to the mediastinal structures is also likely to result in serious hemorrhage, hypovolemia, and shock. Look for intercostal and suprasternal retractions as well as external jugular vein distention. Remember, JVD is normally present in supine normotensive patients and may be exaggerated or may continue if the patient is moved to a seated position if venous pressure is elevated. Jugular veins are usually flat in hypovolemic chest trauma patients.

Watch chest movement carefully during respiration. The chest should rise and abdomen fall smoothly with inspiration and return to their positions during expiration. Any limited motion, either bilaterally or unilaterally, suggests a problem. Watch for the paradoxical motion of flail chest. That movement will be limited because of muscle spasm during early care, but continued respiration further damages surrounding soft tissue and intracostal muscles fatigue. This leads to progressive and more obvious paradoxical motion and greater respiratory embarrassment. Look, too, for any hyperinflation of one side of the chest and any deformity that may exist from rib fracture, sternal fracture or dislocation, or subcutaneous emphysema. Assess air volume effectively moved with each breath and ensure that minute volume is greater than 6 liters. If not, consider gentle overdrive ventilation with the bag-valve mask. Assess pulse oximetry and, should saturation begin to drop, consider more aggressive airway and respiratory support. Examine any open wound for air movement in or out, which is indicative of an open pneumothorax. Observe the general color of the patient. If a patient's skin is dusky, ashen, or cyanotic, suspect respiratory compromise. Suspect traumatic asphyxia if a patient's head and neck are swollen and red, dark red, or blue.

Question

Question a patient about any pain, pain on motion, pain with breathing effort, or dyspnea. Note if the pain is crushing, tearing, or is described otherwise by the patient. Have the patient describe the exact pain's location, its severity, and any pain radiation. Question about other sensations and carefully monitor the patient's consciousness and orientation levels. Gain a complete patient history and identify any serious preexisting conditions, especially those affecting respiration like COPD or asthma.

Palpate

Palpate the thorax carefully and completely, feeling for any injury signs (Figure 17 ●). Feel for any swelling, deformity, crepitus, or crackling. Compress the thorax between your hands with pressure directed inward. Then apply downward pressure on the midsternum. Such pressure will flex the ribs and should elicit pain from any fracture site along the thorax. (Apply pressure only if you have found no signs or symptoms of chest injury. If you suspect rib or sternal fracture, provide appropriate care but do not aggravate the injury.) Rest your hands on the lower thorax and let the chest lift your hands with inspiration and let them fall with expiration (Figure 18 ●). The motion should be smooth and equal. If not, determine the nature of any asymmetry. If appropriate, have the patient take a deep breath and ask him about any discomfort or pain.

Auscultate

Auscultate all lung lobes, both anteriorly and posteriorly (Figure 19 ●). Listen for both inspiratory and expiratory air movement and note any crackles, indicating edema from pulmonary contusion or congestive heart failure, or any diminished breath sounds, suggesting hypoventilation. Compare one

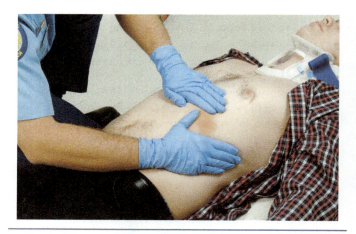

● **Figure 17**   Carefully palpate the thorax of a patient with a suspected injury to the region.

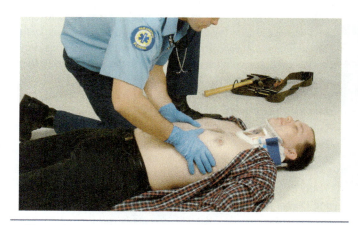

● **Figure 18**   Place your hands on the lower thorax and let them rise and fall with respiration.

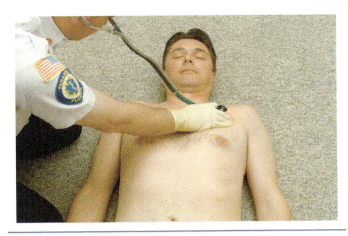

● **Figure 19**   Auscultate all lung lobes, both anteriorly and posteriorly.

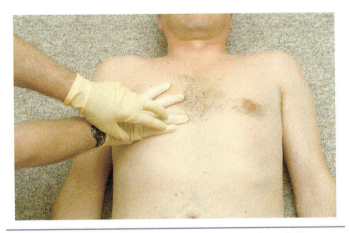

● **Figure 20**   Percuss all lung lobes, listening for a dull response or hyperresonance.

side to the other and one lobe to another. Be sensitive for distant or muffled heart sounds or decreased breath sounds.

Percuss

Percuss the chest and note the responses (Figure 20 ●). Determine if the area percussed is normal, hyperresonant, or dull. A dull response suggests collecting blood or other fluid, while hyperresonance suggests air under pressure as in tension pneumothorax.

Blunt Trauma Assessment

In blunt trauma, you commonly find slight chest surface discoloration reflective of contusions. Contusions also cause pain, generally in an area or region, and somewhat limit respiration. As impact energy increases, it may cause fractures of ribs 4 through 8 and a greater possibility of underlying injury. If upper ribs or ribs 9 through 12 fracture, suspect very serious underlying injury. Sternal fracture also takes great energy and is associated with a higher incidence of internal injury. Rib fractures generate point-specific pain (at the fracture site) and crepitus on deep breathing or your flexing of the patient's chest during

rapid trauma assessment. That pain may further limit chest excursion during respiration. As energy of trauma and chest trauma seriousness increases, more ribs may fracture, causing a flail chest. Remember that a flail chest's paradoxical motion is initially limited by muscular splinting and grows more noticeable and causes more respiratory distress as time since the collision increases.

In blunt chest injury, you must anticipate and assess for additional signs suggesting internal injury. Signs specific for lung injury include increasing dyspnea, signs of hypoxemia, accessory muscle use, and intracostal and suprasternal retractions. Auscultation will help you differentiate between pulmonary contusion and pneumothorax. Contusions demonstrate progressively increasing crackles, while pneumothorax presents with diminishing breath sounds on the ipsilateral side. Further, with pneumothorax the affected side may be hyperinflated and resonant to percussion. If pneumothorax progresses to tension pneumothorax, you will likely note progressing dyspnea and hypoxia, hemodynamic compromise, accessory muscle use, distended jugular veins, tracheal shift toward the contralateral side (a late finding), and ipsilateral chest hyperresonance on percussion. Subcutaneous emphysema may develop, especially if a lung defect was caused by, or is associated with, rib fracture that disturbs parietal pleura integrity. Hemothorax is noticeable more because of vascular loss than from the pathology's respiratory component. Suspect it if you find hypovolemia signs associated with blunt chest trauma. Hemothorax, when sizeable, may cause dyspnea and a lung field that is dull to percussion.

Blunt mediastinal injury will probably affect the heart, great vessels, and trachea. Heart injury may present with chest pain similar to a myocardial infarction and, if serious enough, with heart failure or cardiogenic shock signs. An ECG may reveal tachycardia, bradycardia, PVCs, and, in cases of severe cardiac contusion, may demonstrate ST elevation. Cardiac rupture presents with sudden death, while pericardial tamponade is unlikely in blunt chest trauma. Injury to great vessels (dissection) is most frequently associated with lateral impacts or feet-first high falls and may produce a tearing chest pain and pulse deficits in the extremities. If dissection ruptures, rapidly progressing hypovolemia, hypotension, shock, and death ensue. Tracheobronchial injury results in rapidly developing pneumomediastinum or pneumothorax and possible subcutaneous emphysema, hemoptysis, dyspnea, and hypoxia. Positive-pressure ventilations may increase sign development and severity. Traumatic asphyxia presents with jugular vein distention, head and neck discoloration, severe dyspnea, and possible hypovolemia and shock signs.

Penetrating Trauma Assessment

Penetrating injury displays a different set of signs associated with different injuries. Inspect a chest wound for frothy blood or air exchange sounds with respirations (open pneumothorax). Remember that a wound needs to be rather large (high-velocity bullet exit wound or close-range shotgun blast) for these signs to occur. A penetrating wound, however, commonly induces a simple pneumothorax with its associated signs and symptoms. A hyperinflated chest, distended jugular veins, tracheal shift away from the injury, distant or absent breath sounds, hyper-resonance to percussion, and severe dyspnea and hypotension suggest tension pneumothorax. Tension pneumothorax may push air outward through a penetrating wound or cause subcutaneous emphysema around the wound.[11] Some degree of hemothorax is likely to be associated with penetrating chest trauma and, if extensive, may present with diminished or absent breath sounds and a chest region that is dull to percussion. Hemothorax also causes, or significantly contributes to, hypovolemia and shock.

Penetrating heart trauma is likely to cause pericardial tamponade and present with jugular vein distention, distant heart sounds, and hypotension (Beck's triad). Pulsus paradoxus (pulse weakening or blood pressure falling by more than 10 mmHg with inspiration) may be present and jugular filling may occur with inspiration (from a paradoxical rise in venous pressure during inspiration, known as Kussmaul's sign, that is associated with pericardial tamponade). Both pulsus paradoxus and jugular filling are indicative of pericardial tamponade. Additionally, with pericardial tamponade, heart sounds are distant, pulses are weak, and the patient experiences increasing hypotension and shock (Figure 21 ●). Penetrating heart trauma may also cause myocardial rupture and immediate death (Figure 22 ●). This patient demonstrates vital signs that fall precipitously as vascular volume is lost into the mediastinum.

Reassessment

Reassessments simply repeat primary assessment elements and vital signs, and reexamine injury signs discovered during earlier assessment. Reassessment takes on great importance for the chest trauma patient. With any serious chest impact or any penetrating chest injury, observe respiratory depth, rate, and symmetry of effort. Auscultate both lung fields for equality and crackles and monitor distal pulses, oxygen saturation, skin color, and blood pressure for progressing hypovolemia signs (Figure 23 ●). If any signs change between reassessments,

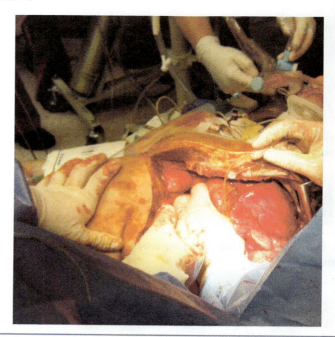

● **Figure 22** Stab wound to the chest. (© *Michael Casey, MD*)

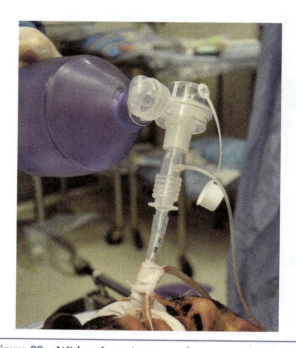

● **Figure 23** With pulse oximetry and capnography, you can continuously monitor the patient's oxygenation and ventilation status. (© *Edward T. Dickinson, MD*)

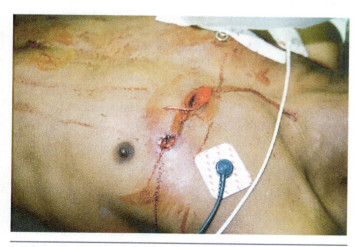

● **Figure 21** Gunshot wound to the chest. (© *Edward T. Dickinson, MD*)

search out a cause and rule out or care for progressing chest injury. Be especially suspicious of developing tension pneumothorax, pericardial tamponade, extensive and evolving pulmonary contusion, and hypovolemia associated with hemothorax. If any of these is suspected, institute the appropriate management steps.

MANAGEMENT OF THE CHEST INJURY PATIENT

General patient management for significant chest injury focuses on ensuring good oxygenation and adequate respiratory volume and rate. Administer supplemental oxygen if the patient is hypoxic. Ensure that the airway is patent and consider endotracheal intubation if the Glasgow Coma Scale score is ≤ 8 or if there is significant ventilatory impairment. Consider intubation early in your care, as patients with thoracic trauma are likely to get worse with time. Rapid sequence intubation may be needed for the combative patient. Endotracheal intubation also makes ventilation of the flail chest or pulmonary contusion patient easier.

Carefully evaluate minute volume (breaths per minute times volume), and if it is less than normal consider assisted ventilation. Bag-valve-mask a conscious patient with severe dyspnea at a rate of 10 to 12 breaths per minute, trying to match the patient's respiratory rate. Closely monitor pulse oximetry, level of consciousness, and skin color. Also monitor capnography to ensure physiologic end-tidal CO_2 levels. Bag-valve-mask ventilation may also be beneficial for patients with serious rib fractures and flail chest. Positive pressure displaces the chest outward, reducing fracture site movement and moving the flail segment with the chest. It may also be beneficial to the patient who is exhausted from increased breathing effort associated with pulmonary contusion. In this case, positive pressure of assisted ventilations helps push any fluids back into the vascular system, relieving edema. Remember, however, that positive-pressure ventilations change respiration dynamics from a less-than-atmospheric to a greater-than-atmospheric process and may exacerbate respiratory problems like tracheobronchial injury, pneumothorax, and tension pneumothorax. Positive-pressure ventilation may also impair venous return to the heart.

Anticipate heart and great vessel compromise with thoracic injury and be ready to support the patient's cardiovascular system. Initiate at least one large-bore IV site if the patient has a serious chest trauma mechanism and place two lines if there are any hypovolemia or compensation signs. Be prepared to administer fluids quickly (in 250 to 500 mL boluses) if the patient's systolic blood pressure drops below 80 mmHg.

IV fluid infusion for the chest trauma patient must be titrated carefully. Excessive fluid administration may increase the blood loss rate and dilute clotting factors, prolonging and possibly increasing any hemorrhage. Additional fluid also increases edema associated with pulmonary contusion, increasing the rate and extent of its development. Anytime you administer fluids to the chest trauma patient, do so incrementally, periodically auscultating all lung fields carefully and slow or stop fluid resuscitation whenever you hear crackles or dyspnea increases. The technique of hypotensive resuscitation also demands careful titration of fluid boluses to keep the systolic BP at or below 80 mmHg.

Care is specific for thoracic injuries including rib fractures, sternoclavicular dislocation, flail chest, open pneumothorax, tension pneumothorax, hemothorax, blunt cardiac injury, pericardial tamponade, aortic dissection, tracheobronchial injury, and traumatic asphyxia.

Rib Fractures

Rib fractures, either isolated or associated with other respiratory injuries, may produce pain that significantly limits respiratory effort and leads to hypoventilation. In these patients you may consider administering analgesics to afford greater patient comfort and improve chest excursion. Ensure that the patient is hemodynamically stable, that there is no associated abdominal or head injury, and that a patient is fully conscious and oriented. Consider administration of morphine sulfate, fentanyl, or meperidine. Note that nitrous oxide use is contraindicated in chest trauma as nitrous oxide may migrate into a pneumothorax or tension pneumothorax, making them worse.

Sternoclavicular Dislocation

Supportive therapy with oxygen is usually all that is required for an isolated sternoclavicular dislocation. However, hemodynamic instability indicates associated injuries requiring rapid transport to a trauma center with aggressive resuscitation measures instituted en route. If you suspect posterior sternoclavicular dislocation and note the patient to be in significant respiratory distress that is not effectively treated with initial airway maneuvers and supplemental oxygen, if needed, then consider dislocation reduction. Place the patient in the supine position with a sandbag between his shoulder blades. A sandbag helps to pull the shoulders backward and moves the clavicle head laterally and away from the trachea. Do not perform this procedure for multiple-trauma patients because of the risk of spine injury. An alternative field-expedient method of reducing impingement is to place the patient supine and grasp the clavicle near the sternum. Pull it upward and laterally, directly perpendicular to the sternum. This distracts the clavicle forward, alleviating its airway impingement.

Flail Chest

Place a flail chest injury patient on the injured side if spinal immobilization is not required. If spinal injury is suspected, secure a large and bulky dressing with bandaging against the flail segment to stabilize it. Administer supplemental oxygen, if needed, and monitor oxygen saturation with pulse oximetry, and monitor cardiac activity with the ECG. If there is significant dyspnea, underlying pulmonary injury evidence, or respiratory compromise signs, these measures will not suffice. Then consider an advanced airway and mechanical ventilation. Positive-pressure ventilations internally splint the flail segment, expand atelectatic lung areas, and also treat underlying pulmonary contusion. Monitor end-tidal CO_2 if possible. Use of sandbags to support a flail segment is not indicated because they may diminish chest movement, adding to hypoventilation, atelectasis, and subsequent hypoxemia. Rapid transport to the trauma center is indicated as this injury, its complications, and associated injuries are often life threatening.

Open Pneumothorax

Support a patient with open pneumothorax by administering high-concentration oxygen and monitoring oxygen

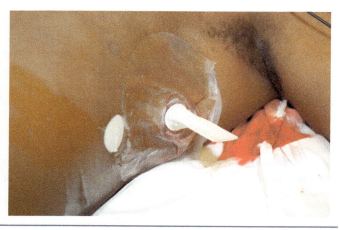

● **Figure 24**   An Asherman chest seal in place on a patient. (© Edward T. Dickinson, MD)

saturation and respiratory effort. If you find a penetrating injury, cover it with a sterile occlusive dressing (sterile plastic wrap) taped on three sides or with a commercially available one-way valve dressing such as the Asherman Chest Seal (Figure 24 ●). This process converts an open pneumothorax into a closed pneumothorax, prevents further air aspiration, and relieves any building pressure (tension pneumothorax) through the valvelike dressing. If dyspnea diminishes somewhat but still continues, provide positive-pressure ventilations and intubate as needed. Carefully monitor the patient when you employ intermittent positive-pressure ventilation because its use may lead to a tension pneumothorax. If, after a dressing has been applied, the patient has progressive breathing difficulty, appears to be hypoventilating and hypoxemic, has decreasing breath sounds on the injured side, and has increasing jugular distention, remove the occlusive dressing. If you hear air rush out and the patient's respirations improve, reseal the wound, monitor breathing carefully, and again remove the dressing if any dyspnea redevelops. If removing a dressing does not relieve increasing signs and symptoms, suspect and treat for tension pneumothorax using needle decompression.

Tension Pneumothorax

Confirm possible tension pneumothorax by auscultating lung fields for diminished breath sounds, percussing for hyperresonance, and observing for severe dyspnea, chest hyperinflation, and jugular vein distention.[12] Successful treatment depends on rapid recognition and then pleural decompression. As you prepare to decompress the affected (ipsilateral) side, administer supplemental oxygen as needed if the airway is intact and the patient is able to demonstrate adequate ventilatory effort. Pleural decompression should be employed only if the patient demonstrates significant dyspnea and distinct signs and symptoms of tension pneumothorax.

Provide ventilations with a bag-valve mask and supplemental oxygen and intubate if the patient is unable to maintain an airway or continues to show hypoxemia signs/symptoms while on high-concentration oxygen. Perform needle thoracentesis by inserting a long (e.g., 3 inch or longer) large-bore

(14-gauge intravascular or larger) catheter into the second intercostal space, midclavicular line on the side of the thorax with decreased breath sounds and hyperinflation (Figure 25 ●).[13,14] In the supine patient, this location is most appropriate for pleural decompression, as any air in the thorax will migrate to the anterior regions of the thorax. This location is easy to identify by finding the Angle of Louis and palpating the intercostal space just lateral to it. Then advance the catheter in a straight posterior trajectory (in the supine patient this is straight toward the floor) through the chest wall. Ensure that you enter the thoracic cavity by passing the needle just over the rib. The intercostal artery, vein, and nerve pass just under each rib and may be injured if the needle's track is too high. As you enter the pleural space, you will feel a pop and may hear a rush of air. Advance the catheter into the chest and then withdraw the needle.[15,16]

If the patient remains symptomatic, place a second or third catheter in the third or fourth intercostal space, midaxillary line to ensure proper decompression. Secure the catheter in place with tape, being careful not to block the port or kink the catheter. Leaving the catheter open to air converts tension pneumothorax into a simple pneumothorax and stabilizes the patient. Monitor patient respirations and breath sounds for a recurring tension pneumothorax. If signs and symptoms again appear, decompress the chest again. Frequently, the initial catheter clogs or kinks and necessitates replacement by another.

Rapidly transport the patient to the trauma center for definitive treatment (usually a chest tube). Avoid infusing IV crystalloid boluses if the patient is hemodynamically stable. An underlying pulmonary contusion may lead to edema, which is made worse with overaggressive fluid therapy. If your patient remains significantly hypotensive (SBP < 80 mmHg) after chest decompression and respirations do not become adequate, consider possible internal hemorrhage and a need for fluid resuscitation. If respirations do not dramatically improve, assess for a contralateral tension pneumothorax or pericardial tamponade as the cause.

Hemothorax

Treat a patient with suspected hemothorax with oxygen administration and ventilatory support, as needed. Initiate two large-bore intravenous catheters, readied to infuse fluid in 250 to 500 mL boluses. (For newborns <30 days old, administer a 10 mL/kg bolus while children >30 days old should receive a 20 mL/kg bolus.) Be conservative in fluid administration. Maintain a systolic blood pressure of 80 mmHg but do not attempt to return it to preinjury levels. Carefully listen to breath sounds during any infusion because increasing vascular volume may increase edema and pulmonary contusion congestion. It may also increase the pressure, rate, and volume of internal hemorrhage. If pulmonary contusion is extensive and the patient cannot be adequately oxygenated by high-concentration oxygen, positive-pressure ventilations are indicated and may limit further edema that contributes to the injury. Positive end expiratory pressure (PEEP) and more likely continuous positive airway pressure (CPAP) may also benefit a patient experiencing hemothorax. Increased intrathoracic pressure may serve to expand collapsed alveoli, slow hemorrhage, push edema fluid back into the circulatory system, and increase oxygen partial pressure.

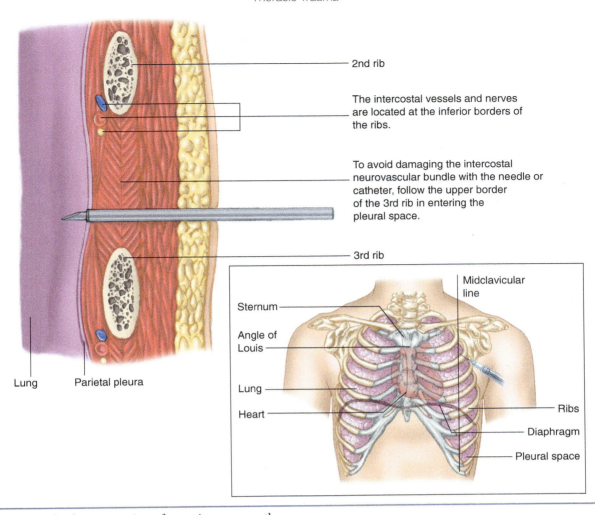

● Figure 25 Needle decompression of a tension pneumothorax.

Blunt Cardiac Injury

In serious frontal impact collisions, suspect blunt cardiac injury and supplemental oxygen, if needed. Monitor cardiac electrical activity and watch for tachycardias, bradycardias, ectopic beats, and conduction defects. Establish an IV line in the event that antiarrhythmics (such as amiodarone) are needed, and monitor the patient for great vessel injury. Employ pharmacological care measures recommended for advanced cardiac life support. Rapidly transport the patient to the trauma center for further evaluation and continued monitoring.

Pericardial Tamponade

Maintain a high index of suspicion for pericardial tamponade in the patient with central thoracic penetrating trauma. Appropriate prehospital care is oxygen administration and IV fluid administration to maximize oxygenation and venous return. Definitive care is to remove some of the accumulating pericardial fluid through pericardiocentesis. This action is rarely permitted in the field; hence, the patient needs to be transported as rapidly as possible to the emergency department. Note that

a relatively simple procedure can relieve this problem and can be adequately administered by an emergency physician. If a physician-staffed emergency department is significantly closer to you than a trauma center, it may be the best choice for a patient with isolated pericardial tamponade. After pericardiocentesis is performed, the patient may then be directed to the closest trauma center.

Aortic Dissection

Care for a patient with aortic dissection is performed through gentle but rapid transport to the trauma center. Any jarring during extrication, assessment, care, packaging, or transport increases the risk of rupture and rapidly fatal exsanguination. Initiate IV therapy en route, but be very conservative in fluid administration. Mild hypotension may be protective of the injury site. Titrate IV fluids to keep the systolic blood pressure at 80 mmHg. If a dissection ruptures, as indicated by an immediate deterioration in vital signs, provide rapid administration of fluids and cardiovascular resuscitation. Anxiety and its effect on cardiac output and blood pressure may increase the likelihood of dissection rupture. Place a special emphasis on calming and reassuring the patient during very gentle care and transport.

Tracheobronchial Injury

Support a tracheobronchial injury patient with high-concentration oxygen and clear the airway of blood and secretions. If you are unable to maintain a patent airway or adequately oxygenate the patient, then intubate the trachea and provide positive-pressure ventilations. Observe the patient carefully for tension pneumothorax development, which may result as a complication of positive-pressure ventilations, and treat as previously prescribed. Provide rapid transport as soon as the patient can be extricated and stabilized. This is important because these patients can rapidly destabilize and then require emergency surgical intervention.

Traumatic Asphyxia

Administer oxygen and support the airway and respiration of the traumatic asphyxia patient. This may require using positive-pressure ventilations with the bag-valve mask to ensure adequate ventilation during entrapment and possibly thereafter.

Establish two large-bore IV lines for rapid crystalloid infusion in anticipation of rapidly developing hypovolemia with chest decompression. Monitor the ECG for evidence of arrhythmias. Once compressing force is removed, the direct effects of traumatic asphyxia spontaneously resolve; however, serious internal hemorrhage may begin. Prepare to transport immediately after release from entrapment because the patient will likely have severe coexisting injuries.

If a patient remains entrapped for a prolonged time, consider sodium bicarbonate administration. Prolonged stagnant blood flow and a hypoxic cellular environment may cause metabolic acid accumulation. As compression is released, this blood returns to the central circulation, much as it does with the release of entrapped limbs during crush injury. Consider the administration of 1 mEq/kg of sodium bicarbonate just before or during decompression of the chest if entrapment has lasted more than 20 minutes.

CHAPTER REVIEW

SUMMARY

Thoracic trauma by either blunt or penetrating mechanisms has a great potential for posing a threat to a patient's life. In fact, 25 percent of all traumatic deaths are secondary to thoracic trauma injuries. In assessing these patients, the mechanism of injury, when considered along with the clinical findings, may help in differentiating among the many possible injuries. Assessment, in turn, helps guide your interventions and determines the need for rapid extrication and transport. Aggressive airway management, oxygenation, ventilation, and fluid resuscitation, when indicated, can make the difference between patient survival or death. Specific interventions, such as pleural decompression or flail segment stabilization, can also affect mortality and morbidity from chest trauma. Understanding the pathological processes affecting the chest during trauma and employing proper assessment and care measures will ensure the best possible outcome for your patients.

YOU MAKE THE CALL

Medic 101 responds to the interstate where they are called to a crash scene. An older pickup truck has struck a bridge abutment, apparently after the driver fell asleep while driving home from the night shift. The scene survey reveals that the State Patrol has deployed appropriate warning flares and controlled traffic to allow safe access to the scene. The paramedics approach the truck and find a 20-year-old male patient unconscious behind the wheel. The paramedics note that no seat belt has been worn and no air bag has deployed. The steering wheel is displaced somewhat upward and bent inward against the dash. The windshield is starred.

The primary assessment reveals an unconscious male patient with central cyanosis, poor air exchange, and no peripheral (radial) pulses palpable. With in-line stabilization, the patient is rapidly extricated to a long board, the airway is opened by a jaw thrust (with cervical precautions), and an oral airway is then placed with respiratory assistance provided via BVM with high-concentration oxygen. Little improvement is noted in the patient's color, air exchange, level of consciousness, and peripheral pulses. The trachea appears midline, but jugular vein distention is present. As the patient's clothes are cut away, subcutaneous emphysema is palpable along the left anterior and lateral chest wall. There is a pronounced inward movement of a section of anterior chest wall with the patient's inspiratory efforts.

1. Considering the mechanism of injury and what is known about the patient, what thoracic pathophysiology may explain the patient's presentation?

2. As the treating paramedic, what is your next step in stabilizing this patient?

3. What further emergency treatment is likely indicated by the absence of breath sounds on the left side and a relatively normal abdominal exam?

See Suggested Responses at the back of this chapter.

REVIEW QUESTIONS

1. The union between the xiphoid process and the body of the sternum is called the _____.
  a. manubrium
  b. thoracic duct
  c. costal margin
  d. xiphisternal joint

2. During a football game, a 17-year-old male is tackled and knocked to the ground. Although he reports hearing a "bone crack," he initially appears to be stable. The team manager summons the paramedics. By the time they arrive, the patient states that he is "feeling funny" and having difficulty breathing. On primary assessment, a rapid, weak pulse and a low BP are noted. The patient's appearance suggests that he may be developing shock. You suspect a fractured rib and possibly _____.
  a. traumatic asphyxia
  b. pericardial tamponade
  c. tension pneumothorax
  d. traumatic aortic rupture

3. Secondary to a severe chest wall contusion, which of the following signs/symptoms is most commonly seen?
  a. retractions
  b. hypoventilation
  c. deep, gasping respirations
  d. use of accessory muscles

4. You have elected to apply an occlusive dressing to your patient who has sustained a stab wound to the chest. You realize that you should secure the dressing _____.
  a. on two sides
  b. on four sides
  c. on three sides
  d. loosely over the wound

5. Your patient has received significant deceleration trauma to his chest. He presents with absent radial and brachial pulses in the left upper extremity and severe hypotension. He reported that he felt a tearing sensation in his chest before quickly losing consciousness. He most likely has experienced a _____.
  a. severe rib fracture
  b. pericardial tamponade
  c. pulmonary contusion
  d. traumatic aortic dissection

6. The type of crash impact most commonly associated with aortic rupture when the patient has been involved in a motor vehicle collision is _____.
  a. lateral   c. rollover
  b. frontal   d. rotational

7. The following mechanism of injury that is most likely to cause traumatic asphyxia is _____.
  a. blunt trauma, low impact
  b. penetrating trauma, low velocity
  c. penetrating trauma, high velocity
  d. blunt trauma, compressive force

8. You and your partner are called to the scene of a motor vehicle collision. When you arrive, you note that a car has struck a parked vehicle. Your 30-year-old female patient complains of difficulty breathing and you note that breath sounds are diminished bilaterally. The patient states that, at the last minute, she anticipated the impending crash and held her breath. You suspect "paper-bag syndrome" in which the sudden pressure exerted on her expanded lungs, with closed glottis preventing the escape of air, caused the rupture of _____.
  a. alveoli
  b. arteries
  c. the spleen
  d. the diaphragm

9. The most appropriate prehospital management for a patient with a flail segment and no other suspected underlying injury is judicial use of _____.
  a. chest tube insertion
  b. positive-pressure ventilation
  c. needle decompression
  d. sandbag placed on the injured side

10. The most appropriate prehospital management for a patient with a traumatic rupture of the aorta is to _____.
  a. initiate a large-bore IV prior to transport
  b. delay transport to complete application of the PASG garment
  c. begin a rapid IV drip of plasma expanders bilaterally, prior to transport
  d. expedite transport to a trauma center; administer conservative IV fluids en route

See Answers to Review Questions at the back of this chapter.

REFERENCES

1. Eckstien, M. and S. Henderson. "Thoracic Trauma." *Emergency Medicine: Concepts and Clinical Practice.* 7th ed. St. Louis: Mosby, 2009.

2. Vukich, D. and V. Markovchick. "Thoracic Trauma." *Emergency Medicine: Concepts and Clinical Practice.* 4th ed. St. Louis: Mosby, 1998.

3. Buchman, T., B. Hall, W. Bowling, and G. Kelen. "Thoracic Trauma." *Emergency Medicine: A Comprehensive Study Guide.* 7th ed. New York: McGraw-Hill, 2008.

4. Hubble, M. and J. Hubble. "Chest Trauma." *Principles of Advanced Trauma Care.* Albany: Delmar, 2002.

5. Campbell, John E. *International Trauma Life Support for Prehospital Care Providers.* 6th ed. Upper Saddle River, N.J.: Pearson/Prentice Hall, 2008.

6. Montagnana, M., et al. "Sudden Cardiac Death in Young Athletes." *Internal Medicine* 47(2008): 1373–1378.

7. Markovchick, V. and R. Wolfe. "Cardiovascular Trauma." *Emergency Medicine: Concepts and Clinical Practice.* 4th ed. St. Louis: Mosby, 1998.

8. Kanowitz, A. and V. Markovchick. "Esophageal and Diaphragmatic Trauma." *Emergency Medicine: Concepts and Clinical Practice.* 4th ed. St. Louis: Mosby, 1998.

9. "Thoracic Trauma." *Advanced Trauma Life Support Course: Student Manual.* 8th ed. Chicago: American College of Surgeons, 2008.

10. Kidler, E., et al. "The Effect of Prehospital Time Related Variables in the Mortality following Severe Thoracic Trauma." *Injury* (May 2011).

11. Leigh-Smith, S. and G. Davies. "Tension Pneumothorax: Eyes May Be More Diagnostic than Ears." *Emerg Med J* 20 (2003): 495–496.

12. Leigh-Smith, S. and T. Harris. "Tension Pneumothorax–Time for a Re-Think?" *Emerg Med J* 22 (2005): 8–16.

13. Stevens, R. L., et al. "Needle Thoracostomy for Tension Pneumothorax: Failure Predicted by Chest Tomography." *Prehosp Emerg Care* 13(1) (Jan–Mar 2009): 14–17.

14. Ball, C. G., et al. "Thoracic Needle Decompression for Tension Pneumothorax: Clinical Correlation with Catheter Length." *Can J Surg* 53(3) (Jun 2010): 184–188.

15. Eckstein, M. and D. Suyehara. "Needle Thoracostomy in the Prehospital Setting." *Prehosp Emerg Care* 2(2) (Apr–Jun 1988): 132–135.

16. Holcomb, J. B., J. G. McManus, S. T. Kerr, and A. E. Pusateri. "Needle versus Tube Thoracostomy in a Swine Model of Tension Pneumothorax." *Prehosp Emerg Care* 13(1) (Jan–Mar 2009): 18–27.

FURTHER READING

American College of Surgeons, Committee on Trauma. *Advanced Trauma Life Support Course: Student Manual.* 8th ed. Chicago: American College of Surgeons, 2008.

Bates, Barbara, and Peter G. Szilagyi. *A Guide to Physical Examination and History Taking.* 9th ed. Philadelphia: J. B. Lippincott, 2007.

Bledsoe, B. E., and D. Clayden. *Prehospital Emergency Pharmacology.* 7th ed. Upper Saddle River, NJ: Pearson/Prentice Hall, 2011.

Bledsoe B. E., B. J. Colbert, and J. E. Ankney. *Essentials of A & P for Emergency Care.* Upper Saddle River, NJ: Pearson/Prentice Hall, 2010.

Campbell, John E. *International Trauma Life Support for Emergency Care Providers.* 7th ed. Upper Saddle River, NJ: Pearson/Prentice Hall, 2012.

Clemente, C. D. *Anatomy: A Regional Atlas of the Human Body.* 5th ed. Baltimore: Lippincott, Williams & Wilkins, 2006.

Hall-Craggs, E. C. B. *Anatomy as a Basis for Clinical Medicine.* 3rd ed. Baltimore: Lippincott, Williams & Wilkins, 1995.

Martini, Frederic. *Fundamentals of Anatomy and Physiology.* 7th ed. San Francisco: Benjamin Cummings, 2011.

McSwain, N. E., and S. B. Frame, eds. *Prehospital Trauma Life Support.* 6th ed. St. Louis: Mosby, 2007.

Rosen, P., and R. Barkin, eds. *Emergency Medicine: Concepts and Clinical Practice.* 7th ed. St. Louis: Mosby, 2009.

SUGGESTED RESPONSES TO "YOU MAKE THE CALL"

The following are suggested responses to the "You Make the Call" scenarios presented in this chapter. Each represents an acceptable response to the scenario but should not be interpreted as the only correct response.

1. *Considering the mechanism of injury and what is known about the patient, what thoracic pathophysiology may explain the patient's presentation?*

   The patient struck his chest on the steering wheel of the vehicle, resulting in a "flail" segment of chest which has also caused a tension pneumothorax.

2. *As the treating paramedic, what is your next step in stabilizing this patient?*

   Secure the airway as necessary. Then provide for more effective ventilatory support by securing the flail segment. Finally, determine which side (if not both) needs to be decompressed and provide a chest decompression.

3. *What further emergency treatment is likely indicated by the absence of breath sounds on the left side and a relatively normal abdominal exam?*

   A chest decompression is likely to be indicated along with a chest tube to help remove any blood and air caught in the pleural space.

ANSWERS TO REVIEW QUESTIONS

1. d
2. c
3. b
4. c
5. d
6. a
7. d
8. a
9. b
10. d

GLOSSARY

aneurysm   a weakening or ballooning in the wall of a blood vessel.

atelectasis   collapse of a lung or part of a lung.

commotio cordis   Lethal cardiac arrhythmia caused by a sharp nonpenetrating blow to the sternum.

electrical alternans   alternating amplitude of the P, QRS, and T waves on the ECG rhythm strip as the heart swings in a pendulum-like fashion within the pericardial sac during tamponade.

epicardium   serous membrane covering the outer surface of the heart; the visceral pericardium.

flail chest   defect in the chest wall that allows for free movement of a segment. Breathing will cause paradoxical chest wall motion.

great vessels   large arteries and veins located in the mediastinum that enter and exit the heart; the pulmonary artery, the aorta, the inferior vena cava, and the superior vena cava.

hemopneumothorax   condition where air and blood are in the pleural space.

hemoptysis   coughing of blood that originates in the respiratory tract.

hemothorax   blood within the pleural space.

ligamentum arteriosum   cordlike remnant of a fetal vessel connecting the pulmonary artery to the aorta at the aortic isthmus.

pericardial tamponade   a restriction to cardiac filling caused by blood (or other fluid) within the pericardial sac.

pericardium   fibrous sac that surrounds the heart.

pneumothorax   a collection of air in the pleural space. Air may enter the pleural space through an injury to the chest wall or through an injury to the lungs. In a tension pneumothorax, pressure builds because there is no way for the air to escape, causing lung collapse.

precordium   area of the chest wall overlying the heart.

pulmonary hilum   central medial region of the lung where the bronchi and pulmonary vasculature enter the lung.

pulsus alternans drop of greater than 10 mmHg in the systolic blood pressure during the inspiratory phase of respiration that occurs in patients with pericardial tamponade.

pulsus paradoxus alternating strong and weak pulse.

rhabdomyolysis acute pathological process that involves the destruction of skeletal muscle.

tension pneumothorax buildup of air under pressure within the thorax. The resulting compression of the lung severely reduces venous return, cardiac output, and the effectiveness of respirations.

tracheobronchial tree the structures of the trachea and the bronchi.

xiphisternal joint union between xiphoid process and body of the sternum.

Head, Face, Neck, and Spinal Trauma

Robert S. Porter, MA, EMT-P

STANDARD
Trauma (Head, Facial, Neck, and Spine Trauma)

COMPETENCY
Integrates assessment findings with principles of epidemiology and pathophysiology to formulate a field impression to implement a comprehensive treatment/disposition plan for an acutely injured patient.

OBJECTIVES

Terminal Performance Objective
After reading this chapter you should be able to integrate knowledge of anatomy, physiology, pathophysiology, and treatment principles to assess and provide prehospital management for patients with injuries of the head, face, neck, and spinal column.

Enabling Objectives
To accomplish the terminal performance objective, you should be able to:

1. Define key terms introduced in this chapter.

2. Describe the epidemiology of injuries to the head, face, neck, and spinal column.

3. Describe the anatomy and physiology of:
   a. the structures that make up the head.
   b. the structures that make up the face.
   c. the structures that make up the neck and spinal column.

4. Anticipate specific types of injuries to the head, face, neck, and spinal column based on mechanisms of injury.

5. Discuss the pathophysiology of:
   a. scalp and cranial injuries.
   b. facial and eye injuries.
   c. blunt and penetrating trauma to the neck.
   d. spinal column injuries.

6. Demonstrate assessment of patients with head, face, neck, and spinal column injuries.

7. Demonstrate proper techniques of manually stabilizing and immobilizing the spine.

8. Demonstrate proper techniques of handling, moving, and positioning patients with injuries to the head, face, neck, and spinal column.

9. Describe criteria that can be used as part of a spinal clearance protocol.

10. Given a variety of scenarios, develop treatment plans for patients with injuries to the head, face, neck, and spinal column.

KEY TERMS

acute retinal artery
   occlusion
ankylosing spondylitis
aqueous humor
bamboo spine
bilateral periorbital
   ecchymosis
cervical vertebrae
coccyx
conjunctiva
cornea
cranium
diplopia
galea aponeurotica
hyphema

intervertebral disc
intracranial pressure (ICP)
iris
kyphosis
lacrimal fluid
Le Fort criteria
lumbar vertebrae
mandible
maxilla
nares
orbit
pinna
pupil
retina
retinal detachment

retroauricular ecchymosis
sacrum
sclera
scoliosis
semicircular canals
spinal canal
spinal clearance
   protocols
sutures
thoracic vertebrae
vertebra
vertebral column
vertebral foramen
vitreous humor
zygoma

CASE STUDY

Paramedics Fred and Lisa are providing standby service at a local high school football game. Just before the end of the third quarter, they are called onto the field when a player is thrown to the ground and "can't get up."

On arrival at the player's side, they find a well-developed teenager who is oriented to person but not to time and place. He states that he was hit hard from the side and now has a burning sensation (commonly called a "stinger") in his arms and neck. On further questioning, the player complains of some localized pain just above the shoulders in his central lower neck. His medical history is unremarkable. He has no allergies and his tetanus vaccination is up to date.

The paramedics' physical exam reveals a patient clothed in protective football gear and helmet without external signs of physical injury. The patient's airway is clear, and the rate, strength, and quality of his breathing and pulse are within normal limits. Physical examination of the head is limited by the helmet, but palpation of the posterior neck reveals some localized midline tenderness at or slightly above the first thoracic vertebra. Respiratory excursion and diaphragm movement seem unaffected by the injury. Paresthesia appears to affect the entire chest, abdomen, and lower extremities, as well as the posterior surface of the upper extremities. The patient's upper extremity grip is strong, while the strength of foot dorsiflexion and plantar flexion appears diminished. The patient is able to maintain both bowel and bladder control.

Fred feels it will be very difficult to immobilize the player with the helmet and shoulder pads in place. He has the athletic trainer hold the helmet while he and Lisa release the air pressure in the bladder, remove the face shield, and begin its removal. Lisa stabilizes the player's head, while Fred gently and carefully negotiates the helmet around the patient's face. Once the helmet is removed, Fred assumes manual stabilization of the player's head, which is well above the surface of the playing field because the shoulder pads raise his shoulders more than an inch off the ground. Lisa proceeds to cut off the patient's shirt and the webbing that holds the pads in place and gently removes the pads. Then, using a rope sling, Fred, Lisa, and the athletic trainer gently slide the player with axial control onto the spine board. After the torso is immobilized to the board, they use padding and a cervical immobilization device to immobilize his head about 1 inch above the board to maintain neutral alignment.

The patient's blood pressure, pulse rate and strength, and respiratory rate and volume have all remained relatively normal during these procedures. Fred notes no differences in skin temperature or capillary refill in any extremity, which reduces the likelihood of neurogenic shock from spinal cord injury. The pulse oximeter reads 98 percent, and the ECG displays a normal sinus rhythm at 68 as the paramedics load him into the ambulance and begin transport to the regional trauma center.

Fred and Lisa learn from the local paper that the unfortunate player suffered a compression fracture of the seventh cervical vertebra and will miss the rest of the season. The injury may limit Bill's athletic career but is not expected otherwise to affect his life.

INTRODUCTION TO HEAD, FACE, NECK, AND SPINAL COLUMN TRAUMA

Head, face, neck, and spinal column injuries are common with major trauma.[1] Approximately 1.54 million people experience a significant head impact each year, with 1 in 5 requiring hospitalization.[2] While most of these hospitalizations are due to relatively minor injuries, severe head injury is the most frequent cause of trauma death. It is especially lethal in auto crashes and frequently produces significant long-term disability in patients who survive them. Gunshot wounds that penetrate the cranium occur less frequently but result in a mortality of about 75 to 80 percent. Sports injury and falls, especially in the elderly, account for a significant number of head, face, neck, and spinal column injuries as well. Injuries to the face and neck threaten critical airway structures, sensory organs, and the significant vasculature found in these regions. They are also suggestive of injury to the central nervous system.

The populations most at risk for serious head and spinal column injury are males between the years of 15 and 24, infants and young children, and the elderly.[3] Educational programs promoting safe practices in many different fields and the use of head protection, seat belts, and air bags have had major effects in reducing head injury mortality and morbidity. The use of helmets for bicycling, rollerblading, skateboarding, and motorcycling and in contact sports such as football and hockey has also significantly reduced the incidence of serious head injury. Once a head injury occurs, however, time becomes a critical consideration. Intracranial hemorrhage and progressing edema can increase the intracranial pressure, hypoxia, and the internal and permanent damage done.[4]

Despite the dangers posed by these injuries, head, face, neck, and spinal column injury severity is often difficult to recognize in the prehospital setting. As a result, subtle and unforeseen problems associated with injuries to these regions may cause a patient to quietly deteriorate while caregivers direct attention toward more apparent and gruesome injuries that are not as critical. Even if a life-threatening injury is recognized, you as a paramedic can provide important supportive field care while directing the patient toward the hospital and definitive care. To lessen the chances of death and disability, you must learn to recognize the signs and symptoms of head, face, neck, spinal column, and central nervous system injury early in your assessment; maintain a clear airway and adequate respirations; maintain the patient's blood pressure; and provide rapid transport to a facility that can administer proper care.

HEAD, FACE, NECK, AND SPINAL COLUMN ANATOMY AND PHYSIOLOGY

This chapter will consider injuries to four areas: the head, which contains the brain; the facial region, which contains the beginning of the airway, the beginning of the alimentary canal, and sense organs of sight, taste, hearing, and smell; the neck, which contains the blood vessels, the midportion of the airway, and other vital structures that link the head and torso; and the spinal column, specifically its structure and function. Let us begin by looking at the relevant anatomy and physiology of these four areas.

Anatomy and Physiology of the Head

The head is made up of three structures that cover and protect the brain: the scalp, the cranium, and the meninges. Each of these structures provides essential protection from environmental extremes and from trauma.

The Scalp

The scalp is a strong and flexible layer of skin, fascia (bands of connective tissue), and muscle tissue that is able to withstand and absorb tremendous kinetic energy. The scalp is also extremely vascular in order to help maintain the brain at the body's core temperature. Scalp hair further insulates the brain from environmental temperatures and, to a lesser degree, from trauma.

The scalp is only loosely attached to the skull and is made up of the overlying skin and a number of thin muscle layers and connective tissue underneath. Directly beneath the skin and covering the most superior surface of the head is a fibrous connective tissue sheet called the **galea aponeurotica**. Connected anteriorly to it and covering the forehead is a flat sheet of muscle, the frontal muscle. Connected posteriorly and covering the posterior skull surface is the occipitalis muscle. Laterally, the auricularis muscles cover the areas above the ears and between the lateral brow ridge and occiput. A layer of loose connective tissue beneath these muscles and the galea and just above the periosteum is called the areolar tissue. It contains emissary veins that permit venous blood to flow from the dural sinuses into the venous scalp vessels. These emissary veins also exist in the upper reaches of the nasal cavity. These veins become potential infection routes in scalp wounds or nasal injuries. A helpful way to remember the layers of skin protecting the scalp is the mnemonic SCALP: S—skin; C—connective tissue; A—aponeurotica; L—layer of subaponeurotica (areolar) tissue; P—the skull's periosteum (the pericranium).

The Cranium

The bony structure supporting the head and face is the skull. It can be subdivided into two components: the vault for the brain, called the **cranium**, and facial bones that form the skeletal base for the face (Figure 1 ●). The cranium actually consists of several bones fused together at pseudojoints called **sutures**. These bony plates are constructed of two narrow plates of hard compact bone, separated by a layer of spongy cancellous bone. The plates form a strong, light, rigid, and spherical container for the brain. The cranium is, therefore, quite effective in protecting its contents from the direct effects of trauma. This cranial vault, however, provides very little space for internal swelling or hemorrhage. Any expanding lesion within the cranium displaces other contents or results in an increase in **intracranial pressure (ICP)**. This reduces cerebral perfusion and can severely damage the delicate brain tissue.

The cranial bones form regions that are helpful in describing the cerebral regions beneath. The anterior or frontal bone begins at the brow ridge and covers the upper and anterior surface of the brain. The parietal bones, one on either side, begin just behind the lateral brow ridge and form the skull above the external portions (pinnae) of the ears. The occipital bone forms the posterior and inferior aspect of the cranium, extending to and forming the foramen magnum. The temporal bones form the lateral cranial surfaces anterior to the ears; they are the thinnest bones of the skull and are prone to fracture. The ethmoid and sphenoid bones, which are very irregular in shape, form the portion of the cranium concealed and protected by the facial bones.

The base of the skull consists of portions of the occipital, temporal, sphenoid, and ethmoid bones. This area is important during trauma because the openings, or foramina, for blood

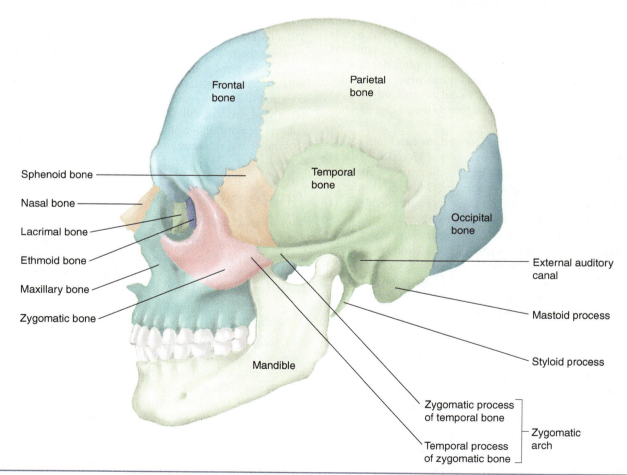

● **Figure 1**   Bones of the human skull.

vessels, spinal cord, auditory canal, and cranial nerves pass through it. These openings weaken the area, leaving it prone to fracture with serious trauma.

Other anatomic points of interest within the cranium are the cribriform plate and the foramen magnum. The cribriform plate is an irregular portion of the ethmoid bone and a portion of the cranium's base. It and the remainder of the cranial base have rough surfaces against which the brain may abrade, lacerate, or contuse during severe deceleration. The foramen magnum is the largest opening in the skull. It is located at the base of the skull where it meets the spinal column and is where the spinal cord exits the cranium.

Facial Anatomy and Physiology
The Face, Nasal Cavity, and Oral Cavity

Facial bones make up the anterior and inferior structures of the head and include the zygoma, maxilla, mandible, and nasal bones (Figure 2 ●). The **zygoma** is the prominent bone of the cheek. It protects the eyes and muscles controlling eye and jaw movement. The **maxilla** comprises the upper jaw, supports the nasal bone, and provides the lower border of the orbit. The nasal bone is the attachment for the nasal cartilage as it forms the shape of the nose. The last of the facial bones is the **mandible**, or jawbone. It resembles two horizontal "L's," which join anteriorly and hinge underneath the posterior zygomatic arch. Besides forming the beginning of the airway and the alimentary canal, the facial bones form supporting and protective structures for several sense organs, including the tongue (taste), eye (sight), and olfactory nerve (smell).

The facial region, like most other areas of the body, is covered with skin that serves to protect the tissue underneath from trauma and against adverse environmental effects. In the facial region, the skin is very flexible and relatively thin. It also has a very good vascular supply and hemorrhages briskly when injured. Beneath the skin is a minimal layer of subcutaneous tissue; beneath that, there are many small muscles that control facial expression and the movements of the mouth, eyes, and eyelids.

Circulation for the facial region is provided by the external carotid artery as it branches into the facial, temporal, and maxillary arteries. The facial artery crosses the mandible, then travels up and along the nasal bone. The maxillary artery runs under the mandible and zygoma, then provides circulation to the cheek area. The temporal artery runs anterior to

the ear just posterior to the zygoma. Each major artery has an associated vein paralleling its path.

The most important cranial nerves traversing this area are the trigeminal (CN-V) and the facial (CN-VII). The trigeminal nerve provides sensation for the face and some motor control over eye movement as well as enabling the chewing process. The facial nerve provides motor control to facial muscles and contributes to the sensation of taste.

The nasal cavity is formed by the juncture of the ethmoid, nasal, and maxillary bones. It is a channel running posteriorly with a bony septum dividing it into left and right chambers and plates protruding medially from the lateral sides. These plates, called turbinates, form support for the vascular mucous membranes that serve to warm, humidify, and collect particulate matter from the incoming air. The lower nasal cavity border is formed by the bony hard palate and then, posteriorly, by the more flexible cartilaginous soft palate. The soft palate moves upward to close off the posterior nasal cavity opening during swallowing. The nasal bone lies anterior and inferior to the eyes and provides a base for the nasal cartilage. Nasal cartilage defines the shape of the nose and divides the nostrils and their openings, which are called the **nares**.

The oral cavity is formed by the concave shape of the maxillary bone, the palate, and the upper teeth meeting the mandible and the lower teeth. The floor of the chamber consists of musculature and connective tissue that span the mandible and support the tongue. The tongue is a large muscle that occupies much of the oral cavity, provides the taste sensation, moves food between the teeth during chewing (mastication),

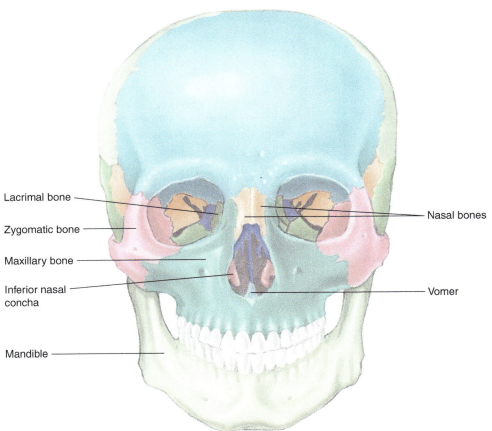

Lacrimal bone

Zygomatic bone

Maxillary bone

Inferior nasal concha

Mandible

Nasal bones

Vomer

● **Figure 2** The facial bones.

and propels chewed food posteriorly, then inferiorly during swallowing. The tongue connects with the hyoid bone, a free-floating U-shaped bone located inferiorly and posteriorly to the mandible. The mandible articulates with the temporal bone at the temporomandibular joint, under the posterior zygoma, and is moved by the very strong masseter muscles. The lip muscles (orbicularis oris) are responsible for sealing the mouth during chewing and swallowing.

Special structures are found in and around the oral cavity. Salivary glands provide saliva, the first of the digestive juices. These glands are located just anterior and inferior to the ear, under the tongue, and just inside the inferior mandible. Specialized lymphoid nodules, the tonsils, are located in the posterior pharynx wall.

Prominent cranial nerves serving the oral area include the hypoglossal, the glossopharyngeal, the trigeminal, and the facial nerves. The hypoglossal nerve (CN-XII) directs swallowing and tongue movement. The glossopharyngeal nerve (CN-IX) controls saliva production and taste. The trigeminal nerve (CN-V) carries sensations from the facial region and assists in chewing control. The facial nerve (CN-VII) controls the muscles of facial expression and taste.

Posterior and inferior to the oral cavity is a collection of soft tissue called the pharynx. The process of swallowing begins in the pharynx once a bolus of food has been propelled back and down by the tongue. The epiglottis moves downward while the larynx moves up, sealing the lower airway opening. Food or liquid moves into the esophagus where a peristaltic wave begins its trip to the stomach. This area is of great importance because it maintains the critical material segregation between the digestive tract and the airway.

Sinuses are hollow spaces within the bones of the cranium and face that lighten the head, protect the eyes and nasal cavity, help give the face its shape, and help produce the voice's resonant tones. They also strengthen this region against the forces of trauma.

The Ear

The outer, visible portion of the ear is termed the **pinna**. It is composed of cartilage and has a poor blood supply. It connects to the external auditory canal, which leads to the eardrum. The external auditory canal contains glands that secrete wax (cerumen) for protection. The ear's important structures are interior and exceptionally well protected from nearly all trauma (Figure 3 ●). Only trauma involving great pressure differentials (e.g., blast and diving injuries), objects inserted directly into the auditory canal, or basilar skull fractures are likely to damage this area.

The ear provides the body with two very useful functions, hearing and positional sense. The middle and inner ear contain structures needed for hearing. Hearing occurs when sound waves cause the tympanic membrane (eardrum) to vibrate. The eardrum transmits these vibrations through three very small bones (the ossicles) to the cochlea, the organ of hearing. These vibrations stimulate the auditory nerve, which in turn transmits a signal to the brain.

The **semicircular canals** are responsible for sensing position and motion. They are three hollow, fluid-filled rings set at different angles. When the head moves, fluid in these rings shifts. Small cells with hairlike projections sense the motion and signal the brain to help maintain balance. This positional sense is present even when the eyes are closed. If injury or illness disturbs this area, it transmits excess signals to the brain. Patients then experience a continuous moving sensation known as vertigo.

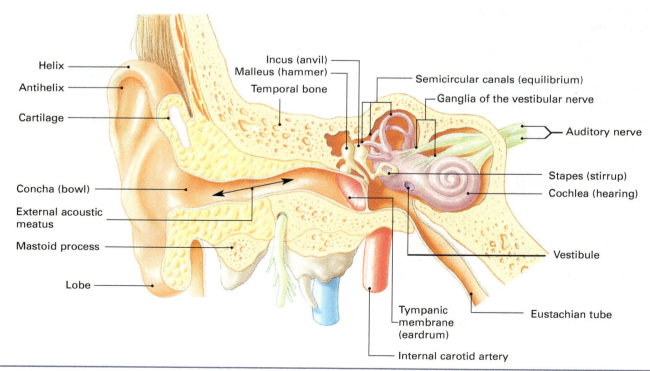

● **Figure 3** The anatomy of the ear.

The Eye

The eyes provide much of the input we use to interact with our environment. Although they are placed prominently on the face, the eyes are well protected from trauma by a series of facial bones. The frontal bones project above the globe of the eye, while the nasal bones and cartilage protect medially. The bone of the cheek, or zygoma, completes the physical protection both laterally and inferiorly. These bones collectively form the eye socket or **orbit**. The soft tissue of the eyelid and eyelashes give additional protection to the very sensitive and critical ocular surface.

The eye is a spherical globe, filled with liquid (Figure 4 ●). Its major compartment (the posterior chamber) contains a crystal-clear gelatinous fluid called **vitreous humor**. Lining the compartment's posterior is a light- and color-sensing tissue known as the **retina**. Images focused on the retina are transmitted to the brain via the optic nerve. The eye's lens separates the posterior and anterior chambers. The lens is responsible for focusing light and images on the retina by the action of small muscles that change its central thickness. A fluid called **aqueous humor**, which is similar to vitreous humor, fills the anterior chamber. The anterior chamber also contains the **iris**, the muscular and colored portion of the eye that regulates the amount of light reaching the retina. Light enters the eye through the dark opening in the center of the iris called the **pupil**.

By examining the eye, you can easily identify several of its components such as the colored iris and the central black pupil. Bordering the iris is the **sclera**, the white and vascular area that forms the remaining, underlying surface of the exposed eye. The **cornea**, a very thin, clear, and delicate layer, covers both the pupil and iris. Contiguous with the cornea and extending out to the eyelid's interior surface is the **conjunctiva**, another delicate, smooth layer that slides over itself and the cornea when the eye closes or blinks.

The eye is bathed in **lacrimal fluid**, which is produced by almond-shaped lacrimal glands located along the brow ridge just lateral and superior to the eyeball. Lacrimal fluid flows through lacrimal ducts and then over the cornea. Because the cornea does not have blood vessels, the fluid provides crucial lubrication, oxygen, and nutrients. If injury or some other mechanism—for example, a contact lens left in an unconscious patient's eye—prevents this fluid from reaching the cornea, the surface of the eye may be damaged. The lacrimal fluid is drained from the eye into the lacrimal sac, located along the medial orbit, and empties then into the nose.

The last major functional elements of the eyes are the muscles that move them and their controlling cranial nerves. These

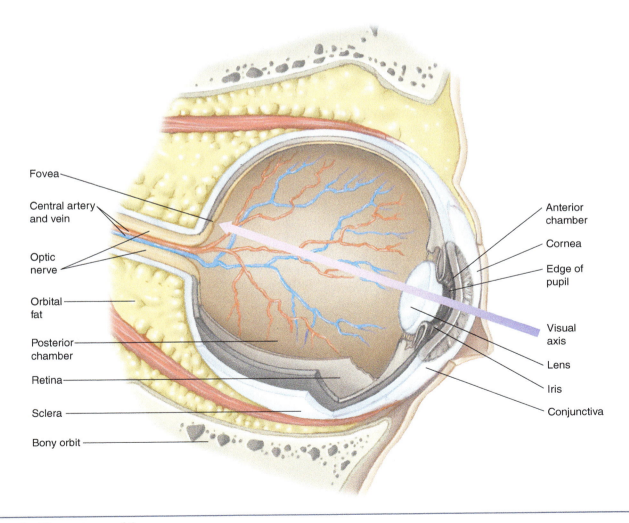

● **Figure 4**   The anatomy of the eye.

CONTENT REVIEW

▶ Anatomic Components of the Neck

- Larynx
- Trachea
- Esophagus
- Carotid arteries
- Jugular veins
- Cranial nerves
- Lymphatic and thoracic ducts
- Thyroid gland
- Brachial plexus
- Muscles, fascia, soft tissues

small muscles are attached to the eyeball in the region of the conjunctival fold and are hidden within the eye socket and under the zygomatic arch. The oculomotor (CN-III), trochlear (CN-IV), and abducens (CN-VI) nerves control these muscles, which in turn control the eye's motion. The oculomotor nerve controls pupil dilation, conjugate movement (movement of the eyes together), and most of the eye's travel through its normal range of motion. The trochlear nerve moves the eye downward and inward, while the abducens nerve is responsible for eye abduction (outward gaze).

Anatomy and Physiology of the Neck

The neck is the anatomic region between the inferior occiput and mandible and the thoracic outlet. It links the head to the rest of the body. Traveling through this region is blood for the facial region and brain, air for respiration, food for digestion, and neural communications to sense body surfaces and organs and to control voluntary and involuntary muscles and organ and gland function. The neck also contains some important muscles permitting head and shoulder movement as well as the endocrine system's thyroid and parathyroid glands.

Vasculature of the Neck

The major blood vessels traversing the neck are the carotid arteries and jugular veins. The carotid arteries arise from the brachiocephalic artery on the right and the aorta on the left. They travel upward and medially along the trachea and split into internal and external carotid arteries at about the level of the larynx's upper border. At this split are the carotid bodies and carotid sinuses, which are responsible for monitoring carbon dioxide and oxygen levels in the blood and the blood pressure, respectively. Jugular veins are paired on each side of the neck. The internal jugular vein runs in a sheath with the carotid artery and vagus nerve, while the external jugular vein runs superficially just lateral to the trachea. The jugular veins join the brachiocephalic veins just beneath the clavicles.

Airway Structures

The airway structures of the neck begin with the larynx. It is a prominent hollow cylindrical column made up of the thyroid and cricoid cartilages, atop the trachea. The thyroid opening is covered during swallowing by a cartilaginous and soft-tissue flap, the epiglottis. The vocal cords, two folds of connective tissue sitting atop the laryngeal opening, further protect the airway. These cords vibrate with air passage and form sounds; they may also close during swallowing to prevent foreign bodies from entering the lower

airway. The cricoid cartilage is a circular ring between the thyroid cartilage and the trachea. The trachea is a series of C-shaped cartilages that maintain the tracheal opening. The posterior trachea shares a common border with the anterior esophageal surface. The trachea extends inferiorly to just below the sternum, where it bifurcates into the left and right mainstem bronchi at the carina.

Other Neck Structures

Other structures within the neck include the esophagus, cranial nerves, lymphatic and thoracic ducts, thyroid and parathyroid glands, and brachial plexus. The esophagus is a smooth muscle tube located behind the trachea that carries food and liquid to the stomach. Its anterior border is continuous with the posterior tracheal border. Some cranial nerves, including the glossopharyngeal (CN-IX) and the vagus (CN-X), traverse the neck. The vagus nerve is essential for many parasympathetic activities including speech, swallowing, and cardiac, respiratory, and visceral function. The glossopharyngeal nerve innervates the carotid bodies and carotid sinuses, monitoring blood oxygen levels and blood pressure. The right lymphatic and left thoracic ducts deliver lymph to the venous system at the juncture of the jugular and subclavian veins. The thyroid gland sits over the trachea just below the cricoid cartilage. It controls cellular metabolic rate as well as systemic calcium levels. The brachial plexus is a network of nerves in the lower neck and shoulder responsible for lower arm and hand function. Lastly, numerous muscles (including the sternocleidomastoid, platysma, and upper trapezius), fascia, and soft tissues are found in the neck. Most of the anterior and lateral neck is covered by the thin platysma muscle. Penetration of this muscle suggests injury to the important structures beneath it. The neck muscles, like those of the extremities, are contained within fascial compartments. In the presence of soft-tissue injury, rapid swelling may increase pressure within a compartment and restrict blood flow.

The neck can be divided into three zones: Zone I is below the cricoid ring; Zone II is above the cricoid ring and below the angle of the jaw; Zone III is above the angle of the jaw (Figure 5 ●). Zone I injuries carry the highest mortality, as they involve the great vessels and the trachea. Zone II injuries are more common, because of the limited protection offered by anterior neck structures, and frequently involve the carotid arteries or larynx. Zone III injuries are also of concern since

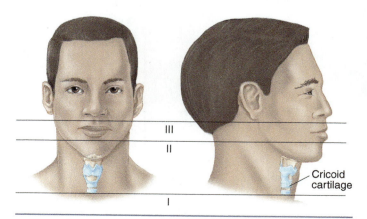

● **Figure 5** Zones of the neck.

they may involve both cranial nerves and larger vascular structures and are often hidden from view.

Anatomy and Physiology of the Spine

Vertebral Column

The **vertebral column**, also called the *spinal column*, consists of 33 bones and provides the main support for the axis of the body. Each bone of the vertebral column is called a **vertebra**. By adulthood, 9 of the lower vertebrae have fused forming the **sacrum** and the **coccyx**, respectively (Figure 6 ●). This leaves a total of 26 bones (24 separate vertebrae, the sacrum, and the coccyx). The vertebral column extends from the skull to the pelvis. The weight supported by each vertebra progressively increases as you move inferiorly down the spine. Thus, the **cervical vertebrae** are much smaller in width than the **thoracic vertebrae** and the **lumbar vertebrae**. An **intervertebral disc** separates each pair of vertebrae except the first and second cervical vertebrae and the fused vertebrae of the sacrum and coccyx. The intervertebral discs account for 25 percent of the total spinal column height and serve to absorb energy and cushion the vertebrae. The intervertebral disc contains an inner sphere called the *nucleus pulposus,* which is surrounded by an outer collar called the *annulus*

fibrosus. The nucleus pulposus is gelatinous and absorbs compressive stress, whereas the purpose of the annulus fibrosus is primarily to contain the nucleus pulposus. The vertebral column, when examined from an anterior or posterior perspective, is relatively straight. However, when examined laterally, curvatures are noted. These curvatures are normal and are referred to as the *cervical concavity,* the *thoracic convexity, the lumbar concavity,* and the *sacral convexity* (Figure 7 ●). The body's weight is eventually transmitted through the spine, then the pelvis, to the lower extremities.

Each vertebra is different, yet they share common features. Anteriorly, the vertebra consists of a *vertebral body* (or body). Posteriorly, each vertebra has a *vertebral arch.* Together, the vertebral body and the vertebral arch form the **spinal canal**, also called the **vertebral foramen**, which contains and protects the spinal cord. The vertebral arch is formed by two *pedicles* and two *laminae.* The pedicles protrude superiorly and contain the *superior articular processes* and *facets,* which help to form the joint between the vertebra and the vertebra immediately above it. The *laminae* are lower and consist of the *spinous process,* the *transverse processes,* and the *inferior articular facets.* The inferior articular facets form the joint between the vertebra and the vertebra immediately below it (Figure 8 ●).

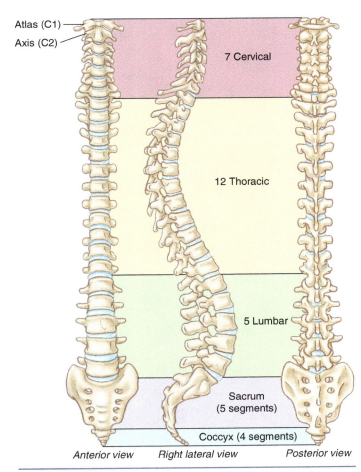

Atlas (C1)
Axis (C2)
7 Cervical
12 Thoracic
5 Lumbar
Sacrum (5 segments)
Coccyx (4 segments)

Anterior view   *Right lateral view*   *Posterior view*

● **Figure 6**   The anatomic dimensions of the vertebral column (anterior, right lateral, and posterior).

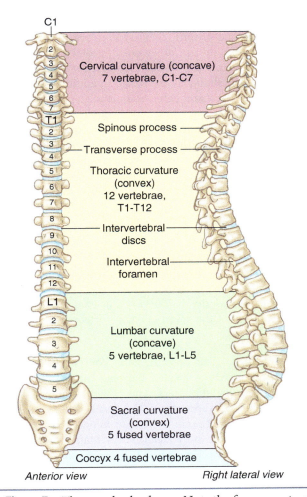

C1
2
3
4
5
6
7
Cervical curvature (concave) 7 vertebrae, C1-C7
T1
2
3
4
5
6
7
8
9
10
11
12
Spinous process
Transverse process
Thoracic curvature (convex) 12 vertebrae, T1-T12
Intervertebral discs
Intervertebral foramen
L1
2
3
4
5
Lumbar curvature (concave) 5 vertebrae, L1-L5
Sacral curvature (convex) 5 fused vertebrae
Coccyx 4 fused vertebrae

Anterior view   *Right lateral view*

● **Figure 7**   The vertebral column. Note the four curvatures of the spine in the right lateral view.

CONTENT REVIEW

▶ Divisions of the Vertebral Column

- Cervical spine
- Thoracic spine
- Lumbar spine
- Sacral spine
- Coccygeal spine

The vertebral column is held in place by various ligaments. The major supporting ligaments are the *anterior longitudinal ligament* and the *posterior longitudinal ligament* (Figure 9 ●). The anterior longitudinal ligament runs vertically along the anterior surfaces of the vertebrae from the sacrum to the first cervical vertebra and onto the occipital bone of the skull. This ligament helps to prevent hyperextension of the vertebral column. The posterior longitudinal ligament is narrower and weaker than the anterior longitudinal ligament. It runs vertically along the posterior surfaces of the vertebral bodies in the vertebral canal from the sacrum to the second cervical vertebra. The posterior longitudinal ligament helps to prevent hyperflexion of the vertebral column.

Other ligaments help to support the vertebral column. These are primarily located posteriorly and connect the vertebrae together. The strongest of these is the *ligamentum flavum*. The ligamentum flavum helps to maintain the normal curvatures of the spine and helps to straighten the spine after flexing. The *interspinous ligament* is a thin ligament that connects the spinous processes of two adjoining vertebrae together. The *supraspinous ligament* runs posteriorly along the spinous processes from the seventh cervical vertebra to the sacrum. A similar ligament, the *nuchal ligament*, protects and supports the neck. It runs from the seventh cervical vertebra to the occipital bone of the skull (Figure 10 ●). In addition to the ligaments, the back, chest and pelvic muscles also provide support for the vertebral column. The physical shape of each vertebra, the intervertebral joint surfaces, and the ligaments holding the intervertebral joints together permit significant spinal column motion, especially in the cervical region. This joint structure also provides anatomic barriers to motion beyond the normal range of motion and protects the spinal cord from injury.

Vertebral Column Divisions

The vertebral column can be divided into five specific anatomic regions: the cervical spine, thoracic spine, lumbar spine, sacrum, and coccyx. The individual vertebrae of the column are identified by the first letter of their region and numbered from superior to inferior. For example, the most inferior of the seven cervical vertebrae is identified as C-7.

Cervical Spine The cervical spine consists of seven cervical vertebrae located between the base of the skull and the shoulders. The cervical spine is the sole skeletal support for the head, which weighs about 16 to 22 pounds (7 to 10 kilograms). The cervical vertebrae are wider laterally than they are in an anteroposterior width. With the exception of C-7, the spinous process is short and bifid (split). The spinal canal is triangular in shape. Each transverse process contains a hole, called the

transverse foramen, that contains the vertebral blood vessels (Figures 11 ● and 12 ●).

The first two cervical vertebrae have a unique relationship with the head and each other that permits rotation to left and right and nodding of the head. The first cervical vertebra, C-1, is called the atlas, named after the mythical Greek Titan who was condemned by Zeus to support the heavens on his shoulders. It has

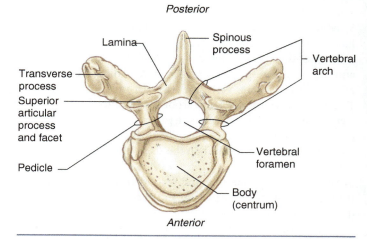

● **Figure 8** Structure of a typical vertebra (superior view).

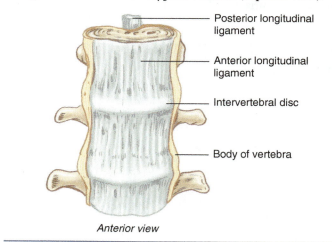

● **Figure 9** Anterior view of the spinal column showing anterior and posterior longitudinal ligaments.

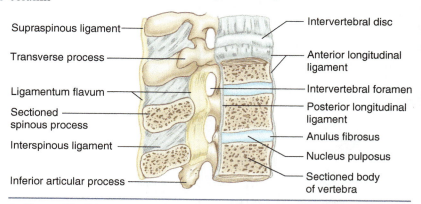

● **Figure 10** Ligaments and intervertebral discs of the spine. Lateral view of the spinal column (anterior to the right). The lower vertebrae have been cut sagittally to reveal the spinal canal and some of the ligaments.

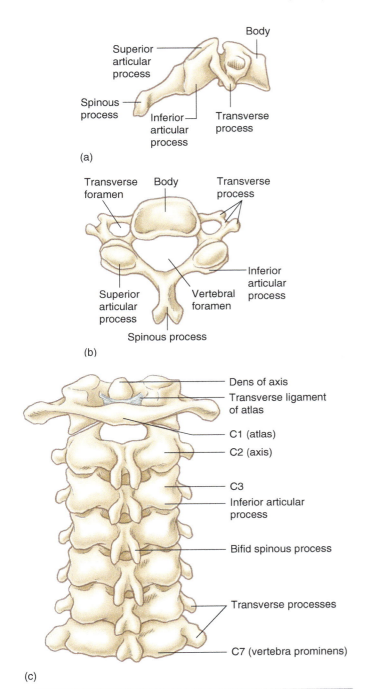

(a)

(b)

(c)

● **Figure 11** The cervical vertebrae: (a) right lateral view of vertebra; (b) superior view of vertebra; (c) cervical spine articulations.

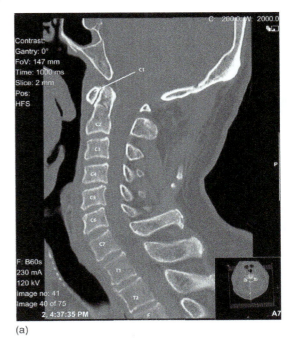

(a)

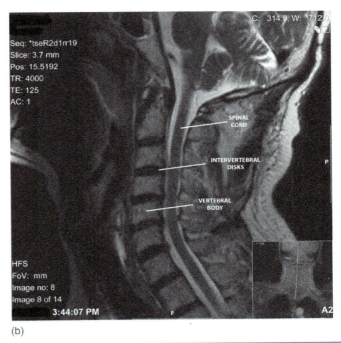

(b)

● **Figure 12** (a) Sagittal CT of the cervical spine. (b) Sagittal MRI of the cervical spine. *(Both: © Dr. Bryan E. Bledsoe)*

no spinous processes or vertebral body. This ring-shaped bone supports the head. This is the atlanto-occipital joint. It is securely affixed to the occipital and permits nodding but does not accommodate any twisting or turning motion (Figure 13 ●). The highest percentage (approximately 50 percent) of neck flexion and extension occurs at the atlanto-occipital joint. The atlas and the next vertebra, C-2, differ from most vertebrae in not having discernible vertebral bodies. Vertebra C-2, called the axis, is the strongest of the cervical vertebrae and has a small bony tooth, called the *odontoid process* or *dens*, that projects upward (Figure 14 ●).

This projection provides a pivotal point around which the atlas and head can rotate from side to side (Figure 15 ●).

The remaining cervical vertebrae permit some rotation as well as flexion, extension, and lateral bending. The range of motion provided by the cervical spine is greater than allowed by any other portion of the spinal column, despite the fact that the portion of the spinal cord traveling through this region is critical to virtually all body functions. The last cervical vertebra (C-7) is quite noticeable as its spinous process, called the *vertebra prominens*, is quite pronounced and can be felt as the first bony prominence along the spine and just above the shoulders. The

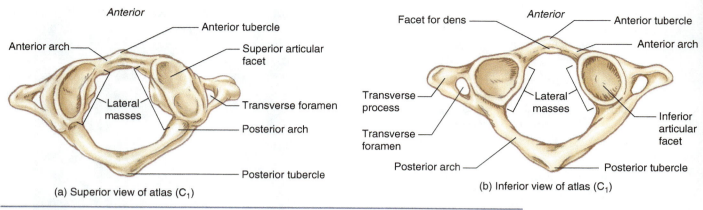

Figure 13   The atlas (a) superior view; (b) inferior view.

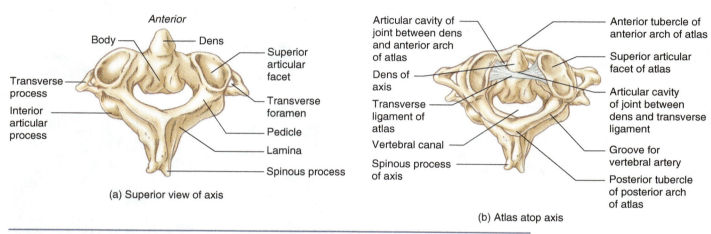

Figure 14   (a) The axis (superior view); (b) the atlas seated on the axis.

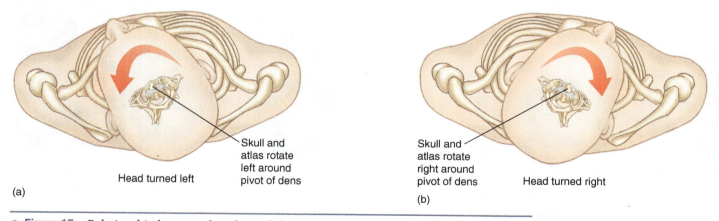

Figure 15   Relationship between the atlas and the axis. The dens of the axis provides a pivotal point around which the atlast and head can rotate (a) left and (b) right.

spinal canal diameter in the cervical region is normally 17 mm. The cord becomes compromised when the diameter is reduced to less than 13 mm as occurs in trauma such as when the spinal foramina of two vertebrae become displaced against each other or when bleeding and swelling of the cord increase its size.

Thoracic Spine   The thoracic spine consists of 12 vertebrae. The thoracic vertebrae contain a readily identifiable vertebral body that is heart-shaped. Because the thoracic spine supports more of the human body than the cervical spine, the thoracic vertebral bodies are larger and stronger. The vertebral foramen in this region is circular in shape. The spinous and transverse processes are also larger and more prominent because they are associated with the musculature holding the upper body erect and with thoracic cage movement during respiration.

On each side of the thoracic vertebral bodies are specialized facets, called *demifacets*, that articulate with the ribs. Generally, the head of the rib articulates with the demifacets on two adjoining vertebrae. The T-1 vertebra differs in that its body has a full facet with the first rib and a demifacet for the second rib. The vertebral bodies of T-10 through T-12 have only a single facet for the three floating ribs (ribs 10–12). This system of fixation limits rib movement and increases the strength and rigidity of the thoracic spine (Figure 16 ●).

Lumbar Spine The five bones of the lumbar spine each carry the weight of the head, neck, upper extremities, and thorax above them. They also bear the forces of bending and lifting above the pelvis. The vertebral bodies are largest in this region of the spinal column, and the intervertebral discs are also the thickest and bear the greatest stress. In addition, the anterior parts of the vertebral bodies are higher than the posterior parts causing the normal lumbar spine curvature (lordosis). The lumbar pedicles and laminae are shorter and thicker. The spinous processes are short, flat, and hatchet-shaped and project straight posteriorly. Thus, they are stouter than those in the thoracic spine. The vertebral foramen is largest in the lumbar region and is triangular in shape (Figure 17 ●).

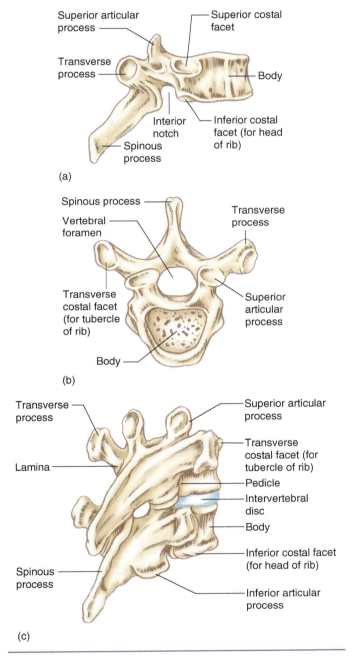

● **Figure 16** The thoracic vertebrae: (a) right lateral view of vertebra; (b) superior view of vertebra; (c) thoracic spine articulations.

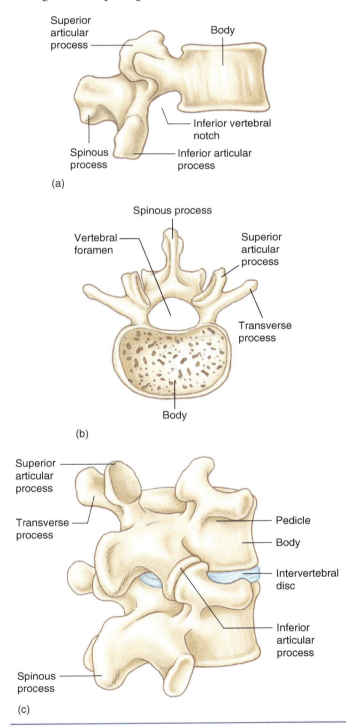

● **Figure 17** The lumbar vertebrae: (a) right lateral view of vertebra; (b) superior view of vertebra; (c) lumbar spine articulations.

Sacral Spine The sacral spine consists of five sacral vertebrae that fuse and form the posterior wall of the pelvis. Superiorly it articulates with L-5. Inferiorly it is connected to the coccyx. The anterosuperior margin of the first sacral vertebral remnant projects into the pelvic cavity and is called the *sacral promontory*. The body's center of gravity is approximately 1 centimeter posterior to this landmark. The sacrum, in conjunction with the bones of the pelvis, protects the urinary and reproductive organs. It also serves as the points of attachment between the spinal column and the lower extremities. The articulation with the pelvis is called the *sacroiliac joint* and is very strong. The sacroiliac joint is normally fused and does not allow movement (Figure 18 ●).

Coccygeal Spine The coccygeal spine, commonly called the coccyx, is made up of four fused vertebrae that represent the evolutionary remnants of a tail. It is small and triangular in shape and comprises the short skeletal end of the vertebral column. The coccyx serves no major function. It is, however, occasionally fractured during a fall or with childbirth.

Blood Supply to the Spine

Blood to the spinal cord is primarily supplied by the anterior spinal artery and the two posterior spinal arteries. The anterior spinal artery arises from branches of the vertebral arteries and supplies the anterior two-thirds of the spinal cord. Each posterior artery primarily arises from a branch of the vertebral arteries and perfuses the posterior one-third of the spinal cord. The anterior spinal artery and the posterior spinal arteries primarily supply blood to the superior part of the spinal cord. The anterior two-thirds of the lower aspects of the cord are also perfused by the great anterior segmental medullary arteries (medullary artery of Adamkiewicz). The posterior one-third is perfused by the posterior segmental medullary artery. An occlusion or damage to any of these arteries can result in spinal cord infarction which will give signs and symptoms virtually identical to those of spinal cord injury.

HEAD, FACE, NECK, AND SPINAL COLUMN PATHOPHYSIOLOGY

Head, face, neck, and spinal column injuries are difficult to assess in the prehospital setting, yet commonly threaten life or may expose victims to lifelong disability. A clearer appreciation of the injury mechanisms affecting these regions and of the specific pathological processes related to head, facial, neck, and spinal column injury can help you anticipate, assess, and then manage these injuries and their effects on the human system.

General Mechanisms of Injury to the Head, Face, Neck, and Spinal Column

Injuries to the head, face, and neck are divided by mechanisms of injury into blunt (closed) and penetrating (open).

Blunt Injury

Head, face, neck, and spinal column structures protect their associated anatomic regions very well against most blunt trauma. At times, however, forces producing blunt trauma overcome this protection and can cause serious injury. The most serious of these injuries affect the central nervous system—the brain and spinal cord. Injury, however, may also affect the head, face, neck, and spinal column and the airway, alimentary canal, and sense organs located in and protected by the structures of these regions. For example, trauma to the head (brain) most frequently results from auto and motorcycle crashes and accounts for more than half of vehicle crash mortality. Sports-related impacts, falling objects, explosions, falls, and acts of violence, like assault with a club, are less common, but are still significant mechanisms associated with injury to these areas (Figure 19 ●).

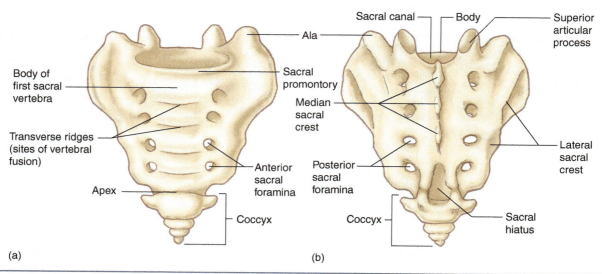

● **Figure 18** The sacrum and coccyx: (a) anterior view; (b) posterior view.

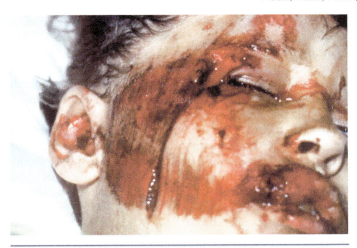

● **Figure 19**   Blunt injury to the face can produce hemorrhage, soft-tissue injuries, internal fractures, and brain injuries.

The head is a frequent recipient of blunt trauma because it is anatomically prominent at the top of the body. The victim of trauma may flex the neck to protect the face but then exposes the head to impact. The head is the frequent point of impact in auto collisions where an occupant impacts the windshield or steering wheel or in diving mechanisms or frontward or backward falls. Blunt trauma can be more focused when caused by blunt-force instruments (clubs, sticks, pipes, or other objects) wielded by an assailant. Because of the structure of the scalp, a glancing blunt blow can tear the borders of the scalp and result in an open wound with a resulting flap of tissue. Head injury is especially prevalent in very young patients. The size of the head relative to the rest of the body, the flexibility of the neck, and the inability of very young patients to protect themselves all contribute to the incidence and severity of blunt head trauma in the pediatric patient.

The face is an area frequently subjected to blunt trauma. Significant facial injury occurs less frequently than head injury in auto impacts because the head's frontal or parietal regions are more likely to impact the windshield than the face. The same holds true for falls, as the arms, chest, or head absorb energy as the conscious victim tries to protect the facial area and head from injury. Intentional violence is less likely to spare the facial region. The face is often the target of blows from a fist or from impact-enhancing objects like sticks or clubs. The middle and inner ears and the eyes are very well protected against most blunt trauma, though ear injury may be caused by the pressures associated with diving or explosions. The eyes may occasionally be injured by impacts from smaller blunt objects like a racquetball, baseball, or tennis ball.

The neck is anatomically well protected from most blunt trauma because the head, face, and chest protrude more anteriorly. Laterally, the neck is protected as the shoulders protrude a significant distance from the neck. The neck is, however, a point of impact in special situations. For example, during an auto crash the neck may strike the steering wheel or be injured by a shoulder strap that is worn without a lap belt. During a rear impact vehicle collision the neck may be injured by extremes of extension or flexion. The region may also be impacted by objects during fights or traumatically constricted or distracted during an attempted suicide by hanging.

The spine is vulnerable to numerous types of injury. Injurious forces may tear tendons, muscles, and ligaments causing pain and possibly destabilizing the vertebral column. Those forces may cause displacement of the vertebrae from their normal position resulting in a subluxation (partial or incomplete dislocation) or dislocation. The injury process may fracture the spinous or transverse processes, the pedicles, the laminae, or the vertebral body itself. Trauma, especially axial loading, may damage the intervertebral discs and the connective and bony tissues of the vertebral column. They may or may not be associated with injury to the spinal cord itself.

Penetrating Injury

Penetrating injuries to the head, face, neck, and spinal column are not as common as those resulting from blunt trauma, but they can be more severe and life threatening. In addition, a penetrating injury to the head suggests the meninges have been opened, producing a route for potentially serious infection.

Penetrating injuries to the head, face, neck, and spinal column usually result from either gunshots or stabbings. Gunshot wounds are most common and especially hideous because bullets release tremendous energy as they slow during collision with skeletal and central nervous tissue. Similarly, explosions propel projectiles, either intrinsic to the explosive device or from debris produced by the blast, that may penetrate and damage this region. Knife wounds to the head and face tend to be superficial because of the region's extensive skeletal components. The anterior and lateral neck, however, are not as well protected, and wounds there may compromise the airway (larynx and trachea), esophagus, and major blood vessels, quickly threatening patient life.

There are many other types of penetrating injuries that may involve the head, face, neck, and spinal column. Some examples include the "clothesline" impact with a wire fence while a victim is riding an all-terrain vehicle or snowmobile; bites from humans, dogs, and other animals; or a tongue bitten when a victim traps it between the teeth when he lands very firmly on his feet. Infrequently, a fall may impale a person on a fixed object such as a concrete reinforcing bar, producing a penetrating injury.

Spinal injuries can involve the spinal column, spinal cord, peripheral nerve roots as they leave the spinal column, the ligaments that hold the spinal column aligned and together, the musculature of the back and neck, or any combination of these. Spinal injuries can vary significantly from relatively minor compression fractures without spinal cord involvement to significant vertebral fractures with transection of the spinal cord and resultant paralysis. It is important to note that spinal column injury does not, necessarily, mean the cord is injured. Conversely, you can have cord injury without spinal column fracture or displacement. However, spinal column injury reduces the stability of the column and further movement may endanger or further endanger the cord.

Specific Mechanisms of Spinal Column Injury

Numerous mechanisms of injury have been associated with injury to the spinal column. These include extremes of normal anatomic motion such as hyperflexion and hyperextension as well as rotation and lateral bending. In addition, compression (axial loading) or traction (distraction) along the axis of the spine can cause serious spinal injury. As with injuries to the head, face, and neck, spinal column injury may occur as a direct result of either blunt or penetrating trauma.

Extremes of Motion

Hyperextension or hyperflexion bend the spine forcibly beyond its normal range of motion. These injuries occur most commonly in the cervical or lumbar regions. A classic example of a hyperextension injury mechanism is a rear-impact auto collision. The patient's head remains stationary while the upper torso rapidly moves forward as the auto impact accelerates the seat forward. The head moves backward and subsequently hyperextends the unsupported neck. The hyperextension places compressive forces on the posterior vertebral structures (spinous processes, laminae, and pedicles). In addition, it stretches the anterior longitudinal ligament. Hyperextension injuries may cause disc disruption, compression of the interspinous ligaments, and fracture of the posterior vertebral elements. If the forces are great enough, ligaments may tear or the vertebra may fracture, resulting in instability and bone displacement. The bone fragments may penetrate the spinal canal and injure the spinal cord.

In frontal impact crashes, the shoulder strap may restrain the body while the head continues forward. The neck restrains the head and flexes the spine with the movement. The process is frequently forceful enough to hyperflex the spine and cause a patient to literally "kiss the chest" (sometimes demonstrated by the patient's lipstick print on the shirt front). Hyperflexion may lead to anterior vertebral body wedge fractures, posterior longitudinal and interspinous ligament stretching or rupture, compression injury to the cord, pedicle fracture, and disruption of the intervertebral discs with dislocation of the vertebrae.

Excessive rotation beyond normal anatomic barriers may occur in the cervical and lumbar spine. Anatomically, the head is attached to the vertebral column at the foramen magnum, located well posterior of the neck's midline and the head's center of mass. With lateral impact, the head turns toward the impacting force as the body moves to the side and out from under it. The cervical spine attachment restrains its motion and turns the head violently. Rotation injury normally affects the upper reaches of the cervical region, but may also be transmitted to the lumbar spine as, for example, when a tackled football player's thorax twists while his feet are firmly planted. The result is a rotational injury that may include stretching or tearing of the ligaments, rotational subluxation or dislocation, and vertebral fracture. Rotational injury can also occur in a motor vehicle collision where there are multiple impacts and force vectors involved.

Lateral bending beyond the normal anatomic barriers may take place along the entire vertebral column, though it is most common and likely to cause injury in the cervical and lumbar regions. As one body portion moves sideways and the remaining portion remain fixed, the spine bends and absorbs the energy. The movement may compress vertebral structures inducing compression fracture on one side of the column (toward the impact) while it stretches and tears ligaments on the opposite side. The result may be compression of the vertebral pedicles with bone fragments driven into the spinal foramen, torn ligaments, and vertebral instability. An example of this mechanism is a lateral-impact auto crash in which the forces of the crash move the thorax to the side and out from under the head, placing severe lateral stress on the cervical spine. Because of the spine's structure, forces necessary to induce injury from lateral bending are generally less than those needed to cause flexion/extension injury.

Axial Stress

Axial stress occurs when either compression or distraction forces are applied to the spinal axis. Compression stress, most commonly called axial loading, may occur when a person lifts a weight too great for the strength of his lumbar spine. The weight of the upper torso, head, and neck, in addition to the weight of the object being lifted, pushes against the pelvis, legs, and feet. The lumbar spine is compressed and a vertebra is crushed. Similar compression injury can also occur when a person falls from a height and lands on his heels. The resulting force is transmitted up the lower extremities to the pelvis, the sacrum, and the lumbar spine. Axial loading injuries are also common in helicopter crashes where the crash energy is transmitted to the lumbar spine (Figure 20 ●). Another frequent mechanism of axial loading injury is the shallow water dive. In this case, the diver impacts the pool, lake, or river bottom with the head while the weight of the lower body drives the thorax into the head, crushing the cervical spine. This mechanism also occurs in auto crashes, when an occupant is propelled into the windshield by crash forces. With these mechanisms, an impact is likely to compress, fracture, and crush the vertebrae and herniate (rupture) discs. This will often release the gelatinous centers into the vertebral foramina compressing the spinal cord. The most common sites of axial loading injuries are between

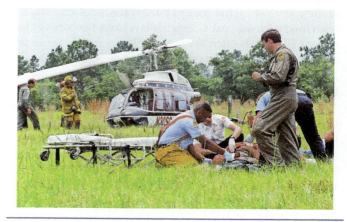

● **Figure 20**   Axial compression injuries are common in falls from a height and in helicopter crashes. (© *Craig Jackson/In the Dark Photography*)

T-12 and L-2 (for lifting injuries and heel-first falls) and the cervical region (for head impacts).

Distraction is the opposite of axial loading. A force, such as gravity applied during hanging or at the end of a bungee jump stretches the spinal column and tears ligaments. The process may also stretch and damage the spinal cord without causing physical damage to the spinal column. The upper cervical region is most commonly affected by this mechanism of injury.

Often the actual spinal injury process involves complicated combinations of the various injury mechanisms previously mentioned. Hanging may suspend the victim from the side of the head, causing injury from distraction and severe lateral bending directed at the C-1/C-2 region (causing a hangman's fracture). The lateral-impact auto crash may produce both lateral bending and rotational injury mechanisms affecting the cervical spine. The shallow water dive may result in both axial loading and hyperflexion as the body pushes against and bends the neck. (Note that the cervical spine is posterior to the midline of both the head and chest. In-line impacts frequently cause the head and neck to flex as the body pushes forward.)

Be aware of the distinctions among connective tissue, skeletal, and spinal cord injuries. Connective tissue and skeletal injuries do not necessarily result in spinal cord injuries. They do, however, represent potential instability of the spinal column and the danger that any subsequent motion, even normal motion, may result in spinal cord injury. Spinal cord injury can also occur without noticeable injury to the ligaments, discs, and vertebrae of the spinal column. This is why a patient who shows any sign of spine injury, or has experienced a mechanism that suggests the possibility of spine injury, should receive immediate manual immobilization and full mechanical immobilization as soon as possible. Maintain immobilization during all of your assessment, care, and transport.

Other Mechanisms of Spinal Column Injury

As already noted, spinal column injuries can also result from both direct blunt and penetrating trauma. A direct blow to the spine may injure the spinal column, cord, or associated structures. Penetrating injuries, caused by objects such as knives, ice picks, or bullets, may also injure the spine, although infrequently. The penetrating object can damage vertebral ligaments, can fracture vertebral structures, can drive bone fragments directly into the spinal cord, or can directly damage the cord itself. However, unlike blunt trauma, penetrating injury infrequently causes spinal cord injury or instability of the vertebral column.

As a result of trauma, tissues adjacent to the spinal cord may swell or otherwise encroach on the vertebral foramen. Because of the close tolerances between the interior surfaces of the vertebral foramen and the cord, this swelling may place pressure on the cord either causing direct compression injury or interrupting blood flow through the compressed tissues. Such an injury may also involve the spinal nerve roots that exit the vertebral column close to the injury.

Electrocution, on rare occasions, can cause spinal injury. The extreme and uncontrolled muscular contractions associated with this mechanism of injury can tear tendons and ligaments

and fracture vertebrae, resulting in column instability and possible spinal cord injury.

A direct injury to the spinal or vertebral blood vessels, or any swelling from soft-tissue or skeletal injury, can interfere with circulation to portions of the spinal cord. This will likely cause tissue ischemia and compromise of spinal cord function.

The coccygeal region of the spinal column can also be injured. Although it contains neither the spinal cord nor many peripheral nerve roots, injury to the region can be painful. Such injuries are usually related to direct blunt trauma, for example, such as a fall on the upper buttocks region. The coccyx is commonly fractured during delivery during childbirth.

Blunt and penetrating injury mechanisms have different impacts depending on the structures they involve. The following sections discuss the pathological processes of injuries as they affect the head, face, neck, and spinal column.

SPECIFIC INJURIES TO THE HEAD, FACE, NECK, AND SPINAL COLUMN

Head Injury

Head injury is defined as a traumatic insult to the cranial region that may result in injury to soft tissues, bony structures, and the brain. Let us look at head injury as it progresses from the exterior to the interior, examining scalp and cranial injuries.

Scalp Injury

The most superficial head injuries involve the scalp (Figure 21 ●). A scalp injury may also be the only overt indication of deeper, more serious injury beneath. The scalp overlies the firm cranium and is very vascular. Its blood vessels lack the ability to constrict as effectively as those found elsewhere in the body; hence, scalp wounds tend to

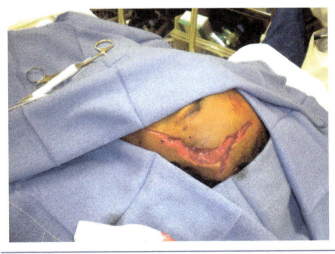

● **Figure 21**   Scalp wounds can bleed heavily. (© *Dr. Bryan E. Bledsoe*)

bleed heavily and persistently. It is said that head injuries do not result in shock. This, however, assumes that the hemorrhage they cause is easy to control. In fact, any serious blood loss from scalp wounds contributes to shock and, if left uncontrolled, may itself cause hypovolemia and shock. Scalp wounds further provide a route for infection because emissary veins drain from the dural sinuses, through the cranium, and into the superficial venous circulation. This structure provides a route during injury for infectious agents to enter the meninges. Because of rich circulation to the area, scalp wounds tend to heal well.

Scalp wounds may present in a manner that confounds assessment (Figure 22 ●). Usually, blunt trauma creates a contusion that, because of the firm skull underneath, expands outwardly in a very rapid and noticeable way. However, blunt trauma may also tear underlying fascia and areolar tissue, causing it to separate. This can leave an elevated border surrounding a depression, mimicking the contour of a depressed skull fracture. However, the scalp's blood vessels may bleed under the skin and into a depressed skull fracture, fill any depression, and conceal the injury's true nature. It is therefore important to assess and record the nature of a head wound early in your assessment.

A common and special type of scalp wound is the avulsion. Areolar tissue is only loosely attached to the skull, and glancing blows can create a shearing force against the scalp's border. Such blows frequently tear a flap of scalp loose and fold it back against the uninjured scalp, exposing a portion of the cranium. The mechanism of injury may also seriously contaminate the wound and may cause moderate hemorrhage unless the avulsed tissue folds back sharply, compressing the blood vessels.

Scalp/Head Injury Presentations

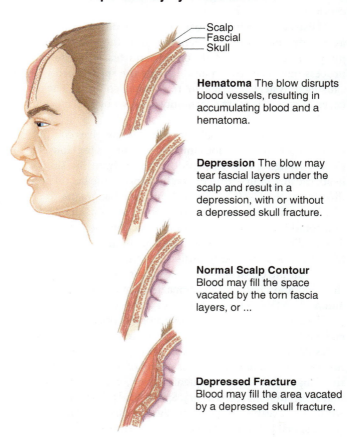

Scalp
Fascial
Skull

Hematoma The blow disrupts blood vessels, resulting in accumulating blood and a hematoma.

Depression The blow may tear fascial layers under the scalp and result in a depression, with or without a depressed skull fracture.

Normal Scalp Contour Blood may fill the space vacated by the torn fascia layers, or ...

Depressed Fracture Blood may fill the area vacated by a depressed skull fracture.

● **Figure 22** Scalp/head injuries can present as a raised hematoma, a depression, or disguised by a normal scalp contour.

Cranial Injury

Because of its spherical shape and skeletal design, the skull does not fracture unless trauma is extreme. Such fractures may present as linear, depressed, comminuted, or basilar in nature (Figure 23 ●). Linear fractures are small cracks in the cranium and represent about 80 percent of all skull fractures. The temporal bone is one of the thinnest and most frequently fractured cranial bones. If there are no associated intracranial or vascular injuries, a linear fracture poses very little danger to the patient. In contrast, a depressed fracture represents an inward skull surface displacement and results in a greater likelihood of intracranial damage. Comminuted fractures involve multiple skull fragments that may penetrate the meninges and cause physical harm to the structures beneath. And, severe traumatic brain injury can occur without skull fracture.

A common type of skull fracture involves the base of the skull. This area is permeated with foramina (openings) for the spinal cord, cranial nerves, and various blood vessels. The basilar skull also has hollow or open structures such as the

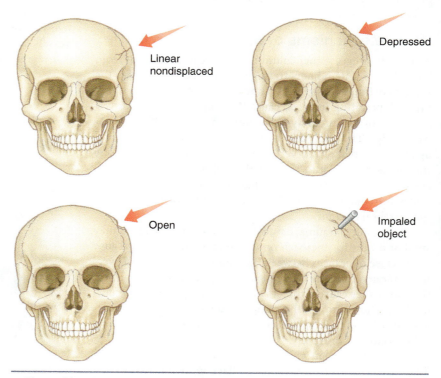

Linear nondisplaced

Depressed

Open

Impaled object

● **Figure 23** Various types of skull fractures.

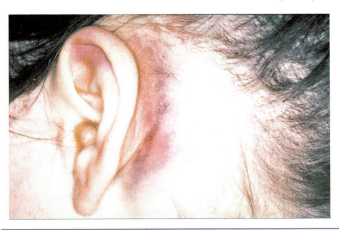

● **Figure 24a**   Retroauricular ecchymosis (Battle's sign). *(© David Effron, MD)*

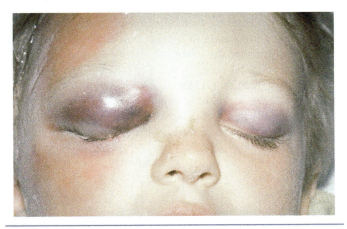

● **Figure 24b**   Periorbital ecchymosis (raccoon eyes). *(© David Effron, MD)*

sinuses, orbits of the eye, nasal cavities, external auditory canals, and middle and inner ears. These spaces weaken the skull and leave the basilar area prone to fracture.

Signs of basilar skull fracture vary with the injury's location (Figure 24 ●). If a fracture involves the auditory canal and lower lateral areas of the skull, hemorrhage may migrate to the mastoid region (just posterior and slightly inferior to the ear). This causes a characteristic black and blue discoloration called **retroauricular ecchymosis** or "Battle's sign." Another classic basilar skull fracture sign is **bilateral periorbital ecchymosis**, sometimes referred to as "raccoon eyes." This is a dramatic discoloration around both eyes associated with orbital fractures and hemorrhage into the surrounding tissue. Both retroauricular ecchymosis and bilateral periorbital ecchymosis take time to develop; neither is likely to be visible during the period after an injury when the patient is under paramedic care. However, you may see these signs if a patient waits some time before summoning EMS.

Basilar skull fracture can tear the dura mater, opening a wound between the brain and the body's exterior. Such a wound may permit cerebrospinal fluid to seep out through a nasal cavity or an external auditory canal and also provide a possible route for infection to enter the meninges. This wound type may also provide an escape for cerebrospinal fluid in the presence of increasing intracranial pressure. Escaping cerebrospinal fluid may mitigate the rise in ICP and somewhat limit damage to the brain. (While cerebrospinal fluid is an important medium, the body can regenerate it quite rapidly.) Although it is not a reliable sign of basilar skull fracture, blood mixed with cerebrospinal fluid and flowing from the nose, mouth, or ears may produce the target or "halo" sign (a dark red circle surrounded by a lighter yellowish ring) when dropped on a pillow or towel.[5,6] Normal blood produces a narrow ring of yellowish coloration around the red circle produced by the less mobile erythrocytes. If cerebrospinal fluid is mixed with the blood, this outer yellowish ring is much larger. Be aware, however, that other fluids, like lacrimal or nasal fluids or saliva, may cause a similar response. Hence, the halo sign is most reliable when associated with fluid leaking from the ear.

Bullet impacts induce specific types of cranial fracture. The entrance wound often produces a small comminuted fracture and sends bone fragments into the brain. Often the bullet's kinetic energy is sufficient to permit the bullet to exit from the cranium and cause a second fracture. This exit wound site is blown outward and is often more severe in appearance than the entrance wound.

In many cases, the energy of projectile passage through the cranium causes a cavitational wave of extreme pressure, which is contained and enhanced by the rigid cranial container. The result is extreme damage to the cranial contents, and, if the transmitted kinetic energy is strong enough, the skull may fracture and "explode" outward.

Another wound type occurs when a bullet enters the cranium at an angle, is deflected within, and continues to move along the cranium's interior until its energy is completely exhausted. This process does devastating damage to the cerebral cortex and is rarely survivable.

A special type of cranial injury involves an impaled object. As is the case with objects impaled in most other regions of the body, any further object motion may cause additional hemorrhage and tissue damage. When the object is impaled in the cranium, the situation is especially serious. Brain tissue is much more delicate than other body tissue, does not immobilize the object as well, and is easily injured by object motion. As with objects impaled elsewhere, impaled object removal from the cranium may cause further injury and increase the blood loss rate and the amount of blood accumulation.

Note that a cranial fracture is a skeletal injury that will heal with time; it does not, by itself, threaten the brain. Rather, it is the possibility of injury beneath (and suggested by the skull fracture) that is of greatest concern. The forces necessary to fracture the cranium are extreme and likely to cause serious injury within.

Facial Injury

Facial injury is a serious trauma complication, not only because of the cosmetic importance people place on facial appearance, but also because of the region's vasculature and the location of the initial airway and alimentary canal structures and the organs of sight, smell, taste, and hearing present there. Remember, too, that serious facial injuries suggest associated head and spinal injuries.

Facial Soft-Tissue Injury

Facial soft-tissue injury is common and can threaten both the patient's airway and physical appearance. Because of the ample arterial and venous supply, injuries in the region may bleed heavily, contributing to hypovolemia. Facial injuries are often the result of violence (e.g., bullet or knife wounds). Superficial injuries and hemorrhage rarely affect the airway. With deep lacerations, however, blood may accumulate and endanger the airway or enter the digestive tract and induce vomiting. Serious blunt or penetrating injury to the soft tissues and skeletal structures supporting the pharynx may reduce the patient's ability to control the airway, increasing the likelihood of foreign body or fluid aspiration and airway compromise. Aspiration and hypoxia are more likely to involve blood than other fluids or physical obstruction.

Remember, the inspiration process creates a less-than-atmospheric pressure in the lungs to draw air in. This reduced pressure may collapse damaged structures along the airway that are normally held open by bony or cartilaginous formations. Soft-tissue swelling may also rapidly restrict the airway or close it completely. Swelling and deformity from trauma may distort the facial region so landmarks are hard to recognize, making airway control even more difficult. In serious facial soft-tissue injury, always consider the likelihood of associated injury, especially basilar skull fracture and spinal column injury.

Facial Dislocations and Fractures

Trauma may result in open or closed facial fractures with significant associated pain, swelling, deformity, crepitus, and hemorrhage. Common injuries include mandibular, maxillary, nasal, and orbital fractures and dislocations.

Mandibular dislocation occurs as the condylar process displaces from the temporomandibular joint, just anterior to the ear. This dislocation may result in the malocclusion of the mouth, misalignment of teeth, deformity of the facial region at or around the joint, immobility of the jaw, and pain. The patient's ability to control the airway may be decreased, but dislocation is not usually a significant airway or breathing threat.

Mandibular fractures are painful, present with deformity along the jaw's surface, and may result in the loosening of a few teeth. An open mandibular fracture may produce blood-stained saliva. Mandibular fracture may represent a serious life threat if the patient is placed supine. With such a fracture, the tongue is no longer supported at its base and may displace posteriorly, blocking the airway even in a conscious patient. Always look for a second fracture site when you encounter a patient with a mandibular fracture.

Maxillary fractures are classified according to **Le Fort criteria** (Figure 25 ●). A slight instability involving the maxilla alone usually presents with no associated displacement and is classified as a Le Fort I fracture. A Le Fort II fracture results in fractures of

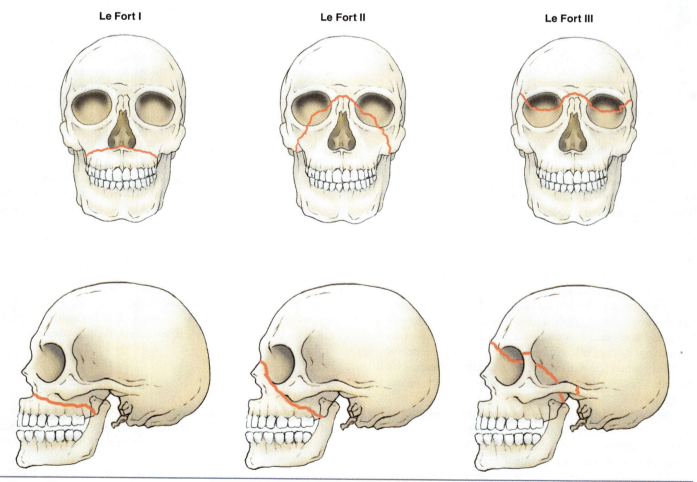

Le Fort I   **Le Fort II**   **Le Fort III**

● **Figure 25**   Le Fort facial fracture classification.

both the maxilla and nasal bones and results in instability of the maxilla and nasal region. Le Fort III fractures characteristically involve the entire facial region below the brow ridge, including the zygoma, nasal bone, and maxilla. The Le Fort II and III fractures usually result in cerebrospinal fluid leakage and may endanger the patency of the nasal and oral portions of the airway.

Dental injury is commonly associated with serious blunt facial trauma. Teeth may chip, break, loosen, or dislodge from the mandible or maxilla. They may then become foreign objects drawn (aspirated) into the airway. Note that a dislodged tooth may be replanted if fully intact and handled properly during prehospital care.

Orbital (blowout) fractures most commonly involve the zygoma or maxilla of the inferior shelf. Zygomatic arch fractures are painful and present with a unilateral depression over the prominence of one cheek. This fracture is most common as pressure on the orbital contents fractures the weakest region, the inferior shelf and into the maxillary sinus. The fracture may entrap the extraocular muscles, reducing the eye's range of motion, and can cause blurred or double vision (diplopia). Zygomatic fracture may also entrap the masseter muscle and limit jaw movement. With maxillary bone fracture, the patient often experiences significant swelling and pain in the maxillary sinus region. Although these injuries are not life threatening, they warrant evaluation by emergency department staff.

Often injury to the facial region is limited to soft-tissue injury. This region is very vascular and is supported by skeletal structures underneath. Swelling tends to be rapid and pronounced, deforming the region very quickly. The area is also prone to rapid and significant hemorrhage.

A special type of facial injury is that associated with a suicide attempt using a rifle or shotgun. The victim places the gun barrel under the chin but, in an effort to push the trigger, stretches and tilts the head back. The gunshot blast is directed under the chin and at the facial region but may be deflected from entering the cranium. The result is a very disrupted facial region with most of the structures of, and supporting, the airway destroyed. The patient may still be conscious, there is usually heavy bleeding, and the remains of the airway are hard to locate. With such a patient, the airway is in serious danger of obstruction and attempts to secure it are very challenging.

Nasal Injury

Nasal injuries are painful and often create a grossly deformed appearance, but they are not usually life threatening. While dislocation or fracture of the cartilage and nasal bone may interfere with nasal air movement, the swelling and associated hemorrhage are more likely threats to the airway. However, the conscious and alert patient is usually very able to control the airway.

Epistaxis (nosebleed) is a common nasal problem associated with facial trauma. Bleeding can be spontaneous as well as traumatic and can be further classified as either anterior or posterior. Anterior hemorrhage comes from the septum and is usually due to bleeding from a network of vessels called Kiesselbach's triangle and plexus. Such hemorrhage bleeds slowly and is usually self-limiting. Posterior hemorrhage may be severe and cause blood to drain down the back of the patient's throat. In epistaxis secondary to severe head trauma

with likely basilar skull fracture, the nasal cavity's posterior wall integrity may be compromised. Attempts at nasal airway, nasogastric tube, or nasotracheal tube insertion may permit the tube to enter the cerebral cavity and directly damage the brain.

Ear Injury

The external ear, or pinna, which is exposed to the environment, is frequently subjected to trauma. It has a minimal blood supply and often does not bleed heavily when lacerated. In glancing blows, the pinna may be partially or completely avulsed. In a folding type of injury, the cartilage may separate. Because of the poor blood supply, external ear injuries do not heal as well as other facial wounds.

The internal portions of the ear—the external auditory canal and the middle and inner ear—are well protected from trauma by the skull's structure. Injury results only from objects forced into the ear or from rapid changes in pressure as in diving accidents, water skiing impacts, or explosions. With an explosion—even with repeated small arms fire—the pinna focuses the rapidly changing air pressure and directs it into the external auditory canal. This enhanced pressure irritates or ruptures the tympanum and, if strong enough, fractures the small bones of hearing (the ossicles). The result can be temporary or permanent hearing loss. In a diving injury, the changing pressure is not equalized by the eustachian tube (also called the pharyngotympanic passage) and eventually builds until the eardrum ruptures. Water floods the middle ear and interferes with the function of the semicircular canals. The patient experiences vertigo, an extremely dangerous sensation when near weightless underwater.

Basilar skull fracture may also disrupt the external auditory canal and tear the tympanum. If the dura mater is torn, cerebrospinal fluid may flood the middle ear and seep outward through the torn tympanum (otorrhea) (Figure 26 ●). As with the other mechanisms described earlier, hearing loss may result.

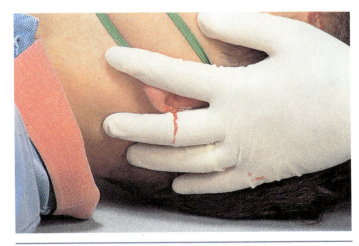

● **Figure 26** Blood or fluid draining from a patient's ear suggests basilar skull fracture.

Tympanic injuries are not life threatening and, in many cases, repair themselves, even with a rupture that tears as much as half the tympanum. However, a victim with an acute hearing loss can be quite apprehensive and anxious. The patient may be frustrated when unable to hear and understand questions or instructions. Such a patient may also be unable to hear sounds of approaching danger such as traffic noise.

Eye Injury

Although the orbit is a very effective protective housing for the eye, penetrating and some blunt trauma may cause serious injury. The anterior eye structures are extremely specialized and, like most specialized tissues, do not regenerate effectively. If significant penetrating injury occurs, especially if accompanied by loss of the eye's fluids—aqueous or vitreous humor—the patient's sight is threatened, possibly with permanent loss. A penetrating object is likely to disturb the integrity of the anterior and possibly the posterior chamber. In addition, removal of the object may allow fluids to leak from the chambers and further threaten the patient's vision. Penetrating injuries may be caused by foreign bodies so small that they are difficult to see with the naked eye. Suspect the presence of such bodies if the patient reports a history of sudden eye pain and the sensation of an impaled foreign body after using a power saw or grinder, especially when working with metal.

Similarly, small foreign particles that land on the eye's surface can also cause ocular injury. The object may embed in the eyelid surface and then drag across the cornea as the eye blinks. Corneal abrasions or lacerations result, often causing intense and continuing pain even after the object is cleared from the eye. These lacerations are usually superficial but can be deep (Figure 27 ●).

Blunt trauma may result in several ocular presentations. Hemorrhage may occur in the anterior chamber and pool, displaying a collection of blood in front of the iris and pupil. This condition, called hyphema, is a potential threat to the patient's vision, requires evaluation by an ophthalmologist, and may result in hospital admission.

A less serious, but equally dramatic, eye injury is a subconjunctival hemorrhage. This may occur after a strong

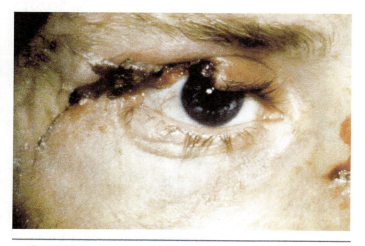

● **Figure 27**   Laceration of the eyelid.

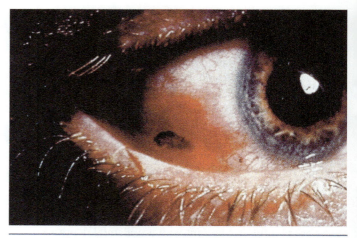

● **Figure 28**   Subconjunctival hemorrhage.

sneeze, vomiting episode, or direct eye trauma, such as orbital fracture. It occurs when a small blood vessel in the subconjunctival space bursts, leaving a portion of the eye's surface blood red (Figure 28 ●). Subconjunctival hemorrhage often clears without intervention and rarely causes any residual scars or impairment.

Blunt trauma may fracture the orbital structures surrounding the eye and produce an injury called eye avulsion. In such a case, the eye is not really avulsed but appears to protrude from the wound as the orbital structure is crushed and depressed. If the eye as well as the nerves and vasculature remain intact, sight in the eye can usually be salvaged. Blunt trauma from such mechanisms as a racket or baseball may compress the orbital contents, fracture the lower orbital wall, entrap the inferior ocular muscles, displace contents into the nasal sinus, and present with a depressed eye, called enophthalmos.

Two other, more serious ocular problems involve the retina. Acute retinal artery occlusion is not an injury but rather a vascular emergency caused when an embolus blocks the blood supply to one eye. The patient complains of sudden and painless loss of vision in the eye. In retinal detachment, which may be traumatic in origin, the retina separates from the eye's posterior wall. The patient complains of a dark curtain obstructing part of the field of view. Both of these conditions are true emergencies in which the patient's eyesight is at risk.

Soft-tissue lacerations can occur around the eye and involve the eyelid. If not properly identified and repaired, such an injury may disrupt lacrimal duct function and interrupt corneal lubrication and oxygenation. Another soft-tissue problem may occur if a contact lens is left in the eye of an unconscious patient. The contact lens will then obstruct the normal lacrimal fluid flow across the eye. This circulation loss may dry out the eye's surface and cause hypoxic injury. The result is usually severe eye pain and possible corneal damage.

Neck Injury

The neck is protected from impact by the more anterior head and chest and by its own skeletal and muscular structures. The neck's major skeletal component is the cervical vertebral column, which is strengthened by interconnecting ligaments. The neck muscles provide additional protection to the vital structures in the neck. They include the muscles that support and move the head through a large range of motion as well as the shoulder muscles that help move the upper extremities and act as auxiliary breathing muscles. The skeletal structures and muscles of the neck protect the airway, carotid and jugular blood vessels, and the esophagus very well from all but anterior blunt trauma and deep penetrating trauma. Such trauma may result in serious injuries to the airway, spine, blood vessels, and other structures in the region.

Trauma to Blood Vessels of the Neck

Blunt trauma to a blood vessel may produce a serious and rapidly expanding hematoma. This hematoma may be trapped within the fascia of the region and apply restrictive pressure to the jugular veins. Laceration of the external jugular vein, or deep laceration involving the internal jugular vein or the carotid arteries, may result in severe hemorrhage as a result of the large vessel size and the blood volume they carry (Figure 29 ●). Their laceration and subsequent hemorrhage can rapidly lead to hypovolemia and shock. Arterial interruption may cause subsequent brain hypoxia and infarct, mimicking signs and symptoms of a stroke. An open neck wound affecting the internal jugular vein may permit formation of an air embolism as the venous pressure drops below atmospheric pressure with deep respirations.

Airway Trauma

Trauma may also injure the larynx and trachea. Severe blunt or penetrating trauma may separate the larynx from the trachea, fracture or crush either of these two structures, or open the trachea to the environment. These injuries may result in serious hemorrhage that threatens the airway, vocal cord contusion or swelling, irritation and trauma to the epiglottis (epiglottitis), destruction of the integrity of the airway and collapse on inspiration, disruption of normal airway landmarks, and restrictive soft-tissue swelling.

Other Neck Trauma

The neck may also demonstrate subcutaneous emphysema from tension pneumothorax (air pushed into the skin from intratho-

racic pressure that migrates to the neck) or from tracheal injury in the neck. Penetrating trauma may involve the esophagus, perforating it and permitting gastric contents or undigested material to enter the fascia. Since the fascia communicates with the mediastinum, this foreign material can physically harm mediastinal structures or provide the medium for infection, which may have devastating results. Deep penetrating trauma may disrupt the vagus nerve, causing tachycardia and gastrointestinal disturbances. More anterior and superficial injuries may damage the thyroid and parathyroid glands.

Spinal Column Injury

Several regions of the spinal column are especially subject to injury. The cervical region accounts for over half of all spinal injuries, with the atlas/axis (C-1/C-2) joint being the site of the majority of fatal spine injuries. This is due to the very delicate nature of these two vertebrae, the mobility of the joint, and the great weight of the head it supports. C-7 is also injured frequently because it is located at the transition between the flexible cervical spine and the more rigid thoracic spine (Figure 30 ●).

Similar injuries can occur at the transition point between the thoracic and lumbar vertebrae (T-12/L-1), again as a result of the differences between the rigid thoracic spine and the flexible lumbar spine. The lumbosacral area (L-5/S-1) likewise can be injured because the pelvis effectively stabilizes the sacral spine. Spinal injuries not associated with the cervical spine are about equally divided between the thoracolumbar and lumbosacral regions.

Remember that the spinal cord ends at the L-1/L-2 region. Below this point, the spinal nerve roots extend until they exit the spinal column (cauda equina). These spinal nerve roots are

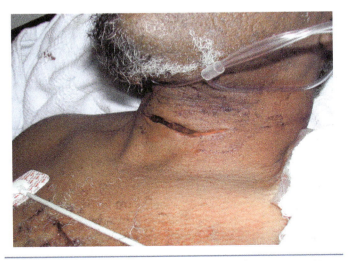

● **Figure 29** Laceration to the neck. (© *Charles Stewart, MD, and Associates*)

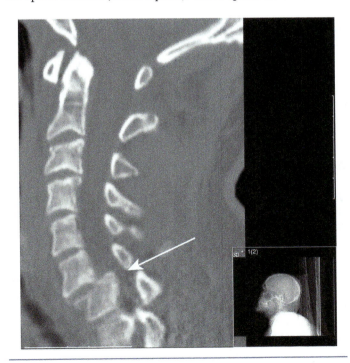

● **Figure 30** Cervical spine injury with a C-1 fracture and a C-7 dislocation (indicated by arrow) with retropulsion into the spinal canal. (© *Dr. Bryan E. Bledsoe*)

more mobile than the cord and less likely to be injured within the spinal foramen during spinal column injury.

HEAD, FACE, NECK, AND SPINAL COLUMN INJURY ASSESSMENT

As with all trauma patients, assessment of a patient with a head, face, neck, or spinal column injury follows the standard assessment process, including the scene size-up, primary assessment, secondary (rapid or focused trauma assessment), detailed assessment, and periodic reassessments, as appropriate. With head, face, neck, and spinal column injuries, pay special attention to ensuring airway patency and monitoring breathing, as well as identifying any specific signs and symptoms of local injury. As a mechanism of injury that causes these injuries is also likely to cause central nervous system injury, carefully monitor your patient's level of consciousness and orientation, pupillary signs, Glasgow Coma Scale score, distal extremity neurologic signs, pulse rate and strength, and blood pressure. With head, face, neck, and spinal column patients, be sure to consider the need for rapid transport to a trauma center specializing in neurologic care.

Scene Size-Up

Mechanism of injury analysis provides the first step in head, face, neck, or spinal column injury patient assessment. During the scene size-up, consider the nature and extent of forces that caused injury. In a vehicle crash, for example, look for evidence of head impact such as the characteristic spider-webbed windshield. Look also for upper steering wheel deformity, which suggests head or neck trauma or shoulder belt use without the lap belt. Identify the direction of forces causing injury and anticipate what body structures these forces may have damaged. In motorcycle impacts, remember that helmet use reduces head injury by about 50 percent but does not spare the neck from cervical spine injury. In shootings, try to determine the caliber and weapon type, the distance from the gun to the patient, and the bullet's approximate angle of entry into the body. Ask yourself if it is possible that the bullet contacted the spinal column.

With other types of impacts, try to determine what forces were involved and how they were directed to the head, face, neck, and spine. Use this information to anticipate injuries to the soft tissues, skeletal structures, airway, and sense organs, and possibly the brain and spinal cord. Remember that many signs of these injuries may be masked by the patient's use of alcohol or other drugs, by the nature of the injury, by other distracting injuries, and/or by the slow development of the wound's signs and symptoms. Consequently, a good MOI analysis and resulting indexes of suspicion are very important. Your thorough analysis must enable you to describe both the incident scene and the mechanism of injury to the attending physician at the emergency department. Remember, however, that a patient's signs and symptoms often give a better indication of injury seriousness than the mechanism of injury.

Examine the scene to determine whether the patient used a helmet or other protective gear. Remember that helmets reduce the likelihood of head injury but neither increase nor decrease the likelihood of neck injury. Also keep in mind that while seat belt use prevents some injuries, it does not preclude spinal injury in strong crashes.

Rule out scene hazards, and request any additional resources needed at the scene as soon as you can. Use of gloves is the minimum Standard Precautions when approaching the potential head, face, and neck injury patient. Serious head injuries pose real exposure risks to blood or other fluids propelled by air movement or by arterial or heavy venous bleeding. Anticipate such exposures, and don splash and eye protection when contacting any patient with significant trauma to the head, face, neck, or spine.

Analyze any effect environmental conditions such as cold temperature or rain will have on your assessment and care. Plan for these contingencies and ensure you and your patient are protected. Effective spinal precautions are time consuming and difficult to provide in an inhospitable environment. Adverse weather can make conditions dangerous for both you and your patient.

Primary Assessment
Spinal Precautions

If the mechanism of injury suggests or, if and when, you find any patient sign or symptom suggesting spine injury, immobilize the head and neck. Gently bring the head and neck into the neutral and in-line position. Maintain this positioning and continue spinal precautions unless you can safely rule out the need for these precautions. The neutral position places the patient's head facing directly forward with the eye directed level and the occiput one to three inches from the plane made by the buttocks and shoulder blades. For obese patients, this distance may be significantly increased. For young children, the occiput should be in-line with that plane, and for infant or very young children the head should be slightly behind the plane.[7]

Firmly apply manual immobilization to hold the patient's head in the neutral, in-line position before proceeding with any remaining assessment and care. In the seated or standing patient, apply just enought lift with your hands not to displace the head upward but just to take some of the head's weight off the spinal column. (Prehospital medicine currently uses terms such as *immobilization*, *stabilization*, and *spinal motion restriction [SMR]* to describe the objective of care techniques used for the spinal injury patient. To limit confusion, we use the term *immobilization* throughout this text.) Manual immobilization should continue from the moment you arrive at the patient's side and suspect spinal injury until the patient receives full mechanical immobilization on a long spine board with a cervical immobilization device or vest-type immobilization device, or is immobilized in a full-body vacuum mattress, or until you can determine that spinal precautions are no longer indicated. It is best if the paramedic responsible for the overall patient assessment and care does not hold manual immobilization. A well-trained EMT or Emergency Medical Responder may best provide this manual immobilization.

Neutral, in-line positioning is very important in spinal injury patient care because it maintains the best spinal column positioning and the greatest clearance between the cord and the spinal foramen interior. This positioning permits the best circulation and thus lessens the impact of local injury and edema. As your assessment progresses, gently and smoothly move any body segment that is out of alignment toward alignment as you examine it. If the patient feels any increase in pain or if you feel a significant resistance to movement, immobilize the head and neck or other portion of the body in the position achieved. Do not continue movement, as doing so may compromise the spinal cord. Maintain a patient's head and body position using manual immobilization until you can secure the position with full mechanical immobilization using the spine board, firm padding, and a cervical immobilization device or full-body vacuum mattress.

Initial Patient Impression

As you begin the primary assessment, form an initial patient impression of his level of consciousness and physical condition. Is the patient alert? Does the patient show any signs of anxiety? Quickly determine the patient's level of consciousness and then orientation to time, place, and person early in the primary assessment. As you gather information about the patient and he responds to your questioning, continue to build and modify your general patient impression and your index of suspicion for head, facial, neck, and spinal column injury and central nervous system (brain and spinal cord) injury.

Spinal Clearance

The decision to continue spinal precautions is predicated on an evaluation of the injury mechanism and of patient findings suggestive of injury. Recent research has demonstrated that prehospital personnel, using a standardized and validated protocol, can reliably identify patients who are likely to have spinal injury, and those who do not. *It should be noted that unstable spinal injury occurs very infrequently, and spinal precautions are not without risk.* Various spinal clearance protocols have been developed and proven reliable, one of the first being the Maine protocol (Figure 31 ●). Many of these spinal clearance protocols are based on a protocol used in emergency departments to determine whether X-rays are required. The protocol was produced through a research project, termed the National Emergency-X-Radiography Utilization Study (NEXUS), and has been used by emergency physicians to determine which patients need spinal X-rays and which do not. It seemed intuitive that if a patient did not meet criteria for emergency department spinal X-rays, prehospital spinal immobilization is probably unwarranted. The NEXUS criteria are essentially the same criteria used in the Maine protocol. International Trauma Life Support (ITLS) recommends a similar protocol (Figure 32 ●). There are several derivations of these protocols, but all have common features.

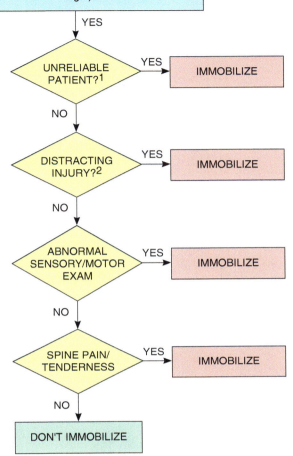

1. Clearance of the spine requires the patient to be calm, cooperative, sober, and alert.
2. Distracting injury includes any injury that produces clinically apparent pain that might distract the patient from the pain of a spine injury—pain would include medical as well as traumatic etiologies of pain.

● **Figure 31** The Maine spinal clearance protocol.

Spinal precautions may be discontinued if the following three criteria are met:

- The patient is alert and fully oriented; is not intoxicated or under the influence of drugs, including alcohol; has a Glasgow Coma Scale score of 15; and is not significantly affected by the "fight-or-flight" response.

- The patient is free of significant distracting injuries such as a significant fracture or joint injury or symptoms like abdominal pain or dyspnea.

- The patient is free of any signs or symptoms of spinal injury.

**Initial Assessment of Spinal Injury
Clinical Criteria**

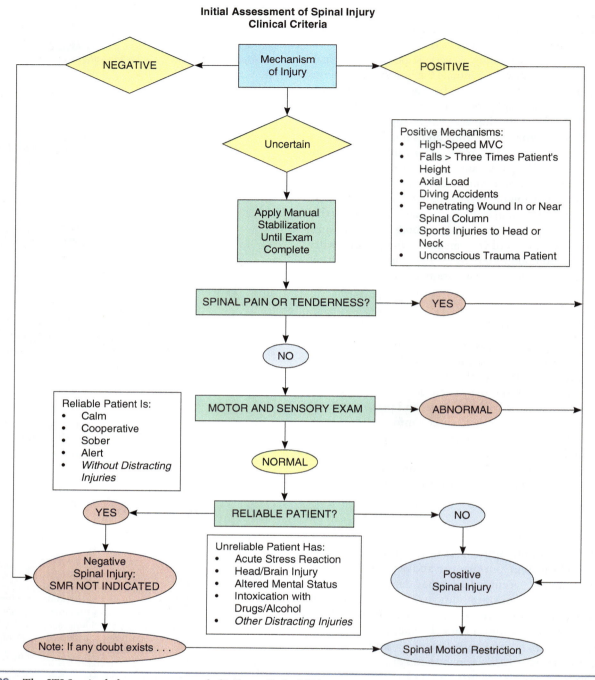

● **Figure 32**   The ITLS spinal clearance protocol. (© Peter Cath, MD)

An additional criterion to consider regarding discontinuance of spinal precautions is the patient's age. Those at both ends of the age spectrum, the very young and the very old, may be unreliable reporters of spinal symptoms. The elderly are not good reporters of spinal symptoms, because preexisting disease and medical problems as well as reduced sensitivity to pain affect their ability to recognize and report pain. The elderly are also more likely to sustain spinal column injury from limited mechanisms of injury, and the clearance between the cord and the spinal column interior may be reduced because of aging and degenerative disease. Very young patients may simply cry as a result of pain or may be too young to accurately articulate spinal

symptoms. Again, consult your protocols to determine if, and under what circumstances, you can discontinue spinal precautions for either the elderly or the very young.

If you have any doubt about the patient's potential for spinal injury or the patient's ability to accurately report any symptoms of such an injury, continue spinal precautions, including full immobilization to the long spine board or full-body vacuum mattress.

If you continue spinal precautions, maintain manual spinal immobilization and apply a properly sized cervical collar after you fully examine the neck for injury and provide any needed emergent care there. Even with the collar in place, maintain manual head immobilization until the patient is fully immobilized to a short spine board, KED, or long spine board with a cervical immobilization device. A new-generation orthopedic stretcher will provide full body and good spinal immobilization as well. While a cervical collar provides some neck immobilization, it does not completely immobilize the region. Its placement may be delayed so long as manual immobilization is continued.

Whenever a patient wearing a helmet sustains moderate or severe head impact, suspect a cervical spine injury and employ spinal precautions. Consider whether or not to remove the helmet as described later in this chapter. A patient's helmet use reduces the likelihood of soft-tissue injury and skull and facial fracture. Helmet use can also significantly reduce the incidence of traumatic brain injury, but do not be lulled into a false sense of security by the absence of a patient's outward trauma signs. Be watchful for the early signs of brain injury, and be sure to inform the emergency department staff that the patient was wearing a helmet. Bring the helmet to the emergency department with the patient or relate any damage it sustained to the emergency physician.

Research is revealing that penetrating trauma is unlikely to injure the spinal cord or cause spinal column instability. Do not initiate spinal precautions for the patient with a penetrating injury mechanism that could involve the spinal column unless there are signs or symptoms of spinal cord injury.

Airway

Move quickly to evaluate the airway. Examine the face and neck for any deformity, swelling, hemorrhage, foreign bodies, or other injury that may threaten the airway. Suction and insert an oral or nasal airway as necessary. Listen for unusual or changing voice patterns as they may be indicative of airway injury and developing edema. Swelling can quickly occlude the airway, and any hemorrhage can complicate airway maintenance, especially if the patient loses consciousness and protective airway reflexes. Anticipate vomiting, possibly without warning. Ensure that the airway is structurally sound and that the mandible supports the tongue well enough to keep it out of the airway. Have a large-bore suction catheter and strong suction ready to remove any fluids, and consider positioning the patient to enhance airway drainage (left lateral recumbent position) if doing so is not contraindicated by injuries. Note that any airway manipulation, as may occur with deep suctioning, oropharyngeal airway use, or endotracheal tube insertion, may increase ICP. Use these procedures as a last resort and have an experienced provider accomplish them quickly.

If there is a serious neck injury, visualize, then palpate the trachea's structural integrity. If the trachea is open to the environment, keep the wound clear of blood to prevent aspiration, and seal the wound unless the patient's upper airway is blocked. If an impaled object obstructs the airway, remove it, anticipating that heavy bleeding may then threaten the airway. It may be prudent to be ready to immediately intubate the patient to secure the airway. Blunt wounds may crush the trachea's cartilage, permitting it to close with the reduced pressure of inspiration. This type of crushing injury may require intubation or opening the trachea by cricothyrotomy to ensure adequate air exchange.

If you are continuing spinal precautions while you assess the airway, be sure that the patient's head remains in the neutral, in-line position. The airway is more difficult to control when you are required to observe spinal precautions. Be ready to carefully log roll the patient if he vomits or if necessary to drain the upper airway of fluids. Have adequate suction ready and anticipate the possible need to clear the airway during transport, should vomiting occur. To prepare for this, secure the patient firmly to a spine board and immobilize him well enough to permit 90-degree rotation of the patient and board. It is also acceptable to raise the head of a patient on a spine board by elevating the head-end of the board. This may help prevent aspiration and can also be a therapeutic maneuver in cases of suspected elevated intracranial pressure from a head injury. Note that firm immobilization to a spine board causes patient discomfort and may make securing the airway more difficult. As spinal instability occurs infrequently, ensure that you apply the long spine board only when you cannot clear a patient with a spinal clearance protocol.

If advanced airway procedures are indicated, consider either an extraglottic airway, orotracheal intubation, or video laryngoscopy with spinal precautions. Neither extraglottic airway insertion nor video laryngoscopy require any movement or special immobilization (beyond spinal precautions) of the patient's head and neck. With endotracheal intubation, have the patient's head held firmly in the neutral, in-line position as you attempt to identify airway features and insert the endotracheal tube. Anticipate that landmarks may be hard to visualize because the head cannot be brought into the sniffing position and the upper airway aligned. During the procedure, be careful not to displace the jaw anteriorly beyond the point at which it begins to lift the neck (extension) or to permit any rotation of the head. Consider employing the laryngeal manipulation to better align the airway structures without displacing the spine.

After performing any advanced airway procedure, especially if it is a difficult one, be very careful to ensure proper initial and continuing airway placement, assessing for the presence of good chest excursion, bilaterally equal breath sounds, and the absence of epigastric sounds with your initial ventilations. It is essential to use capnography and pulse oximetry to ensure proper and continuing tube placement and effective oxygenation and ventilation, especially in patients who received head trauma. If you have placed an endotracheal tube, check the tube's depth of insertion by noting the number on the side of the tube and secure the tube firmly. Monitor the tube's depth, capnography, pulse oximetry, and breath sounds frequently during your care and transport. Reevaluate advanced airway positioning after every patient move and ensure that the tube remains in the trachea. Endotracheal intubation is a high-risk procedure for the patient with head injury. Ensure that you perform it in a short period of time to reduce hypoxia and hypercarbia.

When assessing an infant with head, face, neck, or spinal column injury, pay particular attention to the airway. Infants are obligate nasal breathers and must have a patent nasal passage and pharynx to ensure a clear airway. Hyperextension of the head will obstruct the airway as the tongue pushes the soft palate closed. Ensure proper head positioning, and ventilate using both the mouth and nose.

Breathing

Quickly ensure breathing is adequate. Determine the rate and volume and determine the amount of chest excursion. The chest should gently rise and fall with each breath and this motion should occur between 10 and 16 times per minute. Attach pulse oximetry. If oxygen saturation is less than 96 percent, apply supplemental oxygen and titrate it to maintain at least that saturation. If necessary, ventilate the patient to ensure adequate oxygen saturation and monitor carbon dioxide levels with capnography.

Rapidly evaluate the patient's respiratory effort. In the potential spinal injury patient, watch chest and abdomen motion carefully. They should rise and fall together. Exaggerated abdominal movement and limited chest excursion with motion opposite to that of the abdomen suggest diaphragmatic breathing and high cervical spine injury. For such a patient, provide immediate positive-pressure ventilation coordinated with the patient's respiratory effort (overdrive ventilation) while maintaining spinal precautions. Your assistance will make breathing more effective and less energy consuming. Use pulse oximetry to continuously evaluate the effectiveness of respirations.

Circulation

Monitor the patient's pulse rate and its rhythm early in your care and continue to do so frequently thereafter. Quickly look for any hemorrhage from the head, face, and neck, and control any moderate to severe bleeding with direct pressure and bandaging. Carefully apply direct pressure to the head, especially if you suspect skull fracture. If necessary, apply pressure around the wound to halt any serious blood flow. Direct pressure on an unstable fracture (such as a depressed skull fracture) may worsen brain injury.

Be cautious of open neck wounds because they may present a risk for air embolism. Cover any such wounds quickly with occlusive dressings and secure them in place. Bleeding may be heavy from the neck as blood vessels here are large. Venous hemorrhage may be rather easy to control though arterial bleeding may not. Use direct pressure but do not apply that pressure with circumferential dressings. Use and maintain digital pressure (using a finger or two) to control the blood loss.

Patient Priority

At the end of the primary assessment, you must identify the patient's category for care and transport. Using the CUPS acronym, a critical (C) patient is one who has a problem with airway, breathing, and/or circulation and does not ever make it out of the primary assessment. Unstable (U) and potentially unstable (P) patients receive the rapid trauma assessment while stable (S) patients may receive the focused trauma assessment. With most head, face, and neck injury patients, you will perform a rapid trauma assessment because of the high likelihood of airway, vascular, special sense organ, or central nervous system injuries. If there is no significant mechanism of injury and injuries appear minor and superficial, perform a focused trauma exam directed at the specific location(s) of injury.

Secondary Assessment

Secondary assessment of the trauma patient begins with the physical exam, followed by patient questioning (the history) and vital signs.

Rapid Trauma Assessment

Rapid trauma assessment is performance of a quick and directed head-to-toe examination of a patient with any significant mechanism of injury. When head, facial, neck, or spinal column injury is suggested in such a patient, pay particular attention to the procedures described in the following sections as you carry out this assessment. Manage any life-threatening injuries and conditions as you find them during the rapid trauma assessment. If the patient shows any signs of pathology within the cranium, consider rapid transport. Traumatic brain injury patients can deteriorate quickly, but rapid neurosurgical intervention may alleviate life-threatening problems.

Head Look at, then sweep, each region of the skull, feeling for deformity and bleeding with the more sensitive tips of your fingers. Interlock your fingertips, making sure there is no gap between your fingers, to sweep the posterior head, and look at your gloves to check for any blood that indicates hemorrhage there. If you find any moderate or serious hemorrhage, apply direct pressure unless you suspect skull fracture. If the skull is depressed, control hemorrhage with gentle pressure around the wound and place a loose dressing over it. Palpate gently for any swelling or deformity, being careful, however, not to palpate the interior of open wounds (Figure 33 ●). Remember and record the results of this assessment. Tissue swelling often changes the presentation of head wounds. The initial evaluation may be important in determining just what type of injury has occurred. If assessment identifies a depressed or unstable skull fracture, consider the patient to have a brain injury and prepare for expedited transport.

Shine a penlight into the external auditory canal and look for signs of escaping cerebrospinal fluid. This fluid loss may be difficult to notice early during assessment, so observe carefully. If blood or fluid drains from the auditory canal, cover the ear

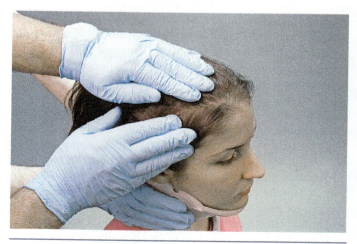

● **Figure 33** Carefully inspect and palpate the head for bleeding and other signs of injury.

with gauze dressings to permit fluid to move outward while providing a barrier to keep contaminants from entering. Examine the ear's pinnae for injury and, after you complete the rapid trauma assessment, bandage and dress as needed.

If you observe a skull deformity, palpate such a closed wound very gently. Try to determine the probability of skull fracture before swelling makes this determination more difficult. Cover any open wounds with dressings to restrict bleeding and prevent further contamination. The signs of basilar skull fracture—bilateral periorbital ecchymosis and retroauricular ecchymosis (raccoon eyes and Battle's sign)—are very late indications of this injury and are not likely to be recognizable during field assessment and care.

Face   Study the patient's facial features carefully, looking for asymmetry, swelling, discoloration, or deformity. Palpate the facial region including the brow ridge, nasal region, cheeks, maxilla, and mandible, searching for any deformity, instability, or crepitus that suggests fracture and for any signs of soft-tissue swelling (Figure 34 ●). Palpate the maxilla and attempt, gently, to move it from left to right. It should be firmly attached to the facial bones and should display no crepitus. Do likewise with the mandible. It should be solid yet very mobile up and down and display modest left-to-right (lateral) motion. Examine for and note any mandibular instability or false motion. Note and investigate any patient report of pain during your palpation and movement. Ensure that the mandible is intact and supports the airway. Open the mouth and examine for any signs of trauma, excessive secretions and bleeding, or swelling. All teeth should be firmly in place (loose teeth may suggest mandibular fracture). Find any displaced teeth and prepare them for transport with the patient (in an approved tooth preservative) or suspect that missing teeth may have been aspirated. Ensure that the zygoma

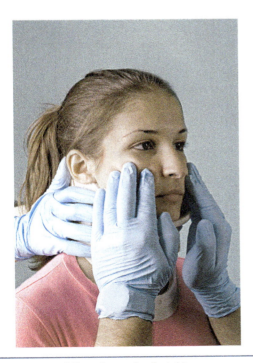

● **Figure 34**   Carefully palpate the facial bones.

(cheekbone) and brow ridge (frontal bone) are prominent, rigid, without crepitus to palpation, and symmetrical.

Carefully examine the eyes. Have the patient, if conscious and alert, follow your finger up and down, left and right, with each eye. Watch for and note any limited eye movement. Restricted eye movement, especially if the patient reports diplopia (double vision), suggests eye muscle entrapment or nerve compression or injury and paralysis. Carefully examine the pupil, iris, and conjunctiva. The pupil and iris should be round, anterior chamber clear, and sclera free of accumulating blood. Check for contact lenses, especially in the unconscious patient. If they are noted, remove them carefully.

Neck   Examine the anterior, lateral, and posterior neck for injury signs including swelling, discoloration, skin disruption, blood loss, or frothy blood. Frothy blood is likely caused by bleeding in association with a tracheal injury and suggests serious airway compromise. Palpate the region, feeling for any changes in skin tension, deformities, or unusual masses underneath. Crepitus beneath the skin may be associated with subcutaneous emphysema from a tracheal or laryngeal fracture or chest injury. These injuries are likely to push air into the subcutaneous tissues and enlarge the region they affect and produce crepitus. Identify the thyroid cartilage, beneath and posterior to the mandible. Palpate it, the cricoid cartilage, then the trachea. Ensure they are not deformed by trauma and remain midline in the neck. Visually examine any neck wound's depth to anticipate those that may involve jugular or carotid blood vessels, and cover any open wounds with occlusive dressings. Watch for any changes in voice and, if so noted, limit your patient questioning.

Spine   Begin your spinal column assessment by observing the natural curvature of the spinal regions, looking for any discoloration and open or closed wounds, and asking the patient about any pain or abnormal sensations along the spine. Then gently palpate the entire posterior spine (Tables 1 and 2). Feel for any deformity, crepitus, and unusual warmth, and ask about pain or tenderness from C-1 through L-5. It may be beneficial to repeat spinal palpation from L-5 to C-1 as pain or tenderness may be difficult to identify in the presence of painful injuries elsewhere when minor tenderness may be the only symptom of significant vertebral column instability. If you find any pain, tenderness, or deformity, continue or institute spinal precautions.

Remember that some patients will have spinal abnormalities that may make it difficult to assess for spinal injury and apply spinal precautions if needed. The most commonly encountered abnormalities are **kyphosis** and **scoliosis**. Kyphosis is an exaggeration of the thoracic convexity. It is most common in the elderly and often results from calcium loss in the spinal vertebrae (osteoporosis). Scoliosis is a condition that results in complex lateral and rotational curvature and deformity of the spine. **Ankylosing spondylitis** is a chronic, painful, progressive inflammatory arthritis that primarily affects the spine and sacroiliac joints. It eventually causes fusion and complete spinal rigidity, a condition known as **bamboo spine**. These patients sometimes cannot lie flat and must have padding

TABLE 1	Cervical Spine Exam Reminder	
Nerve Root	**Muscle Group/Function**
C-5	Deltoid
C-6	Wrist extension
C-7	Wrist flexion
C-8	Finger flexors
T-1	Interossei (flaring of fingers)

TABLE 2	Lumbar Spine Exam Reminder	
Nerve Root	**Muscle Group/Function**
L-2/L-3	Quadriceps muscles
L-4	Ankle dorsiflexion/inversion
L-5	Great toe extension
S-1	Foot plantarflexion and eversion

placed to accomodate their deformity. Attempts to force them to lie flat or to forcibly extend the spine can result in fracture of the brittle spine with resultant cord injury—often transection.

Remember that spinal column injury can occur without cord injury (and spinal cord injury signs) just as cord injury can occur without column injury or injury signs.

Patient Questioning

Question the head, facial, neck, and spinal column injury patient about any painful or unusual sensations. Examine any area of reported paresthesia, anesthesia, weakness, or paralysis, noting the borders of the area and whether it is unilateral or bilateral. Ask if the patient has any unusual fullness in the throat, or has any difficulty swallowing or otherwise maintaining the airway. Also ask about any numbness or tingling and any apparent weakness in a limb or limbs. Ask the patient to move uninjured limbs (presuming there are no signs of spinal column injury) and inquire as to any pain, weakness, or unusual feelings.

Ask about any visual disturbances such as double vision (diplopia) and blurred vision that may indicate eye muscle entrapment. Inquire about visual acuity (the ability to distinguish objects) both near and far, and note reports of any restriction to vision, which the patient might describe as a curtain drawn across the field of view. Patient complaints of eye pain are also important and may suggest conjunctival or corneal injury. Question the patient frequently to identify any increase or decrease in awareness and any changes in injury symptoms.

Conduct a complete patient medical history investigation following the AMPLE elements. Listen carefully for any history of central nervous system problems or the use of medications that impact level of consciousness or the body's response to injury and shock. Also anticipate the impact any preexisting disease may have on assessment or the patient's response to the trauma they have just suffered.

Complete the rapid trauma assessment by examining the rest of the body, paying particular attention to any region where the mechanism of injury suggests serious injury or in which the patient complains of serious symptoms. While examining the extremities, look for any signs of decreased muscle tone, flaccid muscles, or diminished sensation or muscle strength, and determine if any unusual findings are bilateral or unilateral and where the deficit begins. Then gather the balance of the patient history, take a set of the patient's vital signs, and determine the patient's Glasgow Coma Scale (GCS) score or the Simplified Motor Score (SMS).

Vital Signs

Carefully monitor vital signs for evidence of increasing intracranial pressure. Identify and record pulse rate and strength. Note blood pressure and especially pulse pressure. Ensure that your assessment of past medical history investigates and identifies any history of hypertension. This may help you determine whether an elevated blood pressure is due to head injury or a preexisting condition. Lastly, note the respiratory pattern. Vital signs change with increasing ICP or brainstem injury. Be watchful for a slowing pulse rate, increasing systolic blood pressure, and development of irregular respirations (Cheyne-Stokes, central neurologic hyperventilation, or ataxic respirations), which together are known as Cushing's triad.

Blood pressure may also be adversely affected in the patient with spinal injury and loss of vascular control below the injury. The patient may not be able to employ vascular constriction in the lower abdomen and extremities to help compensate for blood loss and hypovolemia. The blood pressure may drop early in the progression of shock. In the setting of head injury, even brief periods of hypotension (generally considered as a systolic less than 80) are known to worsen outcomes. Remain vigilant for any signs of hypotension and move rapidly to correct it.

As you conclude the rapid trauma assessment, reevaluate your patient's CUPS score. If the patient remains unstable or potentially unstable, move quickly but carefully to expedited transport. Remember, unnecessary manipulation of the patient with a potential spinal column injury can result in spinal cord injury and permanent disability. Significant airway threats and uncontrolled hemorrhage are also indicators for rapid transport. Carefully monitor head, face, neck, and spinal column injury patients during reassessments and care for any signs of increasing intracranial pressure or expanding lesions. Identify the wounds and other injuries you have found or suspect and prioritize them for care.

Focused Trauma Exam

If your head, face, neck, or spinal column injury patient has no significant mechanism of injury and no other indications of serious injury, perform a focused trauma assessment, concentrating on the area of injury. During your assessment, however, be alert for any signs of a diminishing level of consciousness or orientation or any evidence of previous unconsciousness or airway or vascular restriction or compromise. It is recommended to perform a Glasgow Coma Scale evaluation to form a baseline. If you discover any evidence of brain or spinal cord injury, complete a rapid trauma assessment and consider the patient for rapid transport to the appropriate facility. Remember, the signs of significant brain injury may not develop for some time or may be masked by drug or alcohol use or by the patient's anxiety. It is always better to err on the side of more intensive patient care and expeditious transport.

Direct the focused trauma exam to areas of specific patient complaint and to areas where the mechanism of injury suggests injury. Use assessment techniques—observation, inspection, palpation, and so forth—to evaluate the area of suspected injury. With superficial wounds to the head, face, and neck, apply dressings and bandages as for minor soft-tissue injuries but be alert for hemorrhage into the airway and vomiting that may follow it and for any signs of progressive swelling that may restrict the airway. Watch also for open neck wounds that may permit air to enter the jugular vein. Cover such wounds with occlusive dressings held firmly in place.

Inspect any soft-tissue head, facial, or neck injury very carefully before bandaging it and be prepared to describe the injury to the attending emergency department physician or nurse so they do not have to remove and replace dressings and bandages unnecessarily.

When you have completed the focused assessment, obtain a set of baseline vital signs and gather a patient history. Then provide emergency care for the injuries you have found and prepare the patient for transport.

Detailed Assessment

You will normally perform a detailed assessment for head, face, neck, and spinal column injury patients during transport and only if and when you have cared for all significant injuries. The detailed assessment is an in-depth, head-to-toe assessment searching for any other signs or symptoms suggestive of injury. Use your skills of questioning, inspection, palpation, and—as appropriate—auscultation to search out these additional injuries. Look for signs of neurologic deficit in the extremities, including flaccidity, paresthesia, anesthesia, weakness, and paralysis. Remember that early in the course of trauma, serious injuries may be masked by other more painful ones, by patient anxiety, by the fight or flight response, and by drug and alcohol use. Careful evaluation is required to identify injuries at this stage of patient care.

Reassessment

During reassessments, repeat the primary assessment elements, take vital signs, review Glasgow Coma Scale scoring, and reevaluate any spinal cord injury signs or symptoms every 5 minutes (Figure 35 ●). Carefully monitor for any changes in neurologic status, including the levels of orientation, responsiveness, sensation, and motor function. Look for any improvement or deterioration. Watch for a slowing pulse rate or a constant pulse rate in the presence of falling blood pressure. Also, be observant for a falling blood pressure without signs of shock compensation. Remember that spinal column injury may not produce any overt neurologic signs or symptoms yet may still threaten the spinal cord if the patient is moved without proper spinal precautions.

For the patient who did not receive spinal immobilization following application of a spinal clearance protocol, periodically question the patient about pain along the spinal column and other symptoms of spinal injury. Also perform frequent sensory and motor evaluations of the distal extremities to ensure that evidence of spinal injury has not developed undetected. If it does, employ full spinal precautions.

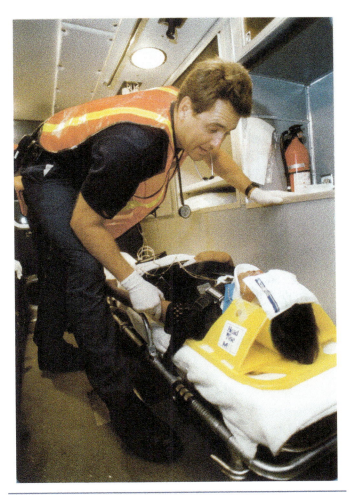

● **Figure 35**   Repeat the ongoing assessment every 5 minutes with seriously injured patients. (© *Craig Jackson/In the Dark Photography*)

HEAD, FACE, NECK, AND SPINAL COLUMN INJURY MANAGEMENT

Management priorities for a patient sustaining head, face, neck, or spinal column trauma include care directed at protecting the spinal cord from injury through spinal immobilization (discussed later in this chapter) and maintaining the airway, breathing, circulation.

Airway

Vigilant airway monitoring and aggressive care are the only means of ensuring that the head, facial, neck, and spinal column injury patient's airway remains protected and patent. Airway management techniques appropriate for such patients include suctioning, oropharyngeal and nasopharyngeal airways, cricoid pressure/laryngeal manipulation, advanced airways (e.g., extraglottic airways, endotracheal intubation, directed intubation), and cricothyrotomy.

Suctioning

Maintaining a clear airway in the head injury patient is critical to patient survival. Airway tissues are extremely vascular, bleed profusely, and swell quickly. Soft-tissue injury may cause significant hemorrhage that can compromise the airway in two ways. First, the sheer blood volume may physically obstruct the airway. Secondly, blood is a gastric irritant that frequently induces emesis. In addition, vomiting is a frequent result of brain injury or increasing intracranial pressure. Here, vomiting often occurs without warning (without nausea) and can be projectile in nature. Emesis is especially dangerous with brain injury patients because they commonly have depressed or absent protective airway reflexes. Gastric contents are very acidic and will quickly damage the lower airway tissues if aspirated. Aspiration of gastric contents is associated with a high patient mortality.

Be ready to immediately turn the patient (if possible and with spinal precautions as needed) to allow gravitational drainage, and suction aggressively with severe airway hemorrhage or vomiting. Suctioning may increase ICP and interrupts ventilation, so limit it to just that which is needed to clear the airway in the brain injury patient. Use a large-bore catheter or a suction hose without a tip to clear the airway of any blood or emesis. Assure good ventilation after suctioning and monitor oxygen saturation and capnography during the procedure.

Oropharyngeal and Nasopharyngeal Airways

Oro- and nasopharyngeal airways each have advantages and disadvantages when used with head, face, neck, and spinal column injury patients. The nasal airway does not trigger protective airway reflexes (the gag reflex) as easily as an oral airway and is better tolerated by the patient who is not completely unconscious. Because there is less stimulation of the airway reflexes, there is also a reduction in transient increases in intracranial pressure. One hazard of nasal airway use is possible insertion of the tube

directly into the cranium through a fracture of the posterior nasal cavity (cribiform plate). Do not use this device when the patient has been subjected to serious blunt force trauma to the face or who is suspected of basilar skull fracture. Always insert the nasal airway straight back along the floor of the nasal cavity, and use only gentle force in its introduction. You may also consider a second nasopharyngeal airway insertion into the other nostril, as needed. If you suspect basilar skull fracture, use an oral or an advanced airway to establish and maintain the airway.

While oro- and nasopharyngeal airways help to keep the respective pharynxes open, they can represent threats to the airway. The end of the airway sits just superior to the laryngeal opening. If a patient vomits, which frequently happens with brain injury, the airway restricts outward movement of vomitus through and around the airway. With the next ventilation, the patient can aspirate gastric contents. Whenever an oral or nasal airway is in place, monitor the patient's airway carefully and continuously and be prepared to remove the airway and suction any emesis, immediately.

Cricoid Pressure/External Laryngeal Manipulation

When ventilating a patient with a bag-valve mask, and when you have sufficient personnel, consider using cricoid pressure (also called the Sellick maneuver) to limit vomiting and emesis. With a supine patient, the person performing the maneuver applies pressure to the cricoid ring of the trachea with the thumb and index finger, directed posteriorly, to move the cricoid ring toward the vertebral column. This compresses the esophagus, which lies behind the trachea, thus reducing the likelihood of emesis being able to enter the upper airway during ventilations. Exercise caution to prevent the pressure from flexing the cervical spine. If the patient should actively vomit, release the pressure immediately and suction the airway. Continuing to hold the esophagus closed during active vomiting could result in its rupture. Be aware that cricoid pressure often will not align the airway enough to permit visualized oral intubation. Using cricoid pressure during intubation has come under scrutiny recently, and there is scientific evidence questioning its effectiveness.

When intubating, if cricoid pressure does not move airway landmarks into view, have the person applying cricoid pressure ease or release the pressure. If that does not allow you to visualize the airway landmarks, move the person's hand to the larynx (thyroid cartilage). While trying to visualize the glottic opening, place your free hand on top of the hand on the larynx and gently displace the larynx downward until the landmarks become more visible. Have your assistant maintain that position while you grasp the endotracheal tube and insert it into the trachea.

Another technique that may better align the airway landmarks and increase the ease and success rate for endotracheal intubation is external laryngeal manipulation (ELM). (See the discussion of ELM in Volume 2, Chapter 5.) In many EMS systems ELM is becoming a firstline choice to align the airway for intubation.

Advanced Airways

Advanced airway insertion is the method of choice to ensure a clear and patent airway in the head injury patient. Use one of these devices early in the care of an unresponsive patient (GCS of

8 or <8 or SMS <1). Advanced airway techniques useful in caring for head injury patients include extraglottic airway, and orotracheal and directed intubation.[8]

Extraglottic Airways Improvements in extraglottic airways (those that do not enter the space between the vocal folds and the trachea) have made them easy to use and more effective in airway control than earlier models. Their insertion does not involve airway landmark visualization, and they can be inserted quickly without any additional equipment or patient positioning. Extraglottic airways can be either retroglottic or supraglottic. Retroglottic airways include the Combitube, King LT, and pharyngeotracheal lumen (PTL) airways. Supraglottic airways include laryngeal airways (including newer versions of the laryngeal mask airway (LMA)) and the CookGas, AirQ, and Ambu Laryngeal Mask airways, plus the Supra-glottic Airway Laryngopharynx Tube (S.A.L.T.). The use of these devices requires careful airway assessment and ventilation to ensure the extraglottic airway is placed properly and successfully isolates the lower airway. Carefully monitor chest rise and breath sounds, and monitor both pulse oximetry and capnography to ensure proper and continuing airway placement and appropriate ventilation for the head injury patient.

Orotracheal Intubation Orotracheal intubation is commonly used to secure the airway (Figure 36 ●). It does, however, pose some hazards for head, face, and neck injury patients. Many patients who sustain serious injuries in these regions require spinal immobilization. Immobilization limits patient head and neck positioning during intubation attempts and restricts your ability to visualize the vocal folds and watch the endotracheal tube pass into the trachea. This may prolong the intubation attempt and the time between ventilations, thus exposing the patient to greater hypoxia.

If spinal precautions are in place, maintain head and neck positioning while the collar is removed from the anterior neck and the provider stabilizing the head and neck displaces the jaw anteriorly (jaw thrust). Consider the ELM (as described earlier) to improve visualization during intubation. If ELM is unsuccessful in permitting airway landmark visualization consider a technique

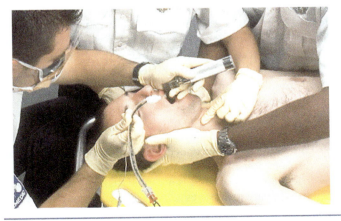

● **Figure 36**   Oral intubation is difficult in the patient with facial trauma because landmarks may be distorted, blood may flow into the airway, and the head must remain in the neutral position.

called the BURP maneuver. Using your thumb and first finger, displace the larynx **B**ackward (posteriorly), **U**pward (cephalad), and just slightly to the patient's **R**ight with slight **P**ressure.

Keep in mind that prolonged attempts at endotracheal intubation can induce hypoxia and hypercarbia, both very detrimental to the head injury patient. Therefore, if you choose endotracheal intubation, carry it out rapidly. If possible, have the most experienced care provider attempt the procedure to reduce intubation time and increase the likelihood of success. Optical and video laryngoscopy can also be of great benefit for the patient with probable spine injury as you do not need to reposition the head and neck to successfully visualize airway landmarks and place an endotracheal tube.

Directed Intubation In serious facial or upper neck trauma, as in a shotgun blast, the landmarks of the upper airway may be disrupted or destroyed. In such cases, obtaining and maintaining an airway may be extremely difficult, yet of maximum importance. Use strong suction over the area to clear fluid accumulation and use the laryngoscope to visualize the elements of the oro- and laryngopharynx.

A form of directed intubation uses a device called the gum-elastic bougie. The bougie is a long, malleable, gum-rubber stylet, inserted into the trachea while visualizing it with the laryngoscope or video laryngoscope. The endotracheal tube is then inserted over the bougie and into the trachea. The bougie is withdrawn and the patient is ventilated through the endotracheal tube. The bougie can be placed by digital intubation techniques (See Volume 2, Chapter 5) with endotracheal tube introduction then guided by the bougie. However, you must then be especially careful to confirm proper endotracheal tube placement.

Retrograde intubation is a process in which a wire is introduced through the cricothyroid membrane into the larynx, then the pharynx, and then out through the mouth. The process begins with catheter placement through the cricothyroid membrane, directed superiorly. A flexible wire is advanced through the catheter toward the oral opening. A laryngoscope is used to identify the advancing wire and then a McGill forceps is used to retrieve it. The endotracheal tube is then advanced over the wire down to the thyroid cartilage. When the tube reaches the larynx, the wire is withdrawn and the tube is advanced into the trachea. Retrograde intubation is more complicated and time-consuming than oral tracheal intubation. However, in some circumstances, it may be the only effective technique for intubation when the normal landmarks are disrupted by severe facial and airway trauma.

If you cannot see airway landmarks themselves, look for bubbling air escaping from the trachea with expirations. If you believe you are close to the tracheal opening and can visualize the area, have an assistant compress the chest to induce bubbling. Attempt to pass the endotracheal tube quickly along the route of bubbles and into the trachea. With this technique, it is critically important to confirm proper placement of the endotracheal tube.

Medication-assisted intubation, including rapid sequence induction (RSI), will be discussed in the next chapter, "Nervous System Trauma."

Confirmation of Airway Placement Once an advanced airway is inserted using one of the techniques previously described, confirm its proper placement. Auscultate, at a minimum, the axillae and over the epigastrium. (Good breath sounds at both axillae reflect good ventilation to the distal alveoli.) Watch carefully for good, symmetrical chest wall excursion with each ventilation. If you hear good breath sounds bilaterally, detect no epigastric sounds, and see the chest wall move equally with each breath, your airway is properly placed. Use capnography, pulse oximetry, and patient skin color observation to confirm and monitor proper and continuing airway placement. Remember that the advanced airway may dislodge during any patient movement, as from the ground to the stretcher or as the stretcher is loaded into the ambulance. Reconfirm proper tube placement frequently.

Confirm—and document—proper airway placement using at least three of the following methods with the device placement and after every time you move the patient: Auscultate bilateral breath sounds, observe symmetrical chest rise, monitor capnography readings, and monitor oxygen saturation readings. The use of continuous waveform capnography provides a graphic and almost irrefutable record of patient ventilation and, thereby, proper airway placement and ventilation on a breath-to-breath basis. Waveform capnography is the gold standard for confirmation of initial and continuing airway placement and to guide ventilation, especially in the head injury patient.

Cricothyrotomy

In some cases of face and neck trauma, the region may be so distorted or the airway so blocked that advanced airway placement is impossible. Here the only potential for providing a lifesaving airway may be opening a pathway for ventilation through the neck, the cricothyrotomy. Consult your protocols and medical direction to identify whether this advanced airway procedure or the other procedures already described may be used in your system.

Cricothyrotomy is the surgical entry through the cricothyroid membrane for the purpose of providing an alternate and temporary airway. Devices such as the Quicktrach and Pertrach are commercially available cricothyrotomy devices that make the procedure simple and effective.

Cricothyrotomy is a procedure of last resort, when the airway cannot be secured by any other way. (However, if it is clear that airway landmarks have been devastated by massive trauma or your visualization of the airway with the laryngoscope reveals a grossly disrupted or distorted pharynx, it may be prudent to move quickly to cricothyrotomy.) The optimal patient position for cricothyrotomy is supine with the neck in hyperextension. This is contraindicated for many head and spinal injury patients. In these patients, the head should be maintained firmly in the neutral position while the procedure is attempted. Locate the cricothyroid membrane by feeling with a gloved hand for the thyroid cartilage in the upper central anterior neck. Find the small depression along its anterior surface, the thyroid notch. Slide your finger inferiorly to the next depression, the cricothyroid membrane. You will notice a small cartilage ring just below this notch, the cricoid cartilage. (Alternatively, locate the membrane by palpating upward along the trachea from the sternal notch. The first, slightly larger, and firm ring you feel is the cricoid cartilage. Immediately above it, and before the next firm and even larger cartilage (thyroid cartilage), is the cricothyroid

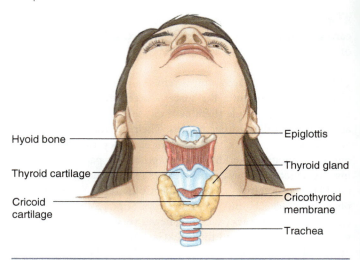

● **Figure 37** Anatomic landmarks associated with the cricothyroid membrane.

membrane (Figure 37 ●). Firmly immobilize the trachea in a midline position with one (the nondominant) hand and move your fingers apart to stretch the skin and permit easier insertion. Firmly grasp the device with the other hand and insert it in accordance with the manufacturer's instructions.

It is likely that cricothyrotomy device insertion will cause moderate hemorrhage around the insertion site. This can usually be controlled by moderate direct pressure; however, do not attempt to control bleeding until ventilations are effective. Improper device placement will increase the pressure necessary to ventilate and may result in air driven into the subcutaneous tissue (subcutaneous emphysema).

Ventilate the patient with a bag-valve mask connected to the tube and seal the wound area with sterile dressings as necessary. You may have to close the patient's mouth and nose or otherwise seal the upper airway opening to ensure that the air reaches the lungs. If the airway obstruction is partial, open the mouth and nose during expiration to enhance outward airflow, especially when using cricothyrotomy.

Breathing

Adequate ventilation becomes extremely critical with head injury patients. Not only is reduced air exchange a frequent problem, but excessive air exchange and the excessive depletion of carbon dioxide can also endanger the patient. Providing carefully monitored supplemental oxygenation and appropriate ventilation are essential with such patients.

Oxygenation

Any patient who has sustained a significant head injury or who displays any indication of lowered level of consciousness, orientation, or arousal is a candidate for oxygen administration. If a patient displays an oxygen saturation of less than 96 percent, administer oxygen titrated carefully to maintain at least 96 percent saturation. If the patient is not breathing adequately, supplement any positive-pressure ventilations with oxygen via reservoir, flowing at a rate to obtain an oxygen saturation of at least 96 percent.

Ventilations

Provision of a good supply of oxygen is critical to the head injury patient, but so too is the removal of carbon dioxide. Hyperventilation removes too much carbon dioxide and causes profound cerebral vasoconstriction and reduced cerebral perfusion. Hyperventilation also may increase intrathoracic pressure, thereby decreasing venous return and the effectiveness of circulation. Hypoventilation increases the circulating CO_2 levels, causing cerebral vasodilation and an increase in ICP. Either condition can be very dangerous for the head injury patient. Use both capnography and pulse oximetry to guide your ventilations and oxygen administration.

Assess the patient's respiratory status and, if the patient is not moving a normal volume of air, ventilate. Ventilations for the serious head injury patient (GCS = 8) are guided by capnography. For the head injury patient without signs of herniation, adjust ventilation rates to maintain an end-tidal CO_2 reading of between 35 and 40 mmHg (adults at about 10 breaths per minute, children at about 20 breaths per minute, and infants at about 25 breaths per minute). For patients with signs of herniation (declining level of consciousness, increasing blood pressure, decreasing heart rate, and irregular respirations), the capnography reading should range between 30 and 35 mmHg, using ventilation rates about 10 breaths per minute faster than for patients without herniation (guided by capnography). Also ensure the oxygen saturation level is at least 96 percent for any serious head injury patient.

If your patient is breathing on his own yet not moving an adequate volume of air and not maintaining an oxygen saturation of 96 percent or greater, try to synchronize any ventilation to his own breathing efforts. However, it may be preferable to paralyze the patient, as their fighting ventilations may increase ICP.

Circulation

Your care of the head, facial, neck, and spinal column injury patient includes both control of any serious hemorrhage and support of the body's attempts to maintain blood pressure and cerebral circulation. Research clearly demonstrates that any period of hypotension adversely affects the outcome of patients with traumatic brain injury.

Hemorrhage Control

Head and facial hemorrhage is usually easy to control because most of these injuries are to the tissues that lie over facial and cranial bones. Direct pressure is commonly an effective means of controlling such bleeding, though you should take care not to put pressure directly on suspected skull or facial fractures. Wrap bandaging circumferentially, but be careful to keep the airway clear and give the patient the freedom to rid himself of vomitus should emesis occur. Watch the airway and be prepared to suction aggressively to limit danger from aspiration. Suctioning can also ensure that a patient does not swallow large blood volumes, stimulating emesis. Permit the conscious and alert patient with no suspected spinal injury who is suffering epistaxis to sit leaning forward, allowing the blood to drain. This positioning keeps blood from flowing down the pharynx and entering the esophagus. Moderate pressure applied to the side of the nose on either side of the nares, against the maxilla and medially, may compress the arteries feeding the medial nasal cavity and help control epistaxis.

An open neck injury may carry the risk of air entering the external jugular vein during strong inspiration, leading to cerebral embolism with stroke-like symptoms. Seal any open neck wound with an occlusive dressing held firmly in place by bandaging and tilt the patient's body—head down on a backboard or stretcher, if possible. Carefully evaluate any other open wounds for frothy blood suggestive of tracheal involvement, seal those wounds on three sides with occlusive dressings, and monitor respirations.

Blunt trauma to the neck may produce the equivalent of compartment syndrome. Fasciae in the region compartmentalize muscle and anatomic structures and permit pressures to rise with rapid edema or blood accumulation. Any sign of neck edema or hematoma is an indication for rapid transport. Monitor the patient's skin tension and level of consciousness while en route to the hospital.

Severe hemorrhage associated with open neck wounds can lead quickly to hypovolemia and shock. Control the blood loss by using a dressing and gloved fingers to apply direct pressure to the source of bleeding. You may have to maintain digital pressure throughout prehospital care because application of circumferential bandaging to apply direct pressure may restrict the airway and circulation.

IMMOBILIZATION OF THE SPINAL INJURY PATIENT

Spinal injury care steps (spinal precautions) performed during the primary assessment include moving the patient to the neutral, in-line position, maintaining that position with manual immobilization until the patient is fully immobilized by mechanical means, and applying the cervical collar once the neck assessment is complete. The remaining steps in spinal injury patient management are related to maintaining the neutral, in-line position while moving the patient to the long spine board or orthopedic stretcher and then firmly securing him for transport to the hospital. Spinal immobilization can be very uncomfortable for the patient and can make airway maintenance more difficult. Furthermore, an unstable spinal injury occurs very infrequently. Employ full spinal precautions only when the patient cannot be cleared by your spinal clearance protocol.

These skills have but one major objective: maintaining the neutral, in-line position. Although this might seem a simple objective, it is not. Remember that the spine is a chain of 24 small bones, which are attached to other skeletal structures only at the base of the head, posterior thorax, and superior border of the posterior pelvis. These skeletal attachments may transmit forces that may flex, extend, rotate, compress, distract, and laterally bend the spine during any patient movement. The procedures and devices discussed in the following text are intended to ensure that the patient remains in the neutral, in-line position throughout assessment, care, movement, and transport.

Constantly calm and reassure a patient with suspected spinal injury. Spinal injury can produce extreme anxiety in patients because of the severity of its effects and their potentially lifelong implications. Application of spinal precautions can compound this anxiety. The patient must endure complete immobilization on a rigid and relatively uncomfortable device, the long spine board. He will be unable to move and protect himself during the processes of immobilization, assessment, care, and transport to the hospital. To alleviate some anxiety, be sure to communicate frequently with the patient. Tell the patient why you are employing spinal precautions and explain, in advance, what you will be doing in each step of the process. Do what you can to make the patient comfortable and to provide assurance that you and your team are caring for his needs.

Spinal Alignment

The first step in the spinal precautions process is to bring a patient from the position in which he is found into a neutral, in-line position adequate for assessment, airway maintenance, and spinal immobilization. This process involves moving an adult patient to the supine position with the head facing directly forward and elevated 1 to 2 inches above the ground. Remember that the spine curves in an "S" shape through its length. This leaves the head displaced forward when the posterior thorax and buttocks (supporting the pelvis) rest on a firm, flat surface. Also remember that the neutral position (also known as the position of function) is generally with the joints halfway between extremes of their motion. In spinal positioning, this means the hips and knees should be somewhat flexed for maximum comfort and minimum stress on the muscles, joints, and spine. For complete spinal immobilization, consider placement of a tightly rolled blanket under the knees.

It is also important to ensure that there are no distracting or compressing forces on the spine. If the patient is seated or standing, support the head in order to leave only a portion of the head's weight on the spine. Be careful not to lift the entire head as this places a distracting force on the cervical spine. Finally, bring the spine into line by aligning the nose, navel, and toes to ensure that there is no rotation along the spine's length. The head must face directly forward and the shoulders and pelvis must be in a single plane with the body. This neutral, in-line positioning allows for the greatest spacing between the cord and inner lumen of the spinal foramen. Neutral, in-line positioning both reduces pressure on the cord and increases circulation to and through it, an especially important consideration in the presence of injury. There are many techniques for moving and immobilizing the potential spine injury patient. Regardless of the technique you employ, always focus on obtaining and then maintaining neutral, in-line positioning. Doing this ensures the best opportunity to protect the patient's vertebral column and spinal cord during your time at his side.

The only contraindications to moving the potential spine injury patient from the position in which he is found to the neutral, in-line position are the following:

- When movement causes a significant increase in pain,
- When you meet with noticeable resistance during the procedure,

- When you identify an increase in neurologic signs as you move the head, or
- When the patient's spine is grossly deformed.

Both pain and resistance suggest that the alignment process may be moving the injury site and thus may be causing further injury. When you meet with resistance or increased pain during any positioning of the head or spine, immobilize the patient as found. The same rule applies when you note an increase in the signs of neurologic injury in the patient with movement of the spine. Finally, in cases of a severe deformity of the spine, do not move the patient because any movement may further compromise the spinal column and cord. Use whatever padding and immobilization devices are necessary to accommodate the patient's positioning and ensure that no further movement occurs.

Ensure that any patient movement during assessment or care is toward alignment. If, for example, the patient is lying twisted on the ground when you find him, first assess the exposed areas. Then, move the patient toward alignment. If the patient is found prone, assess the patient's posterior surfaces before you log roll him (to a long spine board) for further assessment and care. Never move a patient twice before you complete your mechanical immobilization, if possible.

Manual Cervical Immobilization

The typical trauma patient is found either seated (as in an auto) or lying on the ground. For the seated patient, initially approach from the front and carefully direct the patient not to move or turn his head. It is an almost reflexive act to turn to listen when we hear someone speak to us from behind. Such movement is dangerous for the potential spine injury patient. Ask the patient to keep his head immobile and explain that a provider is going to position himself behind him to immobilize the spine.

The assigned provider should then move behind the patient and bring his hands up along the patient's ears, using the little fingers to catch the mandible and the medial aspect of the heels of the hand to engage the mastoid region of the skull. Gentle pressure inward engages the head and prevents it from moving. A gentle lifting force of a few pounds helps take some of the head's weight off the cervical spine, but care should be taken not to lift the head or apply any traction to this critical region. The patient's head should then be moved slowly and easily to a position in which the eyes face directly forward and along a line central to and perpendicular to the shoulder plane.

If there is no access to the seated patient from behind, employ the same techniques of movement and immobilization from in front with the little fingers engaging the mastoid region while the heels of the hand support the mandible. When approaching from the patient's side, place one hand under the mandible while using the other to support the occiput.

If the patient is supine, support the head by placing your hands along the lateral and inferior surfaces of the head. Position the little fingers and heels of the hands just lateral to the skull's occipital region to support the head. With gentle inward pressure, hold the patient's head immobile and prevent flexion/extension, rotation, and lateral bending motion. Lift the head gently off the ground to approximately the neutral position, usually 1 to 3 inches for the adult. (If the surface on which the patient is found is not flat, adjust the height accordingly.) Position a small adult's or a large child's head at about ground level. Elevate the shoulders of infants or very small children because of their proportionally larger heads. Do not apply an axial pressure and do not pull the head toward or away from the body.

If a patient is found prone or on his side, position your hands according to the patient's position. If it will be some time until the patient can be moved to the supine position, place your hands so that they are comfortable during cervical immobilization. You should then reposition your hands just before the patient is moved to the final position. If it will be a short time until moving the patient to the supine position, place your hands so they will be properly positioned at the move's conclusion. This may involve initially twisting your hands into a relatively uncomfortable position.

Assessment, care, and patient movement may require the provider holding immobilization to reposition his hands. To accomplish this, another provider supports and immobilizes the patient's head and neck by bringing his hands in from an alternate position. This provider places one hand under the patient's occiput while the other hand holds the jaw. Once the head is stable, have the original provider reposition his hands, reassume immobilization, and then have the second provider remove his hands.

Cervical Collar Application

After a potential spinal injury patient has been manually immobilized, apply a cervical collar. The collar should be applied as soon as the neck is fully assessed, generally during the rapid trauma assessment. The cervical collar is only an adjunct to full cervical immobilization and should never be considered to provide significant immobilization by itself. The collar does limit cervical spine motion and reduce compression forces (axial loading), but it does not completely prevent flexion/extension, rotation, or lateral bending.

To apply a cervical collar, size it to the patient according to the manufacturer's recommendations. Position the device under the chin and against the chest. Contour it over the shoulders and secure it firmly behind the neck. Be sure the Velcro closures remain clear of sand, dirt, fabric, or the patient's hair and make a secure seal behind the neck. The collar should fit snugly around the neck but not place pressure against its anterior surface (carotid and jugular blood vessels and trachea). Be sure the mandible does not slip inside the collar. The collar should direct a limiting force against the jaw and occiput to restrict any flexion or extension of the head and neck. Ensure that the collar does not seriously limit the movement of the jaw, as this could prevent the patient from expelling vomitus. Once the cervical collar is in place, do not release or relax manual cervical immobilization until the patient is fully immobilized either with a vest-type immobilization device or to a long spine board or orthopedic stretcher with a cervical immobilization device.

Standing Takedown

Often at vehicle crash sites, you will find patients walking around when the mechanisms of injury suggest the potential for spinal injuries. If you cannot rule out spinal injury—a reliable reporter of spinal symptoms and no distracting injury (and the patient is not very young or old)—provide spinal precautions, even though they are found standing. The objective in such cases is to bring the patient to a fully supine position for further assessment, care, immobilization, and transport.

To accomplish this, employ a standing takedown procedure that maintains the spine in axial alignment. Have the patient remain immobile while a provider approaches from the rear and assumes manual cervical immobilization. Quickly assess any areas that will be covered by the cervical collar or long spine board. Apply a cervical collar and place a long spine board behind and against the patient, with the provider holding immobilization spreading his arms to accommodate the board. Position two other providers, one on each side of the spine board, and have each place a hand under the patient's axilla while they grasp the closest (preferably next highest) handhold on the board. The team should then move the upper patient and spine board backward, tilting the patient on his heels until the patient and board are supine (Figure 38 ●).

During the move, hand position in the handholds supports the axillae and thorax while the provider holding cervical immobilization rotates his hands against the patient's head without either flexing or extending the head and neck as the patient moves from standing to supine. During this maneuver, the hands holding the patient's head must move from grasping the mastoid and mandible (standing) to grasping the lateral occiput (supine). This is not easy, because the head must rotate while the provider's hands remain in the same relative position. As with all movement procedures, the provider at the patient's head should be in control and direct the process.

Once the patient and board are on the ground, continue to maintain manual immobilization while assessing and caring for the patient. Then provide mechanical immobilization to the long spine board before moving the patient to the ambulance.

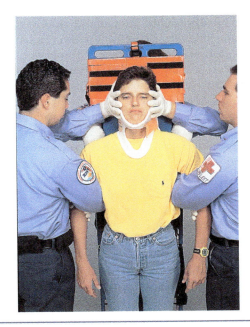

● **Figure 38**   The standing takedown.

287

Helmet Removal

Helmet use in contact sports, bicycling, skateboarding, in-line skating, and motorcycling has increased over the past decade. While these devices offer significant head protection during impact, they have not been proven to reduce spine injuries. Their use, in some cases, also complicates spinal injury care for prehospital providers. Many helmets are of the partial variety (such as those worn while bicycling and skateboarding) and are easy to remove at the scene. Some motorcycle and sports helmets, however, fully enclose the head and are very difficult to remove. These helmets are also difficult to secure to the spine board because of their spherical shapes. Furthermore, some full helmets do not hold the head firmly within. Thus, even fixing the helmet securely to the spine board does not result in effective cervical immobilization. Newer contact sport helmets contain air bladders that expand and firmly hold the head in position within the helmet. These helmets immobilize the head well, but they are still difficult to firmly secure to a spine board. Consequently, you must carefully evaluate full-enclosure helmets to determine if it would be in the patient's best interest to remove the helmet or leave it in place. Procedures considered acceptable for sport helmet removal vary among the athletic trainer community. Consult your local athletic trainers, sports medicine practitioners, and your system medical director.

The helmet must be removed if you find any of the following conditions:

- The helmet does not immobilize the patient's head within.
- The helmet cannot be immobilized to the long spine board.
- The helmet prevents airway care.
- The helmet prevents assessment of anticipated injuries.
- There is a current or anticipated airway or breathing problem.
- Helmet removal will not cause further injury.

During helmet removal, have a provider initially stabilize the cervical spine by manually immobilizing the helmet. Remove the face mask, if present, either by unscrewing it or by cutting it off, if possible. Remove or retract any eye protection or visor and unfasten or cut away any chin strap as well. Often sports trainers will have special equipment to remove the face guard. Be careful not to manipulate the helmet or otherwise transmit movement to the patient through the helmet. Then have another provider immobilize the head by sliding his hands under the helmet and placing them along the sides of the head, supporting the occiput, or by placing one hand on the jaw and the other on the occiput. This provider should choose hand placement that works best for him and can be accommodated by the helmet. The provider holding the helmet should then grasp the helmet and spread it slightly to clear the ears by pulling laterally just below and anterior to the ear enclosure. That provider then rotates the helmet to clear the chin, counter rotates it to clear the occiput, and then rotates it to clear the nose and brow ridge. The clearance is usually very tight with a well-fitted helmet.

Complete the previous procedure slowly and carefully to prevent head and neck motion and to minimize patient discomfort. For helmets with air bladders, use the same procedure, but empty the bladder after someone stabilizes the head and before you begin the removal. Helmet removal is a complicated skill that you must practice frequently before you can employ it successfully in the field.

MOVING THE SPINAL INJURY PATIENT

Once a patient with potential spinal injury has been assessed and immobilized, plan movement to a long spine board carefully. Recent design improvements in the orthopedic stretcher have made it a rigid movement device, effective in immobilizing the patient with potential spine injury.[9] It can now be considered an acceptable alternative to the long spine board. If any assessment step or patient care requires patient movement, consider moving the patient onto a long spine board. Movement techniques suitable for moving the spinal injury patient to the long spine board include the log roll, straddle slide, rope-sling slide, orthopedic stretcher lift, application of a vest-type device (or short spine board), and rapid extrication. Choose a technique that affords the least spinal movement for the conditions and equipment at hand. Also select your movement technique and adjust its steps to accommodate the patient's particular injuries and the care they prescribe.

A key factor in all movement techniques for the patient with potential spinal injury is the coordination of the move. It is essential that you move the patient as a unit with his head facing forward and in a plane with the shoulders and hips. This can best be accomplished if the provider at the head controls and directs the move. He is able to see other rescuers and has a focused and limited function (holding the head), which permits that person to evaluate what other providers are doing. The provider at the head directs the move by counting a cadence such as, "Move on four—one, two, three, four." A four-count is preferable because it gives the other providers a good opportunity to anticipate the actual start of movement. All moves must be slowly executed and well coordinated among providers.

Consider what the final patient positioning will be when you choose a spinal movement technique. Most spinal injury patients are best served with supine positioning on a long spine board. However, a patient with a thoracic spine injury is frequently placed in a prone position on a soft stretcher. With this patient, other positioning, such as supine on a firm spine board, puts pressure on the injury site from the body's weight and any movement is more likely to cause injury site motion and compound any damage.

Log Roll

The log roll can be used to rotate the patient 90 degrees, insert the long spine board, and then roll the patient back. It can also be used to roll the patient 180 degrees from prone to supine or vice versa.

As you begin the 90-degree roll, ensure manual spinal immobilization and apply a cervical collar. Notice that anatomically the shoulders are wider than the hips and legs. To provide a uniform roll, extend the patient's arm above his head. Then place a rolled bulky blanket between the legs (with its bulkiest portion between the feet) and tie the legs together. This reduces pelvic movement and lateral bending of the lumbar spine.

It takes four providers to properly perform the log roll for a spinal injury patient. One provider holds the head, while one kneels at the patient's shoulder with the knees tight against the patient's chest. A third provider kneels at the patient's hip with the knees tight against the patient's hip. The last provider kneels at the patient's knees with his knees tight against the patient's knees. If you only have three providers available for the move, the one at the knees is least critical to the move.

The providers reach across the patient and around the opposite shoulder, hip, and knee, respectively, and grasp the patient firmly. On a count initiated by the provider at the head, the team, in unison, rolls the patient against their knees and up to a 90-degree angle. With a free hand, the provider at the knees (or an additional provider) slides a long spine board under the patient from the patient's side or the foot end. The board should be positioned tightly against the patient so that the head, torso, and pelvis will eventually rest solidly on the board. Then, at the count of the provider at the head, the team rolls the patient back 90 degrees onto the board.

The 180-degree log roll begins with placement of the long spine board between the providers and the patient, with the board resting at an angle on the providers' thighs. The providers reach across the board and grasp the patient as for the 90-degree log roll. The provider at the head must be careful to anticipate the turning motion and position his hands so they will be comfortably positioned at the end of the roll. On the provider at the head's count, the team rolls the patient past 90 degrees until they are positioned against the tilted long spine board. Then the providers reposition their hands against the other (lower) side of the patient and slowly back their thighs out from under the patient until the board rests on the ground.

Straddle Slide

Another technique effective for moving the patient with potential spinal injury is the straddle slide. With this procedure, three providers are positioned at the patient's head, shoulders, and pelvis, while a fourth prepares to insert the long spine board from either the patient's head or feet. The provider at the head holds cervical immobilization and guides the lift with a cadence. A second provider straddles the patient (facing the patient's head) and grasps the shoulders. A third provider straddles the patient (facing the head) and grasps the pelvis. All providers keep their feet planted widely enough apart to permit insertion of the long spine board. At the direction of the provider at the head, the three providers lift the patient just enough to permit the fourth provider to negotiate the long spine board underneath the patient. (Note: If the board is to be inserted from the patient's feet, the provider inserting the board lifts the patient's feet with one hand and slides the board into place with the other.) On a signal from the provider at the head, the team gently lowers the patient to the long spine board.

Rope-Sling Slide

A continuous ring or length of thick rope or other material can be used to help slide a supine patient, using axial traction, onto a long spine board. One provider holds cervical immobilization from the side of the patient or with his feet spread far enough apart to accommodate the spine board. Another provider places the rope across the patient's chest and under his arms. The rope is tied together (with a cravat) behind the patient's neck and a long spine board is placed from the patient's head to contact his shoulders. The second provider positions himself at the head end of the spine board with the board resting on his thighs (this provides a small angle to more easily drag the patient onto the board). The second provider then pulls on the two strands of rope, guiding the patient onto the spine board as directed by the provider at the head. The provider holding cervical immobilization moves with the patient as he is moved onto the spine board. (The provider at the head may crouch or kneel to the patient's side to hold immobilization.) The provider at the head must be careful to move smoothly with the provider pulling axial traction. That person must ensure that the head moves with the body and does not pull against it.

Orthopedic Stretcher

The orthopedic stretcher, also known as the scoop stretcher, is a valuable device for positioning the patient on the spine board or helping to secure the patient to the long spine board.[9,10] Newer designs of this device are sufficiently rigid to provide spinal immobilization. To apply the device, lengthen it to accommodate the patient's height and then separate it into its two halves. Maintain cervical immobilization while you gently negotiate each half of the stretcher under the patient from the sides and connect them at the top, then bottom. Be careful not to pinch the patient's skin or body parts while positioning the stretcher, especially on uneven ground. It may be necessary to use your fingers, slid along the patient's body, to lift the shoulders and buttocks as the leaves of the stretcher are inserted. Once the device is connected, you may use the stretcher to lift the patient to the waiting spine board or immobilize the patient to the stretcher.

Vest-Type Immobilization Device (and Short Spine Board)

A specialized piece of EMS equipment that may be used with some spinal injury patients is the vest-type immobilization device. This device immobilizes the patient's head, shoulders, and pelvis to a rigid board so that you can move the patient from a seated position, as in an automobile, to a fully supine position. The vest-type device comes as a commercially made device that usually has the needed strapping already attached. The device is usually constructed of thin, rigid wood or plastic strips embedded in a vinyl or fabric vest. It is then wrapped and secured around the patient to provide immobilization. An alternative to the vest-type device is the short spine board, a cut-out piece of rigid plywood to which you attach strapping and padding. The basic principles of application are the same with both short-spine-board and vest-type devices. It is essential to be well practiced with both types of devices because in the multi- or mass-casualty incident the vest-type device may not be available in adequate numbers.

To apply the vest-type device, manually immobilize the patient's cervical spine and apply a cervical collar while the device is being readied for application. If the patient is positioned against a soft seat (as in an automobile), gently move the patient's shoulders and head a few inches forward to permit vest insertion. The provider holding cervical immobilization directs and coordinates the move while a second provider guides and controls shoulder motion. Place the device behind the patient by either inserting the head portion under and through the arms of the provider providing cervical immobilization, or angling it, base first, then moving it behind the patient's back. Position the device vertically so the chest appendages fit just under the arms. This positioning allows you to fasten the straps and secure the shoulders without any upward or downward device movement. First, secure the device to the chest and pelvis with strapping and ensure that the vest is immobile. Tighten the straps firmly, but be sure that they do not inhibit respiration. Secure the thigh straps as they hold the hips and thighs in the flexed position, limiting lumbar motion. Then fill the space between the occiput and the device with non-compressible padding to ensure neutral positioning. Secure both the brow ridge and chin to the device with straps, but be very careful to allow for vomiting by the patient and subsequent airway clearing or be prepared to release the chin strap immediately if vomiting occurs. Tie the patient's wrists together.

The vest-type immobilization device is not meant to lift the patient but rather to facilitate rotating him on the buttocks and then to tilt him to the supine position for further spinal immobilization. Once the patient is positioned on the long spine board, gently and carefully release the thigh straps and slowly and gently extend the hips and knees. If, after transfer to the spine board, the patient's head remains firmly affixed to the vest-type device, leave the vest on the patient and secure the vest to the long spine board since doing this effectively secures both head and torso. If the head becomes loose during the transfer, reapply manual cervical immobilization, secure the torso with strapping, and secure the head with a cervical immobilization device.

Rapid Extrication

Applying a vest-type immobilization device is a time-consuming process. Sometimes scene circumstances, either issues of scene safety or the need for rapid transport to a trauma center, preclude spending the time required for standard spinal immobilization. In such cases, use a rapid extrication procedure.[11,12]

With whatever personnel are available, stabilize the patient's spine, shoulders, pelvis, and legs with the patient's nose, navel, and toes kept in line. Ensure that providers are coordinated and understand what movement is to take place. One provider, usually at the patient's head, should direct the move, counting a cadence to permit the crew to work together (Figure 39 ●). Ensure that personnel involved in the extrication move the patient while maintaining patient alignment of the nose, navel, and toes. Then, on the leader's count, they should move the patient from a seated or other position to a waiting spine board.

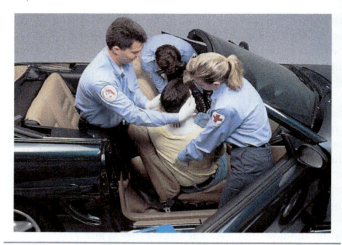

● **Figure 39** Rapid extrication of a patient with a spinal injury.

Remember the objectives of spinal movement and stabilization: Keep the spine in the neutral, in-line position by keeping the patient's eyes facing directly forward and keeping the shoulders and pelvis in a plane perpendicular to that of the gaze. Be sure to prevent any flexion/extension, rotation, or lateral bending.

While the rapid extrication technique does not provide maximum protection for the spine, it does permit rapid movement of the patient with a spinal injury when other considerations demand it. Use the procedure only when the patient is unstable and cannot afford the time it would take for normal spinal movement techniques. Rapid extrication from the confined space of a wrecked automobile is difficult at best. Plan your move carefully and execute rapid extrication by carefully explaining the process and individual responsibilities to your team members.

Final Patient Positioning

Once the patient is on the long spine board, consider positioning for proper mechanical immobilization. Centering the patient on the board is essential to ensuring that the patient's spine remains in-line and he is effectively immobilized. Accomplish this by placing team members at the patient's head, shoulders, pelvis, and feet. The providers then place one hand on each side of the patient and prepare to move the patient toward the board's centerline. On a cadence signaled by the provider at the head, they slide the portion of the patient that is out of alignment to an in-line position, centered on the long spine board.

Long Spine Board

The long spine board is simply a reinforced flat, firm surface designed to facilitate patient immobilization in a supine or prone position. While the board may immobilize patients with multisystem trauma, pelvic and lower limb fractures, and many other types of trauma, it is primarily designed for patients with spine injuries. The board has several hand and strap holes along its lateral borders for lifting and to ensure effective strapping and patient immobilization. Using nylon web strapping, you can immobilize a patient with almost any combination of injuries to the board firmly enough to permit rotating the patient and board 90 degrees to clear the airway in case of vomiting.

Secure the patient to the board with the strapping, immobilizing and holding the shoulders and pelvis firmly to the board. Such strapping may cross the body and capture the shoulder and pelvic girdles. Ensure that you firmly immobilize the patient to prevent lateral motion as well as cephalad (headward) and caudad (tailward) motion. Be sure that the pressure created by strapping does not come to bear on the central abdomen. That would cause forced extension of the lumbar spine. Immobilize the lower legs and feet with strapping or cravats. Tie the legs together and place a rolled blanket under the patient's knees to immobilize them in a somewhat flexed position. Once you have firmly immobilized the patient's body to the board, you can move on to immobilizing the head.

Long spine board immobilization is made more effective by use of the cervical immobilization device (CID). This device is made up of two soft, padded, lateral pieces that bracket the patient's head, maintaining its position, and a base plate that permits you to easily secure the device to the board. The base plate is affixed to the long spine board before the patient is moved to it. Once you position the patient on the board, fill the void between the occiput and the CID base plate with firm, non-compressible padding. Use limited or no padding for the small adult or older child, and pad the shoulders in the very young child or infant to ensure proper spinal positioning. While a provider maintains manual head immobilization, bring the lateral CID components against the sides of the patient's head. Use medial pressure to hold them against the head and keep the head in position. Then affix the lateral CID components to the Velcro of the CID base plate. Secure the head in position and to the long spine board using forehead and chin straps or tape. Make sure the strapping catches the brow ridge and the mandible or the upper portion of the collar. The properly secured CID must hold the patient's head in the neutral position without movement while not placing undue pressure on the neck or restricting jaw movement (in case of vomiting). Be careful that the straps do not flex, extend, or rotate the head. This procedure results in quick and effective immobilization of the head. Bulky blanket rolls, placed on each side of the head and secured both to the head and the board, will also effectively immobilize the head to the long spine board.

While the long spine board is almost universally accepted for spinal immobilization, it does have drawbacks. The use of a long spineboard in the immobilization of the potentially spine injured patient is likely to cause respiratory compromise, pain, and, in some cases, pressure sores (when applied for more than 30 minutes). Because of its firm surface, the long board places extreme pressure on the skin and tissues covering the ischial tuberosities (the pelvic protuberances we sit on) and the shoulder blades.

The board also tends to encourage providers to immobilize the patient directly to it in a non-neutral position. In a proper neutral position, the head should be elevated about 1 to 3 inches above the board's surface and the knees should be bent at 15 to 30 degrees. This positioning relieves pressure on the cervical spine, lumbar spine, hips, and knees and increases patient

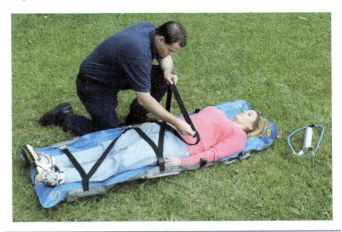

● **Figure 40** A full-body vacuum mattress can adequately immobilize the spine injury patient.

comfort. You can obtain proper knee positioning by placing folded or rolled blankets under the patient's knees. You can also increase patient comfort by placing some padding under the curves of the back. Do not overpad; just fill the voids at the small of the back and neck with bulky soft dressing material.

Research is demonstrating that carefully sliding or log rolling the patient from a long spine board to a stretcher can afford adequate spinal immobilization for transport to the hospital. In the future, the use of the rigid long spineboard may be limited to extrication and transport from where the victim is found to where a stretcher can be placed at the scene. As always, consult with your protocols and medical direction regarding long spineboard use.

A device that is now showing merit for spinal immobilization is the full-body vacuum mattress (Figure 40 ●), also known as a full-body vacuum splint.[13] The full-body vacuum mattress uses small plastic beads that maintain their position in the reduced pressure after air is evacuated from the splint. To apply the vacuum mattress, place the patient on the device and shape it around him. Evacuating the air causes the device to form to the contours of the patient's body and maintain immobilization. It is more difficult to position the patient in the vacuum mattress than on a long spine board, but use of this device can adequately immobilize the spine injury patient.

Diving Injury Immobilization

Patients injured in shallow water dives are often paralyzed from the impact. They must rely on others to protect their airway and remove them from the water. When carried out by untrained bystanders, however, these activities may compound any spinal injury. If you are present when such an incident occurs, be sure to carefully control any patient motion while he is still in the water. If necessary, turn the patient to a supine position, ensuring that the nose, navel, and toes remain in a single plane and that the eyes face directly forward. You can accomplish this by sandwiching the patient's chest between your forearms while your arms and shoulders cradle the head. Once the patient is in the supine position, water provides neutral buoyancy and, if the water is calm, helps to immobilize the patient. Move the patient by pulling on the shoulders while you cradle the head, in the neutral position, with the forearms. Float a long spine board under the patient, strap him firmly to the board, and then lift and carry him from the water.

MEDICATIONS

Several medications, including oxygen, may be useful in the care of the head injury patient. Other medications that may be useful for patients with central nervous system injury include diuretics (furosemide), paralytics (succinylcholine, atracurium, vecuronium), sedatives (diazepam, lorazepam, etomidate, midazolam, morphine, fentanyl), atropine, dextrose, and thiamine.

Oxygen

Oxygen is essential in the care of patients with suspected head, face, neck, and spinal column injury. When needed, administration of supplemental oxygen increases the inspired oxygen level and facilitates both diffusion through the alveolar and capillary walls and efficient oxygen uptake by the hemoglobin of the red blood cells. Oxygen saturation is important for the head injury patient because the brain is acutely dependent on a good oxygen supply. It is well established that hypoxia in the traumatic brain injury greatly increases morbidity and mortality. However, recent research is revealing that routine oxygen administration may have some negative effects if the patient becomes hyperoxic. This is causing us to guide our oxygen administration by observing oxygen saturation, aiming for normal oxygen levels (neither hypoxic nor hyperoxic). It appears that if a patient is adequately saturating hemoglobin on his own, there is no need for supplemental oxygen.

Administer supplemental oxygen to maintain an oxygen saturation (SpO_2) of greater than 96 percent. Titrate the oxygen flow via a nasal cannula or nonrebreather mask as needed for the patient who is breathing adequately and has an oxygen saturation at or below 96 percent. Also monitor skin color, respiratory excursion, orientation, and anxiety to ensure the patient is well oxygenated. If the patient is receiving positive-pressure ventilations, supplement the ventilations with 15 liters per minute of oxygen flowing into the reservoir if saturation is at or below 96 percent. Continue to monitor oxygen administration using the pulse oximeter, and keep the saturation level above 96 percent.

TRANSPORT CONSIDERATIONS

There are special considerations to observe when transporting the patient with serious head injury to the hospital. Some suggest that the use of red lights, siren, rough ride (high speed), and other patient stimulation may agitate the patient, increase intracranial pressure, and induce seizures. While there is little evidence to support this claim, it is probably prudent to reduce speed and use red lights and siren sparingly.

Be cautious in considering head injury patients as candidates for air medical service transport. While the time saved by helicopter transport may be very important, the head injury patient is prone to seizures, especially with physical stimulation (noise and vibration) associated with this mode of transport. Seizures aboard any type of aircraft are very dangerous. If you elect to transport by air, ensure that the patient is firmly secured to a long spine board (including feet and hands) and that his airway is protected by endotracheal intubation.

EMOTIONAL SUPPORT

Identify someone to remain with the patient with the specific role of calming and reassuring him during care and transport. Have that care provider continuously reorient the patient to his environment. Remember, head injury patients may have trouble remembering events preceding and immediately following the incident as well as have difficulty laying down short-term memory. The person assigned this role should describe what happened to the patient and help the patient remain oriented to his current location and what is happening. This simple step aids greatly in reducing the patient's anxiety and in helping to return to a normal level of orientation.

Head injury patients may be very confused, distressed, abusive, or even combative. Do not take their behavior personally. Maintain a professional demeanor and provide emotional support during assessment, care, and transport.

SPECIAL INJURY CARE

There are certain types of head, face, and neck trauma that deserve special care. They include scalp avulsion, injury to the pinna of the ear, eye injury, dislodged teeth, and impaled objects.

Scalp Avulsion

Avulsion occurs when a glancing blow tears the scalp's border and releases a flap of scalp. The flap may remain in anatomic position, fold back exposing the cranium, or may be torn completely free. If the avulsion uncovers the cranium, cover both the open wound and the undersurface of the exposed scalp flap with a large bulky dressing. Also place padding under the fold of the scalp to prevent a sharp kinking along its border. If the region is seriously contaminated, remove gross contamination and rinse the area with normal saline before applying dressings. Scalp avulsions tend to heal very well unless grossly contaminated or when circulation to the flap is severely disrupted.

Pinna Injury

Serious injury to the pinna, or exposed portion of the ear, often results from glancing blows and trauma, like a tearing or avulsion injury. Such an injury is best treated by placing the pinna in as close to its anatomic position as possible. Then place a dressing between the head and medial surface of the injured ear and cover the exposed ear with a sterile dressing. Finally, bandage the dressed injury firmly to the head.

Eye Injury

Care for eye injuries involves careful assessment and protective care. Most eye wounds or injuries are best cared for by applying soft dressings to cover the closed, injured eye. In cases of severe eye injury, the other eye, even if uninjured, is also dressed and the dressings on both eyes are held in place with gentle bandaging. This technique prevents sympathetic motion (one eye moving with the other), which may cause additional damage to the injured eye. (It is not necessary to cover the uninjured eye in cases of mild to moderate injury to the other eye.) If the eye injury is an open wound or torn eyelid, consider using a sterile dressing soaked in normal saline to reduce the pain and discomfort and prevent evaporative loss of lacrimal fluid. Local cooling may serve to reduce edema and pain. Place the patient in the supine position if other injuries do not prevent it.

If the patient complains of eye pain without apparent injury, suspect corneal abrasion or laceration, possibly caused by an object embedded in the conjunctiva or sclera. Gently invert the eyelid and examine the inside of the lid for any small embedded object. If you observe one, you may attempt to remove it with a saline-moistened cotton swab. Avoid trying to remove an object on the cornea, as you may cause more damage. Even if you successfully remove the object from the inside of the lid, the patient is likely to continue reporting pain and the sensation of a foreign body still in place. Cover the affected eye with soft dressings and loose bandaging.

If the eye is contaminated by the residue from an air bag or other material, consider irrigation. Place a nasal cannula with one prong pointing into each side of the nose and into the corners of the eyes. Run a liter or two to rinse material from the eye. Turn the head (if not contraindicated) if a single eye is involved to permit a freer flow of the fluid and contaminated material away from the eye. The Morgan lens may make this flushing more effective. The lens—which is a concave, soft plastic device—is gently placed on the eye's surface. Saline solution runs through a small outlet and flows outward from the center of the lens.

If an eye is avulsed or has an impaled object in it, cover the eye and object with a cup or other protective material and again dress and bandage both eyes. If the patient is combative or has a significantly reduced level of consciousness, secure his hands together and then to his waist or belt. This prevents accidental dislodging of the protective dressing and possible aggravation of the eye injury.

Eye injuries and the loss of eyesight in one or both eyes will create anxiety in most patients. Be sure to calm and reassure the patient and explain in advance your actions as you move the patient from the scene to the ambulance and to the hospital.

If, during the assessment, you observe that the patient is wearing contact lenses and there is any risk that he may become unresponsive, have the patient remove the lenses. If the patient is already unresponsive, try removing the lenses yourself with a contact removal suction cup. This miniature suction cup seals against the contact lens and allows easy removal. Alternatively, lift the eyelid, which may cause the lens to dislodge, or, with the eye closed, gently push the lens into the corner of the eye.

Dislodged Teeth

Locate any teeth that may have been dislodged by trauma and transport them to the hospital with the patient. Rinse the teeth in normal saline and place them in an approved tooth preservative solution. If tooth preservative solution is not available, wrap them in saline-soaked gauze for transport to the emergency department. If a tooth is largely intact, it may be successfully replanted.

Impaled Objects

Any object impaled in the head, face, or neck should be left in place and dressed and bandaged to ensure that it does not move about during care and transport. Use bulky dressings to stabilize the object. Secure the patient's hands if there is a danger that he may dislodge the object. Only if the object obstructs or seriously threatens the airway should you consider its removal. In such cases, removal will likely increase the associated hemorrhage and possibly damage adjoining structures, but the patency of the airway is absolutely essential.

Removal of objects that pass through the patient's cheek pose the least danger for removal. With such a wound, you have ready access to both of its sides, and the wound involves no critical structures or organs. Nevertheless, expect increased hemorrhage from the wound, have dressings ready, and be prepared to apply direct pressure as soon as the object is removed.

SUMMARY

The head, face, neck, and spinal column contain very special and important structures—key elements of the central nervous system, the airway, the alimentary canal, and major organs of sensation. Serious trauma to the region endangers these structures and demands special assessment and care. During the scene size-up, identify possible mechanisms of injury and the injuries they suggest. If a MOI suggests spine injury, provide spinal precautions unless you have a reliable reporter (fully conscious and alert, without any intoxication or distracting injury, not elderly or very young) and without any spinal cord injury signs. Establish a general patient impression and his level of consciousness and orientation early. Ensure the airway is clear and protected from aspiration and physical obstruction. Administer high-concentration oxygen, titrated to oxygen saturation and ventilate, as necessary, being careful not to under- or overventilate the patient. Guide ventilation by capnography. Secure rapid transport for the patient with possible intracranial hemorrhage or serious lesion.

Once the central nervous system, the airway, and breathing are protected, address skeletal structure fractures, minor bleeding, and open wounds. Provide complete immobilization for the potential spine injury patient and careful movement. During all your care for the patient with injury to the head, face, neck, or spinal column, provide emotional support and help orient the patient to what happened, to where he is, and to what will be happening during prehospital care.

YOU MAKE THE CALL

You are called to a scene where a young woman, in an attempt to end her life, has deeply lacerated her anterior and lateral neck. The wound is deep and produces severe flowing hemorrhage with bubbling on expiration. She also has blood gurgling and spattering from her mouth with expiration.

1. What structures are most likely injured?

2. What care would you employ?

3. What are serious life threats associated with this injury?

See Suggested Responses at the back of this chapter.

REVIEW QUESTIONS

1. Retroauricular ecchymosis over the mastoid bone, indicating a basilar skull fracture, is called _____.
   a. Battle's sign
   b. raccoon eye
   c. Goblet's sign
   d. periorbital ecchymosis

2. Battle's sign and raccoon eyes indicate _____.
   a. tension pneumothorax
   b. basilar skull fracture
   c. abdominal injury
   d. impending shock

3. A sight-threatening injury, involving hemorrhage into the anterior chamber pools, is known as _____.
   a. ecchymosis
   b. blepharospasm
   c. erythema
   d. hyphema

4. Your patient has been involved in serious trauma and has received an open wound to the neck and blood vessels. Your concern should be directed toward the danger of exsanguination and _____.
   a. pulmonary edema
   b. tension pneumothorax
   c. air embolism
   d. subcutaneous emphysema

5. Sudden painless loss of sight in one eye is most generally associated with _____.
   a. ocular trauma
   b. acute retinal artery occlusion
   c. retinal detachment
   d. increasing intracranial pressure

6. A classic sign of increasing intracranial pressure, which includes slowing pulse, increasing systolic blood pressure, and irregular respirations, is referred to as _____.
   a. Cheyne-Stokes
   b. Cushing's triad
   c. Kernig's sign
   d. medullary syndrome

7. The connective tissue sheet covering the superior aspect of the cranium is called the galea _____.
   a. pericranium
   b. periosteum
   c. aponeurotica
   d. subaponeurotica

8. The most common sites of axial loading for lifting injuries and heel-first falls are located between _____.
   a. T-12 and L-2
   b. C-1 and C-7
   c. C-5 and T-4
   d. L-3 and L-5

9. Your patient has presented with a facial injury secondary to blunt trauma. You note left facial abrasions and lacerations, depression over the prominence of the left cheek, diminished movement of the left ocular muscles, and diplopia. This injury pattern is consistent with _____.
   a. Le Fort I fracture
   b. mandibular dislocation
   c. basilar skull fracture
   d. orbital fracture

10. All of the following are primary functions of the intervertebral discs except _____.
   a. limiting bone wear
   b. absorbing shock
   c. accommodating motion of adjacent vertebrae
   d. elevating the diaphragm during inspiratory efforts

11. The major weight-bearing component of a vertebra is the _____.
   a. pedicle
   c. vertebral body
   b. laminae
   d. spinal canal

12. Which of the following statements regarding cervical collars is true?
   a. They serve as an adjunct to full cervical immobilization.
   b. They serve to accentuate axial loading and prevent flexion/extension.
   c. They serve to immobilize the cervical, thoracic, and lumbar spine.
   d. They serve to prevent axial loading when utilized before manual stabilization.

13. Which of the following articulates with the ribs and serves as the site for muscle attachment?
   a. spinous process
   b. vertebral pedicle
   c. intervertebral disc
   d. transverse process

See Answers to Review Questions at the back of this v.

REFERENCES

1. Trafton, P. G. "Spinal Cord Injuries." *Surg Clin North Am* 62(1) (Feb 1982): 61–72. [Medline]

2. Biros, M. and W. Heegaard. "Head Injury." *Rosen's Emergency Medicine: Concepts and Clinical Practice.* 7th ed. St. Louis: Mosby, 2009.

3. Kirsch, T. and C. Lipinski. "Head Injury." *Emergency Medicine: A Comprehensive Study Guide.* 7th ed. New York: McGraw-Hill, 2008.

4. Rasouli, M. R., et al. "Preventing Motor Vehicle Crashes Related Spine Injuries in Children." *World J Pediatr* 7(4) (Nov 2011): 311–317.

5. Dula, D. J. "The Ring Sign: Is It a Reliable Indicator for Cerebral Spinal Fluid?" *Ann Emerg Med* 22(4) (Apr 1993): 718–720.

6. Ray, A. M. "Halo Sign Is Neither Sensitive nor Specific for Cerebrospinal Fluid Leak." *Ann Emerg Med* 53(2) (Feb 2009): 288.

7. Pimentel, L. and L. Diegelmann. "Evaluation and Management of Acute Cervical Spine Trauma." *Emerg Med Clin North Am* 28(4) (Nov 2010): 719–738.

8. El-Orbany, M. and L. A. Connolly. "Rapid Sequence Induction and Intubation: Current Controversy." *Anesth Analg* 110(5) (May 2010): 1318–1325.

9. Del Rossi, G., G. R. Rechtine, B. P. Conrad, and M. Horodyski. "Are Scoop Stretchers Suitable for Use on Spine-Injured Patients?" *Am J Emerg Med* 28(7) (Sep 2010): 751–756.

10. Krell, J. M., et. al. "Comparison of the Ferno Scoop Stretcher with the Long Backboard for Spinal Immobilization." *Prehosp Emerg Care* 10 (2006): 46–51.

11. Brown, J. B., et al. "Prehospital Spinal Immobilization Does Not Appear to Be Beneficial and May Complicate Care following Gunshot Injury to the Torso." *J Trauma* 67(4) (Oct 2009): 744–748.

12. Haut, E. R., et al. "Spine Immobilization in Penetrating Trauma: More Harm than Good?" *J Trauma* 68(1) (Jan 2010): 115–120.

13. Johnson, D. R., M. Hauswald, and C. Stockhoff. "Comparison of a Vacuum Splint Device to Rigid Backboard for Spinal Immobilization." *Amer J Emerg Med* 14 (1996): 369–372.

FURTHER READING

American College of Surgeons, Committee on Trauma. *Advanced Trauma Life Support Course: Student Manual.* 8th ed. Chicago: American College of Surgeons, 2008.

Bates, Barbara, and Peter G. Szilagyi. *A Guide to Physical Examination and History Taking.* 9th ed. Philadelphia: J. B. Lippincott, 2007.

Bledsoe, B. E. and D. Clayden. *Prehospital Emergency Pharmacology.* 7th ed. Upper Saddle River, NJ: Pearson/Prentice Hall, 2011.

Bledsoe, B. E., B. J. Colbert, and J. E. Ankney. *Essentials of A & P for Emergency Care.* Upper Saddle River, NJ: Pearson/Prentice Hall, 2010.

Campbell, John E. *International Trauma Life Support for Emergency Care Providers.* Upper Saddle River, NJ: Pearson/Prentice Hall, 2011.

Martini, Frederic. *Fundamentals of Anatomy and Physiology.* 9th ed. San Francisco: Benjamin Cummings, 2011.

Rosen, P., and R. Barkin, eds. *Emergency Medicine: Concepts and Clinical Practice.* 7th ed. St. Louis: Mosby, 2009.

Tintinalli, J. E., ed. *Emergency Medicine: A Comprehensive Study Guide.* 7th ed. New York: McGraw-Hill, 2011.

SUGGESTED RESPONSES TO "YOU MAKE THE CALL"

The following are suggested responses to the "You Make the Call" scenarios presented in this chapter. Each represents an acceptable response to the scenario but should not be interpreted as the only correct response.

1. *What structures are most likely injured?*

The bubbling with expiration indicates her trachea has been perforated along with several major vessels in the neck.

2. *What care would you employ?*

Immediately cover the bleeding areas with occlusive dressings and attempt to control the hemorrhage. An ET tube could be placed into the trachea through the neck if the wound is large enough; otherwise, securing her airway with a conventional ET tube would be acceptable.

3. *What are serious life threats associated with this injury?*

The serious life threats include airway compromise, air embolus to the brain, and hemorrhagic shock.

ANSWERS TO REVIEW QUESTIONS

1. a
2. b
3. d
4. c
5. b
6. b
7. c

8. a
9. d
10. d
11. c
12. a
13. d

GLOSSARY

acute retinal artery occlusion   a nontraumatic occlusion of the retinal artery resulting in a sudden, painless loss of vision in one eye.

ankylosing spondylitis   a form of inflammatory arthritis that causes inflammation of the joints between the vertebrae of the spine and the sacroiliac joints in the pelvis and may also cause inflammation and pain in other parts of the body.

aqueous humor   clear fluid filling the anterior chamber of the eye.

bamboo spine   development of bony bridges between vertebrae, causing the spine to become stiff and inflexible, effectively fusing the spine.

bilateral periorbital ecchymosis   black-and-blue discoloration of the area surrounding the eyes. It is usually associated with basilar skull fracture. (Also called raccoon eyes.)

cervical vertebrae   the seven vertebrae that form the top of the vertebral column, supporting the neck.

coccyx   small bone, formed from four fused vertebrae, that lies below the sacrum at the base of the vertebral column.

conjunctiva   mucous membrane that lines the eyelids.

cornea   thin, delicate layer covering the pupil and the iris.

cranium   vault-like portion of the skull encasing the brain.

diplopia   double vision.

galea aponeurotica   connective tissue sheet covering the superior aspect of the cranium.

hyphema   blood in the anterior chamber of the eye, in front of the iris.

intracranial pressure (ICP)   pressure exerted on the brain by the blood and cerebrospinal fluid.

iris   pigmented portion of the eye. It is the muscular area that constricts or dilates to change the size of the pupil.

kyphosis   exaggerated convectivity in the curvature of the thoracic spine as viewed from the side.

lacrimal fluid   liquid that lubricates the eye.

Le Fort criteria   classification system for fractures involving the maxilla.

lumbar vertebrae   the five vertebrae that lie between the thoracic vertebrae and the sacrum, helping to support the lower back.

mandible   the jawbone.

maxilla   bone of the upper jaw.

nares   the openings of the nostrils.

orbit   the eye socket.

pinna   outer, visible portion of the ear.

pupil   dark opening in the center of the iris through which light enters the eye.

retina   light- and color-sensing tissue lining the posterior chamber of the eye.

retinal detachment   condition that may be of traumatic origin and presents with patient complaint of a dark curtain obstructing a portion of the field of view.

retroauricular ecchymosis   black-and-blue discoloration over the mastoid process (just behind the ear) that is characteristic of a basilar skull fracture. (Also called Battle's sign.)

sacrum   triangular bone, formed from five fused vertebrae, that lies between the fifth lumbar vertebra and the coccyx.

sclera   the "white" of the eye.

scoliosis   lateral deviation of the normally straight vertical line of the spine.

semicircular canals   the three rings of the inner ear. They sense the motion of the head and provide positional sense for the body.

spinal canal   opening in the vertebrae that accommodates the spinal cord; also called the vertebral foramen.

spinal clearance protocol   set of criteria for discontinuing spinal precautions.

sutures   pseudojoints that join the various bones of the skull to form the cranium.

thoracic vertebrae   the 12 vertebrae that lie between the cervical and lumbar vertebrae, helping to support the thorax.

vertebra   one of 33 bones making up the vertebral column.

vertebral column   the main support for the axis of the body, consisting of 33 bones (vertebrae); also called the spinal column.

vertebral foramen   *see* spinal canal.

vitreous humor   clear watery fluid filling the posterior chamber of the eye. It is responsible for giving the eye its spherical shape.

zygoma   the cheekbone.

Burn Trauma

Robert S. Porter, MA, EMT-P

STANDARD
Trauma (Soft-Tissue Trauma)

COMPETENCY
Integrates assessment findings with principles of epidemiology and pathophysiology to formulate a field impression to implement a comprehensive treatment/disposition plan for an acutely injured patient.

OBJECTIVES

Terminal Performance Objective
After reading this chapter you should be able to integrate knowledge of anatomy, physiology, pathophysiology, and treatment principles to assess and provide prehospital management for patients with burns.

Enabling Objectives
To accomplish the terminal performance objective, you should be able to:

1. Define key terms introduced in this chapter.
2. Describe the epidemiology of burn injuries.
3. Describe the anatomy and physiology of the skin.
4. Describe the pathophysiology and complications of:
    a. thermal burns.
    b. electrical burns.
    c. chemical burns.
    d. radiation injury.
    e. inhalation injury.
5. Demonstrate the assessment of patients with burn injuries, including particular attention to the patient's airway, and determination of burn depth and extent of body surface area involved.
6. Anticipate and take measures to minimize systemic complications of burns.
7. Recognize indications that burns may have resulted from abuse.
8. Identify patients whose burns are considered critical.
9. Given a variety of scenarios, develop management plans for patients with:
    a. thermal burns.
    b. inhalation injury, including suspicion of carbon monoxide and cyanide poisoning.
    c. electrical burns.
    d. chemical burns.
    e. radiation injuries.

KEY TERMS

alpha radiation

ampere

Baux score

beta radiation

blepharospasm

body surface area (BSA)

coagulation necrosis

current

denature

emergent phase

eschar

extravascular space

fluid shift phase

full thickness burn

gamma radiation

Gray

hypermetabolic phase

intravascular space

ionization

Jackson's theory of thermal
  wounds

Joule's law

liquefaction necrosis

neutron radiation

ohm

Ohm's law

partial thickness burn

rad

resistance

resolution phase

rule of nines

rule of palms

subglottic

superficial burn

supraglottic

voltage

zone of coagulation

zone of hyperemia

zone of statis

CASE STUDY

Ben and Ronny, Fire Rescue paramedics, respond with trucks 23 and 56 to a working structural fire. On arrival, they find two fire units already deployed, with firefighters engaging a wood frame home fully engulfed in flames. As Ronny positions their vehicle, she and Ben see the structure's south exterior wall collapsing on a firefighter. Within minutes, other firefighters extinguish the burning wall and free the firefighter. They also douse their comrade with water to extinguish any smoldering embers in contact with him and stop the burn process.

When firefighters have secured the scene, Ben and Ronny proceed to the patient and begin their primary assessment. The patient is a male who is lying supine with his turnout gear burned and charred in places, indicating that he has received serious burns. Because of the wall's collapse onto the firefighter, they provide manual in-line cervical immobilization while proceeding with assessment. The downed firefighter's respirations appear adequate, although he is coughing up sooty sputum and is slightly hoarse. The firefighter, who gives his name as Karl, is conscious and alert. His airway seems clear except for the hoarseness. However, the sooty sputum and hoarseness indicate possible airway burns, making Karl a priority for rapid transport.

Ben proceeds to perform the rapid trauma assessment. On removal of Karl's turnout gear, Ben exposes dark, discolored burns to the patient's posterior thorax and lower back as well as circumferential burns of the left upper extremity. Despite the burn severity, Karl denies much pain. Ben also finds angulation, false motion, and pain to the right forearm. Vital signs reveal normal breathing in terms of volume and rate and a strong, regular pulse at a rate of about 100. Distal pulses are also strong, and capillary refill is timed at 2 seconds. Karl is fully conscious and oriented and is joking about the incident.

The rescue crew now takes some initial care steps. Ben cuts away Karl's clothing and then covers the burn site with a dry, clean sheet and starts an IV line, running normal saline at a to-keep-open rate. Ronny applies oxygen via a nonrebreather mask and observes an oximetry reading of 97 percent. They package Karl and quickly load him into the ambulance for rapid transport. En route to the hospital, Ben checks Karl's blood pressure (120/88) and respirations (30 and shallow), noting that he displays increasing respiratory effort.

While Ronny is splinting the right upper limb, Karl begins to cough deeply and experiences severe dyspnea. The dyspnea progresses, and Karl's level of consciousness drops. Oxygen saturation falls to 86 percent. Ben begins to provide supplemental oxygen via a bag-valve mask, while Ronny prepares intubation equipment.

Medical direction orders the crew to intubate, and they attempt to do so during transport. The airway is edematous, and vocal cord visualization is difficult. After the first attempt, Ronny withdraws the tube when auscultation of breath sounds, failure to obtain chest rise, absent end-tidal CO_2 levels, and a dropping oxygen saturation indicate esophageal placement. Ben reventilates Karl using a bag-valve-mask device while Ronny prepares for another intubation attempt. She is again unsuccessful.

As they withdraw the tube, the ambulance arrives at the emergency department. The ED physician quickly views the airway and finds it severely swollen. She then decides to insert a Quick-trach into the cricothyroid membrane and attempts ventilation. The technique is successful. Karl begins spontaneous respirations and maintains a strong pulse. His level of consciousness does not improve, however, and the hospital staff transfers him to the burn unit for definitive care.

INTRODUCTION TO BURN TRAUMA

The incidence of burn injuries in the United States and other developed countries has been declining for several decades. Despite this decline, an estimated 450,000 Americans are treated for burns annually and 45,000 are hospitalized. Some 3 to 5 percent of these burns are considered life threatening. Persons at greatest risk for serious burns are the very young and old, the infirm, and workers, such as firefighters, metal smelters, and chemical workers, who are exposed to occupational combustion and chemical sources. Burn injuries remain the second leading cause of death in children under 12 years of age and the fourth overall cause of trauma death after vehicular crashes, penetrating trauma, and falls. Males account for 70 percent of burn mortality.[1]

Much of the national decline in burn mortality is attributed to improved building codes, safer construction techniques, sprinkler systems, and smoke detector use. Smaller but still important effects are attributed to educational campaigns aimed primarily at schoolchildren. Other simple and inexpensive measures that have helped prevent burns include keeping cigarette lighters and matches away from children and reducing household hot-water temperatures to below scalding levels. Half of all scald burns occur in children under five years old.[1] Merely adjusting the hot-water temperature to below 48.9°C (120°F) can prevent most scalding burns.

Burns are a specific subset of soft-tissue injuries with a specific pathologic process. While the term "burn" suggests combustion, the actual process producing burn injuries is much different. The human body is predominantly water and does not support combustion. Instead, body tissues change chemically, evaporating water and denaturing proteins that make up cell membranes. The result can be widespread damage to the skin, also known as the integumentary system.

To effectively assess and treat burns, you must have a good understanding of the structures and functions of the integumentary system as well as of thermal, chemical, electrical, and radiologic pathologies that may affect it. This understanding ensures that you can provide the best possible assessment and care for patients who sustain burn injuries.

ANATOMY AND PHYSIOLOGY OF THE SKIN

The skin is one of the largest, most important, and least appreciated human organs. Covering the entire body, the skin protects it from fluid loss and bacterial invasion. The skin also provides a massive surface for sensation and is a natural radiator for dissipating excess body heat. With all these functions, the skin still remains durable, flexible, and very able to repair itself.

Layers of the Skin

Skin comprises three layers of tissue: the epidermis, dermis, and subcutaneous tissue (Figure 1 ●). Together they form the body's outermost shell.

Epidermis

The first and outermost skin layer is the epidermis. It is an area of dying and dead cells being pushed outward by new cells growing from beneath. As these cells reach the surface, they abrade away during everyday activity. The constant movement outward provides a barrier that is difficult for bacteria and other pathogens to penetrate.

Glands beneath the epidermis secrete an oil called sebum. This oil coats the outer skin layers and makes the epidermis pliable. In addition, sebum provides a barrier to water and other fluid flow through the skin.

Dermis

Directly below the epidermis is a tissue layer called the dermis. It contains many different structures, including blood vessels, glands, and nerve endings. It is in this layer that sebaceous glands produce sebum and secrete it directly onto the skin's surface and into hair follicles. Sudoriferous glands in the dermis secrete sweat and direct it to the skin's surface. As water in sweat evaporates, passing air carries the vapor and associated heat energy away with it. The change of a fluid to a vapor (evaporation) is an efficient method of skin cooling. This process helps the body maintain a normal temperature

CONTENT REVIEW

► Layers of the Skin
  • Epidermis (outermost layer)
  • Dermis (layer beneath the epidermis)
  • Subcutaneous tissue (fatty layer beneath the dermis)

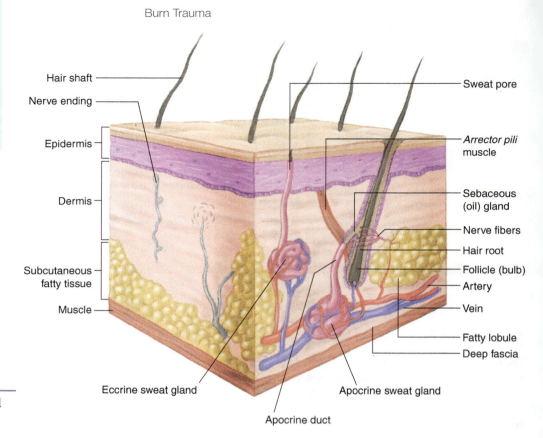

● Figure 1 The cross-sectional anatomy of the skin.

even when ambient temperatures are greater than 100°F (as long as evaporation is possible). The primary mechanism for maintaining body temperature uses the skin as a radiator of excess body heat. Warm blood from the body's core travels either through blood vessels in the dermis (close to the skin surface) or through the subcutaneous tissues.

Subcutaneous Tissue

Subcutaneous tissue, which is composed of adipose (fat) and connective tissues, serves as a stratum of insulation against both trauma and heat loss. Heat moves two to three times more slowly through adipose tissue than through muscle. When blood is directed to, and beneath, subcutaneous tissues, it takes longer for heat to move to the skin, the skin's surface cools, and heat loss slows. If warm core blood is directed to the dermis, skin temperature increases as does the rate of heat loss. This causes body cooling.

Underlying Structures

Although they are not part of the integument, it is important to identify the structures underneath the skin. These structures include the muscles and their thick, fibrous capsules of fascia, nerves, tendons, bones, and, of course, the vital organs such as the heart, lungs, and brain. Each of these structures is sensitive to the effects of thermal, chemical, electrical, and radiation injury.

Functions of the Skin

The skin varies in thickness from almost a centimeter on the heel of the foot to microscopic dimensions on the surface of the

eye. This durable container for the body provides a number of valuable functions:

● Skin protects the human body from infection by bacteria and other microorganisms.

● Skin functions as an organ of sensation, perceiving temperature, pressure (touch), and pain.

● Skin contains vital body fluids and controls their loss to the environment as well as the movement of fluids into the body when it is exposed to water or other fluids.

● Skin aids in temperature regulation through secretion of sweat and shunting of blood.

● Skin provides insulation from trauma.

● Skin is flexible to accommodate free body movement.

Although the skin and its functions are often taken for granted, burn injury can lead to severe fluid loss, infection, hypothermia, and death. Therefore, as a paramedic, you must be familiar with burn pathophysiology.

BURN PATHOPHYSIOLOGY

Burns result from protein disruption in the cell membranes. Burns can be caused by several different mechanisms including thermal, electrical, chemical, or radiation energies, as well as a combination of these. Being able to understand burn mechanisms and to determine the degree and area of a burn helps you assess the seriousness of the burn and thus guide your care.

Types of Burns

Soft-tissue burns can occur from thermal (heat), electrical, chemical, or radiation insults to the body. While the resulting burns are much the same, the damage process differs with the various mechanisms. The following sections describe each of these four types of burns.

Thermal Burns

A thermal burn causes damage by increasing the rate at which the molecules within an object move and collide with each other. Heat is a measure of the speed of the molecules that make up an object. The more rapidly molecules move and the more frequently they collide with one another, the greater the object's temperature. This phenomenon explains why, as we heat ice and increase the speed of its molecules, it changes character to become water and then steam. At absolute zero, the molecules within a substance are at rest. As the molecules begin to move, the object's temperature rises. If an object feels cool, it is because the object has less of this molecular movement (and temperature) than you do. If an object feels warm, it is because its molecules have greater movement (and temperature) than you do. If you contact something hotter than you, its molecular movement is transferred rapidly to your skin, heating it, and if the transfer of molecular movement is great enough, it may cause a burn.

Heat energy may also cause chemical changes. As temperature increases, substances such as gasoline may combine with oxygen. The nature of matter may change as well. Water, for example, may change into ice (with decreasing heat energy) or steam (with increasing heat energy). In addition, the chemical structure of proteins can be affected by heat. An egg changes its nature as the proteins break down, or **denature**, in a hot frying pan. This is why cooked eggs take on a rubbery consistency.

Similar changes also take place in burned tissue. As molecular speed increases, cell components, especially membranes and proteins, begin to denature (break down) just like with the egg in a frying pan. The result of extreme heat exposure is progressive injury and cell death.[2]

The extent of burn injury is related to the amount of heat energy transferred to the patient's skin. The amount of that heat energy in turn depends on three components of the burning agent: its temperature, the concentration of heat energy it possesses, and the length of its contact time with the patient's skin.

Obviously, the greater an agent's temperature, the greater its potential to cause damage. However, it is also important to consider the amount of heat energy possessed by the object or substance. Receiving a blast of heated air from an oven at 350°F is much less damaging than contact with hot cooking oil at the same temperature. In general, water, oils, and other liquids tend to have a high heat energy content. This content is roughly related to the material's density. In a similar fashion, solids also usually have a high heat content. Gases, however, usually have less capacity to hold heat owing to their being less dense.

The duration of exposure to a heat source is obviously important in determining burn severity. A patient's momentary contact with hot oil would result in less damage than if the oil were poured into his shoe with his foot in it.

A burn is a progressive process, and the greater the heat energy transmitted to the body, the deeper the wound. Initially, the burn damages the epidermis through an increase in its temperature. As contact with the substance continues, heat energy penetrates deeper into body tissue. Thus, a burn may involve the epidermis, dermis, and subcutaneous tissue as well as muscles, bone, and other internal tissues.

At the local tissue level, thermal burns cause a number of effects collectively described by **Jackson's theory of thermal wounds**. This theory helps us understand the physical effects of high heat and helps explain a number of clinical effects (Figure 2 ●).

With a burn, the skin nearest the heat source suffers the most profound changes. Cell membranes rupture and are destroyed, blood coagulates, and structural proteins denature. This most-damaged area is the **zone of coagulation**. If the zone of coagulation penetrates the dermis, the resulting injury is termed a full thickness or third-degree burn. Adjacent to the zone of coagulation is a less-damaged yet still inflamed region where blood flow decreases. This burn region is called the **zone of stasis**. Even more distant from the burn source is a broader area where inflammation and changes in blood flow are limited. This is the **zone of hyperemia**; this zone accounts for the erythema (redness) associated with some burns.

CONTENT REVIEW

► Basic Types of Burns

- Thermal
- Electrical
- Chemical
- Radiation

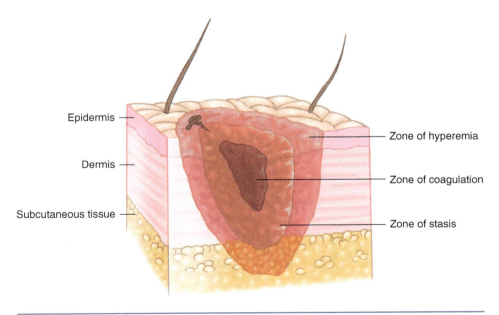

Epidermis

Dermis

Subcutaneous tissue

Zone of hyperemia

Zone of coagulation

Zone of stasis

● **Figure 2** The zones of injury commonly caused by a thermal burn.

CONTENT REVIEW

► Effects of Heat according to Jackson's Theory of Thermal Wounds

- Zone of coagulation—most damaged area nearest heat source; cell membranes rupture and are destroyed, blood coagulates, structural proteins denature
- Zone of stasis—adjacent to most damaged region; inflammation present, blood flow decreased
- Zone of hyperemia—area farthest from heat source; limited inflammation and changes in blood flow

Large burns have profound pathological effects on the body as a whole. In general, these effects are important in any burn that covers more than 15 to 20 percent of the patient's body surface area. To understand these effects and the resulting burn shock, you must first learn a little about the progression of burns.

The body's response to burns occurs over time and can usefully be classified into four phases. The first phase occurs immediately following a burn and is called the **emergent phase**. This is the body's initial reaction to the burn. This phase includes a pain response as well as an outpouring of catecholamines in response to the pain and the physical and emotional stress. During this stage, the patient displays tachycardia, tachypnea, mild hypertension, and mild anxiety.

The **fluid shift phase** follows the initial phase and can last up to 24 hours. It occurs in those with thermal burns larger than 15 to 20 percent total body surface area and is unlikely to occur in those with smaller burns. The fluid shift phase begins shortly after the burn and reaches its peak in 6 to 8 hours. You are therefore likely to see only the beginning of it in the prehospital setting. In this phase, damaged cells release agents that initiate an inflammatory response. This increases blood flow to capillaries surrounding the burn and increases capillary permeability. The response results in a large fluid shift away from the **intravascular space** into the **extravascular space** (massive edema). Note that capillaries leak plasma (water, electrolytes, and some dissolved proteins) and not blood cells. Red blood cell loss from burns uncomplicated by other trauma is usually minimal.

After the fluid shift phase comes the **hypermetabolic phase**, which may last many days or weeks depending on burn severity. This phase is characterized by a large increase in the body's demands for nutrients as it begins the long process of repairing damaged tissue. Gradually this phase evolves into the **resolution phase**, in which scar tissue is laid down and remodeled, and the burn patient begins to rehabilitate and return to normal function.

Electrical Burns

Electricity's power is the result of an electron flow from a point of high concentration to one of low concentration. The difference between the two concentrations is called **voltage**. It is helpful to envision voltage as the "pressure" of the electric flow. The rate or amount of flow in a given time is termed **current** and is measured in **amperes**. With direct current, electrons flow in one direction, while alternating current reverses the flow in short intervals. Standard house current is alternating at 60 cycles per second.

Another factor affecting electricity flow is **resistance**, which is measured in **ohms**. Copper electrical wire has very little resistance and allows a free flow of electrons. Tungsten (the filament in a light bulb) is moderately resistant and heats, glows, and emits light as more and more current is applied to it.

The relationship between current (*I*), resistance (*R*), and voltage (*V*) is well known as **Ohm's law**:

$$V = IR \text{ or } I = V/R$$

Like tungsten, internal human tissues vary in conductivity and are moderately resistant to electron flow. Skin, however, is highly resistant to electrical flow. Moisture or sweat on the skin lowers this resistance. Nerve tissue on the other hand conducts electricity very easily. If the human body is subjected to voltage, tissue initially resists the flow. If the voltage is strong enough, the current begins to pass into and through the body. As it does, heat energy is created. The heat produced by the electrical current (power, or P) is equal to the product of the square of the current (I^2), the resistance of the conductor (*R*), and the time during which it flows, as expressed in **Joule's law**:

$$P = I^2Rt$$

The highest heat occurs at the points of greatest resistance, often at the skin. This accounts for the severe "entry" and "exit" wounds sometimes seen in electrical injuries. Dry, callused skin can have enormous resistance values, ranging from 500,000 to 1,000,000 ohms/cm. Wet skin, particularly the thin skin on the palm side of the arm or on the inner thigh, can have values as low as 300 to 10,000 ohms/cm. Mucous membranes have very low resistance (100 ohms/cm) and allow even small currents to pass. This accounts for the relative ease with which household current can cause lip and oral burns in children who accidentally bite electrical cords (Figure 3 ●).

With small currents, heat energy produced is of little consequence. But if the voltage or current is high, profound damage can occur. The longer the duration of contact, the greater will be the potential for injury. Electrical burns can be particularly damaging because the burn heats the victim from the inside out,

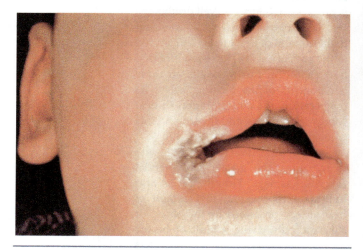

● **Figure 3** Electrical burns to a child's mouth caused by chewing on an electrical cord. *(Photo courtesy of Scott & White Healthcare)*

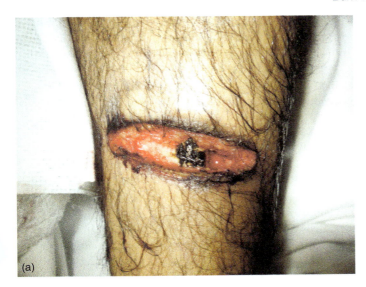

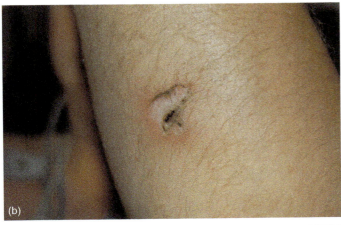

● **Figure 4** Injuries from electrical shock: (a) Electrical entrance wound. (b) Electrical exit wound. *(Photo a: © Dr. Bryan E. Bledsoe; Photo b: © Edward T. Dickinson, MD)*

causing great damage to internal organs and structures while possibly leaving little visible surface damage, save for the entry and exit wounds (Figure 4 ●).

Thermal injury due to electrical current occurs as energy travels from the point of contact to the point of exit. At both these points, the concentration of electricity is great, as is the degree of damage you might expect. The smaller the area of contact, the greater will be the concentration of current flow and the greater the injury. Between the entrance and exit points, the energy spreads out over a larger cross-sectional area and generally causes less injury. Electrical current may follow blood vessels and nerves because they offer less resistance than muscle and bone. This may lead to serious vascular and nervous injury deep within the involved limbs or body cavity.

Electrical contact also interferes with the nervous control of muscle tissue. Current passage, especially alternating current, severely disrupts the complicated electrochemical reactions that control muscles. If contact with a current as small as 18 to 30 milliamperes (mA) is maintained for a period of time, the muscles of respiration may be immobilized. The result is prolonged respiratory arrest, anoxia, hypoxemia, and—eventually—death.

Electrical currents greater than 70 mA may also disrupt the heart's electrical system, causing ventricular fibrillation accompanied by ineffective pumping action.[3] Alternating electrical current such as that found in household current can also cause tetanic convulsions or uncontrolled contractions of muscles. If the victim is holding a wire at such a time, the victim may be unable to let go, thereby prolonging exposure and increasing the injury severity. This can occur with as little as 9 mA of current.

Electrical injury may also physically injure muscle and other tissue, leading to its degeneration. As the tissue dies, it releases materials toxic to the human body. These materials may damage the liver and kidneys, leading to failure.

At times, electrical energy may cause flash burns secondary to the heat of current passing through adjacent air. Air is very resistant to electrical current passage. If the current is strong enough and the space through which it passes is small, the electricity arcs, producing tremendous heat. If the patient's skin is close by, heat may severely burn or vaporize tissue. In addition, heat may ignite articles of clothing or other combustibles and produce thermal burns.

Chemical Burns

Chemical burns denature the biochemical makeup of cell membranes (primarily the proteins) and destroy the cells. Such injuries are not transmitted through the tissue as are thermal injuries. Instead, a chemical burn must destroy the tissue before it can chemically burn any deeper. This fact generally limits the "burn" process unless very strong chemicals are involved (Figure 5 ●). Agents that can cause chemical burns are too numerous to mention. However, the most common causes of these burns are either strong acids or alkalis (bases).

Both acids and alkalis burn by disrupting cell membranes and damaging tissues on contact. As they cause damage, acids usually form a thick, insoluble mass, or coagulum, at the point

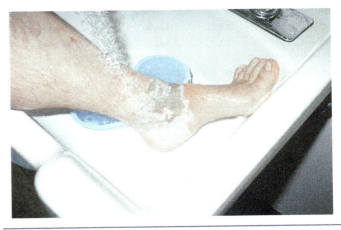

● **Figure 5** An acid burn to the ankle. *(© Roy Alson, PhD, MD, FACEP, FAAEM)*

CONTENT REVIEW

► Processes of Chemical Burns

- Acids—usually form a thick, insoluble mass where they contact tissue through coagulation necrosis, limiting burn damage
- Alkalis—usually continue to destroy cell membranes through liquefaction necrosis, allowing them to penetrate underlying tissue and causing deeper burns

of contact. This process is called **coagulation necrosis** and helps to limit acid burn depth. Acid burns usually cause immediate pain. Alkalis, however, have limited pain and do not form a protective coagulum. Instead, the alkali continues to destroy cell membranes, releasing intercellular and interstitial fluid, destroying tissue in a process called **liquefaction necrosis**. Liquifaction necrosis progressively denatures protiens and collagen, disolves fats (saponification), dehydrates tissues, and damages blood vessels. This process allows the alkali to rapidly penetrate underlying tissue, causing progressively deeper burns. For this reason, alkali burns can be quite serious. Alkalis are commonly used as oven and drain cleaners, agricultural fertilizers, and in industry.

Radiation Injury

Ionizing radiation has bombarded Earth since long before recorded time. It is a daily, natural phenomenon arising from the sun and the distant cosmos. Natural radiation also occurs from radioactive rocks and gases found throughout our planet. In most cases this natural background radiation is inconsequential. Radiation becomes a danger when people are exposed to synthetic sources that greatly increase radiation intensity. Medicine and industry use radioactive materials for diagnostic testing and treatment and for energy production. Deaths from exposure to radiation are extremely rare, as are serious injuries, because of safety measures commonly used with the handling of nuclear materials. However, the possibility of a large risk of injury typically comes from accidents associated with improper handling, either in the on-site environment or during transport.

Radiation causes damage through a process known as **ionization**, in which a radioactive energy particle travels into a substance and changes an internal atom (Figure 6 ●). In the human body, the affected cell either repairs the damage, dies, or goes on to produce damaged cells (cancer). The cells most sensitive to radiation injury are the cells that reproduce most quickly, like those responsible for erythrocyte, leukocyte, and platelet production (bone marrow); cells lining the intestinal tract; and cells involved in human reproduction.

We commonly encounter four types of ionizing radiation. These are:

- **Alpha radiation.** The unstable atomic nucleus releases **alpha radiation** in the form of a small helium nucleus. Alpha radiation is a very weak energy source and can travel only inches through air. Paper or clothing can easily stop alpha radiation. This radiation also cannot penetrate the epidermis. On the subatomic scale, however, alpha particles are massive and can cause great damage over the

short distance they travel. Alpha radiation is a significant hazard only if the patient inhales or ingests contaminated material, thus bringing the source in proximity to sensitive respiratory and digestive tract tissue.

- **Beta radiation.** A second type of radiologic process produces **beta radiation**. Its energy is greater than that of alpha radiation. However, the beta particle is relatively lightweight, with the mass of an electron. Beta radiation can travel 6 to 10 feet through air and can penetrate a few layers of clothing. Beta particles can invade the first few millimeters of skin and thus have the potential for causing external as well as internal injury.

- **Gamma radiation.** **Gamma radiation**, also known as X-rays, is the most powerful type of ionizing (atom-changing) radiation. It can travel through the entire body or ionize any atom within. Its lack of mass or charge (it is pure electromagnetic energy, or photons) helps give it great penetrating power. Gamma radiation evokes the greatest concern for external exposure. It is the most dangerous and most feared type of radiation because it is difficult to protect against. Many feet of concrete or many inches of lead are needed to shield against the highest-energy gamma rays. Fortunately, exposure to high-energy gamma rays occurs only in individuals who are exposed to nuclear blasts, are near nuclear reactor cores, or are very close to highly radioactive materials. More modest amounts of concrete, steel, or lead can provide shielding from the more common and lower energy X-rays and gamma rays encountered in medicine and industry.

- **Neutron radiation.** Neutrons are small, yet moderately massive subatomic particles with no charge. Their small size and lack of charge account for their great penetrating power. Fortunately, strong **neutron radiation** is uncommon outside of nuclear reactors and bombs.

Exposure to radiation and the effects of ionization can occur through two mechanisms. In the first, an unshielded person is directly exposed to a strong radioactive source—for example, an unstable material such as uranium. The second exposure mechanism is contamination by dust, debris, or fluids that contain very small particles of radioactive material. These contaminants give off weaker radiation than a direct radioactive source like uranium. However, the proximity of these contaminants to the body and their longer contact times with it may result in greater exposure and contamination. Note that most substances, including human tissue, do not give off radiation. The patient is not the danger in a radiologic exposure incident. Any danger comes from the radioactive source, such as the contaminated material on the patient.

Three factors are important to keep in mind whenever you are called to radiation exposure incidents. They are the duration of exposure; the distance from the radioactive source; and the shielding between you, the patient, and the source. Knowledge of these three factors can limit your exposure and potential for injury.

- **Duration.** Radiation exposure is an accumulative danger. The longer you or the patient remain exposed

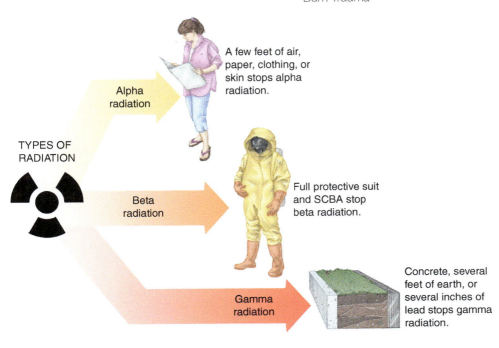

TYPES OF RADIATION

Alpha radiation

A few feet of air, paper, clothing, or skin stops alpha radiation.

Beta radiation

Full protective suit and SCBA stop beta radiation.

Gamma radiation

Concrete, several feet of earth, or several inches of lead stops gamma radiation.

CONTENT REVIEW

► Types of Radiation

- Alpha—very weak, stopped by paper, clothing, or the epidermis
- Beta—more powerful than alpha; can travel 6 to 10 feet through air; can penetrate some clothing and the first few millimeters of skin
- Gamma—most powerful ionizing radiation; great penetrating power; protection requires thick concrete or lead shielding
- Neutron—great penetrating power, but uncommon outside nuclear reactors and bombs

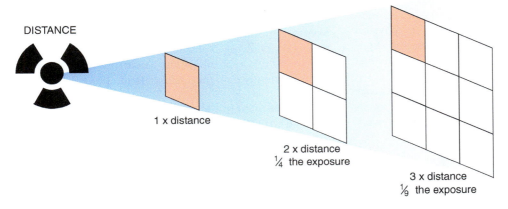

DISTANCE

1 x distance

2 x distance
¼ the exposure

3 x distance
⅑ the exposure

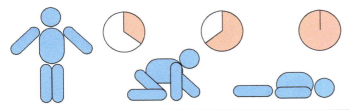

TIME (EXAMPLE SHOWS 300 r/hr)

● **Figure 6**   The injury considerations associated with nuclear radiation.

to the source, the greater the injury potential. The realtionship is linear; for example, twice the exposure doubles the risk.

- *Distance.* Radiation strength diminishes quickly as you travel farther from the source. The effect is similar to that of a light bulb's intensity. At a few feet, you can easily read by it, while at a few hundred feet the light barely casts a shadow. Mathematically, the relationship is inverse and squared. As you double your distance from a radioactive source, its strength drops to one-fourth of the original

strength. As you triple the distance, its strength diminishes to one-ninth, and so on.

- *Shielding.* The more material between you and a radioactive source, the less exposure you experience. With alpha and beta radiation, shielding is very easy to provide and reasonably effective. With gamma and neutron sources, dense objects such as earth, concrete, metal, and lead are needed to provide any real protection. Shielding generally follws a linear relationship; for example, three times the shielding thickness will yield one-third the radiation exposure.

Radiation emission, usually in units-per-hour, is measured with a Geiger counter, while cumulative exposure is recorded by a device called a dosimeter (Figure 7 ●). Both devices record units of radiation expressed as either the **rad** or the **Gray** (Gy), with 1 Gray equal to 100 rads.

Radiation effects vary with different tissues. As little as 0.2 Gy can cause cataracts in exposed eyes and damage blood-cell-producing bone marrow (also called hematopoietic) tissue. The radiation dose that is lethal to about 50 percent of exposed individuals is approximately 4.5 Gy.

With whole-body exposure, and as the radiation dose increases, signs and symptoms of exposure appear earlier and become more severe. The first signs of serious exposure are slight nausea and fatigue, occurring between 4 and 24 hours after exposure. As radiation doses move toward the lethal range, nausea severity increases and is joined by anorexia, vomiting, diarrhea, and malaise. Erythema may be present, and fatigue becomes more intense. These signs appear within 2 to 6 hours. With exposure to even higher, fatal doses, the patient displays all radiation exposure signs almost immediately and soon thereafter experiences confusion, watery diarrhea, and physical collapse. Note that the signs and symptoms of radiation exposure and the injuries associated with it vary because individual sensitivity to radiation exposure varies greatly.

Prolonged exposure to even small radiation amounts may produce long-term and delayed problems. Infertility is a potential injury, because the cells producing eggs and sperm are very susceptible to ionization damage. Cancer is another delayed and severe side effect. It may occur years or even decades after a radiation exposure.

Inhalation Injury

The burn environment, on occasion (10 to 25 percent of the time), produces inhalation injury. This occurs most commonly if the patient is trapped or unconscious in an enclosed space, but it can occasionally occur even in an open field if the smoke is dense enough. A victim will eventually inhale gases, heated air, flames, or steam. This inhalation results in airway and respiratory injury.

As you approach a burn environment, protect yourself and anticipate the following inhalation conditions (Figure 8 ●). Keep them in mind as you survey the scene, take the necessary protective measures, and begin your assessment.

Toxic Inhalation   Modern residential and commercial construction use synthetic resins and plastics that release toxic gases as they burn. Combustion of these materials can form agents such as cyanide, hydrogen sulfide, and other toxic or caustic substances. If a patient inhales these gases, they either react with the lung tissue, causing internal chemical burns, or they diffuse across the alveolar-capillary membrane, enter the bloodstream, and interfere with delivery to or the cell's use of oxygen. Signs and symptoms of these injuries may present immediately following exposure or their onset may be delayed for an hour or two after inhalation. Toxic inhalation injury occurs more frequently than thermal inhalation burns.

Carbon Monoxide Poisoning   A significant concern associated with the fire/burn environment is carbon monoxide (CO) poisoning. Carbon monoxide is the product of incomplete hydrocarbon combustion. It is a tasteless, odorless, and otherwise unrecognizable gas. There is a very small amount of carbon monoxide in ambient air but, as that concentration increases by more than 100 times, the danger of carbon

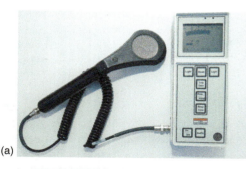
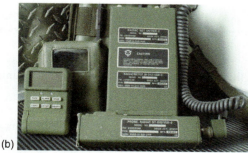

● **Figure 7**   (a) A Geiger counter measures the radiation exposure level; (b) A dosimeter records cumulative exposure. *(Photo a: © Jeff Forster; Photo b: Equipment courtesy of Ogunquit Maine Fire-Rescue)*

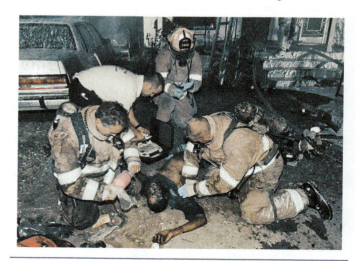

● **Figure 8**   There are numerous hazards associated with fire in an enclosed environment. These include heat, toxic chemicals (carbon monoxide, hydrogen sulfide, cyanide), and others. *(© Glen E. Ellman)*

monoxide poisoning begins. This poisoning risk exists with improperly ventilated open flame in a contained area (house fires, faulty fuel-fired heating units, nonelectric stoves and ovens, gas and charcoal grills and camp stoves, improperly ventilated fireplaces) and internal combustion engines (auto exhaust fumes, home generators, propane-fueled vehicles, boat exhaust fumes). Each year, as many as 6,000 people die from carbon monoxide poisoning, and it accounts for 40,000 emergency department visits yearly.

Carbon monoxide is a stable molecule consisting of one carbon and one oxygen atom firmly bonded to each other. It competes for the four oxygen-bonding sites on each hemoglobin molecule. Hemoglobin has an affinity for carbon monoxide that is greater than 200 times its affinity for oxygen. Carbon monoxide bound to hemoglobin prevents oxygen from attaching and, thereby, prevents hemoglobin from transporting oxygen from the alveoli to the tissue capillaries. As carbon monoxide concentrations increase, and as the time of exposure increases, more and more hemoglobin is saturated with carbon monoxide (carboxyhemoglobin), while less and less hemoglobin is saturated with oxygen (oxyhemoglobin).

Carbon monoxide also attaches to myoglobin. Myoglobin is another iron-containing protein that serves as an oxygen storage site in muscles, including those of the heart. The resulting reduction in oxygen availability can induce cardiac ischemia and arrhythmias.

Recognizing carbon monoxide poisoning is a challenge, as the signs and symptoms of toxicity are very nonspecific. The victim of this poisoning presents with a general ill feeling (malaise) and CNS symptoms: headache, dizziness, blurred vision, nausea, and vomiting. As the exposure increases, the victim may present with confusion, weakness, syncope, dyspnea, tachypnea, tachycardia, and chest pain. With extreme exposure, the victim may present with hypotension, cardiac ischemia, arrhythmias, pulmonary edema, seizures, coma, pulmonary arrest, cardiac arrest, and death. As a paramedic, you should carry a high index of suspicion for this poisoning as temperatures drop (causing heating units to function) in the late fall or early winter and especially when a group of people who work or live together suffer flu-like symptoms.

Carbon monoxide poisoning is of special concern for the young, the elderly, patients with preexisting heart disease, and the fetuses of pregnant patients. Young pediatric patients are susceptible to CO poisoning because of alterations in their physiology. The elderly are more likely to have preexisting disease, including COPD and other respiratory problems, as well as reduced respiratory reserves. This leaves them more adversely affected by CO poisoning. Patients with cardiac problems are at special risk because the myocardium does not store oxygen, and CO poisoning reduces oxygen transport by the blood. The myocardium is then even more prone to hypoxia. Finally, fetal hemoglobin is different from normal hemoglobin and has an increased affinity for carbon monoxide. With exposure, the fetus may suffer ill effects well before they appear in the mother.

Airway Thermal Burn   Another, though less frequent, injury is the airway thermal burn. Very moist mucosa lines the airway and helps insulate it against heat damage. Because of this mucosa,

supraglottic, or upper airway, structures may absorb the heat and prevent lower airway burns. High levels of thermal energy are required to evaporate the fluid and injure cells. Inspiration of hot air or flame rarely produces enough heat to cause significant thermal burns to the lower airway.

Superheated steam has greater heat content than hot, dry air and can cause subglottic, or lower airway, burns. Superheated steam is created under great pressure and can have a temperature well above 212°F. A common hazard to firefighters, superheated steam develops when a stream of water strikes a hot spot and vaporizes explosively. The blast can dislodge the mask of a firefighter's self-contained breathing apparatus, exposing him or her to superheated steam inhalation. Steam contains enough heat energy to severely burn the upper airway. It also may damage the lower respiratory tract, although this happens less frequently.

Risk factors for inhalation injuries associated with burns include standing in the burn environment (hot gases rise), screaming or yelling there (the open glottis allows toxic gases to enter the lower airway), and being trapped in a closed burn environment.

With any thermal or smoke-related chemical burn injury to the respiratory tract, there is the danger of airway restriction, severe dyspnea, and possible respiratory arrest. The airway is a narrow tube lined with extremely vascular tissue. If damaged, this tissue swells rapidly, seriously reducing the size of the airway lumen. The patient presents with minor hoarseness, followed precipitously by dyspnea. Stridor or high-pitched "crowing" sounds on inspiration are ominous signs of impending airway obstruction. Other clues leading you to suspect potential airway burns include singed facial and nasal hair, black-tinged (carbonaceous) sputum, and facial burns. The airway injury may be so extensive that it induces complete respiratory obstruction and arrest. Accurate assessment is important because 20 to 35 percent of patients admitted to burn centers and some 60 to 80 percent of burn patients who die have an associated inhalation injury.

Burn Depth

After you determine the burn source and assess the possibility of associated inhalation injury, you need to assess the burn's severity. One element in determining the severity of a burn is the depth of damage it causes. Depth of burn damage is normally classified into three categories (Figure 9 ●).

Superficial Burn

The superficial burn, also termed a first-degree burn, involves only the epidermis and upper dermis. It is an irritation of the

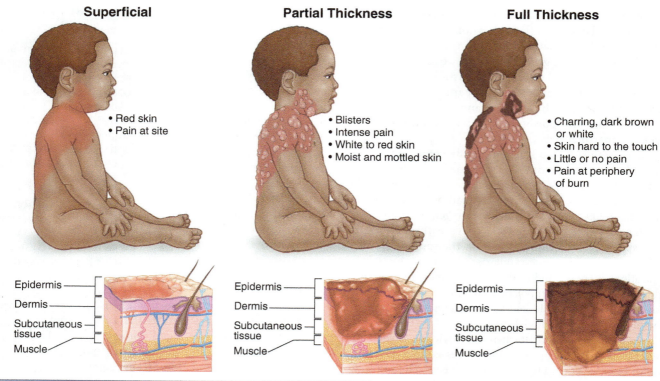

Superficial
- Red skin
- Pain at site

Epidermis
Dermis
Subcutaneous tissue
Muscle

Partial Thickness
- Blisters
- Intense pain
- White to red skin
- Moist and mottled skin

Epidermis
Dermis
Subcutaneous tissue
Muscle

Full Thickness
- Charring, dark brown or white
- Skin hard to the touch
- Little or no pain
- Pain at periphery of burn

Epidermis
Dermis
Subcutaneous tissue
Muscle

● **Figure 9** Classification of burns by depth.

living cells and nerve endings in this region and results in some pain, minor edema, and erythema. It normally heals without complication.

Partial Thickness Burn

The **partial thickness burn**, also termed a second-degree burn, penetrates slightly deeper than a superficial burn and produces blisters. Heat energy travels into the dermis, involving more of the tissue and resulting in greater destruction. The partial thickness burn is similar to a superficial burn in that it is reddened, painful, and edematous. You can differentiate it from the superficial burn only after blisters form. Because there are many nerve endings in the dermis, both superficial and partial thickness burns are often very painful. With both superficial and partial thickness burns, the dermis is still intact and complete skin regeneration is very likely.

The sunburn is a common, but specialized type of burn. Ultraviolet radiation causes the burn rather than normal thermal processes. The radiation penetrates superficially and damages the uppermost layers of the dermis. Sunburn can present as either a superficial or partial thickness burn.

Another similar type of burn occurs as someone watches an arc welder without proper protection. In this injury, called ultraviolet keratitis, the outermost parts of the eye (cornea) trap the ultraviolet radiation, causing injury to the layer. This causes delayed eye pain and, possibly, transient blindness. The injury usually heals completely within 24 hours.

Full Thickness Burn

The **full thickness burn**, or third-degree burn, penetrates both the epidermis and the dermis and extends into the subcutaneous layers or even deeper, into muscles, bones, and internal organs. These burns destroy the tissue's regenerative properties and the peripheral nerve endings. Injury is painless because of nerve destruction, but the margins of full thickness burns are frequently partial thickness burns, which can be quite painful. Full thickness burns take on various colorations depending on the nature of the burning agent and the damaged, dying, or dead tissue. They can be white, brown, dark red, or a charred color and typically have a dry, leather-like appearance. Because the burn destroys the entire dermis, skin grafting is usually required.

Body Surface Area

Another factor affecting burn severity is how much of a person's **body surface area (BSA)** the burn involves. There are two approaches to estimating the BSA involved in a burn. The first, the rule of nines, is useful in estimating large burn areas. The second method, the rule of palms, is helpful in assessing smaller burns more accurately.

Rule of Nines

The **rule of nines** identifies 11 topographical adult body regions, each of which approximates 9 percent of the patient's BSA (Figure 10 ●). These regions include the entire head and neck, the anterior chest, the anterior abdomen, the posterior chest, the lower back (the posterior abdomen), the anterior surface of each lower extremity, the posterior surface of each lower extremity, and the entirety of each upper extremity. The genitalia make up the remaining 1 percent of BSA.

Because infant and child anatomy differs significantly from that of adults, you must modify the rule of nines to maintain an accurate approximation of BSA. Divide the head and neck area into the anterior and posterior surface and award 9 percent for

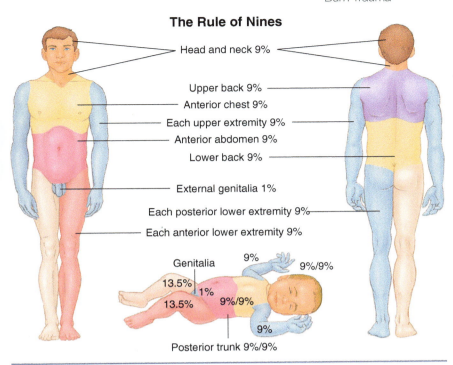

The Rule of Nines

Head and neck 9%

Upper back 9%
Anterior chest 9%
Each upper extremity 9%
Anterior abdomen 9%
Lower back 9%

External genitalia 1%

Each posterior lower extremity 9%
Each anterior lower extremity 9%

Genitalia 9%
13.5% 9%/9%
1%
13.5% 9%/9%
9%
Posterior trunk 9%/9%

● **Figure 10** The rule of nines.

each. Reduce the surface area of each lower extremity by 4.5 percent to ensure the total body surface area remains at 100 percent. The rule of nines is at best an approximation of the area burned. It is, however, an expedient and useful tool to help measure a burn's extent.

Rule of Palms

The **rule of palms** is an alternative system for approximating a burn's extent. It uses the palmar surface as a point of comparison in gauging the size of the affected body area (Figure 11 ●). The patient's palm (the hand less the fingers) represents about 1 percent of the BSA, whether the patient is an adult, a child, or an infant. If you can visualize the palmar surface area and apply it to the burn area mentally, you can then obtain an estimate of the total BSA affected.

The rule of palms is easier to use for local burns of up to about 10 percent BSA, while the rule of nines is simpler and more appropriate for larger burns. Many other burn approximation techniques exist that are both more specific to age and, in general, more accurate such as the Lund and Browder chart (Figure 12 ●). However, these techniques are more complicated and time consuming to use. Both the rule of nines and the rule of palms provide reasonable approximations of BSA when used properly in the field.

Systemic Complications

Burns cause several systemic complications. These can affect the overall severity of a burn. Typical complications include hypothermia, hypovolemia, eschar formation, and infection.

Hypothermia

A burn may disrupt the body's ability to regulate its core temperature. Tissue destruction reduces or eliminates the skin's ability to contain fluid within. The burn process releases plasma

and other fluids, which seep into the wound. There they evaporate and rapidly remove heat energy. Injured skin has increased blood flow, enhancing the heat loss, and the burn injury does not have the reflex vasoconstriction that normally protects against excessive heat loss. If the burn is extensive, uncontrolled body heat loss induces rapid and severe hypothermia.[4]

Hypovolemia

Hypovolemia also may complicate the severe burn. In patients with thermal burns greater than 15 to 20 percent total body surface area, the inability of damaged blood vessels to retain plasma causes a fluid and electrolyte shift into burned tissue. Additionally, loss of plasma protein reduces the blood's ability, via osmosis, to draw fluids from uninjured tissues. This in turn compromises the body's natural response to fluid loss and may produce a profound hypovolemia. Although this is a serious and life-threatening complication of extensive burns, it takes hours to develop. Modern aggressive fluid resuscitation can effectively counteract this aspect of the burn process.

A related complication is electrolyte imbalance. With the massive fluid shift to the interstitial space, the body's ability

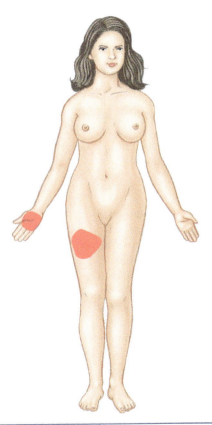

● **Figure 11** Using the rule of palms, the surface of the patient's palm represents approximately 1 percent of BSA and is helpful in estimating the area of small burns.

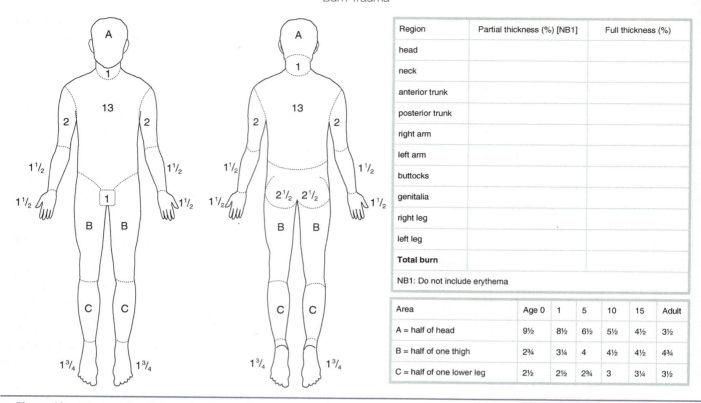

Region	Partial thickness (%) [NB1]	Full thickness (%)
head		
neck		
anterior trunk		
posterior trunk		
right arm		
left arm		
buttocks		
genitalia		
right leg		
left leg		
Total burn		
NB1: Do not include erythema		

Area	Age 0	1	5	10	15	Adult
A = half of head	9½	8½	6½	5½	4½	3½
B = half of one thigh	2¾	3¼	4	4½	4½	4¾
C = half of one lower leg	2½	2½	2¾	3	3¼	3½

● **Figure 12**   The Lund and Browder chart takes into consideration that proportions of the head and lower extremities vary at different ages from infancy to adulthood and provides age-appropriate percentages for calculating the burn area.

to regulate sodium, potassium, and other electrolytes becomes overwhelmed. In addition, large thermal and electrical burns can lead to massive tissue destruction with a resultant release of breakdown products into the bloodstream. Potassium is one such breakdown product and its oversupply, or hyperkalemia, can lead to life-threatening cardiac arrhythmias. Careful ECG monitoring and appropriate fluid resuscitation can help prevent hyperkalemic complications.

Eschar

Skin denaturing further complicates full thickness thermal burns. As the burn destroys dermal cells, they become hard and leathery, producing what is known as an eschar. Skin as a whole constricts over the wound site, increasing the pressure of any edema beneath and restricting the flow of blood (Figure 13 ●). If an extremity burn is circumferential, constriction may be severe enough to occlude all blood flow into the distal extremity. In the case of a thoracic burn, eschar may drastically reduce chest excursion and respiratory tidal volume.

Infection

Although infection is the most persistent killer of burn victims, its effects do not appear for several days following an acute injury. Pathogens invade the wound shortly after the burn occurs and continue to do so until the wound heals. These pathogens pose a hazard to life when they grow to massive numbers, a process that takes days or weeks. To reduce a patient's exposure

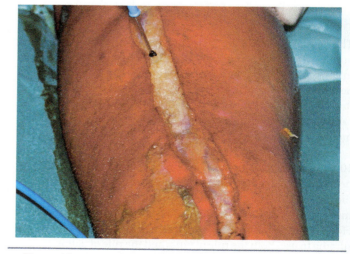

● **Figure 13**   The constriction created by an eschar can limit chest excursion or cut off blood flow to and from a limb. (© *Michael Schurr, MD, Professor, University of Denver*)

to infectious pathogens, carefully employ Standard Precautions, use clean or sterile dressings and clean equipment, and avoid gross contamination of the burn.

Organ Failure

As previously noted, the burn process releases material from damaged or dying body cells into the bloodstream. Myoglobin, released from the muscles in patients with severe electrical injuries, clogs the tubules of the kidneys and, with hypovolemia, may cause kidney failure. Hypovolemia and the circulating by-products of cellular destruction may also induce liver failure. In addition, the release of cellular potassium into the bloodstream affects the heart's electrical system, causing arrhythmias and possible cardiac arrest.

Special Factors

Certain factors involving the burn patient's overall health and age will also affect the patient's response to a burn and should influence your field decisions regarding treatment and transport. Geriatric and pediatric patients and patients who are already ill or otherwise injured have greater difficulty coping with burn injuries than do healthy individuals. The pediatric patient has a high body surface area to body weight ratio, which means the fluid reserves needed for dealing with the burn effects are low. Geriatric patients have reduced mechanisms for fluid retention and lower fluid reserves. They are also less able to combat infection and more apt to have underlying diseases. Ill patients are already using body energy to fight their diseases; with burns, these patients have additional medical stresses to combat. The fluid loss that accompanies a burn also compounds the effects of blood loss in a trauma patient. This patient now must recover from two injuries.

Physical Abuse

When assessing any burn, particularly in a child or an elderly and infirm adult, be alert for any signs of potential physical abuse. Look for mechanisms of injury that don't make sense, such as stove burns on an infant who cannot yet stand or walk. Certain burn patterns should also give rise to suspicion. Multiple circular burns each about a centimeter in diameter may reflect intentional cigarette burns. Infants who have been dipped in scalding hot water will have characteristic circumferential burns to their buttocks as they raise their feet and legs in an attempt to avoid the burning water or "stocking" burns if their feet and legs have been dipped into the scalding water (Figure 14 ●). Branding is an unusual form of abuse and is sometimes seen in

ritualistic or hazing ceremonies in some cultures and organizations. In all cases of suspected abuse, document your findings objectively and accurately, report them to the person assuming patient care in the emergency department, and notify the proper authorities as state and local laws require.

ASSESSMENT OF THERMAL BURNS

Skin evaluation tells more about the body's condition than any other aspect of patient assessment. Not only is the skin the first body organ to experience the effects of burns, but it is the first and often the only organ to display them. Therefore, assessment of the skin and associated burns must be deliberate, careful, and complete.

Burn assessment is simple and well structured. Assess burn patients carefully and completely to ensure that you establish the nature and extent of each injury. This helps you to assign burns the appropriate priority for care.

Assessment of thermal burns follows established procedures for performing the scene size-up, the primary assessment, the rapid or focused trauma assessment, the detailed physical exam, and reassessments.

Scene Size-Up

The safety of your patients, fellow rescuers, and yourself depends on a complete and thorough scene size-up. Look around carefully as you arrive at the scene to ensure there is no continuing danger to you or your patient. Examine the scene to ensure it is safe for you to enter. If there is any doubt, do not enter until the scene is made safe by appropriate emergency personnel (Figure 15 ●).

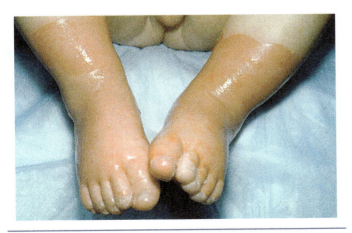

● **Figure 14** Burn injury from placing a child's feet and legs into hot water as punishment. (© Roy Alson, PhD, MD, FACEP, FAAEM)

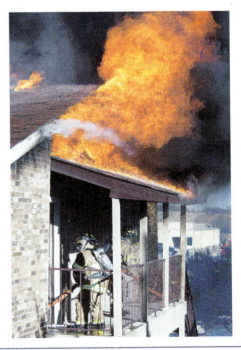

● **Figure 15** Never enter a fire scene until it has been safely contained by appropriately trained personnel. (© Glen E. Ellman)

On calls involving burn patients, be wary of entering enclosed spaces, such as a bedroom or a garage, if there is recent evidence of a fire. Even small fires can cause intense heat in small, enclosed spaces. This can rapidly lead to a near-explosive process (called flashover) in which the contents of a room rise in temperature to the point of rapid ignition. Flashover is frequently fatal to victims caught in the immediate area.

Another significant hazard at fire-ground scenes is the buildup of toxic gases. Carbon monoxide, cyanide, and hydrogen sulfide are common by-products of combustion and can be produced in large quantities in some fires. Cyanide, in particular, can kill after as little as 15 seconds of exposure, a time short enough to fell any would-be rescuer without proper protection.

Never enter any potentially hazardous scene. Instead, ensure that the fire is thoroughly extinguished or that the patient is brought to you by persons skilled in working in hazardous environments who are using proper personal protective equipment. Ensure that the area where you will be caring for the patient is free from dangers such as structural collapse, contamination, electricity, and any other hazards.

Once at the burn patient's side, stop the burning process so it no longer threatens you or the patient. Extinguish any overt flame using copious irrigation, as water is available. As an alternative, a heavy wool or cotton blanket (avoid most synthetics such as nylon or polyester) will smother flames.

Quickly survey the patient for other materials he is wearing that may continue the burn process. Remember that burn patients may be an actual hazard both to themselves and to you. Leather articles, such as shoes, belts, or watchbands, can smolder for hours and continue to induce thermal injury. Watches, rings, and other jewelry may also hold and transmit heat or may restrict swelling tissue and occlude distal circulation. Synthetics (such as a nylon windbreaker) produce great heat as they burn and leave a hot, smoldering residue once the overt flames are out. Remove materials like those previously described as soon as possible. Be careful as you check for and remove these items. They may be hot enough to burn you.

Once the scene is safe and there are no further dangers to you or others, consider the burn mechanism. Ask yourself: "Is there any possibility that the patient was unconscious during the fire or trapped within the building?" If so, be ready to place a special emphasis on your assessment and management of the patient's airway and breathing. Watch for any signs of airway restriction, and be alert to possible poisoning from carbon monoxide or other toxic gases.

Also consider and examine for other mechanisms of injury associated with the burn. Remember that the victim, in attempting to escape the flames, may have fallen down a flight of stairs or jumped from a second- or third-story window. Anticipate skeletal and internal injuries. In cases of electrical burns, consider the possibility that muscle spasms caused by contact with high voltage may also have caused skeletal or spinal fractures. Be aware that trauma injuries will increase the severity of the burn's impact on your patient.

Conclude the scene size-up by considering the need for other resources to manage the scene and treat the patient. Request additional EMS, police, and fire personnel and equipment as necessary. Assess for any impact the environment might have on your assessment and care and integrate with scene oversight (incident command). If you suspect serious airway involvement or carbon monoxide poisoning, do all that is possible to reduce transport time to the hospital or burn/trauma center.

Primary Assessment

Start your primary assessment by forming a general impression of the patient. Rule out any danger of associated trauma or the possibility of head and spine injury. Evaluate the patient's level of consciousness, and, if the patient displays an altered state of consciousness, consider toxic inhalation as a cause. Anticipate and rule out spinal injury or provide spinal immobilization.

Next, ensure the airway is patent. If it is not, protect it. You must give a burn patient's airway special consideration. Look for the signs of any thermal or inhalation injury during your primary airway exam (Figure 16 ●). Look carefully at facial and nasal hairs to see if they have been singed. Examine any sputum and areas around the mouth and nose for carbonaceous residue or any other evidence of inhalation burns. Listen for airway sounds, such as stridor, hoarseness, or coughing, that indicate irritation or inflammation of the mucosa. Such sounds should alert you to possible airway inhalation injury and, likely, progressive airway swelling and restriction. Stridor, in particular, is a serious finding. Consider a patient with any signs of respiratory involvement as a potential acute emergency, and provide immediate care and transport.

With patients in whom respiratory involvement is suspected, provide high-concentration oxygen and prepare the equipment for endotracheal intubation. High-concentration oxygen (at levels approaching 100 percent) is especially important for burn patients because they may be suffering from carbon monoxide poisoning. Very high oxygen concentrations more effectively provide oxygen to body cells and may reduce the half-life of carbon monoxide on the hemoglobin molecule by up to two-thirds.

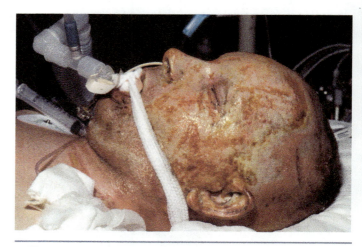

● **Figure 16**   Facial burns or carbonaceous material around the mouth and nose suggest the potential for chemical and thermal burns to the airway. (*© M. English, MD/Custom Medical Stock Photo*)

Pulse oximetry is a very useful tool in evaluating respiratory and cardiovascular effectiveness in the burn patient. However, carbon monoxide replaces oxygen in the red blood cell and colors it much as oxygen does. This leads the oximeter to display high saturation readings when the blood actually has greatly reduced oxygen-carrying capacity. Do not rely on pulse oximetry readings alone for the patient who is suspected of suffering from carbon monoxide poisoning, who has been burned in an enclosed space, or who has inhaled significant amounts of smoke.

Pulse CO-oximetry monitors are now available that monitor oxygen saturation (SpO_2), the amount of total hemoglobin (SpHb), carboxyhemoglobin (SpCO), and methemoglobin (SpMET). Consider their use when there is any reason to suspect inhalation of smoke or the by-products of combustion (Figure 17 ●). Normal carbon monoxide levels should be less than 5 percent in nonsmokers and less than 10 percent in smokers. Consider carbon monoxide poisoning to exist when levels exceed 10 to 12 percent. Care includes high-concentration oxygen, positive-pressure ventilation as needed, and rapid transport.

Cyanide poisoning is a significant risk associated with the burn environment and toxic inhalation. It is often found in combination with CO poisoning. Whenever CO poisoning is suspected, consider the administration of hydroxocobalamin (a precurser to vitamin B_{12}). Hydroxocobalamin chelates cyanide from cytochrome oxidase to form cyanocobalamin (vitamin B_{12}), a harmless compound easily excreted by the kidneys. Hydroxocobalamin is marketed as a cyanide antidote—Cyanokit®.

Burn patients may progress rapidly from mild dyspnea to total respiratory arrest. While intubation of a respiratory burn patient may be difficult in the field, there are distinct advantages to performing it early. Edema associated with airway burns is progressive and rapidly reduces the airway lumen. If intubation is delayed until the patient becomes extremely dyspneic or goes into respiratory arrest, the airway may be so edematous that it will be difficult, if not impossible, to intubate.

If you elect field intubation for the burn patient, perform it quickly and carefully. The airway is already narrowing, and the normal trauma associated with intubation could make matters worse. Intubation can be more complicated if the patient is conscious and fights the process. Consider using rapid sequence intubation techniques and pharmacological adjuncts including sedatives and paralytics. Use succinylcholine cautiously, if at all, since it may worsen the hyperkalemia sometimes associated with severe burns. You may also find nasotracheal intubation useful. In any case, select the crew member with the most experience to ensure that intubation is completed quickly and with the least amount of associated airway trauma.

As with all intubation, it is best to maintain an airway using the largest endotracheal tube possible. Be sure, however, to have several tubes smaller than you would normally use ready, because edema may have reduced the size of the airway. Select the largest tube that you think will easily pass through the cords. In extreme cases, creation of a surgical airway by percutaneous cricothyrotomy may be a lifesaving necessity; in such cases, follow local protocols or on-line medical direction. Confirm tube placement with at least three methods, including capnography.

Ensure that the patient's breathing is adequate in both volume and rate. Carefully assess tidal volume if there are circumferential chest burns, because developing eschar may restrict chest excursion. Ventilate as necessary via bag-valve mask using the reservoir and high-concentration oxygen.

Secondary Assessment

Begin your secondary assessment of the burn patient with either a rapid or focused trauma assessment and proceed to determining baseline vital signs, Glasgow Coma Scale score, and a patient history. With a burn patient, however, you must also accurately approximate the burn surface area and depth. This approximation guides your care and helps emergency department personnel prepare for patient arrival.

Except in cases of very localized burns, examine a patient's entire body surface, both anterior and posterior. Remove any clothing that was or could have been involved in the burn. If any of the clothing adheres to the burn or resists removal, cut around it as necessary.

Apply the rule of nines to determine the total body surface area (BSA) burned. Add 9 percent if the burn involves an entire "rule of nines" region. If it only involves a portion, add that proportion of 9 percent. For example, if one-third of the upper extremity is burned, the surface area approximation is 3 percent ($1/3 \times 9$ percent = 3 percent). For small burns, use the rule of palms to approximate the affected BSA. It is helpful in burn assessment to identify the relative burn BSA that is full thickness and the relative burn BSA that is not full thickness.

Burn injury depth is also an important consideration. Identify areas of painful sensation as partial thickness burns (Figure 18 ●). Consider those that present with limited or absent pain as probable full thickness burns (Figure 19 ●). This differentiation is difficult because partial thickness injury and its associated pain commonly surrounds a full thickness burn (Figure 20 ●). See Table 1 for the characteristics of the different types of burns.

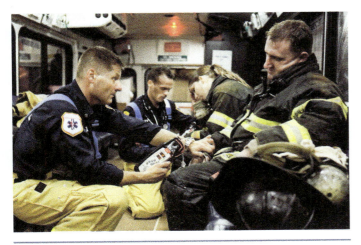

● **Figure 17** Pulse CO-oximetry now allows for the rapid and accurate determination of carbon monoxide exposure in the prehospital setting. (© Dr. Bryan E. Bledsoe)

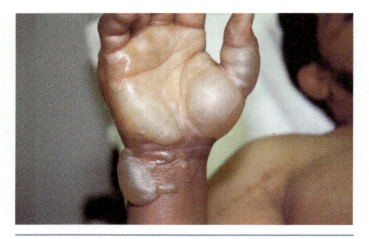

● **Figure 18**   A partial thickness burn. (© Edward T. Dickinson, MD)

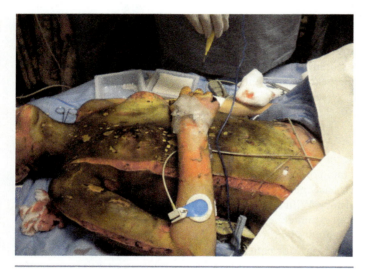

● **Figure 19**   A deep full thickness burn. (© Dr. John P. Brosious)

A third consideration in determining the burn severity is the body area affected. The face, hands, feet, joints, genitalia, and circumferential burns deserve particular consideration. Each presents with special problems to patients and their recovery.

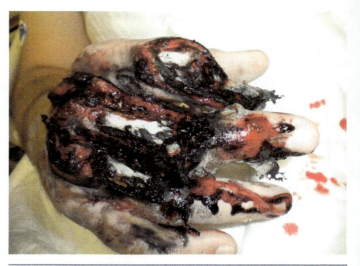

● **Figure 20**   A hand wound displaying both partial and full thickness burns. (© Dr. John P. Brosious)

You have already assessed the face for burns to eliminate respiratory involvement. But this area also needs special consideration for aesthetic reasons. Facial damage and scarring may be more socially debilitating than a joint or limb burn. Carefully assess and give a high priority to these injuries, even if you do rule out airway and respiratory involvement.

Consider full thickness burns involving feet or hands as serious. These areas are critical for much of the patient's daily activities. Serious burns and resulting scar tissue make thermal hand or foot injuries very debilitating. Assess these areas and communicate the precise injury location and the burn degree to the receiving physician. Joint burns can likewise be debilitating for patients. Scar tissue replaces skin, leading to loss of joint flexibility and mobility.

Also pay particular attention to burns that completely ring an extremity, thorax, abdomen, or neck. Due to the nature of a full thickness burn, the area underneath the burn may be drastically compressed as an eschar forms. The resulting constriction may hinder respirations, restrict distal blood flow, or cause hypoxia of the tissues beneath. Carefully assess any burn encircling a part of the body for distal circulation or other signs of vascular compromise. Once you note such

TABLE 1 | Characteristics of Various Depths of Burns

	Superficial (First Degree)	Partial Thickness (Second Degree)	Full Thickness (Third Degree)
Cause	Sun or minor flame	Hot liquids, flame	Chemicals, electricity, hot metals, flame
Skin Color	Red	Mottled red	Pearly white and/or charred, translucent, and parchment-like
Skin	Dry with no blisters	Blisters with weeping	Dry with thrombosed blood vessels
Sensation	Painful	Painful	Anesthetic
Healing	3–6 days	2–4 weeks	May require skin grafting

an injury, perform reassessments to monitor distal circulatory status.

Finally, assign a higher priority to any burns affecting pediatric or geriatric patients or patients who are ill or otherwise injured. Serious burns cause great stress for these patients. The massive fluid and heat loss as well as infection often associated with burns challenge the ability of body systems to perform adequately. Consider a burn more serious whenever it is accompanied by any other serious patient problem.

Once you determine the depth, extent, and other factors that contribute to burn severity, categorize the patient as having either minor, moderate, or severe burns. Use the criteria in Table 2 as a guide.

Burn severity should be increased one level with pediatric and geriatric patients and patients suffering from other trauma or acute medical problems. Also consider burns as critical with a patient who shows any signs or symptoms of respiratory involvement.

A newer scoring system for burn severity is the **Baux score**. The score takes into account the burn victim's age and the percentage of surface area burned. It also adds 17 if there is any significant respiratory involvment. The resulting score reflects seriousness/mortality with a score of 130 to 140 generally approaching a mortality of 100 percent. The scale works well except for those very young and those over 75 years of age.

Seriously burned patients require immediate transport to a burn (or trauma) center, if possible (Table 3). A burn center is a hospital with a special commitment to providing burn patient treatment. That commitment includes intensive patient care focused on reducing infection risk presented by serious burns, providing skin grafting to replace lost skin, and providing extensive rehabilitation services to help restore joint function. While immediate transport to a burn center is not as critically time dependent as transport for other seriously injured patients to a trauma center, burn center resources can optimize a patient's recovery prospects. Review your local protocols for criteria regarding patient transport to a burn center.

Conclude the rapid or focused trauma assessment by prioritizing your patient for transport. Rapidly transport any patient with full thickness burns over a large portion of the BSA. Patients with associated full thickness injuries to the face, joints, hands, feet, or genitalia are also candidates for immediate transport. Other cases needing rapid transport include patients who have experienced smoke, steam, or flame inhalation, or any geriatric, pediatric, otherwise ill, or trauma patient. Direct these patients to the nearest burn center as described by your local protocols or by on-line medical direction.

LEGAL CONSIDERATIONS

Transporting a Burn Patient

Burn patients require highly specialized care in a facility specifically designed for burn injuries. Burn centers offer a multidisciplinary approach to burn care utilizing plastic surgeons, general surgeons, orthopedic surgeons, rehabilitation specialists, pain management specialists, and others. In addition, burn centers provide nutritional counseling (very important to burn healing), pastoral care, and psychological care. Burn care facilities are expensive to operate and patients tend to remain in them for prolonged periods of time. The American Burn Association (ABA) has published guidelines for determining which patients might benefit from treatment in a burn center.

Most burn centers are regional facilities, and frequently patients must be transported some distance to them. Personnel who routinely transport burn patients should be familiar with burn care including dressings, fluid therapy, and escharotomy (if required). In addition, continued adequate analgesia should be provided according to local protocols and interhospital transfer orders. Burn care should be addressed in any trauma system plan.

TABLE 2 | Burn Severity

Minor

Superficial: BSA < 50 percent (sunburns, etc.)

Partial thickness: BSA < 10 percent

Moderate

Superficial: BSA > 50 percent

Partial thickness: BSA < 30 percent

Full thickness: BSA > 10 percent

Any partial or full thickness burns involving hands, feet, joints, face, or genitalia

Critical

Partial thickness: BSA > 30 percent

Full thickness: BSA > 10 percent

Inhalation injury

Source: *American College of Surgeons.*

TABLE 3 | Injuries That Benefit from Burn Center Care

Partial thickness (second-degree) burn greater than 10 percent of BSA

Full thickness (third-degree) burn

Significant burns to the face, feet, hands, perineum, or major joints

High-voltage electrical burns

Inhalation injuries

Chemical burns

Associated significant injuries or medical conditions

Source: *American College of Surgeons.*

Reassessment

Conduct reassessments for all burn patients every 15 minutes for minor burns and every 5 minutes for moderate or critical burns. Although the burn injury mechanism has been halted, the nature of the burn will continue to affect the patient. In addition to monitoring vital signs, watch for early signs of hypovolemia and airway problems. Also be cautious of aggressive fluid therapy. Monitor for lung sounds and respiratory effort suggestive of pulmonary edema, and slow fluid resuscitation if any signs develop. Also carefully monitor distal circulation and sensation with any circumferential burn. Finally, monitor the ECG to identify any abnormalities, which may be caused by electrolyte imbalances secondary to fluid movement and tissue destruction.

MANAGEMENT OF THERMAL BURNS

Once you complete your burn patient assessment and correct or address any immediate life threats, you can begin certain burn management steps, either in the field or en route to the hospital. These include preventing shock, hypothermia, and any further wound contamination.[5]

Thermal burn management can be divided into two categories: that for local and minor burns and that for moderate to severe burns.

Local and Minor Burns

Use local cooling to treat minor soft-tissue burns involving only a partial thickness injury and a small proportion of the body surface area. Provide this care only for partial thickness burns that involve less than 15 percent of the BSA or very small full thickness burns (less than 2 percent BSA). Cooling of larger surface areas may subject the patient to the risk of hypothermia. Cold or cool water immersion has some effect in reducing pain and may limit the depth of the burning process if applied immediately (within 1 or 2 minutes) after the burn.

If you have not already done so, remove any article of clothing or jewelry that might possibly act to constrain edema. As body fluids accumulate at the injury site, the site begins to swell. If the swelling encounters any constriction, it increases pressure on other tissue and may, in effect, serve as a tourniquet. This pressure may result in the loss of pulse and circulation distal to the injury. Evaluate distal circulation and sensation frequently during care and transport.

Also provide a burn patient with comfort and support. Even rather minor burns can be very painful. Calm and reassure your patient; in moderate to severe cases, consider fentanyl or morphine sulfate for pain. Encourage the patient, as much as practical, to keep the burn elevated.

Standard in-hospital treatment for minor burns can vary, depending on the clinical circumstances. Therapies may include the application of topical (not systemic) antibiotic ointments and sterile dressings. Other options such as biological dressings may be appropriate. This is why it is important to cover burns only with a clean, nonadherent dressing or sheet until a definitive management decision has been reached. For example the early use of silver sulfadiazine may preclude the use of biological dressings. Full thickness burns are open wounds, so any patient without an up-to-date tetanus immunization is given a booster of tetanus-diphtheria toxoid.

Moderate to Severe Burns

Use dry, clean (not necessarily sterile), nonadherent dressings or simply a clean sheet to cover partial thickness burns that involve more than 15 percent BSA or full thickness burns involving more than 5 percent of the BSA. Dressings keep air movement past the sensitive partial thickness burn to a minimum, and thereby reduce pain. Bulky dressings also provide padding against minor bumping and other trauma. In full thickness burns, they provide a barrier to possible contamination.

Keep the patient warm. When burns involve large surface areas, the patient loses his ability to effectively control body temperature. If a burn begins to seep fluid, as in a full thickness burn, evaporative heat loss can be extreme. Cover such an area with dry dressings, cover the patient with a blanket, and maintain a warm environment.

When treating full thickness burns to the fingers, toes, or other locations where burned surfaces may contact each other, place soft, nonadherent dressings between the burned skin areas.

If the surface area of the burn is great, medical direction may ask you to provide aggressive fluid therapy during prehospital care. While hypovolemia is not an early development after a burn, fluid migration into the wound later during the burn evolution eventually leads to serious fluid loss. Early and aggressive fluid therapy can effectively reduce the impact of this fluid loss.

If burns cover all the normal IV access sites, you may place the catheter through tissue with partial thickness burns, proximal to any more serious injury. (Full thickness burns usually damage blood vessels or coagulate the blood, making intravenous cannulation difficult and possibly impeding effective fluid flow.) Be careful with insertion. The skin may be leathery, but the tissue underneath is very delicate. Adhesive tape may not stick to burn tissue or may injure skin when it is removed. Try to secure the intravenous needle and lines by alternative means (as with gentle circumferencial bandaging), when possible. Also consider intraosseous access.

Establish intravenous routes in any patient with moderate to severe burns. Introduce two large-bore catheters and hang 1,000-mL bags of either normal saline or lactated Ringer's (preferred) solution. Current fluid resuscitation formulas recommend 4 mL of fluid for every kilogram of patient weight multiplied by the percentage body surface area sustaining full thickness burns:

$$4 \text{ mL} \times \text{Patient weight in kg} \times \text{BSA of full thickness burns} = \text{Amount of fluid over 24 hours}$$

Thus, for a 70-kg patient with 30 percent BSA full thickness burns, the calculation is

$$4 \times 70 \times 30 = 8{,}400 \text{ mL}$$

The patient needs half this amount of fluid in the first 8 hours after the burn. This particular fluid resuscitation protocol is known as the Parkland formula. Other variations exist and may be in use in your local area. In most prehospital situations where transport time is short (less than 1 hour), an initial fluid bolus of 0.25 mL of fluid for every kilogram of patient weight multiplied by the percentage of BSA burned is reasonable:

$$0.25 \text{ mL} \times \text{Patient weight in kg} \times \text{BSA burned} = \text{Amount of fluid}$$

Thus, for an 80-kg patient with 20 percent BSA burned, the calculation is

$$0.25 \times 80 \times 20 = 400 \text{ mL}$$

You may repeat this infusion once or twice during the first hour or so of care.

Be cautious and conservative when administering fluids to the burn patient if there is any possibility of airway or lung injury. Rapid fluid administration may worsen airway swelling or edema that accompanies toxic inhalation. Carefully monitor the airway and auscultate for breath sounds frequently whenever you administer fluid to a burn patient.[6]

Burns are quite painful, yet the pain is often paradoxical to burn severity. Less severe superficial and partial thickness (first- and second-degree) burns are very uncomfortable, while extensive full thickness (third-degree) burns are often almost without pain. Provide patients in severe pain with narcotic analgesia. Fentanyl or morphine should be administered as needed. Consider morphine in 2 mg IV increments every 5 minutes until suffering is relieved. Use morphine with caution as it may depress the respiratory drive and increase any existing hypovolemia. With fentanyl, start with a loading dose of 25 to 50 mcg IV and administer repeat doses of 25 mcg IV as needed.

Infection is another classic and deadly problem associated with extensive soft-tissue burns. This life-threatening condition does not develop until well after prehospital care is concluded. However, proper field care can significantly reduce mortality and morbidity. Providing a clean environment and dressings can lessen the bacterial load for the patient. Avoid prophylactic antibiotics because their early use has been shown to actually worsen outcomes for burn patients.

In dire circumstances medical direction may request you to perform an emergency escharotomy. To do this, you incise the burned tissue through the eschar, perpendicular to the constriction. Be certain to incise about 1 cm deeper than the developing eschar to ensure pressure release. If adequate respirations or distal pulses do not return after the escharotomy consider hypovolemia as the cause. Alternatively, medical direction may request you to repeat the escharotomy a short distance from the first incision.

Emergency department personnel will continue fluid resuscitation for serious burn patients according to the Parkland or another suitable formula. They will perform arterial blood gas evaluation to determine oxygen tension, carbon monoxide concentration, and cyanide poisoning levels. Urine output and cardiac monitoring are instituted as well. The staff will ensure adequate administration of parenteral narcotic analgesia and provide tetanus immunization if necessary. They will closely evaluate severe circumferential burns for eschar development. If the blood flow in an extremity is impaired, the physician may perform an escharotomy.

Inhalation Injury

If you suspect thermal (or chemical) airway burns and airway compromise is imminent, intubation can be lifesaving. Monitor the airway carefully as swelling can quickly restrict it and result in extreme hypoxemia and, possibly, respiratory arrest. A cricothyrotomy, using a Quick-Trach or similar device, may be required. Once you ensure the patient's airway, provide high-concentration oxygen titrated to an oxygen saturation of 96 percent. Oxygen not only counters hypoxia but is also therapeutic in carbon monoxide and cyanide poisoning.[6]

If there is reason to suspect carbon monoxide poisoning, administer 100 percent oxygen regardless of the pulse oximetry reading. A standard pulse oximeter cannot distinguish between hemoglobin carrying oxygen and hemoglobin carrying carbon monoxide. When carbon monoxide poisoning is suspected (or confirmed by a pulse CO-oximeter) oxygen will serve to reduce carbon monoxide's half-life on the hemoglobin molecule. The use of CPAP will increase this effect as the continuous airway pressure forces more oxygen into the bloodstream and displaces carbon monoxide more rapidly.[7]

In some EMS systems, protocols call for possible CO poisoning patients to be transported to facilities able to provide hyperbaric oxygen (HBO) therapy. The HBO chamber provides oxygen under the pressure of two or more atmospheres. This pushes oxygen into the patient's bloodstream, carrying it directly to the body's cells. HBO also drives carbon monoxide from the hemoglobin, shortening carbon monoxide's half-life and the patient's time to recovery. HBO therapy also appears to aid with tissue ischemia. However, despite its widespread use, there is no scientific evidence that HBO benefits the carbon monoxide–poisoned patient.[8]

Cyanide should be suspected in any environment where carbon monoxide is present. Suspect cyanide toxicity in patients with severe symptoms such as dyspnea, chest pain, altered mental status, seizures, and unconsciousness. To be effective, antidotal treatment of serious cyanide poisoning must be started early. Vapor exposures are likely to result in severe respiratory distress or apnea in addition to unconsciousness. Rapid airway intervention with endotracheal intubation and ventilatory support with a bag-valve mask are initial priorities. However, a rapid shift to antidotal therapy is essential to save the patient.

There are two cyanide antidote regimens available: the older cyanide kit (amyl nitrite, sodium nitrite, and sodium thiosulfate) and the newer antidote Cyanokit® (hydroxocobalamin).

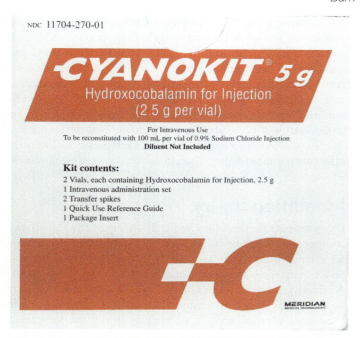

● **Figure 21** The Cyanokit® (© *Dr. Bryan E. Bledsoe*)

Hydroxocobalamin, marketed as Cyanokit® (Figure 21 ●), is now available in the United States and is much safer than the older nitrite-based cyanide kit. Hydroxocobalamin is a precursor to vitamin B_{12} (cyanocobalamin). When hydroxocobalamin is administered intravenously it binds cyanide by freeing it from the cytochrome$_{a3}$ enzyme (an enzyme necessary for oxygen processing by cells), allowing the resumption of cellular metabolism and energy processing via the electron transport chain. Cyanocobalamin is nontoxic and is excreted in the urine.

Administration of the older cyanide antidote, the cyanide kit, is a two-stage process, first using a nitrite compound, followed by a sulfur-containing compound (Figure 22 ●). The nitrite acts by converting hemoglobin (the primary oxygen-carrying protein in blood) to methemoglobin. Methemoglobin then binds to cyanide, removing it from the cytochrome$_{a3}$. The sulfur-containing antidote then removes the cyanide by forming a nontoxic compound (thiocyanate), which is excreted in the urine. The administration of the cyanide antidote should be reserved for patients with a history of acute cyanide inhalation and frank signs and symptoms of serious

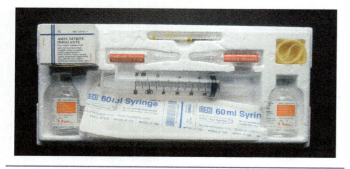

● **Figure 22** An older cyanide antidote kit. (© *Jeff Forster*)

exposure. Nitrite administration is not without risk because methemoglobin cannot carry oxygen and acts much like carbon monoxide.

If an IV is already established, administer 300 mg sodium nitrite over 2 to 4 minutes for adults. Otherwise, crush one amyl nitrite ampule and place it under an oxygen mask with high-concentration oxygen running or in the bag or oxygen reservoir of a bag-valve mask. Do not let the ampule fall into the patient's mouth or down the endotracheal tube. Always follow inhaled amyl nitrite with intravenous sodium nitrite, and do not use amyl nitrite if the patient has already received sodium nitrite. Use care in the administration of sodium nitrite or amyl nitrite as they may induce hypotension. They also bind to the hemoglobin, reducing its ability to carry oxygen.

Following administration of IV sodium nitrite, administer 12.5 g of sodium thiosulfate for the adult. In addition to antidotal therapy, keep the patient supine and administer high-concentration oxygen.

ASSESSMENT AND MANAGEMENT OF ELECTRICAL, CHEMICAL, AND RADIATION INJURIES

Electrical Injuries

Be certain that the power has been shut off before you approach the scene of a suspected electrical injury. Until it is, do not allow anyone to approach the patient or the proximity of the electrical source. Remember that an energized power line need not spark or whip around to be deadly; a power line simply lying on the ground can still present a significant danger. Note also that some utility lines have breakers that will try to reestablish power periodically. Establish a safety zone if there is any question about the status of lines that are down. Keep vehicles and personnel at a distance from downed lines or the source pole that is greater than the distance between power poles. Also be aware that downed power lines may energize metal structures such as buildings, vehicles, or fences.

Once the scene is secure, assess the patient and prepare him or her for transport. Search for both an entrance and an exit wound. Look specifically for possible contact points with both the ground and the electrical source. In some circumstances, multiple entrance and exit wounds are present. Remember that electrical current passes through the body and therefore may result in significant internal burns, especially to blood vessels and nerves, while the assessment reveals only minimal superficial findings. Rapidly progressive cardiovascular collapse can follow contact with an electrical source. Also, examine the patient for any fractures resulting from forceful muscle contractions caused by the current's passage and check distal sensation for signs of nervous system injury. Suspect spinal injury caused by muscle spasm in any significant electrical contact and provide appropriate spinal precautions.

As with thermal burns, look for smoldering shoes, belts, or other clothing items. Such items may continue the burning process well after the current is shut off. Also remove rings, watches, and any other constrictive items from the fingers, limbs, and neck.

Perform ECG monitoring for possible cardiac disturbances in victims of electrical burns. Electrical current may induce arrhythmias, including bradycardias, tachycardias, ventricular fibrillation, and asystole. Ensure that emergency department personnel examine any patient who has sustained a significant electrical shock. Damage the current causes may be internal and not apparent to you or your patient during assessment. Consider any significant electrical burn or exposure patient as a high priority for immediate transport.

Lightning strikes to humans occur more than 300 times each year in the United States and result in over 100 deaths. Strikes to people riding tractors, on open water, on golf courses, and under trees are most common, and men are the victims of 75 percent of all strikes. A lightning strike is a high-voltage (up to 100,000 volts), high-current (10,000 amperes), and high-temperature (50,000°F) event that lasts only a fraction of a second. A direct strike will impart this energy to the patient (Figure 23 ●). However, the lightning will often strike a nearby object with some current traveling sideways (sideflash) or current may radiate outward in alternate pathways from the strike point, thus diminishing the voltage (step voltage).

By the time anyone reaches a victim of a lightning strike, the electricity has long since dissipated. (There will be, however, a continued risk of further strikes as long as the storm remains nearby.) There is no danger of electrical shock from touching someone who has been struck by lightning. The person's clothing, however, may continue to smolder, so remove it as necessary. Among other serious effects, lightning can produce a sudden cessation of breathing. Despite being apneic and perhaps pulseless, these patients frequently survive with prompt prehospital intervention.

Treat visible burns ("entrance" and "exit" wounds) just as any thermal burn with cooling, if necessary, followed by the application of a dry, clean sheet or dressings.. Do not focus too much on the visible burns, but instead recognize that the electricity has passed through the body, possibly causing widespread internal effects.

Treat cardiac or respiratory arrest in electrical burn patients with aggressive circulatory, ventilatory, and airway management (CAB). Patients in cardiac arrest because of contact with electrical current have a high survival rate if prehospital intervention is prompt. Check immediately for ventricular fibrillation and defibrillate if necessary. Secure the airway with an advanced airway and begin ventilations and chest compressions. The usual resuscitative procedures for cardiac arrest apply equally when the cause of the arrest is electrical injury; they might include the use of vasopressors and antiarrhythmics.

For serious electrical burn injuries, initiate at least two large-bore IVs and administer 1,000 mL of fluid per hour in 20 mL/kg boluses. Consider sodium bicarbonate and mannitol, usually at the discretion of medical direction, to prevent the complications of rhabdomyolysis (the destruction of muscle tissue and the release of toxic elements of that process) and hyperkalemia. The usual starting dose is 1 mEq/kg for sodium bicarbonate and 10 g for mannitol.

Chemical Burns

As you perform the scene size-up, identify the nature of the chemical spill/contamination and, if necessary and possible, approach from uphill and upwind. Identify the chemical's location and ensure that it poses no continuing hazard to you, your patient, other rescuers, or the public. Be wary of toxic fumes and cross-contamination from the patient and the surrounding environment. If necessary, have hazardous material team members evacuate and decontaminate the victim before you begin assessment and care. Seek out personnel on the scene who are familiar with the agent and consult with them regarding dangers posed by the agent and any specific medical care and patient handling procedures required with it.

During your assessment and care, always wear medical examination (preferably nitrile) gloves, but never presume that they protect you from the agent. Take appropriate protective action against airborne dust, toxic fumes, and splash exposure for both yourself and the patient (goggles and mask as needed). Wear a disposable gown if there is danger of the agent contacting your clothing. Make certain the agent is isolated and no longer a danger to the patient or others. Have any of the patient's clothing that you suspect may be contaminated removed, and isolate it from accidental contact. Save the clothing and ensure that it is disposed of properly. Identify the type of agent, its exact chemical name, the length of the patient's contact time with it, and the precise patient body areas affected by it.

As you begin your primary assessment, ensure that the patient is alert and fully oriented and that airway and breathing are unaffected by the contact. If there is any airway restriction or respiratory involvement, consider early intubation. As airway tissue swells, the obstruction worsens and intubation becomes more difficult. Monitor the patient's heart rate and consider ECG monitoring, because many chemicals (for example, organophosphates) may affect the heart. If the patient is stable, begin the rapid trauma assessment.

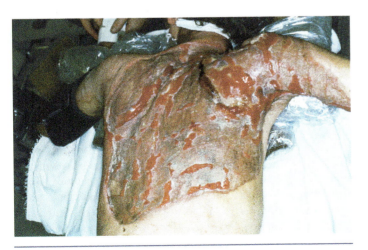

● **Figure 23**   A lightning strike injury. (© 2012 Wellcome *Images/Custom Medical Stock Photo, All Rights Reserved)*

Examine any chemical burn carefully to establish the depth, extent, and nature of the injury. If you suspect phenol, dry lime, sodium, or riot agents, then treat as indicated below.

- **Phenol.** A gelatinous caustic called phenol is used as a powerful industrial cleaner. Phenol is very difficult to remove because it is sticky and relatively insoluble in water. Alcohol, which dissolves it, is frequently available in places where phenol is regularly used. You can use the alcohol to dissolve and help remove the phenol and follow removal with irrigation using large volumes of cool water. In the absence of alcohol for phenol removal, use copious volumes of water to remove the agent.[9]

- **Dry lime.** Dry lime (calcium oxide) is a strong corrosive that reacts with water. It produces heat and subsequent chemical and thermal injuries. Brush dry lime off the patient gently, but as completely as possible. Then rinse the contaminated area with large volumes of cool to cold water. While the water reacts with any remaining lime, it cools the contact area and removes any chemical residue. By rinsing with water, you ensure the lime reacts with that water rather than with water contained within the patient's soft tissues.

- **Sodium.** Sodium is an unstable metal that reacts destructively with many substances, including human tissue. It reacts vigorously with water, creating extreme heat, explosive hydrogen gas, and possible ignition. Sodium is normally stored submerged in oil because the metal reacts with moisture in the air. If a patient is contaminated with sodium, decontaminate him quickly by gentle brushing. Then cover the wound with the oil used to store the substance.

- **Riot control agents.** These agents, which include CS, CN (Mace), and oleoresin capsicum (OC, pepper spray), deserve special mention because people are the targets of their intended use and because that use is frequent. These agents cause intense eye, mucous membrane, and respiratory tract irritation. In general, they do not cause permanent damage when properly deployed. Patients who have contacted them typically present with eye pain, tearing, and temporary "blindness." Coughing, gagging, and vomiting are also common. Treatment is supportive and most patients recover spontaneously within 10 to 20 minutes of fresh air exposure. If necessary, irrigate the patient's eyes with normal saline if you suspect that any riot agent contamination remains in the eye.

If it has not been done earlier, decontaminate the patient who has come in contact with any other chemical capable of causing tissue damage. Stop the damage by irrigating the site with large volumes of cool water. Water rinses away the offending material and dilutes any water-soluble agents. The water also reduces the heat and rate of a chemical reaction and, ultimately, the chemical's effects on the patient's skin. If contamination is widespread, douse the patient with large volumes of water. Use a garden hose or low-pressure water from a fire truck. Ensure that the water is neither warm nor too cold.

When the patient has been thoroughly rinsed for a few minutes, remove any remaining clothing. Take care that the process does not contaminate rescuers. If the agent is dangerous, save all clothing and contain the rinse water for proper disposal at a later time. Next, gently wash the burn with a mild soap (such as ordinary dish detergent) and a gentle brush or sponge. Be careful not to cause further soft-tissue damage. After washing, gently irrigate the wound with a constant flow of water. While the pain and the burning process may appear to subside, it is important to continue irrigation until the patient arrives at the emergency department. If practical, transport the corrosive's container label or a sample of the agent (safely contained and marked) along with the patient. On arrival at the hospital, be sure to describe to emergency department personnel, and enter in your prehospital care report, any first aid given prior to your arrival.

Do not use any neutralizing agent without first gaining approval of medical direction. Neutralizing agents often react violently with agents they neutralize. They may ultimately increase the reaction heat and induce thermal burns. In some cases, the neutralizing agent is more damaging to the skin than the original contaminant.

With chemical burns, pay particular attention to the patient's eyes. Eyes are very sensitive to chemicals and can easily be damaged, even by weak agents. Prompt treatment of chemical eye injury is critical and can reduce damage and preserve eyesight. Ask the patient about chemical contact with the eyes, eye pain, vision changes, and contact lens use. Examine the eyes for eyelid spasm (blepharospasm), conjunctival erythema, discoloration, tearing, and other evidence of burns or irritation.

Irrigate chemical splashes that involve the eye with large volumes of water. Alkali burns are especially damaging and with them you should flush the eye for at least 15 minutes. Irrigate acid burns for at least 5 minutes. Flush splashes of an unknown agent for up to 20 minutes. Do not, however, delay transport while irrigating.

A useful technique for eye irrigation is to hang a bag of normal saline (lactated Ringer's is an acceptable substitute) and use the flow regulator to control the fluid flow into the nasal corner of the eye. Turn the patient's head to the side to facilitate drainage and avoid cross-contaminating the other eye with waste fluid. Be alert for contact lenses in cases where chemicals are splashed into the eyes. Chemicals may become trapped under the lenses, preventing adequate irrigation. Gently remove the lenses before continuing irrigation.

Radiation Burns

An incident involving potential radiation exposure or burns must raise concern during both dispatch and response phases of an emergency call. Because radiation can neither be seen nor felt, it can endanger EMS personnel unless the hazard is anticipated and proper precautions taken. If you suspect radiation exposure, approach the scene very carefully. If the incident occurs at a power generation plant or in an industrial or a medical facility, seek out personnel knowledgeable about the radioactive substance being used. Such persons are always on staff, and frequently on site, at these facilities. Stay a good distance from the scene and ensure that bystanders, rescuers, and patients remain remote from the exposure source. Remember that distance and the nature of shielding materials, like concrete or earth, between you and the radiation source reduce potential exposure. If the exposure may be from dust or fire, approach from and remain upwind of the radiation source.

In radiation exposure incidents, ensure that personnel trained in radiation hazards isolate the source, contain it, and test the scene for safety. If the scene is not deemed safe, move the patient to a site remote from the radioactivity source where you can give care without danger either to yourself or the patient. Plan the removal carefully. Use as much shielding as possible and keep exposure times to a minimum. Remember, the radiation dose you receive is related to three primary factors: duration, distance, and shielding.

If you must carry out a patient removal, consider using the oldest rescuers for the evacuation team. This approach is prudent because many of the radiation exposure effects become evident many years after exposure. If you use older rescuers, they are more likely to be past their reproductive years and have fewer years of life left if and when a problem does surface. This concern is especially important with pregnant females and young adults of both sexes. Remember that radiation damages the reproductive system very easily.

If there is a risk that patients are contaminated, ensure that they are properly decontaminated before you begin assessment and care. If available for this task, use persons knowledgeable in decontamination and monitoring techniques who have the appropriate protective gear. If this is not possible, don goggles, a mask, gloves, and a disposable gown. Direct the evacuation team to place the patients in a decontamination area remote from your vehicle and other personnel and where any contamination can be contained. Have patients disrobe or carefully disrobe them, rinse them with large volumes of water, then wash them with a soft brush and rinse again. Ordinary dish detergent is an effective cleansing agent. Gently scrub, or closely trim (but do not shave) and then gently scrub, any areas of body hair. As in incidents of chemical contamination, save all clothing and decontamination water and dispose of them

safely. Perform decontamination before moving the patients to the ambulance.

Carefully document the circumstances of the radioactive exposure. If possible, identify the source and agent strength. Determine the patient's proximity to the source during the exposure as well as the length of exposure.

Once decontaminated, treat a radiation exposure patient as you would any other patient. Because the human body by itself cannot be a source of ionizing radiation, a decontaminated patient poses no threat to you or your crew. Remember, however, that any contaminated material remaining on the patient or any contamination transferred to you does provide a source of radiation exposure and may contaminate you and your vehicle.

The actual assessment of a patient exposed to radiation is quite simple and usually reveals minimal signs or symptoms of injury. Only extreme exposures result in the classical presentation of nausea, vomiting, and malaise. Burns are extremely rare, although they may occur if the exposure is extremely intense. Even though a patient seems well, delayed consequences of high-dose radiation exposure can be devastating. If you note any early patient complaints, record the findings in the patient's own words and include the time the complaint first was made. This information is helpful in determining the patient's degree of radiation exposure (Table 4).

Treat the radiation injury patient's symptoms, make the patient as comfortable as possible, and offer psychological support. Cover any burns with sterile dressings and, if general symptoms are noticeable, provide oxygen and initiate an IV. Maintain the patient's body temperature and provide transport to the emergency department.

Reassessment

Monitor patients with inhalation, chemical, and electrical burns and radiation exposure for signs of increasing complications associated with their burn mechanisms. Also monitor blood pressure, pulse, and respirations and trend any changes. Perform these evaluations every 15 minutes in stable patients and every 5 minutes in unstable patients.

TABLE 4 | Dose-Effect Relationships to Ionizing Radiation

Whole Body Exposure Dose (RAD)	Effect
5–50	Asymptomatic. Blood studies are normal.
50–75	Asymptomatic. Minor depressions of white blood cells and platelets in a few patients.
75–125	May produce anorexia, nausea, vomiting, and fatigue in approximately 10–20 percent of patients within two days.
125–200	Possible nausea and vomiting. Diarrhea, anxiety, tachycardia. Fatal to less than 5 percent of patients.
200–600	Nausea and vomiting. Diarrhea in the first several hours. Weakness, fatigue. Fatal to approximately 50 percent of patients within six weeks without prompt medical attention.
600–1,000	"Burning sensation" within minutes. Nausea and vomiting within 10 minutes. Confusion, ataxia, and collapse within 1 hour. Watery diarrhea within 1 to 2 hours. Fatal to 100 percent within short time without prompt medical attention.

Localized Exposure Dose (RAD)	Effect
50	Asymptomatic.
500	Asymptomatic (usually). May have risk of altered function of exposed area.
2,500	Atrophy, vascular lesion, and altered pigmentation.
5,000	Chronic ulcer, risk of carcinogenesis.

CHAPTER REVIEW

▰ SUMMARY

Burn injuries may compromise the skin—the protective envelope that protects and contains the human body. Burn damage to the skin may interfere with its ability to contain water within the body and to prevent damaging agents from entering. For these reasons, assessment and care of these soft-tissue injuries are important.

Assess the burn to determine its depth and the body surface area it involves. Be sensitive to any respiratory, joint, hand, foot, or circumferential regions affected by the burn. Give special consideration to pediatric and geriatric burn patients and to burn patients who are also ill or otherwise injured. Consider all these factors in determining the overall burn severity. If the patient's condition warrants, institute aggressive care. Anticipate airway compromise and fluid loss. Secure the airway very early in prehospital care. Initiate IV access, and begin fluid administration.

Electrical, chemical, or radiation burns require special care and assessment. An electrical burn requires careful assessment to determine the area and depth of burn involvement and should be followed by wound site dressing and cardiac monitoring. Chemical burns need rapid and effective decontamination. Radiation burns call for extreme care in removing the patient from the radiation source and in providing decontamination and supportive care.

YOU MAKE THE CALL

A young boy scout on a camping trip ignites his coat and shirt sleeve while attempting to light a campfire. By the time his scoutmaster extinguishes the flames, the arm is seriously burned. Your assessment finds the scout with a relatively painless hand and forearm with some skin discoloration. The upper arm is very painful and reddened with its distal portion just starting to blister.

1. What severity are the burns of the forearm and hand and of the upper arm?

2. What percentage of the body surface area is burned?

3. What level of acuity would you assign this patient?

See Suggested Responses at the back of this chapter.

REVIEW QUESTIONS

1. During the healing process for burns, scar tissue is laid down and remodeled, and the patient begins to rehabilitate and return to normal function. This is called the _____.
a. fluid shift phase
b. resolution phase
c. emergent phase
d. hypermetabolic phase

2. Chemical burns caused by _____ usually continue to destroy cell membranes through liquefaction necrosis, allowing them to penetrate underlying tissue and causing deeper burns.
a. acids
b. alkalis
c. electricity
d. coagulation

3. The type of radiation that can travel through 6 to 10 feet of air, penetrate a few layers of clothing, and cause both external and internal injuries is _____.
a. gamma radiation
b. alpha radiation
c. beta radiation
d. neutron radiation

4. Airway edema is a major concern when dealing with inhalation injuries. To provide the best protection and prevent patient deterioration, it is important to initiate early _____.
a. cardiac monitoring
b. endotracheal intubation
c. intravenous cannulation
d. rapid fluid replacement

5. To reduce the patient's exposure to infectious pathogens, the paramedic must carefully _____.
a. employ Standard Precautions
b. use a dry, clean sheet or dressings and clean equipment
c. avoid gross contamination of the burn
d. all of the above

6. For pediatric or geriatric patients and patients with burns and suffering from other trauma or medical conditions, always _____.
a. increase burn severity one level
b. initiate immediate intubation
c. reduce administered fluids
d. initiate immediate transport

7. Your patient is experiencing airway compromise due to an inhalation injury. You elect to perform rapid sequence intubation to protect the patient's airway. Which of the following paralytics should you use with caution, if at all, because it may worsen hyperkalemia?
a. morphine
b. vecuronium
c. succinylcholine
d. pancuronium

8. Which of the following burns would be classified as a moderate burn?
a. full thickness burns <2 percent body surface area
b. superficial burns <50 percent body surface area
c. partial thickness burns >30 percent body surface area
d. partial thickness burns <30 percent body surface area

9. Fluid replacement is indicated in the care of patients with moderate to severe burns greater than 15 to 20 percent total body surface area. The Parkland formula sets up a calculation for determining the amount of fluid to infuse over 24 hours. Which of the following accurately depicts the Parkland formula?
a. 0.25 mL × patient weight in kilograms × BSA involved
b. 1.25 mL × patient weight in pounds × BSA involved

c. 0.75 mL × patient weight in kilograms × BSA involved

d. 0.15 mL × patient weight in pounds × BSA involved

10. In general, how should dry lime be removed from the skin?
    a. Flush with vinegar, then with water
    b. Brush dry lime away and then flush with water
    c. Apply an oil-based baking soda and a sterile dressing
    d. Cover the wound as is, flush with water, and transport

11. Your 45-year-old male patient was working on his roof, came into contact with power lines, and has experienced possible electrocution. The patient has an irregular pulse of 124 BPM and his respiratory rate is 22 and irregular. The patient's blood pressure is 106/76. You note both entrance and exit wounds. You immediately manage the airway and decide to start an IV. You realize that you should administer an initial fluid bolus of _____.
    a. 20 mL/kg   c. 10 mg/kg
    b. 10 mL/kg   d. 20 mg/kg

12. The burn patient's injured tissue will swell. Therefore, with this knowledge, you realize that it is important to _____.
    a. start IV therapy early
    b. remove restrictive jewelry
    c. administer high-concentration oxygen
    d. cover the injury with a burn sheet

See Answers to Review Questions at the back of this chapter.

REFERENCES

1. American Burn Association, "Burn Incidence and Treatment in the United States: 2011 Fact Sheet." (Available at www.ameriburn.org/resources_factsheet.php)

2. McManus, W. F. and B. A. Pruitt, Jr. "Thermal Injuries," in D. V. Feliciano, E. E. Moore, and K. L. Mattox, eds. *Trauma*. 6th ed. New York: McGraw Hill, 2008.

3. Fish, R, "Electrical Injuries," *Emergency Medicine: A Comprehensive Study Guide,* Tintinalli J, ed. ACEP. New York: McGraw Hill, 2004.

4. Singer, A. J., et al. "The Association between Hypothermia, Prehospital Cooling, and Mortality in Burn Victims." *Acad Emerg Med* 17(4) (Apr 2010): 456–459.

5. Monafo, W. W. "Initial Management of Burns." *New England J Med* 335 (1996): 1581–1586.

6. Eastman, A. L., B. A. Arnoldo, J. L. Hunt, and G. F. Purdue. "Pre-Burn Center Management of the Burned Airway: Do We Know Enough?" *J Burn Care Res* 31 (2010): 701–705.

7. Bizovi, K. E. and J. D. Leikin. "Smoke Inhalation among Firefighters." *Occup Med* 10(4) (Oct–Dec 1995): 721–733.

8. Bledsoe, B. *Carbon Monoxide Poisoning—Student Edition*, Cielo Azul Publications, Midlothian, TX, 2008.

9. Pullin, T. G., M. N. Pinkerton, R. V. Johnson, and D. J. Kilian. "Decontamination of the Skin of Swine following Phenol Exposure: A Comparison of the Relative Efficacy of Water versus Polyethylene Glycol/Industrial Methylated Spirits." *Toxicol Appl Pharmacol* 43(1) (1978): 199–206.

FURTHER READING

American Burn Association National Burn Repository Advisory Committee. *National Burn Repository 2009 Report*. Worldwide 2010.

Bates, Barbara and Peter G. Szilagyi. *A Guide to Physical Examination and History Taking*. 9th ed. Philadelphia: J. B. Lippincott, 2007.

Bledsoe, B. E. and D. Clayden. *Prehospital Emergency Pharmacology*. 7th ed. Upper Saddle River, NJ: Pearson/Prentice Hall, 2011.

Bledsoe, B. E., B. J. Colbert, and J. E. Ankney. *Essentials of A & P for Emergency Care*. Upper Saddle River, NJ: Pearson/Prentice Hall, 2010.

Martini, Frederic. *Fundamentals of Anatomy and Physiology*. 7th ed. San Francisco: Benjamin Cummings, 2011.

Rosen, P., and R. Barkin, eds. *Emergency Medicine: Concepts and Clinical Practice*. 7th ed. St. Louis: Mosby, 2009.

Tintinalli, J. E., ed. *Emergency Medicine: A Comprehensive Study Guide*. 7th ed. New York: McGraw-Hill, 2011.

SUGGESTED RESPONSES TO "YOU MAKE THE CALL"

The following are suggested responses to the "You Make the Call" scenarios presented in this chapter. Each represents an acceptable response to the scenario but should not be interpreted as the only correct response.

1. *What severity are the burns of the forearm and hand and of the upper arm?*

   The forearm and hand are most likely third-degree burns.

2. *What percentage of the body surface area is burned?*

   Nine percent or less. (The entire arm is estimated as 9 percent BSA. If the entire arm is burned, you are looking at a total of 9 percent BSA.)

3. *What level of acuity would you assign this patient?*

   This is a severe/critical burn that should be treated rapidly and transported urgently. It involves the patient's hands and bends of the arm, making this a potentially debilitating injury.

ANSWERS TO REVIEW QUESTIONS

1. b
2. b
3. c
4. b
5. d
6. a
7. c
8. d
9. a
10. b
11. a
12. b

GLOSSARY

alpha radiation   low-level form of nuclear radiation; a weak source of energy that is stopped by clothing or the first layers of skin.

ampere   basic unit for measuring the strength of an electric current.

Baux score   scoring system for burn severity that takes into account the burn victim's age, percentage of surface area burned, and significant respiratory involvement with a resulting score reflecting seriousness/mortality.

beta radiation   medium-strength radiation that is stopped with light clothing or the uppermost layers of skin.

blepharospasm   uncontrolled muscle contraction of the eyelids resulting in tightly closed eyelids.

body surface area (BSA)   percentage of a patient's body affected by a burn.

coagulation necrosis   the process in which an acid, while destroying tissue, forms an insoluble layer that limits further damage.

current   the rate of flow of an electric charge.

denature   alter the usual substance of something.

emergent phase   first stage of the burn process that is characterized by a catecholamine release and pain-mediated reaction.

eschar   hard, leathery product of a deep full thickness burn; it consists of dead and denatured skin.

extravascular space   the volume contained within the cells (intracellular space) and the spaces between the cells (interstitial space).

fluid shift phase   stage of the burn process in which there is a massive shift of fluid from the intravascular to the extravascular space.

full thickness burn   burn that damages all layers of the skin; characterized by areas that are painless and often dry; also called a third-degree burn.

gamma radiation   powerful electromagnetic radiation emitted by radioactive substances with powerful penetrating properties; it is stronger than alpha and beta radiation. Similar to X-rays, which are generally less energetic.

Gray   a unit of absorbed radiation dose equal to 100 rads.

hypermetabolic phase   stage of the burn process in which there is increased body metabolism in an attempt by the body to heal the burn.

intravascular space   the volume contained by all the arteries, veins, capillaries, and other components of the circulatory system.

ionization   the process of changing a substance into separate charged particles (ions).

Jackson's theory of thermal wounds   explanation of the physical effects of thermal burns.

Joule's law   the physical law stating that the rate of heat production is directly proportional to the resistance of the circuit and to the square of the current.

liquefaction necrosis   the process in which an alkali dissolves and liquefies tissue.

neutron radiation   powerful radiation with penetrating properties between that of beta and gamma radiation.

ohm   basic unit for measuring the strength of electrical resistance.

Ohm's law   the physical law identifying that the current in an electrical circuit is directly proportional to the voltage and inversely proportional to the resistance.

partial thickness burn   burn in which the epidermis is burned through and the dermis is damaged; characterized by redness and blistering; also called a second-degree burn.

rad   basic unit of absorbed radiation dose.

resistance   property of a conductor that opposes the passage of an electric current.

resolution phase   final stage of the burn process in which scar tissue is laid down and the healing process is completed.

rule of nines   method of estimating amount of body surface area burned by a division of the body into regions, each of which represents approximately 9 percent of total BSA (plus 1 percent for the genital region).

rule of palms   method of estimating the amount of body surface area burned that sizes the area burned in comparison to the patient's palmar surface.

subglottic   referring to the lower airway.

superficial burn   a burn that involves only the epidermis; characterized by reddening of the skin; also called a first-degree burn.

supraglottic   referring to the upper airway.

voltage   the difference of electric potential between two points with different concentrations of electrons.

zone of coagulation   area in a burn nearest the heat source that suffers the most damage and is characterized by clotted blood and thrombosed blood vessels.

zone of hyperemia   area peripheral to a burn that is characterized by increased blood flow.

zone of stasis   area in a burn surrounding the zone of coagulation that is characterized by decreased blood flow.

Penetrating Trauma

From Chapter 3 of *Paramedic Care: Principles & Practice, Volume 5,* Fourth Edition. Bryan Bledsoe,
Robert Porter, and Richard Cherry. Copyright © 2013 by Pearson Education, Inc. All rights reserved.

Penetrating Trauma

Robert S. Porter, MA, EMT-P

STANDARD
Trauma (Trauma Overview)

COMPETENCY
Integrates assessment findings with principles of epidemiology and pathophysiology to formulate a field impression to implement a comprehensive treatment/disposition plan for an acutely injured patient.

OBJECTIVES

Terminal Performance Objective
After reading this chapter you should be able to relate the kinetics and mechanisms of injury associated with penetrating trauma to patients' potential for injury.

Enabling Objectives
To accomplish the terminal performance objective, you should be able to:

1. Define key terms introduced in this chapter.
2. Apply the laws of inertia and energy conservation to the kinetics of penetrating trauma.
3. Apply the concepts of force and kinetic energy exchange to the potential for injury.
4. Apply principles of ballistics to the prediction of injury patterns.
5. Apply the characteristics of specific weapon types to the prediction of injury patterns.
6. Associate the application of low, medium, and high-velocity penetrating mechanisms to various body tissues with the biomechanical forces produced to predict injury patterns.
7. Describe the forces and characteristics associated with entrance and exit wounds from penetrating trauma.
8. Describe special concerns for EMS provider safety that are associated with penetrating trauma.
9. Given a penetrating trauma scenario, reconstruct events to gain additional information that can help predict injury patterns.
10. Describe medical/legal concerns specific to penetrating trauma situations.
11. Describe the special considerations in assessment and management of penetrating trauma to the face and chest, and of impaled objects.

KEY TERMS

ballistics
caliber
cavitation
drag

percutaneous
 cricothyrotomy
pericardial tamponade
profile
projectile

resiliency
trajectory
yaw
zone of injury

An early morning traffic stop results in a gun battle between a police officer and the armed driver of a car. EMS 7 is dispatched to care for the driver, who has been shot once in the chest. Dispatch informs EMS 7 that officers have the victim in custody and that the weapon has been secured.

On arrival at the shooting scene, paramedic Sandy O'Donnell notices several officers clustered around a male approximately 30 years old, who is seated on the ground and leaning back against an auto. There are several shell casings on the ground near the man, and he appears to be bleeding from a small wound in his left anterior chest. The man's hands are secured behind his back. The man's skin color is somewhat ashen and pale, his facial expression reveals anxiety, and he appears to be breathing shallowly.

The arresting officer states that the man drew a weapon, a small-caliber handgun, pointed it, and fired at the officer several times. In response, the officer drew his weapon (a 9 mm semi-automatic) and fired three times, hitting the victim once in the chest. The victim dropped his weapon and slumped to his current position. The arresting officer took the victim's gun (a .38 caliber revolver), and the weapon is now in that officer's custody.

Sandy asks if the victim was searched for other weapons and the officer replies, "No." An officer performs a quick search, discovering and taking into custody a small knife. He then clears Sandy to care for the victim.

The victim, whose name is Jeffery, seems alert and oriented to time, place, person, and one's own person and does not interrupt speech to breathe. He complains of mild chest pain that increases if he attempts deep breathing. He reports no other pain or injuries. He denies any significant medical history.

Primary assessment reveals a strong pulse with a rate of about 90, respirations about 20, and relatively normal chest excursion. During the rapid trauma exam, Sandy notes a medium-caliber bullet hole in the left anterior chest at about the third intercostal space along the midclavicular line. No air appears to be moving through the wound with respirations, and hemorrhage is very minor. Assessment of the victim's back reveals a larger wound with a more "blown-out" appearance. Again, no air seems to be moving through the wound with respirations, although hemorrhage is more significant than from the anterior wound.

Sandy quickly applies oxygen via nonrebreather mask at 15 liters per minute and listens for breath sounds. The breath sounds are reasonably clear, though there are slight crackles in the left chest near the wounds. Sandy quickly seals both anterior and posterior wounds with occlusive dressings secured on three sides while her partner takes a quick blood pressure. She reports a finding of 122/86 and a regular and strong pulse at a rate of 92. Other findings are normal, except for a pulse oximeter reading of 88 percent. Sandy asks the officers to move the restraints to the patient's front as she moves him to the stretcher. One officer remains with the prisoner during transport.

Sandy alerts the nearby trauma center to the patient's injury mechanism and assessment findings. They request rapid transport with one IV of normal saline run at a to-keep-open rate. Sandy initiates an IV en route with a 14-gauge catheter, blood tubing, and a 1,000-mL bag of normal saline.

During transport to the trauma center, reassessments reveal increasing crackles surrounding the bullet pathway and a slight increase in Jeffery's dyspnea. On arrival at the trauma center, Sandy provides an update on the patient's condition and vital signs to the trauma triage nurse while Jeffery is moved to the trauma suite for evaluation by the trauma surgical team.

INTRODUCTION TO PENETRATING TRAUMA

Modern society is experiencing a significant increase in the number and severity of penetrating trauma injuries, especially gunshot wounds. About 31,500 deaths occur each year as a result of shootings, and the number is increasing. In addition to gunshot wounds, other penetrating trauma includes that caused by knives, arrows, nails, and pieces of glass or wire.[1] There is also an increasing incidence of penetrating trauma due to acts of terrorism using either automatic weapons or explosive devices.

As with blunt trauma, physical principles govern the energy exchange associated with penetrating trauma. The types of weapons and **projectiles** involved and the characteristics of any tissue they strike affect the severity of penetrating injury. Understanding the principles of energy exchange and projectile travel will help you to anticipate the potential for injuries, to recognize the injuries that have occurred, and, ultimately, to provide optimal assessment and care for victims of penetrating trauma.

There are three levels of penetrating trauma: low, medium, and high. Low-velocity penetrating trauma is generally inflicted by mechanisms such as bladed and pointed objects like knives, swords, and ice picks that are thrust into the victim by an assailant; arrows shot from a bow; ski poles impaled during a skiing accident; wire thrown by a lawn mower; a nail stepped on; or a concrete reinforcing rod at a construction site that someone falls on. Medium-velocity penetrating trauma is caused most often by handgun bullets and high-velocity trauma by rifle bullets.

Injury from low-velocity penetrating trauma is generally limited to the tissue actually contacted by the object and restricted to the object's pathway of travel. By contrast, medium- and high-velocity penetrating wounds involve dramatic energy exchanges and more extensive injury pathways. The kinetics of penetrating trauma explain why this occurs.

LEGAL CONSIDERATIONS

Crime, Terrorism, and You

Unfortunately, with the exception of war, the increased incidence of penetrating trauma in the world has been primarily due to an increase in crime, terrorism, and the availability of weapons. Any scene where there is a reported case of penetrating trauma should heighten your awareness of scene hazards and safety. Never approach a scene until law enforcement personnel tell you it is safe to do so. Likewise, if you are providing care to a victim of penetrating trauma and you feel the scene is becoming unsafe, you should retreat immediately to a safe distance—even if that requires you to leave the patient.

Our world is much different than it was 100 years ago, or even 50 years ago for that matter. Crime and terrorism pose real threats to both the public and EMS personnel. Always put personal safety and scene safety above all other priorities. Live to see another day.

KINETICS OF PENETRATING TRAUMA

When a projectile strikes a target, it exchanges its kinetic energy (energy of motion) with the object struck. The kinetic energy of an object (in this case, a penetrating object) is equal to its mass times the square of its velocity, all divided by 2:

$$\text{Kinetic Energy} = \frac{\text{Mass (Weight)} \times \text{Velocity (Speed)}^2}{2}$$

This formula demonstrates that the greater the mass *or* speed of an object, the greater its kinetic energy. The relationship of *mass* to energy is *direct*. If you double an object's mass, it has twice the kinetic energy (if velocity remains the same). If you triple its mass, kinetic energy triples as well, and so on. However, the relationship of *velocity* to energy is *squared*. If you double an object's speed, its kinetic energy increases fourfold (if mass remains the same). If speed triples, kinetic energy increases ninefold, and so on.

This relationship between mass and velocity explains why even very small and relatively light bullets traveling very fast have a potential to do great harm. It also makes clear why different weights of bullets traveling at different velocities can cause differing degrees of damage. For example, handguns, shotguns, and low-powered (.22 caliber—non-magnum round) rifles are considered to be medium-energy/medium-velocity weapons. They deliver bullets, slugs, and pellets much faster than low-energy/low-velocity objects like knives and arrows can be wielded, but they are still slower than bullets fired by high-energy/high-velocity weapons such as hunting and assault rifles. For example, a handgun bullet is generally lighter and much slower (200 to 400 meters per second) than a rifle bullet. Civilian and military rifles, however, commonly fire a heavier bullet at speeds of 600 to 900 meters per second. Hence, a high-energy rifle bullet's kinetic energy is three to nine times that of a medium-energy handgun bullet and can be expected to do significantly more damage. In the urban warfare experience of Northern Ireland (where handguns and rifles were used in about equal proportions), rifle bullets proved to be two to four times more lethal than handgun bullets.[2]

The law of conservation of energy (energy can be neither created nor destroyed—only changed from one form to another) explains why a projectile's kinetic energy is transformed into damage as it slows. If a projectile like a bullet remains within the object it strikes, then all of its kinetic energy is transferred to the object. If a projectile passes completely through an object, the energy transferred to the object is equal to the kinetic energy just prior to entry minus the projectile's remaining energy as it exits the object. The kinetic energy lost by the bullet as it passes through is transformed into tissue displacement, which is converted to physical tissue damage and a small amount of heat.

A final consideration regarding injury caused by penetrating objects is the deceleration rate. The forces causing trauma are related to the force formula: force = mass × acceleration (or deceleration). The more quickly an object slows, the more rapidly it gives up its kinetic energy. This plays a very important role in the study of how a bullet behaves (ballistics) and the damage it causes within human tissue (the biomechanics of penetrating trauma).

Ballistics

The study of projectiles in motion and their effects on objects they impact is called **ballistics**.

Trajectory, Drag, and Cavitation

One aspect of ballistics is **trajectory**, the curved path that a bullet follows after it is fired from a gun. Once a bullet leaves

---

PATHO PEARLS

The Bullet's Travel

When the gun's firing pin strikes the shell casing primer, the resulting flash ignites the powder charge. When the charge ignites, it exerts tremendous force in all directions. Since the barrel prevents any expansion to the side, the only expansion possible occurs as the bullet moves down the barrel. The force of the exploding charge accelerates the bullet rapidly over the length of the barrel. This force gives the bullet great velocity (and kinetic energy to do great damage) as it leaves the end of the barrel. The force that pushes the bullet down the barrel also pushes the rifle in the opposite direction. The energy of the bullet's acceleration down the rifle barrel is exactly matched by the rifle's acceleration in the opposite direction (recoil). Note, however, that the rifle weighs much more than the bullet. It moves only inches while the bullet accelerates over the full length of the barrel.

The rapidly burning powder pressurizes the space behind the bullet and pushes the bullet forward. The gun barrel, which is slightly smaller than the bullet, resists its movement while the explosive pressure behind the bullet grows. As the bullet travels down the barrel, its velocity rapidly increases. The bullet also begins to spin, following the small lands and grooves, called rifling, in the gun's barrel. As it leaves the end of the gun barrel, the bullet is spinning rapidly and is pushed on by the barrel exhaust, often resulting in a slight wobble. For the first several inches beyond the mouth of the barrel, the bullet is followed by the very hot exhaust gases that drove the bullet down the gun barrel and by the residue of the spent explosive charge.

The bullet's spin, induced by the rifling, causes it to track very straight and generally prevents serious wobble, or yaw, during flight. The bullet's speed slows gradually as it meets resistance from the air it must push out of its way. The bullet is also accelerated toward Earth by gravity, dropping faster and faster with time. This effect gives a bullet's trajectory a curved shape. The trajectory of a very fast bullet is flatter or much less curved than that of a slower projectile.

As the bullet impacts its target, it exchanges its energy of motion by deforming the target and creating a shock wave within it. This kinetic energy transfer causes the damage associated with projectile injury.

---

a gun, it is pulled downward by gravity. The faster the bullet and the farther it travels per second, the less gravity is able to change its path and the straighter is its trajectory. When a bullet is fired at close range, gravity has little time to pull it down, and it has a rather flat trajectory. The longer the distance between a gun and an object hit and/or the slower the bullet (from a handgun or lower powered rifle), the more the trajectory curves.

A second, more significant, aspect of projectile travel is the energy exchange as it travels to and into the object it strikes. In addition to velocity, factors that affect this energy exchange include drag, cavitation, profile, shape, stability, expansion, and fragmentation as well as secondary impacts.

As a bullet travels through the air, it meets wind resistance, or **drag**. The faster it travels, the greater the drag that develops and the greater the slowing effect. As a result, the damage caused by a bullet fired at close range is more severe than the damage from one fired at a distance that has been slowed more by drag. Once the bullet arrives at the target, of course, drag increases dramatically, since the density of the object struck is much greater than the density of air.

Objects traveling slowly and without much kinetic energy, such as bladed objects or arrows, tend to damage only tissues they contact. By contrast, medium- or high-velocity projectiles, such as handgun or rifle bullets, set a portion of the semifluid body tissue in motion, creating a shock wave and a temporary cavity. This process is known as **cavitation** and its extent is determined by a bullet's velocity and rate of energy exchange. The rate of energy exchange is related to the size of the projectile's contacting surface which, in turn, is determined by its profile and shape.

Profile

Profile is the portion of the bullet you would see if you looked at it as it traveled straight toward you. That is, it is the cross section of the bullet along its direction of travel. The larger this surface profile, the greater the energy exchange rate, the more quickly the bullet slows, and the more extensive the damage to surrounding tissue. For bullets that remain stable during their travel and do not deform or tumble, the profile is the bullet's diameter, or **caliber**. To increase the energy exchange rate, however, bullets are designed to become unstable in their travel as they pass from air into another medium or to deform through expansion or fragmentation.

Shape

In addition to profile, other aspects of a bullet's shape affect the energy exchange rate and resulting damage. Handgun ammunition is rather blunt, is more resistant to travel through human tissue, and releases kinetic energy more quickly. Rifle bullets are more pointed and cut through soft tissue more

CONTENT REVIEW

▶ Factors Affecting Energy Exchange between a Projectile and Body Tissue

- Velocity
- Profile
- Shape
- Stability
- Expansion
- Fragmentation
- Secondary impacts

efficiently. However, if a rifle bullet tumbles (as it often does), it may exchange energy more rapidly because of an increased presenting profile.

Stability

The location of a bullet's center of mass affects its stability both during its flight and when it impacts a semisolid object, like human tissue. The longer a bullet, the farther its center of mass is from its leading edge. If a bullet is deflected from straight flight—for example, by barrel exhaust or by a gust of wind—lift created by the projectile's tip passing through air at an angle causes the bullet to tumble. If it continues to tumble, the bullet slows rapidly and its accuracy is diminished. To prevent tumbling, bullets are sent spinning through air by gun barrel rifling. This rotation gives a bullet gyroscopic stability like a spinning top. If a spinning bullet is slightly deflected, it wobbles, or yaws, then slowly returns to straight flight.

When a bullet impacts a dense substance, like human tissue, several things occur. If there is already a yaw, this yaw greatly increases as the bullet begins its penetration. This occurs as the bullet's mass tries to overrun its leading edge. Secondly, the gyroscopic spin designed for stability in air becomes insufficient. A bullet needs to spin at a rate 30 times greater in soft tissue than in air to maintain the same stability. The result may be tumbling and a great increase in the bullet's presenting profile.

A handgun bullet's center of mass is not far back from the leading edge, and it is rather stable. Its side profile is slightly greater than its frontal profile and will do only slightly more damage if it tumbles. Since a rifle bullet is generally longer than a handgun bullet and has its center of mass farther back from the leading edge, it is more likely to tumble when it hits body tissue (Figure 1 ●). A rifle bullet's side profile is much greater than its frontal profile. With tumbling and a larger presenting profile, a rifle bullet's kinetic energy exchange rate increases, as does its potential for causing damage. In human tissue, a rifle bullet generally rotates 180 degrees and then continues its travel, base first.

Expansion and Fragmentation

Projectiles also may increase their profile and their energy exchange rate by deforming when they strike a medium that is denser than air. As a bullet's nose contacts the target, it is slowed and then compressed by the bullet's weight behind it. The bullet's nose mushrooms outward as its rear pushes into it, increasing the projectile's diameter, its profile (Figure 2 ●). In some cases, initial impact forces are so great that a bullet separates into several pieces, or fragments. This fragmentation increases the impact energy exchange rate, because the total fragment surface area is much greater than the original bullet's profile (Figure 3 ●).

While handgun bullets are made of relatively soft lead, their velocity, and thus their kinetic energy, is generally insufficient to cause significant bullet deformity. However, some bullets (dumdums or hollow points) are specifically designed to mushroom and/or fragment on impact and cause increased damage. Rifle bullets have much higher velocities than handgun bullets and much more kinetic energy. They are more prone to deform or fragment when contacting human tissue, especially bullets intended for big-game hunting. Most military ammunition is fully

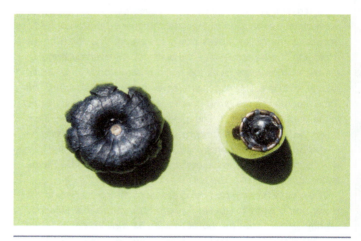

● **Figure 2**   Some bullets are designed to mushroom on impact, thus increasing their profile, energy exchange rate, and damage potential. (*Collection of Robert Porter*)

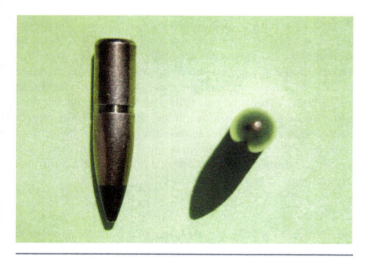

● **Figure 1**   The presenting surface, or profile, of a bullet changes as it tumbles when it contacts human tissue. (*Collection of Robert Porter*)

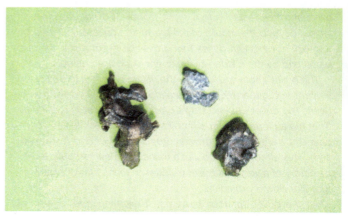

● **Figure 3**   Some firearm projectiles may break apart, or fragment, on contact, greatly increasing their profile and damage potential. (*Collection of Robert Porter*)

jacketed with impact-resistant metal jackets that are resistant to deformity with soft-tissue collision. If a bullet fragments, the irregular shape of the fragments and the increase in profile area means that the projectile gives up its energy more rapidly as well as through more and erratic pathways than a handgun or rifle bullet that remains intact.

Secondary Impacts

The energy exchange between a projectile and body tissue can also be affected by any object the projectile strikes during its travel. Branches, window glass, or articles of clothing may all deflect a bullet and induce yaw and tumble. They may also cause bullet deformity, and thereby increase the energy exchange rate once the bullet impacts the victim.

A special type of secondary impact occurs when a bullet collides with body armor. Kevlar™ and other synthetic fabrics can effectively absorb the kinetic energy of medium-velocity projectiles. The energy that is absorbed by the armor is then distributed to the victim over a relatively large surface area in much the same way that a gun's handgrip or shoulder stock helps distribute the force of recoil to the shooter. A bullet's impact with body armor may produce blunt trauma to the person hit (for example, chest contusions, rib fractures, and/or blunt cardiac injury), but such injury is generally much less severe than injury caused by bullet penetration. High-energy projectiles may pass through body armor, but in doing so they dissipate much of their kinetic energy as blunt trauma, thereby reducing penetrating energy when the bullet strikes body tissue. Bullet deformity caused by body armor may increase the energy exchange rate, but the reduction in bullet velocity and lost kinetic energy reduce overall injury potential. Ceramic or metal inserts for body armor will stop most rifle bullets but permit significant, but less lethal, blunt trauma.

Characteristics of Specific Weapons

Weapons that commonly cause wounds encountered by paramedics include handguns, hunting rifles, assault rifles, shotguns, bladed instruments (knives and swords), and arrows. Each weapon type has certain characteristics associated with the injuries it produces.

Handgun

The handgun is often a relatively short-barreled, medium-velocity weapon with somewhat limited accuracy. It is most effective at close range. Because a handgun does not fire a high-velocity, high-energy projectile (as does a rifle), its potential for causing damage is limited. Blunter bullet shape and, less frequently, softer composition and associated mushrooming and fragmentation may dissipate a bullet's energy more rapidly. Even so, the expected damage is less than that of the higher energy rifle bullet. Injury severity is usually determined by which organs, vessels, and other structures have been directly damaged by the bullet's passage (Figure 4 ●).

Some handguns fire automatically (machine pistols). They continue to discharge bullets until the trigger is released or the magazine empties. While each projectile's energy remains the

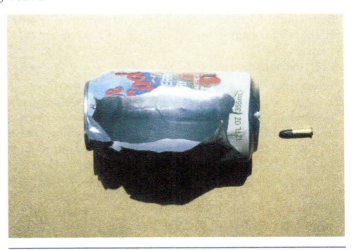

● **Figure 4** The energy of the handgun projectile is limited by low projectile weight and its relatively slow velocity. *(Collection of Robert Porter)*

same, damage potential associated with fully automatic weapons is increased because of an increased likelihood of multiple impacts and/or multiple victims.

Hunting Rifle

The hunting rifle fires a heavier projectile than a handgun through a much longer barrel and with much greater final muzzle velocity. It is either a manually loaded, single-shot weapon with some mechanical loading action to advance the next shell, or a semiautomatic weapon, in which the next shell is fed into the chamber by recoil or exhaust gases. However, no more than one bullet is expelled with each squeeze of the semiautomatic rifle's trigger. High-energy rifle bullets travel much farther, with greater accuracy, and retain much more of their kinetic energy than do handgun projectiles. As a result of the rifle bullet's high speed and energy, it transfers greater damaging energy to its target (Figure 5 ●). This results in extensive wounds with injuries that extend beyond a projectile's immediate track. Hunting ammunition is especially lethal. It is often designed to expand

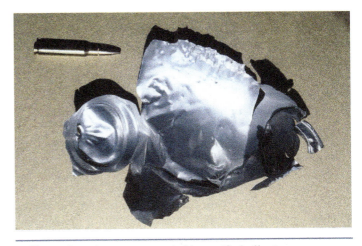

● **Figure 5** The energy carried by a rifle bullet is very damaging because of its heavier weight and very high velocity. *(Collection of Robert Porter)*

dramatically on impact, greatly increasing energy delivery rate and the extent of any injury.

Assault Rifle

Assault rifles differ from hunting rifles in that they generally have a larger magazine capacity and fire in both the semiautomatic and automatic modes. Examples of these weapons include the M16, AR15, and AK47. Resulting injuries are similar to those produced by civilian hunting rifles, although multiple wounds and casualties can be expected. Military ammunition is fully jacketed and specifically designed not to expand; while still very deadly, energy delivery is not as severe as with civilian hunting ammunition. Assault weapons in terrorist hands, however, may be loaded with hunting-type ammunition. This greatly increases their injury potential.

Shotgun

Shotguns can fire a single projectile (slug) or numerous spheres (pellets or shot) at medium velocity. A shell is loaded with a slug or a particular size of lead shot, varying from 00 (about 1/3 inch in diameter) to #9 shot (about the size of a pinhead). Projectile compartment size is approximately the same with various sizes of shot. This means that the larger the shot, the fewer projectiles. Each projectile shares a portion of the total muzzle energy and, free of the gun's barrel, adds to total drag as they move through air. A slug will cause a single entrance wound very similar to that caused by a rifle bullet. Large shot will create multiple wounds that may be deep at a moderate range. Very small shot will cause numerous wounds at close range, but the wound depth falls off very quickly with distance. Shotguns often are equipped with a choke that reduces the exhaust leaving the barrel, just behind the projectiles. This reduces the spreading effect of the exhaust on the shot and keeps the projectiles closer together as they travel toward the target. At very close range, the shot will create an entrance wound that appears as a single bullet wound. Farther out, there may be small entry wounds surrounding a central and larger wound. Beyond 20 to 30 yards, there may be just a pattern of small entry wounds. In addition to the metal projectiles expelled by a shotgun, there will be wadding, material designed to help the shotgun blast propel the shot. This plastic or fiber material may penetrate the wound and contribute to its contamination. A shotgun is limited in range and accuracy; however, injuries sustained at close range can be severe or lethal (Figure 6 ●).

Bladed Instruments and Arrows

In contrast to high- or medium-velocity projectiles such as rifle or handgun bullets, knives, swords, arrows, and other slow-moving, penetrating objects cause low-velocity, low-energy wounds. Because low-velocity objects do not produce either a pressure wave or a cavity, damage is usually limited to physical injury caused by direct contact between the blade or object and the victim's tissue. The penetration can result in serious internal hemorrhage or injury to individual or multiple body organs.

Hunting tips designed for arrows can be especially damaging. These feature three razor-tipped, pointed barbs that are intended to smoothly cut tissue. These tips penetrate deeply and produce severe internal hemorrhage. Also, any arrow movement

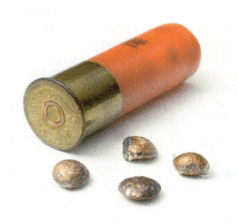

● **Figure 6** A shotgun propels small projectiles with limited velocity, such as the buckshot shown here. However, because of the large number of projectiles, the weapon can be extremely damaging at close range.

while it is impaled in the victim increases both tissue damage and hemorrhage rate.

Other Penetrating Wound Mechanisms

Penetrating wounds can also be caused by mechanisms such as a piece of wire thrown by a lawn mower, a nail stepped on by a child, an air power-gun firing a nail into a roofer rather than the roof, or a worker falling on an exposed concrete reinforcing rod. Injuries such as these are generally low-velocity, low-energy wounds with injury confined to the actual object path. Injury severity is related to the depth of penetration and the organs, blood vessels, and other structures affected. The penetrating object may introduce foreign and infectious material into the wound and complicate transport if the object remains impaled (as with the worker who falls on a reinforcing rod).

Biomechanics of Penetrating Trauma

A high-velocity projectile inflicts a damage pathway related to three injury processes. They are the direct injury, the pressure wave, and cavitation (the creation of a temporary cavity). These three injury processes can also create a permanent cavity and a zone of injury.

Direct Injury

Direct injury is the damage done as a penetrating object strikes tissue, contuses and tears that tissue, and pushes it out of the way. The direct injury pathway is limited to the bullet's profile as it moves through the body or the profiles of resulting fragments as the bullet breaks apart. Except for magnum rounds (generating particularly high velocities), handgun bullet damage is generally limited to direct injury.

Pressure Wave

When a high-velocity, high-energy projectile strikes human tissue, it creates a pressure wave (Figure 7 ●). Since most human

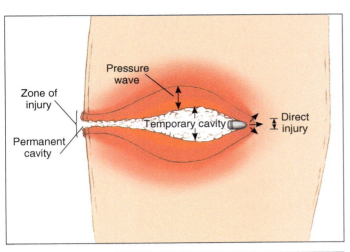

● **Figure 7** As a projectile passes through tissue it creates a pressure wave and temporary cavity, with results that include direct injury, a permanent cavity, and a zone of injury.

PATHO PEARLS

When a Projectile Enters the Body (Biomechanics of Penetrating Trauma)

The spinning bullet contacts the semifluid target (such as human tissue) with great speed and kinetic energy. The tip of the bullet impacts tissue, pushing the tissue forward and to the side along the pathway of its travel. This tissue collides with adjacent tissue, ultimately creating a shock wave of pressure moving forward and lateral to the projectile. This shock wave continues to move perpendicular to the bullet's path as it passes. The rapid compression of tissue laterally and the stretching of the tissue as it moves outward from the bullet path crushes and tears the tissue structure. The motion creates a pocket, or cavity, behind the bullet. The pressure within this cavity is reduced, creating suction. This suction draws air and debris into the cavity from the entrance wound and from the exit wound, if one is present. The body tissue's elasticity then draws the sides of the cavity back together, causing the entrance wound, exit wound, and wound pathway to close completely or remain only partially open.

The bullet's exchange of energy with the body leaves various tissues disrupted and injured. Tissue in the direct pathway of the bullet suffers most. It is severely contused and likely to have been torn from its attachments. In addition to the directly injured tissue, other debris, blood, and air are found along the bullet's pathway. The cavitational wave stretches and tears adjacent tissue, damaging cell membranes and small blood vessels. The adjacent tissue is injured, but will likely regain its normal function slowly. Larger blood vessels torn by the bullet and the cavitational wave bleed heavily into the damage pathway. Over time, this pathway, because of the disruption in circulation and the introduction of infectious material with the drawing-in of debris, may develop severe infection, which will delay the healing process.

tissue is semifluid and elastic, decelerating projectiles transmit the energy of motion forward and outward very quickly. Tissues in front of the bullet are pushed forward and to the side at great speed. They, in turn, push adjacent tissues forward and outward creating a moving wave of pressure and tissue in front of and to the side of a bullet. This effect increases with faster and blunter bullets. With high-velocity rifle bullets, pressures are extreme, approaching 100 times normal atmospheric pressure.

The pressure wave travels very well through fluid, such as blood, and may injure blood vessels distant from the projectile pathway. Air-filled cavities, such as the lung's small air sacs (alveoli), compress very easily and absorb the pressure, quickly limiting the shock wave and resulting temporary cavity. Solid and dense organs, like the liver and spleen, suffer greatly as their dense tissues transmit the pressure wave efficiently and it stretches and tears their inelastic structure. This pressure wave transmission produces serious internal hemorrhage and, in extreme cases, organ fracture. Muscle tissue is also dense but very elastic in nature. It suffers less damage with bullet passage than do solid organs.

Temporary Cavity

The temporary cavity is a space created behind a high-energy bullet as tissue moves rapidly away from a bullet's path. Creation of this temporary cavity is called cavitation. Cavity size depends on the amount of energy transferred during bullet passage. With rifle bullets, the temporary cavity may be as much as 12 times larger than the projectile's profile. After a bullet's passage, tissue elasticity causes the temporary cavity to close.

Cavitation also produces a subatmospheric pressure within the cavity as it expands. This means that air is drawn in from the entrance wound and the exit wound, if one exists. Debris and contamination enter the cavity with the inflow of air, adding to infection risk.

Permanent Cavity

Physical contact with the bullet and movement that creates a temporary cavity crushes, stretches, and tears affected tissues. These processes seriously damage the area in and adjacent to a bullet's path and may also damage tissue elasticity. Tissue thus may not return to its normal orientation, resulting in a permanent cavity that in some cases may be larger than the bullet's diameter. This cavity is not a void but is filled with disrupted tissues, some air, blood and other fluids, and debris.

Zone of Injury

Associated with most projectile wounds is a **zone of injury** that extends beyond the permanent cavity. This zone contains crushed, torn, and contused tissue that does not function normally and may be slow to heal because of cell and tissue damage, disrupted blood flow, and the likelihood of infection.

Heat Injury

A bullet is heated both by the burning of the bullet's propellant and by friction as it is pushed down the gun barrel. As this only takes milliseconds, the bullet's temperature rises only slightly. Some kinetic energy is converted to heat as the bullet impacts the target; however, the bullet's temperature will reach, at most, about 300 degrees Fahrenheit. As it passes tissue rapidly during most of impact, any burn injury is expected to be minimal and mostly associated with the final resting location of the bullet, if at all.

Low-Velocity Wounds

As already noted, penetrating objects such as knives, swords, ice picks, arrows, or flying objects such as blast debris, ski poles in a skiing injury mechanism, nails from a nail gun, or wires thrown by a lawn mower can cause low-velocity penetrating trauma. The object's relatively slow speed limits the kinetic energy exchange rate as it enters a victim's body. Consider, for example, a victim stabbed by a 150-lb attacker who strikes with a knife moving at about 3 meters per second. Although the mass behind the knife blade's penetration is significantly greater than a rifle bullet's mass, the knife's velocity is vastly less. This means that injury is usually restricted to tissue the knife actually contacts (Figure 8 ●).

While injury is limited to a penetrating object's pathway, that object may be twisted, moved about, or inserted at an oblique angle. As a result, the entrance wound may not reflect the object's depth of penetration, extent of its motion within the body, or actual organs and tissues it contacts and injures.

Attacker and victim characteristics are important to keep in mind during assessment of low-velocity, penetrating trauma victims. Knife-wielding males, for example, most often strike with a forward, outward, or crosswise stroke and

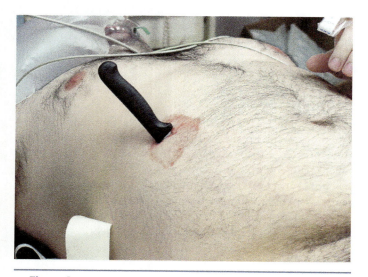

● **Figure 8** Damage caused by a low-velocity wounding process, such as that caused by a knife, is limited to the object's path of travel. (*© Michael Casey, MD*)

carry the knife with the blade protruding from the thumb side of the hand. Females usually strike with an overhand and downward stroke and the blade protruding from the little-finger side of the hand. Attack victims initially attempt to protect themselves by using their hands and arms.[3] This means they often receive deep upper-extremity wounds (commonly called defense wounds). If an attack continues, injuries are often then directed to the chest, abdomen, face, neck, or back.

SPECIFIC TISSUE/ORGAN INJURIES

Damage caused by a projectile varies with the tissue type it encounters. Organ density affects how efficiently a projectile's energy is transmitted to surrounding tissues. The tissue's connective strength and elasticity, called **resiliency**, also influence how much tissue damage occurs with kinetic energy transfer. Structures and tissues within the body that behave differently during projectile passage include connective tissue, solid organs, hollow organs, lungs, and bone.

Connective Tissue

Muscles, tendons, ligaments, skin, and other connective tissues are dense, elastic, and hold together very well. When exposed to cavitational wave pressure and stretching, these connective tissues characteristically stretch and absorb energy while limiting tissue damage. The wound track closes due to this tissue's resiliency and elastic nature, and serious injury is frequently limited to the projectile's pathway.

Organs

Another factor with profound effects on the victim's potential for survival is the particular organ or organs involved in a penetrating injury. Some organs, like the heart and brain, are immediately critical to life, and serious injury may cause immediate death. When large blood vessels are injured, hemorrhage can be rapid and severe. A penetrating injury to the urinary bladder, however, may not threaten the patient's life for several hours or longer. When evaluating a wound's seriousness, anticipate the organs injured and the effect their injury is likely to have on patient condition and survivability.

Solid Organs

Solid organs such as the liver, spleen, kidneys, pancreas, and brain have the density but not the resiliency of muscle and other connective tissues. When struck by a bullet's impact force, these tissues are pushed outward by the pressure wave and cavitation and are compressed and stretched. This results in greater damage more closely associated with the temporary cavity size than with bullet profile. The tissue returns to its original orientation, not because of its own elasticity but because of the resiliency of surrounding tissues or organ capsule. Hemorrhage associated with solid organ projectile damage is often severe.

Hollow Organs

Hollow organs such as the bowel, stomach, urinary bladder, and heart are muscular containers holding liquid. Liquid within them is noncompressible and rapidly transmits impact energy outward. If the container is filled and distended at impact time, energy released can tear the organ apart explosively. (Large blood vessels respond to projectile passage much like hollow, fluid-distended organs.) If the container is not distended or filled with air, it is much more tolerant of cavitational forces. Slower and smaller projectiles may produce small holes in a hollow organ and permit slow leakage of its contents. If this occurs with the heart, it may produce pericardial tamponade (blood filling the pericardial sac, thus limiting heart function) or moderate and slowly life-threatening hemorrhage. Leakage of bowel contents can be particularly troublesome since the contents of this organ are rich in bacteria and can contaminate the wound. If a hollow organ, such as the bowel or stomach, holds air, the air compresses with passage of the pressure wave and somewhat limits the extent of injury.

Lungs

Lungs consist of millions of small, elastic, air-filled sacs called alveoli. As a bullet and its associated pressure wave pass, air within these sacs is compressed, thereby slowing and limiting cavitational wave transmission. Injury to lung tissue in penetrating trauma is generally less extensive than can be expected with any other body tissue. If the projectile, however, strikes the central lung, and the major blood vessels and air passages found there, the injury can be devastating.

A bullet may open the chest wall or disrupt larger airways, thus permitting air to escape into the thorax (pneumothorax) or create a valve-like defect that results in accumulating pressure within the chest (tension pneumothorax). Bullet wounds rarely cause an open pneumothorax (sucking chest wound) because the entrance wound diameter is usually limited to the bullet caliber. Close-range shotgun blasts and explosive exit wounds of high-powered rifles, however, may be large and cause significant disruption of chest wall integrity. In these cases, a sucking chest wound is a possible outcome.

Bone

In contrast to lung tissue, bone is the body's densest, most rigid, and nonelastic tissue. When struck by a projectile or its associated pressure wave, bone resists displacement until it fractures, often into numerous pieces. These bone fragments may then distribute impact energy to surrounding tissue. A projectile's contact with bone may also significantly alter its path through the body and/or cause projectile deformity or fragmentation.[4]

General Body Regions

Several body regions deserve special attention regarding projectile wounds. They include the extremities, abdomen, thorax, neck, and head (Figure 9 ●). A projectile's passage has a special effect on the first and last tissues it contacts, the sites of the entrance and the exit wounds.

Extremities

The extremities consist of skin covering muscles that surround large long bones. An extremity injury may be debilitating but does not immediately threaten life unless it is associated with a vascular injury and severe hemorrhage. Injury severity is often limited by skin and muscle resiliency. However, if bone is involved, there may be increased soft-tissue damage. Injuries above the elbow or knee are more likely to cause significant vascular injury. In recent military experience, extremity injuries account for 60 to 80 percent of all injuries yet result in less than 10 percent of fatalities. (Much of the lower incidence of body cavity injury in the military is due to the protection afforded by body armor.) The remaining 20 to 40 percent of penetrating injuries, divided among wounds to the abdomen, thorax, and head, account for more than 90 percent of mortality.

Abdomen

The abdomen (including the pelvic cavity) is the largest body cavity and contains most organs. The area is not well protected by skeletal structures other than the upper pelvic ring, lower rib cage, and lumbar vertebral column. Passage of a projectile through the abdominal cavity can produce a significant cavitational wave. The bowel fills much of the abdominal cavity and is

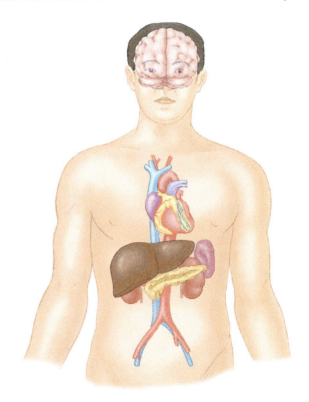

● **Figure 9** Critical structures in which the seriousness of a bullet's impact is increased include the brain, great vessels, heart, liver, kidneys, spleen, and pancreas.

very tolerant to compression and stretching. However, the liver, spleen, kidneys, and pancreas are highly susceptible to injury and hemorrhage. Since these organs occupy the upper abdominal quadrants, you should consider any penetrating projectile injury to this area as serious and to have the potential of causing severe organ injury and internal hemorrhage. Anticipate serious consequences with injuries to the abdominal aorta and inferior vena cava, which are located in the central retroperitoneal space along the spinal column.

If a projectile perforates the small or large bowel, those organs may spill their contents into the abdominal cavity. This spillage results in serious peritoneal irritation due to chemical action or infection, although signs and symptoms take some time to develop. If the injury process disrupts the blood vessels, free blood will result in only limited abdominal irritation. The retroperitoneal space does not display the irritation that is associated with blood in the peritoneal space.

Thorax

Within the chest is a cavity formed by the ribs, spine, sternum, clavicles, and the strong diaphragm muscle. The thoracic cavity houses the lungs, heart, and major blood vessels as well as the esophagus and part of the trachea. A bullet impacting the ribs may induce an extensive energy exchange that injures surrounding tissue with numerous bony fragments. Lung tissue can absorb much of the cavitational energy while sustaining limited injury itself. However, the heart and great vessels, as fluid-filled containers, may sustain significant injury from the energy of the bullet's passage. Damage to these structures and associated massive hemorrhage may cause almost instant death. Because of the pressure-driven dynamics of respiration, any large chest wound may compromise ventilation. Air may pass through a wound instead of through the normal airway (sucking chest wound), may fill the pleural space (pneumothorax), or may build up under pressure (tension pneumothorax). Note that the chest is a dynamic space. With each breath, the abdominal contents move up and down with the diaphragm. Appreciate that a wound to the lower rib border may involve thoracic organs, abdominal organs, or both.

Neck

The neck is an anatomic area traversed by several critical structures. These include the larynx, trachea, esophagus, several major blood vessels (carotid and vertebral arteries and jugular veins), vertebral column, and spinal cord. These structures are packed into a very small space. Penetrating trauma in this area is likely to damage one or more vital structures and lead to airway compromise, severe bleeding, and/or neurologic dysfunction. Associated swelling and formation of a hematoma may further compromise circulation and the airway. Additionally, any large penetrating wound may permit air to be drawn into an open jugular vein, resulting in an immediately life-threatening air embolism. The most commonly injured neck structures are the major blood vessels and the trachea.

Head

The skull is a hollow, strong, and rigid container, housing the brain's delicate semisolid tissue, which is highly susceptible to projectile injury. If a bullet penetrates the skull, cavitational energy is trapped within the cavity and subjects the brain to extreme pressures. If the released kinetic energy is great enough, the skull may rupture outward. In some cases, a bullet may enter the skull and not have enough energy to exit; in such a case, the bullet may continue to travel along the skull's interior, disrupting more and more brain matter. Bullet wounds to the head, particularly those that penetrate the skull, are especially lethal.[5]

Destructive forces released by a projectile that impacts the facial area may disrupt the airway and/or the victim's ability to control his own airway. The head and face are also areas with an extensive blood-vessel supply. Penetrating trauma may damage these vessels and result in serious and at times difficult-to-control hemorrhage.

An occurrence often associated with suicide attempts is severe damage to the facial region. If the individual places a shotgun or rifle under his chin and pulls the trigger, the head tilts up and back. This directs the blast entirely to the facial region, and the projectile(s) may not enter the cranium or strike any immediately life-threatening structures. However, extensive and difficult-to-control bleeding and associated tissue and skeletal damage can make airway control very difficult. In this circumstance, use of an endotracheal tube to secure the airway can be complicated, because many airway structures and landmarks are obliterated by such a blast.

Entrance Wound

Often, entrance wounds are no larger than the bullet's profile. At this point, when the bullet has just impacted the body, cavitational wave energy has not had time to develop and enlarge the wound (Figure 10 ●). The situation is different, however, with bullets that deform or tumble during flight. With these projectiles, initial impact can be especially violent, producing a much larger and more disrupted entry wound than bullet caliber alone would suggest.

Bullet entry wounds sustained at close range, a few feet or less, display special characteristics. Such wounds may be marked

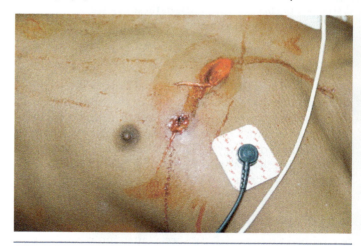

● **Figure 10** The entrance wound is often the same size as the projectile's profile. A bullet's exit wound often has a "blown outward" appearance. Both an entrance and an exit wound are visible on this patient. (*© Edward T. Dickinson, MD*)

by elements of the barrel exhaust and bullet passage. Tattooing from propellant residue may form a darkened circle or an oval (if the gun is held at an angle) around the entry wound and contaminate the wound itself. At the wound site, you may notice a small (usually 1- to 2-mm) ridge of discoloration around the entrance caused by the bullet as it stretches the skin before it tears it. If the gun barrel is held very close or against the skin as the weapon is fired, it may push barrel exhaust into the wound, producing subcutaneous emphysema (air within the skin's tissue) and crepitus to the touch. If the barrel is held a few inches from the skin, you may notice some burns caused by the hot gases of the barrel exhaust.

Exit Wound

Exit wounds are caused by physical damage both from the passage of the bullet itself and from the resulting cavitational wave. Since the pressure wave that causes cavitation moves forward and outward, the exit wound may have a "blown out" appearance. The exit wound may appear stellate, referring to tears radiating outward in a star-like fashion. (Be aware that some entrance wounds may be stellate as well.) Because the cavitational wave has had time to develop by the time the bullet leaves the body, exit wounds may more accurately reflect the probable internal damage than entrance wounds. If a bullet expends all its kinetic energy before it can exit the body, there is no exit wound and the bullet remains within the body. If the bullet does exit, kinetic energy expended within the body is equal to the kinetic energy of the bullet before impact minus the energy that remains in the bullet as it leaves the body. Note that a bullet may be deflected as it travels through the body (as from contact with bone), so there may not be a direct route of travel between the entrance and exit wound.

When you consider entrance and exit wounds, it is important to keep your focus on the medical aspects of any differences in appearance. Whether a wound is an exit or an entrance wound has important implications for crime investigation, but only a thorough forensic examination by a qualified expert can determine with certainty whether a given wound represents a projectile's entrance or exit. Therefore, avoid making assured statements or annotations in the prehospital care report about whether a wound is an exit or entrance wound. Instead, describe the wound and allow investigators to use your description and other evidence in making a valid determination.

SPECIAL CONCERNS WITH PENETRATING TRAUMA

Scene Size-Up

Scene size-up for a shooting or stabbing raises special concerns not associated with most other emergency care situations. The very nature of these injuries should suggest possible danger from further violence and potential injury to you and your crew. Do not approach a shooting or stabbing scene unless and until law-enforcement personnel arrive and secure it and direct you to enter and provide care. If law enforcement personnel are not yet on scene when you arrive, stage your vehicle at least one block away and out of sight of the scene. Once police or other law-enforcement personnel arrive, and on their direction, bring your vehicle closer to the scene but keep the police and their vehicles between you and any shooting or stabbing site. Wait there for police to indicate that it is safe to approach the patient (Figure 11 ●).

Once you reach the patient, carefully survey the area to ensure there are no weapons within the patient's reach. Consider the possibility that a victim (the patient) may be carrying a knife or other weapon. If you have any doubts, request that police search the victim for weapons before you begin your patient assessment and care.

As you carefully survey a shooting scene, try to reconstruct the event. Attempt to determine the victim's original position and his angle to and distance from the shooter. This helps you determine the angle at which a bullet entered the patient (which may not otherwise be revealed by an entrance wound) and whether a wound was received at close range or from a distance. Also try to determine the weapon caliber and type—handgun, rifle, or shotgun.

If your call involves a bladed-weapon injury, attempt to determine the gender and approximate weight of the attacker and the blade length. (You will not be able to determine a wound's depth, but the length of the weapon will likely identify the maximum depth of insertion.) This information will help the emergency physician determine wound severity.

As you move on to patient assessment, do all you can to preserve the crime scene while providing essential patient care. Disturb only those materials around the patient that you must move in order to render care. Cut around, not through, any bullet or knife holes in clothing, and give any clothing you have removed or cut away to police for use as evidence. However, if there is ever any doubt about what to do, err on the side of providing patient care. If a victim is obviously dead, employ your jurisdiction's protocols for handling the body, but try to do so without disturbing evidence that may be crucial in determining what happened.

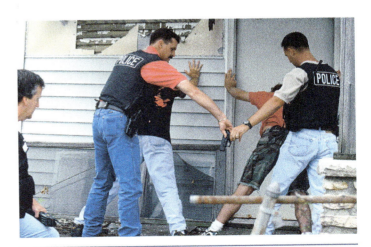

● **Figure 11** Ensure that any potentially violent scene is safe and secured by police before entering. (© *MikaelKarlsson/ Arrestingimages.com*)

Penetrating Wound Assessment

When assessing a penetrating trauma victim, try to determine the penetrating object's pathway and the organs that the wounding process may have affected. Anticipate the impact of potential organ injury, and use this determination in setting priorities for on-scene care or rapid transport. Remember, however, that a bullet may not travel in a straight line between entrance and exit wounds. Often, a very small shift in a bullet's pathway may mean the difference between tearing open a large blood vessel or missing critical organs completely. The human body is also a dynamic place. The diaphragm moves the kidneys, pancreas, liver, spleen, bowel, and heart during respirations, so whether or not these organs are injured may be somewhat dependent on the phase of respiration in which the injury occurs.

It is often hard to anticipate the magnitude of a projectile wound. Injuries to the great vessels, heart, and brain may be immediately or rapidly fatal, while injuries to solid organs (liver, pancreas, kidneys, or spleen) may also be deadly but take more time in working their effects. Consequently, always suspect the worst with bullet wounds that involve the head, chest, or abdomen. Provide rapid transport in these cases, and treat shock aggressively. Appreciate that gunshot wounds account for less than 1 percent of EMS responses, while they account for more than 15 percent of trauma mortality. Treat any gunshot wound as serious if it involves any area of the body other than the distal extremities.

Penetrating Wound Care

Certain penetrating wounds need special attention. These include wounds to the face and chest and those involving impaled objects. Their care is described in the following sections.[6,7]

Facial Wounds

Facial gunshot wounds may endanger the airway and destroy many airway landmarks (Figure 12 ●). With wounds like these, endotracheal intubation may be essential yet is extremely difficult to perform. You might find it helpful to visualize the larynx with a laryngoscope while another rescuer gently presses on the chest. Look for any bubbling during the chest compression, and try to pass the endotracheal tube through the bubbling tissue. Then, very carefully ensure that the endotracheal tube is properly placed in the trachea and that lung ventilation is adequate. Here, carefully assessing breath sounds with ventilations and capnography is essential.

If this approach is not effective, an invasive technique may be essential to restore the airway, at least long enough for the patient to reach more definitive care. This technique is the **percutaneous cricothyrotomy**, in which access is achieved via needle or other approved puncture device (not surgically, as with the use of a scalpel). This emergency airway procedure perforates the membrane between the thyroid and cricoid cartilages, providing a route for ventilation directly into the lower airway.

Chest Wounds

The chest wall is rather thick and resilient. It requires a large wound to create an opening big enough to permit free air movement through the chest wall—an open pneumothorax. Wounds caused by small-caliber handguns usually result in no air movement, while wounds caused by shotgun blasts and exiting high-velocity bullets more commonly cause such injuries. If frothy blood is associated with a chest wound, be alert for a possible tension pneumothorax, in which air builds up under pressure within the thorax. Remember, it takes pressure to push air through the wound and froth blood. If you completely seal the chest wound, you may stop any outward air flow. This can increase both the speed of tension pneumothorax development and its severity. Cover any open chest wound with an occlusive dressing sealed on three sides (Figure 13 ●). If dyspnea is significant, assess for tension pneumothorax and first release any occlusive dressings. If this does not relieve the pressure, perform needle decompression.

Always consider the possibility of heart and great vessel damage with a penetrating chest wound. These injuries may cause severe internal hemorrhage and death. Another serious complication of penetrating chest trauma is pericardial tamponade. This condition occurs when an object or projectile perforates the heart and permits blood to leak into the

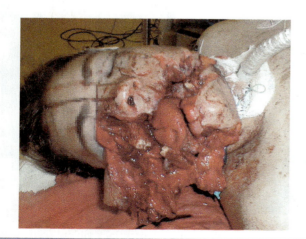

● **Figure 12** Facial wounds may distort or destroy airway landmarks. (© *Dr. Bryan E. Bledsoe*)

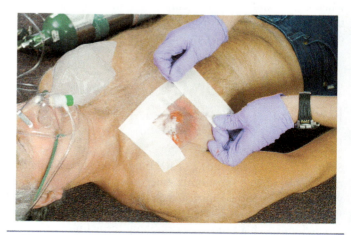

● **Figure 13** Seal open chest wounds and ensure adequate respirations.

pericardial sac. As blood accumulates in the sac, the heart no longer fully fills with blood and circulation slows. If pericardial tamponade is uncorrected, a patient's prognosis is very poor. However, a needle introduced into the pericardial space (pericardiocentesis), a procedure available at the emergency department, can quickly alleviate the life threat.

Therefore, if your patient has a penetrating injury to the central chest, suspect and look for this condition and arrange for rapid transport.

Impaled Objects

If an object that causes a low-velocity wound lodges in the body, removal may be dangerous for the patient. If an object bent as it hit a bone on entry, attempts at removal may cause further injury. If an object is held firmly by soft tissue, it may lie against a severed blood vessel, thereby restricting blood loss; moving or removing the object may then increase hemorrhage.

Immobilize impaled objects in place—where and as they are found—and transport the patient. Use bulky dressings and splinting materials to stabilize the object. Remove only impaled objects that are lodged in the cheek, neck, or trachea that interfere with the airway or those that you must remove to provide CPR. When a patient has fallen on an object that results in impalement, such as a concrete reinforcing rod, carefully cut the object to permit patient transport. If an object is too large to transport with the patient, cut it without subjecting the patient to unnecessary movement; if using a cutting torch, cut it without causing any burn injury.

SUMMARY

Penetrating injuries, especially those associated with gunshot wounds, are responsible for a relatively low incidence of trauma and yet are highly critical injuries, carrying an equally high mortality. Your understanding of the kinetics of trauma and the biomechanics of injury related to these wounds can help you rapidly identify serious life threats (index of suspicion) and ensure that these patients receive rapid transport to a trauma center. Special prehospital care techniques such as sealing an open pneumothorax, recognizing pericardial tamponade, recognizing and decompressing a tension pneumothorax, and managing a difficult airway can also help you stabilize the penetrating-trauma patient in the field and help ensure that he safely reaches definitive care.

YOU MAKE THE CALL

You are dispatched to a large apartment complex for a "domestic disturbance with injuries." As you pull up to the scene, a bystander states that there were shots fired about 5 minutes ago.

1. What is your first concern?

2. What information is important to gain from your scene size-up?

See Suggested Responses at the back of this chapter.

REVIEW QUESTIONS

1. Tissue displacement caused by the pressure wave that accompanies a bullet as it travels through human tissue is called _____.
   a. drag
   b. cavitation
   c. trajectory
   d. ballistics

2. Which of the following would you expect to cause the greatest cavitation?
   a. arrow
   b. ice pick
   c. rifle bullet
   d. handgun bullet

3. Which of the following is considered a high-velocity weapon?
   a. arrow
   b. rifle
   c. shotgun
   d. handgun

4. A bullet's characteristics determine how much damage it creates as it strikes its target. Which of the following would create the most damage?
   a. a bullet that does not tumble
   b. a bullet that mushrooms when it hits
   c. a small-profile bullet
   d. a full-metal-jacket bullet

5. Which of the following abdominal organs is the most tolerant of the cavitational wave associated with penetrating trauma?

   a. liver

   b. bowel

   c. spleen

   d. kidneys

6. In a puncture wound resulting from a knife or gunshot injury, a paramedic must always examine the patient for _____.

   a. an exit wound

   b. epistaxis

   c. powder burns

   d. tattooing

7. Powder burns and crepitus around an entrance wound generally suggest _____.

   a. a gun used at close range

   b. a high-powered rifle

   c. a handgun

   d. the use of a black powder

8. Penetrating trauma is dangerous when it involves the neck because it may cause problems with _____.

   a. severe hemorrhage

   b. the airway

   c. the cervical spine

   d. all of the above

9. The path a bullet follows once it is fired is called _____.

   a. yaw

   b. drag

   c. caliber

   d. trajectory

10. The forces acting on a bullet to slow it down are called _____.

   a. yaw

   b. drag

   c. profile

   d. caliber

See Answers to Review Questions at the back of this chapter.

REFERENCES

1. Laraque, D., B. Barlow, and M. Durkin. "Prevention of Youth Injuries." *J Nat Med Assoc* 91(10) (1999): 557–571.

2. Di Maio, Vincent J. *Gunshot Wounds: Practical Aspects of Firearms, Ballistics, and Forensic Techniques,* 2nd ed. New York: CRC Press, 1999.

3. Butman, Alexander M. and James L. Paturas. *Pre-Hospital Trauma Life Support.* Akron, Ohio: Emergency Training, 2007.

4. Dougherty, P. J., D. Sherman, N. Dau, and C. Bir. "Ballistic Fractures: Indirect Fractures to Bone." *J Trauma* 71(5) (Nov 2011): 1381–1384.

5. Glapa, M., et al. "Gunshot Wounds to the Head in Civilian Practice." *Am Surg* 75(3) (Mar 2009): 233–236.

6. Mabry, R. and J. G. McManus. "Prehospital Advances in the Management of Severe Penetrating Trauma." *Crit Care Med* 36 (2008): S258–S266.

7. Bruner, D., Gustafson C. G., and C. Visintainer. "Ballistic Injuries in the Emergency Department." *Emerg Med Pract* 13(12) (Dec 2011): 1–30.

FURTHER READING

Campbell, John E. *International Trauma Life Support for Emergency Care Providers*. 7th ed. Upper Saddle River, NJ: Pearson/Prentice Hall, 2012.

De Lorenzo, Robert A., and Robert S. Porter. *Tactical Emergency Care: Military and Operational Out-of-Hospital Medicine*. Upper Saddle River, NJ: Pearson/Prentice Hall, 1999.

Di Maio, Vincent J. *Gunshot Wounds: Practical Aspects of Firearms, Ballistics, and Forensic Techniques*. 2nd ed. New York: CRC Press, 1999.

Ivatury, R. R., and C. G. Cayten. *The Textbook of Penetrating Trauma*. Baltimore: Williams and Wilkins, 1996.

NAEMT (N. McSwain, Jr., S. Frame, and J. Salomone, Eds.). *PHTLS: Basic and Advanced Prehospital Trauma Life Support*. 6th ed. St. Louis: Mosby, 2010.

SUGGESTED RESPONSES TO "YOU MAKE THE CALL"

The following are suggested responses to the "You Make the Call" scenarios presented in this chapter. Each represents an acceptable response to the scenario but should not be interpreted as the only correct response.

1. *What is your first concern?*

Your personal safety is the top priority. If law enforcement is not on scene and have not advised that it is safe to enter, LEAVE THE SCENE!

2. *What information is important to gain from your scene size-up?*

In this case, with limited information, the most important thing to determine is the fact that you don't have enough information and it is unsafe for you to be there. All you know is that the call was for a domestic disturbance and someone is reporting shots fired within the last 5 minutes. Without the support of law enforcement, you are in a highly dangerous situation. Evacuate the scene and begin to get an assessment from communications through law enforcement or bystanders who call in. It is important to determine the number of victims, what types of injuries you can suspect, and what type of weapon was used. Most important, determine when the scene is safe for you to enter.

ANSWERS TO REVIEW QUESTIONS

1. b
2. c
3. b
4. b
5. b

6. a
7. a
8. d
9. d
10. b

GLOSSARY

ballistics   the study of projectile motion and its interactions with the gun, the air, and the object it contacts.

caliber   the diameter of a bullet expressed in hundredths of an inch (0.22 caliber = 0.22 inches); the inside diameter of the barrel of a handgun, or rifle.

cavitation   the outward motion of tissue due to a projectile's passage, resulting in a temporary cavity and vacuum.

drag   the forces acting on a projectile in motion to slow its progress.

percutaneous cricothyrotomy   perforation of the membrane between the thyroid and cricoid cartilages and insertion of a needle or commercial cricothyrotomy device to provide an emergency airway.

pericardial tamponade   a restriction to cardiac filling caused by blood (or other fluid) within the pericardial sac.

profile   the cross section of a bullet along its direction of travel; the energy-exchange surface of the bullet when it contacts a target.

projectile   an object hurled or projected by the exertion of force.

resiliency   elasticity; the ability to spring back from a force or impact to resume the original condition.

trajectory   the path a projectile follows.

yaw   swing or wobble around the axis of a projectile's travel.

zone of injury   in association with projectile wounds, the maximum area of injured tissue, usually extending beyond the permanent cavity formed by the projectile.

Blunt Trauma

From Chapter 2 of *Paramedic Care: Principles & Practice, Volume 5,* Fourth Edition. Bryan Bledsoe, Robert Porter, and Richard Cherry. Copyright © 2013 by Pearson Education, Inc. All rights reserved.

Blunt Trauma

Robert S. Porter, MA, EMT-P

STANDARD
Trauma (Trauma Overview)

COMPETENCY
Integrates assessment findings with principles of epidemiology and pathophysiology to formulate a field impression to implement a comprehensive treatment/disposition plan for an acutely injured patient.

OBJECTIVES

Terminal Performance Objective
After reading this chapter you should be able to relate the kinetics and mechanisms of injury associated with blunt trauma to patients' potential for injury.

Enabling Objectives
To accomplish the terminal performance objective, you should be able to:

1. Define key terms introduced in this chapter.
2. Apply the laws of inertia and energy conservation to the kinetics of blunt impact.
3. Apply the concepts of force and kinetic energy exchange to the potential for injury.
4. Associate the application of energy to various body tissues with the biomechanical forces produced to predict injury patterns.
5. Describe the events that occur in motor vehicle impacts.
6. Describe the effects of use of restraints and safety mechanisms on the potential for injuries in vehicle collisions.
7. Describe the association between vehicle damage and injury potential.
8. Describe injury patterns associated with various types of vehicle impacts.
9. Given a variety of scenarios, conduct a vehicle collision analysis.
10. Modify a collision analysis to account for the characteristics of motorcycle and off-road vehicle collisions.
11. Describe the considerations in assessing a patient who has fallen.
12. Describe the mechanisms of blast injury, blast-injury patterns, and special blast-injury care considerations.
13. Describe the considerations in assessing a patient injured during a sporting event.
14. Describe the considerations for assessing crush injuries.
15. Identify mechanisms with a potential for producing compartment syndrome.

KEY TERMS

acceleration
axial loading
blast wind
crumple zone
deceleration
dyspnea
emboli
energy

exsanguination
flechettes
hemoptysis
incendiary
inertia
kinetic energy
kinetics
mass

motion
oblique
ordnance
overpressure
oxidizer
pneumothorax
pressure wave
velocity

CASE STUDY

A call comes in to City Ambulance Unit 2 staffed by paramedic Kris and BLS provider Bob. The dispatcher reports multiple injuries in a two-car collision on the freeway at interchange 20. Because of backed-up traffic, the dispatcher directs the unit to access the scene using the freeway exit ramp.

Police arrive at the scene and provide Unit 2 with an update while en route. A green auto traveling at freeway speed has collided with a red car stalled at the interchange. The wreck involves three injured parties—one in the red car and two in the green.

When Unit 2 reaches the scene, the police have secured it and are directing traffic around the vehicles involved. Kris and Bob approach the vehicles and begin the scene size-up, noting that about 50 feet now separate the two vehicles. The green car has severe front-end damage: two "spider-web" cracks in the windshield, the steering column is deformed, and as an older model car it has no air bags. The police officer in charge reports that both people in the car had failed to wear seat belts. The red car has severe rear-end damage, but the windshield is intact. The driver in this vehicle wore a seat belt and the head rest is in the up position. Before acting, Kris calls for another ambulance to back up Unit 2. Kris and Bob now proceed to the green car, where they expect to find the worst injuries.

Kris and Bob perform primary assessments on the two occupants of that vehicle. The driver has suffered chest trauma caused by impact with the steering wheel. Although she is experiencing difficult and painful breathing, her airway is clear. She is oriented to time, place, and person and denies any period of unconsciousness. Her pulses are strong, regular, and at a moderate rate and she appears to be breathing adequately. The physical exam reveals a forehead contusion, a reddened anterior chest with crepitus, and clear breath sounds bilaterally.

The passenger is unconscious and cannot be aroused. She has shallow, rapid breaths and a rapid, barely palpable pulse. Her forehead is badly contused with minor lacerations and moderate bleeding. There are some contusions to her knees, and her thighs appear noticeably shortened. The rapid trauma assessment reveals instability of the pelvis and both femurs.

A police officer who has been trained as an Emergency Medical Responder indicates that the driver of the red car is conscious and alert. Although "shaken up," he has a blood pressure of 126/84 and a pulse of 86. He is breathing normally at a rate of 20. As the paramedic in charge, Kris asks the officer to stay with the driver until the second ambulance arrives.

Meanwhile, Bob has told the driver of the green car not to move. He then immobilizes the passenger's head manually while Kris applies oxygen, then a cervical collar. Next, Kris prepares a long spine board with straps and a pelvic sling. They place the passenger on the board, strap her securely, firmly apply the sling, and affix her head with a cervical immobilization device. They then load her into the ambulance.

When the second ambulance arrives, Kris briefs that crew and assigns them the remaining patients, the two drivers. Kris and Bob then rush the passenger, who is the most critical patient, to a nearby trauma center. En route, vital signs reveal a blood pressure of 72 by palpation and a weak radial pulse of 130. The legs look ashen, feel cool to the touch, and show no palpable pulses. Capillary refill time is 3 seconds in the upper extremities, longer in the lower ones. The pulse oximeter reading is 82 percent.

Kris gives a brief report to medical direction and receives orders in response. She starts a large-bore IV and quickly administers a 250-mL bolus of normal saline. She will check the patient's response and administer repeat boluses as needed. After administering the first bolus of saline, Kris readies intubation equipment and ventilates the patient using a bag-valve mask. She attempts oral intubation with the patient's head held fixed in the neutral position. When the effort proves unsuccessful, Kris withdraws the tube, ventilates the patient again, and tries to insert an LMA. LMA insertion is successful and Kris infuses another 250-mL bolus of fluid. Lung sounds are clear, chest excursion improves, capnography displays a proper waveform, and oximetry readings begin to rise.

The patient arrives at the trauma center with one more fluid bolus having been administered for a total of 750 mL of fluid infused, an end-tidal CO_2 reading of 35 mmHg, and an oxygen saturation of 96 percent. An orthopedist is called and uses external fixation to stabilize the pelvis. A major bleeding pelvic artery is embolized to halt its hemorrhage. The patient recovers after a few weeks of hospitalization and months of rehabilitation. She will walk again with only slight reminders of the injuries and the care she received.

Based on the speed of impact and the vehicle damage, the second ambulance crew decides to transport the other two patients to the trauma center. The driver of the green car has two fractured ribs, minor pulmonary contusions, a C-spine cleared by CT scan, and no neurologic deficit. She stays overnight for observation and is released the next afternoon with some medication for rib fracture pain. The other driver has a clear C-spine and returns home shortly after the emergency department evaluation.

INTRODUCTION TO BLUNT TRAUMA

Blunt trauma is the most common cause of trauma death and disability. It results from an energy exchange between an object and the human body, without intrusion of the object through the skin (Figure 1 ●). The energy exchange causes a chain reaction within various body tissues that crush, stretch, and tear their structures, resulting in injury at and beneath the skin's surface. Blunt trauma is especially confounding, because the injury's true nature is often hidden, and serious injury evidence is very subtle or even absent.

To properly care for victims of blunt trauma, you must understand the process that brings forces to bear on the human body. The study of this process, called the *kinetics of impact*, gives insight into the events that produce injury, known as the *mechanism of injury*. You also need to appreciate the energy exchange that damages human tissue, referred to as the *biomechanics of trauma*. These insights then help you develop an anticipation of the nature and severity of likely injuries, called the *index of suspicion*. Armed with an index of suspicion, you can better focus your trauma patient's assessment, triage, and care because you know what happened and the injuries the event is likely to produce.

Let us look at the kinetics of impact, biomechanics of trauma, vehicular collisions, blast injuries, and other types of blunt trauma to develop an understanding of these prevalent mechanisms of injury and their effects on human anatomy.

KINETICS OF IMPACT

Kinetics is a branch of physics dealing with objects in motion and energy exchanges that occur as these objects collide. These collisions, or impacts, deliver energy to the patient and thus induce injury. An understanding of kinetics will help you appreciate and anticipate the results of auto and other impacts.[1] The two basic principles of kinetics are the laws of inertia and of energy conservation. Further, kinetic energy and force formulas quantify the energy exchange process between a moving object and the human body. These laws and formulas best describe what happens during impact and help in our understanding of blunt trauma and penetrating trauma.

Inertia

The law of inertia, as described by Sir Isaac Newton and also known as Newton's first law, helps explain how objects in motion behave. The first part of his first law states that a body in

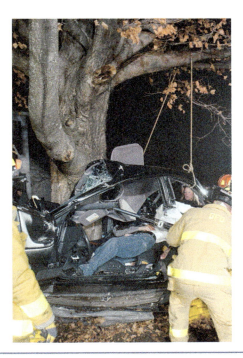

● **Figure 1**   Blunt trauma is the most common cause of injury and trauma-related death. It is a physical exchange of energy from an object or surface transmitted through the skin into the body's interior. (© *Mark C. Ide*)

motion will remain in motion unless acted upon by an outside force. As an example, think of an auto moving at 65 miles per hour. To stop the auto you must apply a force, whether by slowing the car gradually with brake application or by slowing it rapidly as the car collides with a large tree.

The second part of the law states: "A body at rest will remain at rest unless acted upon by an outside force." For example, an auto halted for a stop sign can be propelled forward using the force of the auto engine, engaging the transmission, and turning the wheels, or from the force of another car hitting it from behind and jolting it forward. In both cases, energy from an "outside force" is transferred to the auto, and it moves forward.

Energy Conservation

Energy is defined as the ability to do work in the strict physical sense. The law of energy conservation states: "Energy can neither be created nor destroyed. It can only be changed from one form to another." In an auto crash, this changing of one energy form to another is what deforms the auto and may cause injury to its occupants. By examining this energy transformation we can appreciate the processes and forces that induce injury.

As an auto slows gradually for a stop sign, the brakes develop friction to slow the turning wheels, producing heat. The energy of motion is transformed into heat energy. During an auto crash, however, the energy of motion is converted at a much faster rate and is converted into several forms of energy. This conversion of energy is manifested by the sound of impact, deformation of the auto's structural components, heat released from twisting steel, and forces directed to occupants as they collide with the vehicle interior. As all the energy of motion converts to other energy forms, the auto and its occupants come to rest.

Force

Newton's second law of motion quantifies the forces at work during a collision. It states that force strength is related to an object's weight (mass) and the rate of its change in velocity. (While mass and weight are not identical, we will consider them such for these discussions.) The force formula is summarized below:

$$\text{Force} = \frac{\text{Mass (Weight)} \times \text{Acceleration (or Deceleration)}}{2}$$

The force formula emphasizes the importance of the rate at which an object changes speed, either increasing (**acceleration**) or decreasing (**deceleration**). Gradual changes in speed (low acceleration) generate small forces and are usually uneventful. Normal deceleration, such as slowing for a stop sign, covers about 140 feet (from 65 miles per hour to a stop at a braking rate of 22 feet/10 miles per hour). Because the kinetic energy of a moving vehicle is changed over a great distance (and over several seconds), it rarely results in injury. However, colliding with a large tree and slowing from 65 miles per hour to a stop in a matter of inches and a fraction of a second (and thus high deceleration) produces tremendous force and devastating injuries.

Kinetic Energy

Kinetic energy is the energy of an object in motion. It is a function of the object's **mass** and its **velocity** (Figure 2 ●). The kinetic energy of an object while in motion is measured by the following formula:

$$\text{Kinetic Energy} = \frac{\text{Mass (Weight)} \times \text{Velocity (Speed)}^2}{2}$$

It is important to carefully examine the formula elements. Changes in an object's mass or velocity have different effects on the object's kinetic energy. This formula illustrates that when you double an object's weight, you double its kinetic energy. It is twice as damaging to be hit by a 2-lb ball as to be hit by a 1-lb ball. It is three times as damaging to be hit by a 3-lb ball, and so on (a linear relationship).

As velocity (speed) increases, there is a larger increase in kinetic energy. Being hit with a 1-lb ball traveling at 20 miles per hour is four times as injurious as being hit with the same ball moving at 10 miles per hour. Double the speed, and the energy is quadrupled. If the speed increases to 30 miles per hour (tripling), the energy released (and the expected trauma) is nine times greater. This concept plays a key role in understanding the enormous energy released in high-speed motor vehicle crashes as well as the devastating effects of a gunshot wound in which a small bullet, traveling extremely fast, can do great damage.

Kinetic energy is the measure of how much energy an object in motion has, not necessarily how much injury it will cause. The force formula explains how that energy is delivered to the structure of a vehicle, its occupants, and the occupants' organs and tissues. Once an object has significant kinetic energy, the rate of deceleration (or acceleration) then determines the force of impact and the severity of resultant injuries.

When significant kinetic energy is applied to human anatomy, we call it trauma. Trauma is defined as a wound or injury that is violently produced by some external force. The

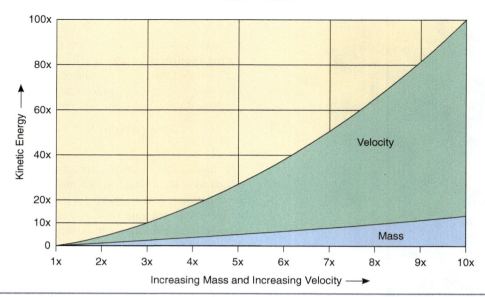

● Figure 2 Increasing mass directly increases kinetic energy, while increasing velocity exponentially increases kinetic energy. Shown here, as mass increases 10 times, kinetic energy increases 10 times, but as velocity increases 10 times, kinetic energy increases 100 times.

biomechanics of trauma—the injury process—is the energy exchange that damages human tissue.

BIOMECHANICS OF TRAUMA

The biomechanics of trauma is an investigation of the injury process. It examines kinetic energy forces as they progress from the body's exterior to the internal organs and structures. As with the kinetics of impact, the biomechanics of trauma are bound by the laws of physics: inertia, force, and energy conservation.

Trauma is divided into two general categories: blunt and penetrating (Figure 3 ●). Penetrating trauma occurs as the object physically enters the body and directly or indirectly injures tissue. Blunt trauma occurs when kinetic energy forces, but not the object, enter the body and damage tissue.

PATHO PEARLS

Compression, Stretch, and Shear

For an example of these biomechanical forces of compression, stretch, and shear at work, let us examine an auto collision. In a frontal impact, the car stops abruptly, setting off the driver-side air bag. While the auto slows, the driver's entire upper body continues to move forward. Unfortunately, in our example, the occupant's forward speed is not reduced by seat belt use. As the driver's chest hits the deployed air bag, the skin's surface drastically slows its forward motion. However, the remaining chest contents—the ribs and intercostal muscles, lungs, heart, great vessels, esophagus, spine, and posterior chest wall—continue their forward motion. As the ribs and intercostal muscles, then the lungs and heart, the great vessels and esophagus, and finally the spine and posterior chest wall collide with one another, kinetic energy of the moving chest changes form, injury may occur, and the chest comes to a rest.

If all body tissue and organs were of a consistent density, elasticity, and strength and were uniformly attached, any injury pattern would be consistent and very predictable.[1] However, this is not the case. Skin and muscle tissue are very strong and well able to withstand compression and stretch. Bone is extremely strong but resists bending and may fracture. Lung tissue consists of delicate microscopic air sacs (alveoli) that are very susceptible to injury by rapid, strong compression, especially when they are filled with air. Finally, hollow organs like the heart, stomach, bowel, and urinary bladder are very tolerant of trauma forces unless they are distended with fluid or air. Then they are more likely to rupture. Solid organs vary in their ability to withstand the forces of trauma. The spleen and brain are very delicate and damage easily. The kidneys, liver, and pancreas are held together rather strongly by the nature of their tissue and by a firm capsule surrounding them. However, as impact energy and the forces directed to these structures increase, there is a greater likelihood of injury.

Organ attachment also plays an important role in the biomechanics of trauma. The heart is a dense muscle filled with a dense fluid, blood. When deceleration forces occur, the heart has more mass and inertia than the less dense lung tissue surrounding it. It easily displaces lung tissue and moves violently against the aorta and venae cavae. Since the thoracic aorta is firmly attached to the posterior thoracic wall, the heart twists against this vessel. This action may rupture the aorta or tear its internal lining and create a dissection. The liver is held firmly in the right upper abdominal quadrant by the ligamentum teres. With strong deceleration, this ligament may lacerate the liver like a wire cheese cutter cutting cheese. Other organs, like the kidneys, are attached by structural regions called pedicles, traversed by blood vessels, which anchor the organ. With severe acceleration or deceleration forces, this attachment may stretch and tear, damaging blood vessels, causing internal hemorrhage, and disrupting blood flow to the organ.

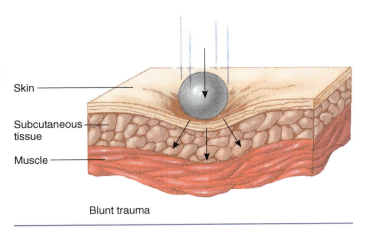

Blunt trauma

● **Figure 3a** Blunt trauma results when an object or force impacts the body and kinetic energy is transferred to the involved body tissues.

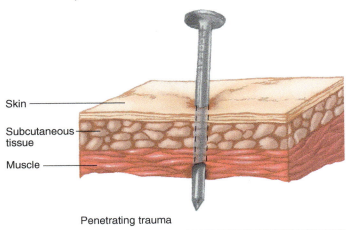

Penetrating trauma

● **Figure 3b** Penetrating injury is produced when an object enters the body resulting in direct injury.

During normal blunt impacts of everyday life, such as sitting in a chair or being jostled in a crowd, little or no damage occurs. However, as an object's kinetic energy and the rate of velocity (acceleration or deceleration) increase, blunt impact begins to cause injury. Blunt trauma can occur when a person in motion contacts a stationary object as at the end of a fall or when a moving object strikes a stationary person as when someone is struck with a baseball.

Blunt trauma involves a continuous series of collisions as outside forces cause body tissue to rapidly accelerate or decelerate. During the process, compressing, stretching, and shearing forces may induce tissue injury. *Compression* injury occurs as blunt impact abruptly halts a portion of the body while inertia causes the remaining anatomy to continue its motion. The result is one tissue or organ being pushed into another, compressing it and damaging small blood vessels, connective tissue, and cell structures within (Figure 4 ●).

Stretch is the opposite of compression. Here, protein fibers that hold tissues together are pulled and injured or torn. Stretch occurs as one part of the body is pulled away from another, as between the vertebrae during a hanging. Another example of stretch is the hollow organ filled with fluid or air. During impact, tissue compression brings the anterior and posterior surfaces of the hollow organ closer together, increasing the pressure within. This pressure is opposed by the decelerating anterior organ wall

and the inertia of the posterior organ wall. However, there are no such opposing forces from the organ's sides. The increasing air or fluid pressure pushes outward, stretching the lateral organ wall. This is much like compressing a fluid-filled plastic bag beneath your foot. With increasing force the side walls of the bag are stressed and may rupture, stretching and tearing the walls and spilling the contents (Figure 5 ●).

CONTENT REVIEW

► Forces of Blunt Trauma

• Compression
• Stretch
• Shear

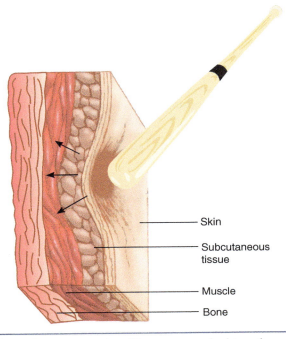

● **Figure 4** Compression. Tissues are pushed together, causing damage.

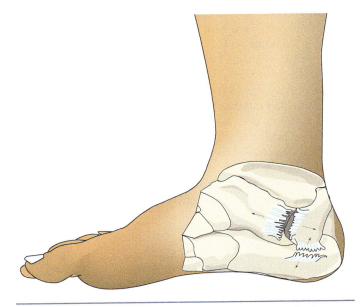

● **Figure 5** Stretch. Drawing shows ligaments attached to ankle and heel bones stretched and torn in a sprain.

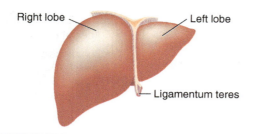

Right lobe   Left lobe

Ligamentum teres

● **Figure 6**   Shear. With rapid deceleration, as in an auto crash, the liver moves forward at the original speed while the supporting ligamentum teres remains in its fixed position, possibly slicing into the liver (a shearing injury).

Shear injury occurs along edges of the impacting force or at organ attachments. As the impacting force slows a part of the body, tissue along the impact border continues its motion. The opposing forces, one slowing the structure, the other (inertia) resisting that slowing, tear the tissue similarly to the opposing blades of a scissors, with tissues sliding in opposite directions along parallel planes (Figure 6 ●). With organ attachment, the attaching ligament resists the motion of the dense organ and tears into its tissue.

Blunt trauma most commonly results from motor vehicle collisions involving automobiles, motorcycles, bicycles, pedestrians, or off-road vehicles (e.g., all-terrain vehicles, watercraft, snowmobiles). It can also result from falls, explosions, crush injuries, and sports injuries. By looking at the biomechanics of injury for each of these mechanisms, we can begin to identify likely injuries (indexes of suspicion).

Vehicular Collisions

Vehicular collisions—sometimes called motor vehicle collisions or motor vehicle crashes (MVCs)—account for a large proportion of paramedic responses. Each year over 100,000 serious collisions occur on U.S. highways and some 34,500 people lose their lives in these collisions, while many more are seriously injured or permanently disabled. As a paramedic, you must be prepared to offer rapid assessment and appropriate care to victims of these collisions.[2] To this end, you must recognize various types of vehicular impacts, identify possible mechanisms of injury, and form an index of suspicion for specific injuries. Analysis of the types of impact and the events associated with them help you arrive at this index of suspicion.

● **Figure 7**   An automobile crash generates four major collisions: (a) the vehicle collision, (b) the body collision, (c) the organ collision, and (d) secondary collisions.

Events of Impact

There are various types of vehicle impacts (frontal, lateral, oblique, rear-end, rollover). Each type generally progresses through a series of five events (Figure 7 ●). These events are:

1. *Vehicle Collision.* Vehicle collision begins when a vehicle strikes an object (or an object strikes the vehicle). The vehicle's kinetic energy causes damage as it converts to mechanical and heat energy and the vehicle comes to a stop. Forces developed in the collision depend on the initial velocity (kinetic energy) and stopping distance (rate of deceleration). If an auto slides into a snow bank and slows gradually, damage is limited. If an auto strikes a concrete retaining wall and stops abruptly, the deceleration rate and vehicle damage are much greater. The degree of auto deformity is an indicator of the strength and direction of forces experienced by its occupants.

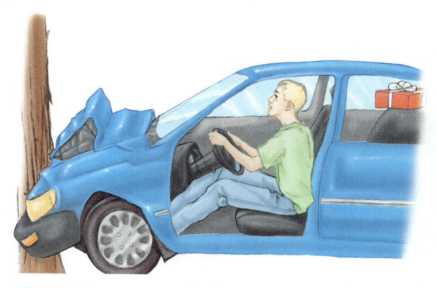

a. Vehicle collision

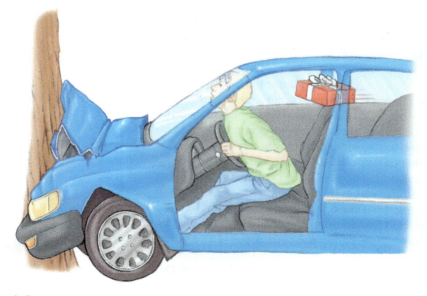

b. Body collision

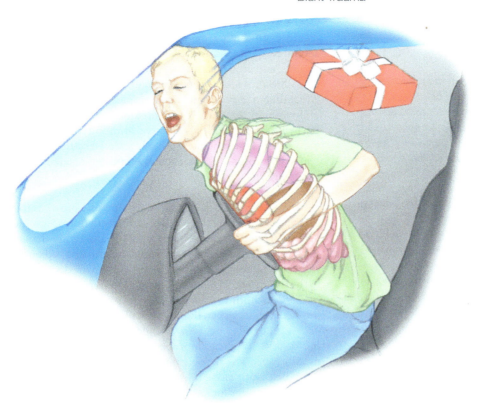

c. Organ collision

CONTENT REVIEW

▶ Events of Vehicle Collision
- Vehicle collision
- Body collision
- Organ collision
- Secondary collisions
- Additional impacts

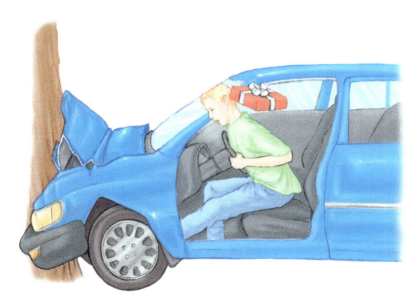

d. Secondary collision

● **Figure 7**   *Continued*

2. ***Body Collision.*** An auto collision slows or stops a vehicle, not necessarily the occupants. Body collision occurs when an occupant strikes the vehicle interior. The vehicle and its interior have slowed dramatically during the collision, but an unrestrained occupant remains at or close to the initial speed. As an occupant contacts the interior, the occupant's kinetic energy is transformed into initial tissue deformity. If the vehicle collision causes intrusion into the passenger compartment, this displacement may further subject occupants to impact forces. Restraints (seat belts and supplemental restraint systems) slow occupants along with the slowing of the vehicle during the collision, thereby decreasing the occupant's rate of deceleration, impact force strength, and seriousness of expected injuries.

3. ***Organ Collision.*** Organ collision results as an occupant contacts the vehicle's interior and/or restraints and slows

Trauma and the Laws of Physics

The laws of physics play a significant role in the pathophysiology of both blunt and penetrating injuries. In blunt trauma, the energy tends to be more widely distributed than with penetrating injuries. Also, as discussed in this chapter, solid organs are at greater risk of injury following blunt trauma than hollow organs because they tend to absorb more of the energy of impact. Whenever a patient has sustained a blunt-force injury to the abdomen, it should increase your index of suspicion of solid-organ injury. Injuries to the liver, spleen, pancreas, or even the kidneys can result in massive blood loss.

It is important to remember, also, that some hollow organs will begin to react in a way similar to solid organs when they are full or distended. For example, the urinary bladder may be full at the time of injury. Blunt-force trauma may result in its rupture with subsequent spillage of urine into the abdomen. Thus, questions about recent meals, alcohol and fluid intake, and similar factors must be taken into consideration when caring for a victim of blunt trauma.

At the trauma center, surgeons may elect to manage some blunt-force injuries conservatively, and others with immediate surgical repair.

or stops. Tissues behind the contacting surface of the occupant's body collide, one into another, as the body comes to a halt. This causes compression, stretching, and shear as tissues and organs violently press into each other. In this process, organs may also twist or decelerate, tearing at their attachments or at blood vessels. The result is blunt trauma.

4. *Secondary Collisions.* Secondary collisions occur when a vehicle occupant is impacted by objects traveling within the auto. During the collision, objects—such as those in the back seat, on the back window ledge, or in the back of a van—or unrestrained passengers may continue to travel at the auto's initial speed. They then impact an occupant who has come to rest within the auto. It is important to consider the possibility of any secondary collisions and their effects on occupants when developing an index of suspicion for injuries.[3]

5. *Additional Impacts.* Additional impacts may occur when a vehicle receives a second impact—for example, when it hits another vehicle, is deflected, then hits a parked car. This second impact may induce additional patient injuries or increase the seriousness of those already received. Consider someone who sustains a femur fracture. It initially takes a great deal of energy to break the bone. Once the bone is broken, however, the energy now needed to move those bone ends around and cause further, possibly more severe, injury to nerves and blood vessels is small. It is important to consider what effect any additional impacts may have on the initial injuries and overall patient condition.

Restraints

Restraints such as seat belts (lap belts, shoulder straps), air bags, and child safety seats have a profound effect on the injuries

associated with auto collisions. They have played a substantial role in significantly reducing collision-related deaths over the past several decades. Consider whether vehicle occupants have used restraints, and used them properly, as you estimate possible injuries.

EMS providers should recognize the value of seat belt use. All ambulance personnel must employ seat belts when driving and while in the patient care area of the vehicle. Securing the lap belt firmly provides positive positioning so drivers and other crew members are not as adversely affected by the gravitational-equivalent forces (G forces) sometimes associated with emergency driving.

Seat Belts Lap belt and shoulder strap use prevents the wearer's continuing and independent movement during a vehicle collision. A belted occupant slows with the auto rather than moving rapidly forward and suddenly impacting the stopped or dramatically slowed interior. An occupant's ultimate deceleration rate is thus reduced, lessening the likelihood of serious injury from collisions within the vehicle. Lap belts and shoulder straps also lessen the chances that the wearer will be ejected from the vehicle.

Although lap belts and shoulder straps significantly reduce injury severity, their improper use may cause some, although usually much less serious, injuries. They must be used together. A lap belt worn alone does not restrain the chest, neck, or head from continuing forward. These body regions may impact the dash, steering wheel, or air bag, resulting in chest, neck, and head injuries. Sudden body folding at the waist during extreme impacts when only a lap belt is worn may result in intra-abdominal or lower spine injuries. If the lap belt is worn too high, abdominal compression and spinal (T12 to L2) fractures may result. If worn too low, it may cause hip dislocations. When used with the lap belt, the shoulder strap restrains the chest and prevents the body from folding at the waist. If the shoulder strap is worn alone, it may cause severe neck contusions, lacerations, possible spinal injury, and even decapitation in more violent collisions.

When both lap and shoulder belts are worn properly, injury may still occur. In very strong impacts, the shoulder strap may induce chest contusions and, in some cases, rib, sternum, and clavicle fractures. Seat belts do not restrict head and neck movement. In rapid deceleration the head's weight may cause the neck to flex well beyond its normal range of motion, causing connective tissue and vertebral injury. The lap belt and shoulder strap do not protect against intrusions into the occupant compartment. In severe collisions, the dashboard may displace into the front seat, crushing and/or trapping an occupant's lower extremities.

Supplemental Restraint Systems (SRS) Supplemental restraint systems (SRS) (also called air bags) work much differently than seat belts and are extremely effective for frontal collisions. They inflate explosively on auto impact, filling a fabric container with gas just prior to occupant impact. This produces a cushion to absorb the energy exchange of rapid deceleration. SRS ignition depends on several detectors sensing a very strong frontal deceleration, as can only occur with serious vehicle impact. Only after these detectors all agree does the explosive agent ignite. Ignition instantaneously fills the bag, slightly before or just as the occupant collides with it. Explosive gases escape quickly as the occupant compresses the bag, cushioning impact

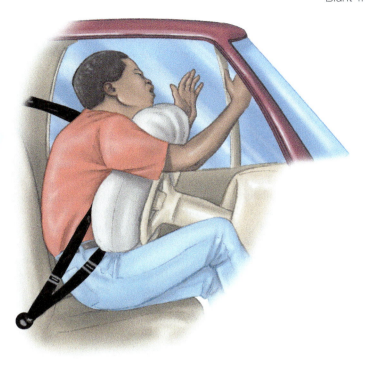

Children secured in safety seats and placed in the front seat may receive serious injury with air bag inflation. Passenger air bags have inflated in minor impacts and pushed infant and child safety seats into the seat back with tremendous force. In some cases, infants and children have been severely injured or killed by air bag inflation. For this reason, it is essential that parents secure child safety seats in the backseat when a passenger SRS is in place (and is not disabled).

Auto manufacturers are installing supplemental restraint systems in the headliners and seat sides, adjacent to the doors, for protection in lateral impact collisions. Lateral impacts account for a very high mortality rate that may be mitigated with lateral-impact and head-protection SRS.

Undeployed driver, passenger, side-door, and headliner air bags may present a hazard at the auto crash scene. Their unexpected inflation may cause serious injury to the patient or rescuer. Fire, rescue, and extrication personnel should be trained in supplemental restraint system deactivation and should deactivate any undeployed devices at the crash scene.

Child Safety Seats   Children's anatomy makes their protection in vehicle collisions difficult. Normal restraint systems are designed for adults and not for children because a child's size changes so quickly with increasing age. Small children should be placed in appropriate child safety seats to ensure their relative safety during an auto impact. With infants and very small children (up to two years of age), the child safety seat is positioned in the rear seating area, facing backward and held firmly to the seat with the lap belt or LATCH child restraint anchoring system. This positioning best distributes frontal impact forces and prevents unrestrained infant movement. As a child grows in size, the child safety seat is turned facing forward and used as a small seat. The lap belt then crosses the child at the waistline with a four point restraint system holding the child firmly in the seat.

Children held in an adult's lap or arms are *not* protected during a collision. The holder may grasp them too tightly during impact or, more likely, will not (or cannot) hold on tightly enough. If not held, the child becomes an unrestrained moving object and impacts the vehicle interior suffering serious, possibly fatal, injury.

Head Rests   Head rests are designed to prevent unopposed rearward motion of the head during a rear-end collision. As a slowed or stopped vehicle is rapidly pushed forward, the torso moves forward with the auto seat. If there is no head rest or the head rest is pushed down, inertia causes the occupant's head to remain still, effectively flinging the head back in relation to the torso. If the head rest is up, however, it causes the head to move with the seat and the rest of the body. This prevents the violent backward head rotation and neck extension. A properly positioned head rest significantly reduces the incidence of injury to the spinal column, neck ligament, and neck muscles (often called "whiplash" injury). In rear-end collisions, always check the head rest position and its relationship to a patient's height.

When evaluating auto impact results, be sure to examine for and ask questions about restraint use. Determine if lap belts and shoulder straps were used and used properly, if any SRS deployed during the collision, if child carriers were properly positioned and secured, and if head rests were in the up position.

● **Figure 8**   Air bags cushion the driver from the forces of impact and significantly reduce mortality and morbidity in frontal impact collisions.

much like the inflated bags used by pole-vaulters and movie stunt performers. Like seat belts, supplemental restraint systems are credited with dramatically reducing vehicular trauma and death (Figure 8 ●).

Supplemental restraint systems are positioned in the steering wheel, and their presence is indicated by an "SRS" insignia on the windshield and/or on the steering wheel itself. Air bags are also located in the dash for the front seat passenger. Some SRS systems permit deactivation of the passenger SRS units to accommodate children or will deactivate the air bag when passenger weight is not detected. Steering wheel and dash-mounted supplemental restraint systems offer significant protection only in frontal impact collisions. This protection is only for the first impact and not subsequent ones.

Supplemental restraint systems may induce injury during their ignition and rapid inflation, especially if seat belts are not properly used. As the bag inflates, especially from the steering wheel, it may impact the driver's fingers, hands, and forearms, possibly causing dislocations and fractures. Air bag inflation may also cause nasal fractures, minor facial lacerations, and contusions in persons of small stature seated very close to the steering wheel (less than 12 inches) or dash (less than 18 inches). Watch for small-stature occupants wearing glasses, because the air bag inflation may cause orbital or eye injuries as the glasses break and are forced into the face and eyes. The residue from SRS inflation may cause some irritation of the eyes, which can be relieved with gentle irrigation. Whenever a supplemental restraint system has deployed, check beneath it for steering wheel or dash deformity, which is indicative of extreme impact forces and more likely injury to the driver or passenger.

CONTENT REVIEW

▶ Types of Vehicle Impact
- Oblique
- Frontal
- Lateral
- Rear-end
- Rollover

Properly employed restraints will likely reduce the severity of vehicle occupant injury.

Occupant Compartment Intrusion Occupant compartment intrusion occurs when collision forces push through the vehicle's structure and deform the occupant compartment. Intrusion suggests that increased kinetic forces may have reached the patient with the likelihood of causing serious injury. Intrusion associated with lateral impact is frequent, because the associated crumple zone (within the vehicle door) is very limited. Lateral impact is also associated with a very high occupant mortality rate.

Types of Impact

There are three general types of auto impacts. They are listed below with frequency percentages in parentheses.

- Frontal (62 percent)
- Lateral (23 percent)
- Rear-end (7 percent)[4]

The listed percentages do not isolate impacts that occur at an angle (oblique impacts) and impacts that cause the vehicle to roll (rollover impacts).

Frontal Impact   Frontal impact is the most common type of impact (Figure 9 ●) and produces four pathways of patient travel. They are:

1. *Restrained Pathway.* Use of lap belts and shoulder straps restrains movement of the wearers and causes them to decelerate with the vehicle. This limits any interior impact and the energy associated with it. As noted earlier, there may be injury associated with lap-belt placement (intra-abdominal injury, lumbar spine injury, and hip dislocation) and with the shoulder belt

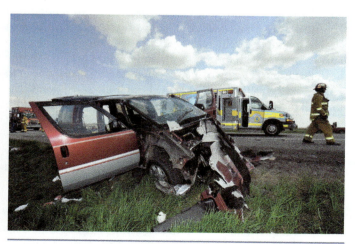

● **Figure 9**   Frontal impact often results in a significant exchange of energy and serious injuries. (© Kevin Link)

(contusions and possible rib fractures). These injuries are far less serious than those expected without restraint use. Supplemental restraint system deployment, likewise, reduces the impact forces and resultant injuries, although they may induce minor hand, arm, and facial injuries.

2. *Up-and-Over Pathway.* In the up-and-over pathway, the unrestrained occupant tenses his legs in preparation for the collision (Figure 10 ●). With vehicle slowing, the unrestrained body's upper half pivots forward and upward. The steering wheel impinges the femurs, possibly causing bilateral fractures. In addition, the steering wheel compresses and decelerates the abdominal contents, causing hollow-organ rupture and liver laceration. Traumatic compression may also force abdominal contents against the diaphragm, causing it to rupture and allowing organs to enter the thoracic cavity. As the body continues forward, the lower chest impacts the upper steering wheel and may account for the same thoracic injuries seen with the down-and-under pathway (see the discussion that follows). Deployment of supplemental restraint systems will mitigate deceleration associated with steering wheel impact and significantly reduce the expected injuries.

   The same forward motion propels the head into the windshield, leading to soft-tissue injury, skull or facial fractures, and internal head injury. Neck injury may result from hyperextension, hyperflexion, or the compression forces of windshield impact. As the body is thrown upward and forward, the head contacts the windshield. The weight and inertia of the rest of the body tries to push the head through the windshield. The result is a compression force on the cervical spine called **axial loading**. This loading may result in collapse of vertebral column support elements. A large proportion of vehicular deaths are attributed to the up-and-over pathway.

3. *Down-and-Under Pathway.* In the down-and-under pathway, the unrestrained occupant slides downward as the vehicle comes to a stop. The knees contact the firewall under the dash and absorb the initial impact. Knee, femur, and hip dislocations or fractures are common. Once the lower body slows, the upper body rotates forward, pivoting at the hip, and crashing against the steering wheel or dash. This resembles the up-and-over pathway, although the points of contact are higher up on the adult anatomy. Chest injuries like flail chest, blunt cardiac injury, and aortic tears result. If the neck contacts the steering wheel, tracheal and vascular injury may occur. An injury process frequently associated with chest-versus-steering-wheel impact is the "paper bag" syndrome (Figure 11 ●). The driver takes a deep breath as impact is imminent; he then closes his glottis, in anticipation of the collision. Impact with the steering wheel compresses the chest and drastically increases pressure within the chest, airway, and alveoli. Lung tissue (alveoli, bronchioles, and larger airways) ruptures much like an inflated paper bag caught

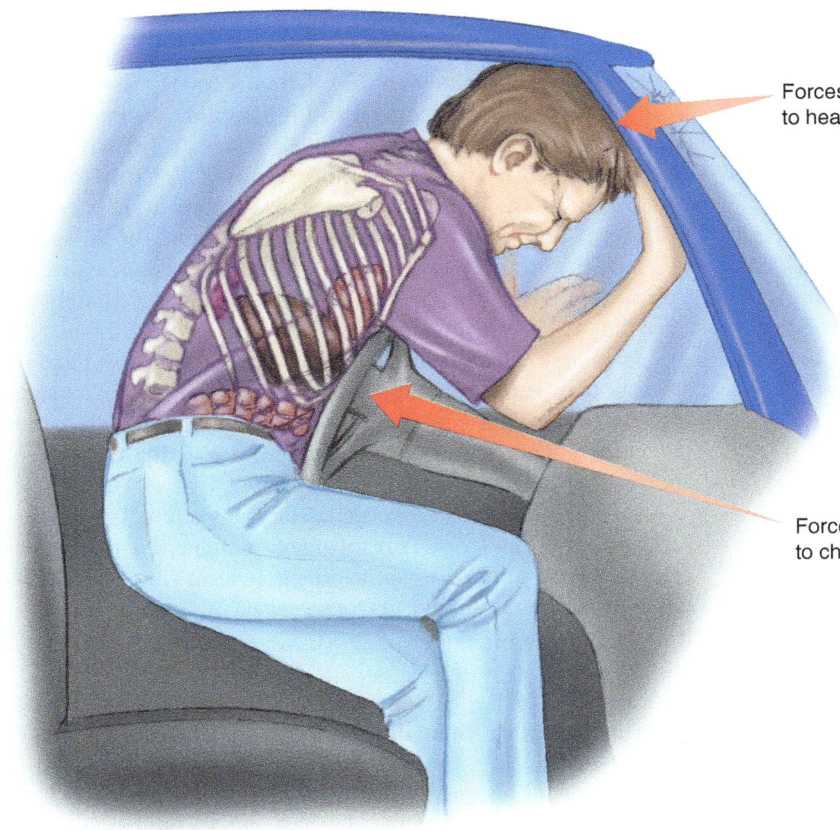

CONTENT REVIEW

▶ Mechanisms Associated with Frontal Impacts

- Restrained pathway
- Up-and-over pathway
- Down-and-under pathway
- Ejection

Forces of impact to head and neck

Forces of impact to chest

● **Figure 10**   The up-and-over pathway is associated with frontal impact collisions if, as shown here, the vehicle does not have frontal air bags or if air bags have been disengaged. (Most vehicles now have frontal air bags which, when deployed, can prevent this pathway.)

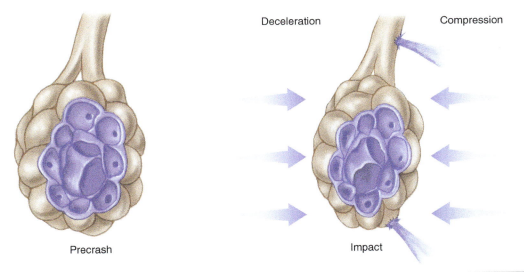

Deceleration   Compression

Precrash   Impact

● **Figure 11**   The "paper bag" syndrome results from compression of the chest against the steering column.

between clapping hands. Pneumothorax and pulmonary contusion may result.

4. *Ejection.* The up-and-over pathway may lead to ejection of an unrestrained occupant. Such a victim experiences two impacts: (1) contact with the vehicle interior and windshield and (2) impact with the ground, tree, or other object. Ejection deprives the occupant of the protections offered by the vehicle design and supplemental restraint systems (SRS). This mechanism of injury is responsible for about 27 percent of vehicular fatalities. While ejection may occur with other types of impact, it is most commonly associated with frontal impact and the unrestrained vehicle occupant.

Environmental Trauma

Bryan Bledsoe, DO, FACEP, FAAEM, EMT-P
Justin Sempsrott, MD

STANDARD
Trauma (Environmental Emergencies)

COMPETENCY
Integrates assessment findings with principles of epidemiology and pathophysiology to formulate a field impression to implement a comprehensive treatment/disposition plan for an acutely injured patient.

OBJECTIVES

Terminal Performance Objective
After reading this chapter you should be able to assess and manage patients with environmental emergencies.

Enabling Objectives
To accomplish the terminal performance objective, you should be able to:

1. Define key terms introduced in this chapter.

2. Identify factors that place patients at particular risk for environmental emergencies.

3. Describe the homeostasis of body temperature, including discussion of the following:
   a. Mechanisms of heat loss and heat production
   b. Physiology of thermoregulation
   c. Factors that can interfere with thermoregulation

4. Describe the pathophysiology of heat-related illnesses.

5. Given a variety of scenarios, assess and manage patients with heat-related illnesses.

6. Describe the pathophysiology of cold-related disorders.

7. Given a variety of scenarios, assess and manage patients with cold-related disorders.

8. Discuss measures to prevent heat-related and cold-related disorders.

9. Describe the pathophysiology of drowning.

10. Given a variety of scenarios, assess and manage patients who have drowned.

11. Describe the pathophysiology of diving emergencies, including the application of gas laws.

12. Given a variety of scenarios, assess and manage patients with diving injuries, including the following:
   a. Surface injuries
   b. Descent injuries
   c. Bottom injuries
   d. Ascent injuries

13. Describe the pathophysiology of high altitude illness.

14. Discuss ways to prevent high altitude illness.

15. Given a variety of scenarios, assess and manage patients with high altitude illnesses.

From Chapter 12 of *Paramedic Care: Principles & Practice, Volume 5*, Fourth Edition. Bryan Bledsoe, Robert Porter, and Richard Cherry. Copyright © 2013 by Pearson Education, Inc. All rights reserved.

KEY TERMS

absolute zero
acclimatization
arterial gas embolism (AGE)
autonomic neuropathy
barotrauma
basal metabolic rate
  (BMR)
conduction
convection
core temperature
decompression sickness
deep frostbite
drowning
environmental emergency
evaporation
exertional metabolic rate

frostbite
heat cramps
heat exhaustion
heat-related illness
heatstroke
homeostasis
hyperbaric oxygen
  chamber
hyperthermia
hypothalamus
hypothermia
J waves
mammalian diving reflex
negative feedback
nitrogen narcosis
pneumomediastinum

pneumothorax
pulmonary overpressure
pyrexia
pyrogens
radiation
recompression
respiration
scuba
superficial frostbite
surfactant
thermal gradient
thermogenesis
thermolysis
thermoregulation
trench foot

CASE STUDY

Today is Sunday and you and your partner are staffing Medic 7. Because of the bad weather, you pick up your partner from his home in your four-wheel-drive sport utility vehicle and ride together to work at the Thunder Bay station. It is another bitterly cold January day, so you warm up with a mug of hot chocolate, awaiting what the day will bring. Suddenly, central dispatch calls in a "priority A" situation at 1050 Ventura Road, a downtown office building in the bar and nightclub district. Apparently, someone on the way to work found an unconscious man lying in the snow. You and your partner depart immediately.

On arrival you find an approximately 20-year-old male huddled and shivering on the ice-covered ground. His breathing is shallow and irregular. He is quite stuporous and confused but manages to tell you that he had been out celebrating his twenty-first birthday last night and early this morning. He thinks he passed out here a couple of hours ago but really is not sure.

Your assessment reveals that the patient is bradycardic and mildly hypotensive. His core temperature is 86°F (30°C). While you are speaking with the patient, he stops shivering and his speech becomes unintelligible. You and your partner gently and slowly put him in the ambulance, remove his wet clothing, apply cardiac and core temperature monitors, and then place warm water bottles at his head, neck, chest, and groin. Your partner notes his core temperature has dropped to 85°F (29.4°C).

En route to Foothills General Hospital, your vehicle passes through a bumpy area of road construction, jostling your patient considerably. The alarms go off, and ventricular fibrillation appears on the monitor. Vitals are absent after checking for 2 minutes. Your partner administers a single 200 J biphasic shock without success. You intubate the patient, ventilate with warmed oxygen, and begin chest compressions. You give no medications through the IV.

In the emergency department, the patient is gradually rewarmed, using active techniques. Once the core temperature is above 86°F (30°C), the usual hypothermia protocol is initiated. The patient is converted from ventricular fibrillation and slowly regains vital signs and is eventually admitted to the ICU. Following admission, he does well and is discharged five days later. The day before his discharge you and your partner stop by to check his progress. He reports that he is doing very well but does not remember the prehospital care or the ambulance ride. The patient is adamant about one thing, however. He vows never to drink alcohol again.

INTRODUCTION

The *environment* can be defined as all of the surrounding external factors that affect the development and functioning of a living organism. Human beings obviously depend on the environment for life, but they also must be protected from its extremes. When factors such as temperature, weather, terrain, and atmospheric pressure act on the body, they can create stresses for which the body is unable to compensate. A medical condition caused or exacerbated by such environmental factors is known as an **environmental emergency**.

Environmental emergencies include a variety of conditions such as heatstroke, hypothermia, drowning, diving accidents or barotrauma, and altitude sickness. Such emergencies often call for special rescue resources.

Although environmental emergencies can affect anyone, several risk factors predispose certain individuals to developing environmental illnesses. These factors include:

- Age—especially very young children and older adults who do not tolerate environmental extremes very well
- Poor general health
- Fatigue
- Predisposing medical conditions
- Certain medications—either prescription or over-the-counter

Environmental factors must also be considered when determining the risk for environmental emergencies. For example, weather in a particular place may vary greatly from moment to moment. Areas where change in temperature can be drastic over the course of the day may catch unwary individuals off guard. For example, desert areas can have temperatures of 105°F during the day but drop below freezing at night, placing unprepared travelers in a difficult situation. As another example, temperatures in parts of southern Alberta can change drastically when the Chinook winds kick up. Other considerations include the current season, local weather patterns, atmospheric pressures (high altitude or underwater), and the type of terrain, which can cause injury or hinder rescue efforts.

As a paramedic, you will frequently be called on to treat medical emergencies related to environmental conditions. It is critical that you understand the particular conditions that prevail in your region. If you live in a mountainous area, near large caves, in an area with swift-moving water, or in a resort area where diving is prominent, you need to be familiar with the specialized rescue resources these situations may require and the particular environmental emergencies they may cause. Understanding their causes and underlying pathophysiology can help you recognize these emergencies promptly and manage them effectively.

Although many environmental factors can result in medical emergencies, this chapter will focus primarily on problems related to temperature extremes, drowning, diving emergencies, and high altitude illness.

HOMEOSTASIS

For the human body to function properly, it must interact with the environment to obtain oxygen, nutrients, and other necessities, but it must also avoid being damaged by extreme external environmental conditions. The process of maintaining constant suitable conditions within the body is called **homeostasis**. Various body systems respond in an effort to maintain the correct core and peripheral temperature, oxygen level, and energy supply to maintain life.

The following sections address how the body attempts to maintain these normal settings and what happens when certain environmental conditions exceed the ability of the body to compensate.

PATHOPHYSIOLOGY OF HEAT AND COLD DISORDERS

Mechanisms of Heat Gain and Loss

The body gains and loses heat in two ways: from within the body itself and by contact with the external environment.

The body receives heat from, or loses it to, the environment via the thermal gradient. The **thermal gradient** is the difference in temperature between the environment (the ambient temperature) and the body. The ambient temperature is usually different from body temperature. If the environment is warmer than the body, heat flows from the environment to the body. If the body is warmer than the environment, heat flows from the body to the environment. Other environmental factors, including wind and relative humidity (the percentage of water vapor in the air), also affect heat gain and loss.

The mechanisms by which heat is generated within the body and by which heat is gained or lost to the environment are discussed in more detail in the following sections.

Thermogenesis (Heat Generation)

In the science of physics, heat is created by molecules in motion. The faster the molecular motion, the higher the heat. Only when molecular motion comes to a stop does the object in question fall to a temperature of **absolute zero** (−273°C or −459°F).

The amount of heat in the body continually fluctuates as a result of the heat generated or gained and the heat lost. The body gains heat from both external and internal sources. In addition to the heat the body absorbs from the environment, the body also generates heat through energy-producing chemical reactions (metabolism).

The creation of heat is called **thermogenesis**. There are several types of thermogenesis. One is *work-induced thermogenesis* that results from exercise. Our muscles need to create heat because warm muscles work more effectively than cold ones. One way muscles can produce heat is by shivering. Another type, *thermoregulatory thermogenesis,* is controlled by the endocrine system. Hormones from the thyroid gland or the hormones norepinephrine and epinephrine from the adrenal gland can cause an immediate increase in the rate of cellular metabolism, which in turn increases heat production. The last type of thermogenesis, metabolic thermogenesis or *diet-induced thermogenesis,* is caused by the processing of food and nutrients. When a meal

CONTENT REVIEW

▶ Comparative Body Temperatures

Celsius	Fahrenheit
40.6°	105°
37.8°	100°
37°	98.6°
35°	95°
32°	89.6°
30°	86°
20°	68°

is eaten, digested, absorbed, and metabolized, heat is produced as a by-product of these activities.

Thermolysis (Heat Loss)

The loss of heat is called **thermolysis**. Heat always flows from the warmer substance to the cooler substance. The heat generated by the body is constantly lost to the environment. This occurs because the body is usually warmer than the surrounding environment. The transfer of heat into the environment occurs through the following mechanisms (Figure 1 ●):

● *Conduction.* Direct contact of the body's surface to another, cooler object causes the body to lose heat by conduction. Heat flows from higher-temperature matter to lower-temperature matter.

● *Convection.* Heat loss to air currents passing over the body. Heat, however, must first be conducted to the air before being carried away by convection currents.

● *Radiation.* An unclothed person will lose approximately 60 percent of total body heat by radiation at normal room temperature. This heat loss is in the form of infrared rays. All objects not at absolute zero temperature will radiate heat into the atmosphere.

● *Evaporation.* The change of a liquid to vapor. Evaporative heat loss occurs as water or sweat evaporates from the skin. Additionally, a great deal of heat loss occurs through evaporation of fluids in the lungs. Water evaporates from the skin and lungs at approximately 600 mL/day.

● *Respiration.* Combines the mechanisms of convection, radiation, and evaporation. It accounts for a large proportion of the body's heat loss. Heat is transferred from the lungs to inspired air by convection and radiation. Evaporation in the lungs humidifies the inspired air (adds water vapor to it). During expiration this warm, humidified air is released into the environment, creating heat loss.

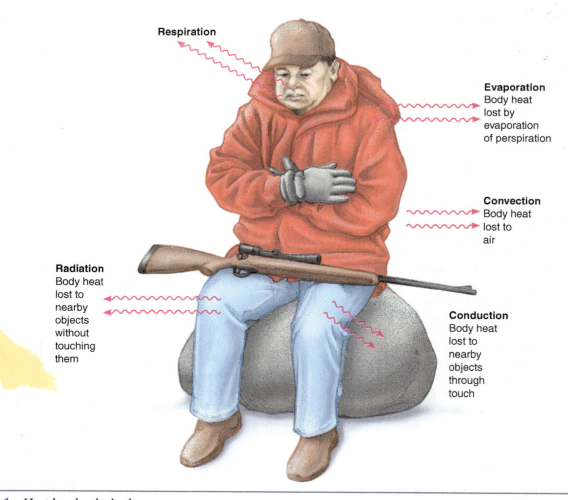

Respiration

Evaporation
Body heat lost by evaporation of perspiration

Convection
Body heat lost to air

Radiation
Body heat lost to nearby objects without touching them

Conduction
Body heat lost to nearby objects through touch

● **Figure 1**   Heat loss by the body.

Thermoregulation

Thermoregulation is the maintenance or regulation of temperature. The body temperature of the deep tissues, commonly called the **core temperature**, usually does not vary more than a degree or so from its normal 98.6°F (37°C). A naked person can be exposed to an external environment ranging anywhere from 55°F (12.8°C) to 144°F (62.2°C) and still maintain a fairly constant internal body temperature. This characteristic of warm-blooded animals is called *steady-state metabolism*. The various biochemical reactions occurring within the cell are most efficient when the body temperature is within this narrow temperature range.

Evaluation of peripheral body temperature can be measured by touch or by taking the temperature by oral or axillary means. Core body temperatures can be measured using tympanic or rectal thermometers.

The body maintains a balance between the production and loss of heat almost entirely through the nervous system and negative feedback mechanisms. The **hypothalamus**, located at the base of the brain, is responsible for temperature regulation. It functions as a thermostat, controlling temperature through the release of neurosecretions (secretions produced by nerve cells). When the hypothalamus senses an increased body temperature, it shuts off the mechanisms designed to create heat, for example, shivering. When it senses a decrease in body temperature, the hypothalamus shuts off mechanisms designed to cool the body, for example, sweating. Because the action involved requires stopping, or negating, a process, it is called a **negative feedback** system.

When the heat-regulating function of the hypothalamus is disrupted, the result can be an abnormally high or low body temperature. At the extremes, such abnormal temperatures can result in death (Figure 2 ●).

Thermoreceptors

Although the hypothalamus plays a key role in body temperature regulation, temperature receptors in other parts of the body also help to moderate temperatures. There are thermoreceptors in the skin and certain mucous membranes (peripheral thermoreceptors) as well as in certain deep tissues of the body (central thermoreceptors). The skin has both cold and warm receptors. Because cold receptors outnumber warm receptors, peripheral detection of temperature consists mainly of detecting cold rather than warmth. Deep body temperature receptors lie mostly in the spinal cord, abdominal viscera, and in or around the great veins. These receptors are exposed to the body's core temperature rather than the peripheral temperature. They also respond mainly to cold rather than warmth. Both peripheral and central thermoreceptors act to prevent lowering of the body temperature.

Metabolic Rate

The **basal metabolic rate (BMR)** is the metabolism that occurs when the body is completely at rest. It is the rate at which the body consumes energy just to maintain itself—the rate of metabolism that maintains brain function, circulation, and cell stability. Any additional activity that the body performs demands energy consumption beyond that supported by the basal rate, metabolizing more nutrients and releasing more calories (units of heat). The rate of metabolism that supports this additional activity is called an **exertional metabolic rate**.

The body continually adjusts the metabolic rate to maintain the temperature of the core (where the crucial structures like the heart and brain are located). The body also achieves temperature maintenance by dilating some blood vessels and constricting others so that the blood carries the excess heat from the core to the periphery where it is close to the skin. This allows heat to dissipate through the skin into the environment.

CONTENT REVIEW

▶ Mechanisms of Heat Dissipation

• Sweating
• Vasodilation

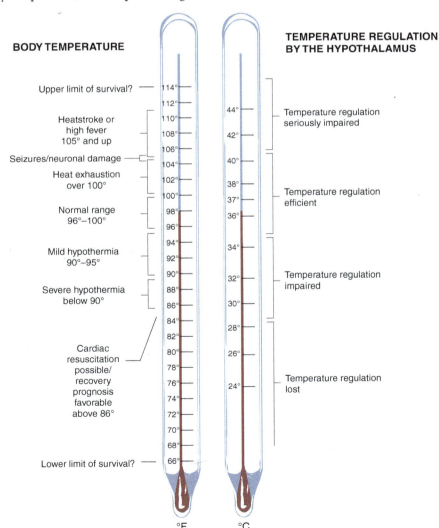

● **Figure 2** Temperature regulation by the hypothalamus.

Conversely, when the environment is too cold, *countercurrent heat exchange* is used to shunt warm blood away from the superficial veins near the skin and back into the deep veins near the core to keep vital structures warm. Another body response that counters a cold environment is shivering, a physical activity that increases metabolism and generates heat.

It is important to note that these various mechanisms can create a difference between the core body temperature and the peripheral body temperature. Core temperature is the crucial measurement since, as noted, the core is where the major organs are located. Therefore, it is important in any heat-related or cold-related emergency to obtain a core temperature reading such as from the rectum. Oral and axillary temperatures may provide convenient approximations in some situations but may lead to incorrect interventions if relied on for treatment of the patient with an environmental illness.

HEAT DISORDERS

Disruption of the body's normal thermoregulatory mechanisms can produce a number of heat illnesses, such as hyperthermia and fever. **Heat-related illness** is increased *core body temperature (CBT)* resulting from inadequate thermolysis (heat loss).[1]

Hyperthermia

Hyperthermia is a state of unusually high body temperature, specifically the core body temperature. Hyperthermia is usually caused by heat transfer from the external environment for which the body cannot compensate. Additionally, it can be caused by excessive generation of heat within the body. Hyperthermia can also occur in conjunction with the use and/or abuse of certain medications (malignant hyperthermia).

As the body attempts to eliminate this excessive heat, you will see the general signs of thermolysis. These signs are caused by the body's two chief methods of heat dissipation, sweating (which leads to evaporative heat loss) and vasodilation (which allows the blood to carry heat to the periphery for dissipation through the skin). These include:

- Diaphoresis (sweating)
- Increased skin temperature
- Flushing

As heat illness progresses, you will also note signs of thermolytic inadequacy (the failure of the body's thermoregulatory mechanisms to compensate adequately):

- Altered mentation
- Altered level of consciousness

Hyperthermia can range from minor heat cramps to heat exhaustion or life-threatening heatstroke, which will be discussed in later sections.

Predisposing Factors

Age, general health, and medications are predisposing factors in hyperthermia. Factors that may contribute to a susceptibility to hyperthermia include:

- *Age of the patient*—Pediatric and geriatric populations can tolerate less variation in temperature, and their heat-regulating mechanisms are not as responsive as those of young adult and adult populations.
- *Health of the patient*—Diabetics can become hyperthermic more easily because they develop **autonomic neuropathy**. This condition damages the autonomic nervous system, which may interfere with thermoregulatory input and with vasodilation and perspiration, which normally dissipate heat.
- *Medications*—Various medications can affect body temperature in the following ways:
  ○ *Diuretics* predispose to dehydration, which worsens hyperthermia.
  ○ *Beta-blockers* interfere with vasodilation and reduce the capacity to increase heart rate in response to volume loss and may also interfere with thermoregulatory input.
  ○ *Psychotropics and antihistamines,* such as antipsychotics and phenothiazines, interfere with central thermoregulation.
- *Level of acclimatization*—**Acclimatization** is the process of becoming adjusted to a change in environment. In response to an environmental change, reversible changes in body structure and function take place that help to maintain homeostasis.
- *Length of exposure*
- *Intensity of exposure*
- *Environmental factors* such as humidity and wind (Figure 3 ●).

Preventive Measures

Ideally, prevention of heat disorders is preferable to treating an illness already in progress. Measures to prevent hyperthermia include the following:

- Maintain adequate fluid intake, remembering that thirst is an inadequate indicator of dehydration.
- Allow time for gradual acclimatization to being out in the heat. Acclimatization results in more perspiration with lower salt concentration and increases body-fluid volume.
- Limit exposure to hot environments.

Specific Heat Disorders

Inevitably, you will be required to respond to heat-related emergencies: heat cramps, heat exhaustion, or heatstroke. Heat cramps and heat exhaustion result from dehydration and depletion of sodium and other electrolytes. Heatstroke, a far more serious, life-threatening condition, results from the failure of the body's thermoregulatory mechanisms.

NOAA's National Weather Service

Heat Index

Temperature (°F)

Relative Humidity (%)	80	82	84	86	88	90	92	94	96	98	100	102	104	106	108	110
40	80	81	83	85	88	91	94	97	101	105	109	114	119	124	130	136
45	80	82	84	87	89	93	96	100	104	109	114	119	124	130	137	
50	81	83	85	88	91	95	99	103	108	113	118	124	131	137		
55	81	84	86	89	93	97	101	106	112	117	124	130	137			
60	82	84	88	91	95	100	105	110	116	123	129	137				
65	82	85	89	93	98	103	108	114	121	128	136					
70	83	86	90	95	100	105	112	119	126	134						
75	84	88	92	97	103	109	116	124	132							
80	84	89	94	100	106	113	121	129								
85	85	90	96	102	110	117	126	135								
90	86	91	98	105	113	122	131									
95	86	93	100	108	117	127										
100	87	95	103	112	121	132										

Likelihood of Heat Disorders with Prolonged Exposure or Strenuous Activity

☐ Caution ☐ Extreme Caution ☐ Danger ☐ Extreme Danger

● **Figure 3** The Heat Index. The Heat Index factors in both temperature and relative humidity and provides information about the condition of the environment and problems related to the duration of exposure.

Signs and symptoms and emergency care procedures for heat cramps, heat exhaustion, and heatstroke are discussed in the following sections and summarized in Procedure 1.

Heat (Muscle) Cramps

Heat cramps are muscle cramps caused by overexertion and dehydration in the presence of high atmospheric temperatures. Sweating occurs as sodium (salt) is transported to the skin. Because "water follows sodium," water is deposited on the skin surface where evaporation occurs, aiding in the cooling process. Since sweating involves not only the loss of water but also the loss of electrolytes (such as sodium), intermittent cramping of skeletal muscles may occur. Heat cramps are painful but are not considered to be an actual heat illness.

Signs and Symptoms The patient with heat cramps will present with cramps in the fingers, arms, legs, or abdominal muscles. He will generally be mentally alert with a feeling of weakness. He may feel dizzy or faint. Vital signs will be stable. Body temperature may be normal or slightly elevated. The skin is likely to be moist and warm.

Treatment Treatment of the patient with heat cramps is usually easily accomplished:

1. *Remove the patient from the environment.* Place the patient in a cool environment such as a shaded area or the air-conditioned back of the ambulance.

In the case of severe cramps:

2. *Administer water or a sports drink.* Do *NOT* administer salt tablets, which are not absorbed as readily and

may cause stomach irritation and ulceration or hypernatremia. *If the patient is unable to take fluids orally, an IV of normal saline may be needed.* Antiemetic medications, such as ondansetron, can be effective in assisting the patient with oral intake.

3. *Educate.* Educate the patient that heat cramps may indicate that he is at risk for heat exhaustion or heatstroke if he continues his current activity without appropriate cooling or hydration.

Some EMS systems recommend massaging the painful muscles. Application of moist towels to the patient's forehead and over the cramped muscles may also be helpful.

Heat Exhaustion

Heat exhaustion, which is considered to be a mild heat illness, is an acute reaction to heat exposure. It is the most common heat-related illness seen by prehospital personnel. An individual performing work in a hot environment will lose 1 to 2 liters of water an hour. Each liter lost contains 20 to 50 milliequivalents of sodium. The resulting loss of water and sodium, combined with general vasodilation, leads to a decreased circulating blood volume, venous pooling, and reduced cardiac output.

Dehydration and electrolyte loss from sweating often account for the presenting signs and symptoms. However, these signs and symptoms are not exclusive to heat exhaustion. Instead, they mimic those of an individual suffering from fluid and sodium loss from any of a number of other causes. A history of exposure to high environmental temperatures is needed to obtain an accurate assessment.

If not treated, heat exhaustion may progress to heatstroke.

Condition	Muscle Cramps	Mental Status	Respirations	Pulse	Blood Pressure	Body Temperature	Other Possible
Heat Cramps	Yes	Alert	Normal	Normal	Normal	Normal	Weakness, dizziness, faintness
Heat Exhaustion	Sometimes	Anxiety to possible loss of consciousness	Rapid, shallow	Weak	Normal	Somewhat elevated	Headache, paresthesia, diarrhea
Heatstroke	No	Confusion, disorientation, or loss of consciousness	Deep, rapid; later shallow, slowing	Rapid, full; later slowing	Low	Very high	Seizures

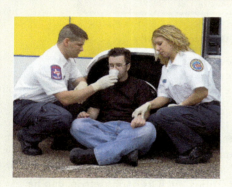

1a ● Heat cramps.

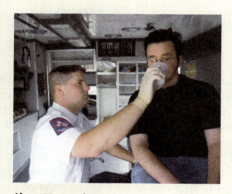

1b ● Heat exhaustion.

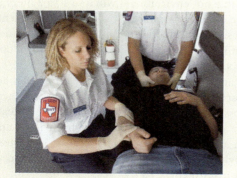

1c ● Heatstroke.

Heat Cramps: Emergency Care

- Remove patient from hot environment. Place in a cool, shaded, or air-conditioned area.
- Administer oral fluids if patient is alert and able to swallow or an IV of normal saline.

Heat Exhaustion: Emergency Care

- Remove patient from hot environment. Place in a cool, shaded, or air-conditioned area.
- Administer oral fluids if patient is alert and able to swallow or an IV of normal saline.
- Place patient in a supine position.
- Remove some clothing and fan the patient. Be careful not to cool to the point of chilling or causing shivering.
- Treat for shock, if suspected; however, do not cover the patient to the point of overheating.

Heatstroke: Emergency Care

- Remove patient from hot environment. Place in a cool, shaded, or air-conditioned area.
- Initiate rapid active cooling en route to the hospital. Remove clothing and cover patient with sheets soaked in tepid water. Lower body temperature to 102°F (39°C). Avoid cooling to a lower temperature.
- Administer supplemental oxygen as needed to correct hypoxia.
- If patient is alert and able to swallow, administer oral fluids. Begin one or two IVs of normal saline, wide open.
- Monitor the ECG.
- Avoid vasopressors and anticholinergic drugs.
- Monitor the body temperature.

Signs and Symptoms Signs and symptoms that you may encounter include increased body temperature (over 100°F, or 37.8°C), skin that is cool and clammy with heavy perspiration, breathing that is rapid and shallow, and a weak pulse. There may be signs of active thermolysis such as diarrhea and muscle cramps. The patient will feel weak and, in some cases, may lose consciousness. If the patient shows any signs of central nervous system (CNS) symptoms such as headache, anxiety, paresthesia, impaired judgment, even psychosis, then the patient should be treated for heatstroke.

Treatment Prehospital management of the patient with heat exhaustion is aimed at immediate cooling and fluid replacement. Steps include:

1. *Remove the patient from the environment.* Place the patient in a cool environment such as a shaded area or the air-conditioned ambulance.

2. *Place the patient in a supine position.*

3. *Administer water or a sports drink.* Do *NOT* administer salt tablets, which are not absorbed as readily and may cause stomach irritation and ulceration or hypernatremia. Anti-emetic medications, such as ondansetron, can be effective in assisting the patient with oral intake. *If the patient is unable to take fluids orally, an IV of normal saline may be needed.*

4. *Remove some clothing and fan the patient.* Remove enough clothing to cool the patient without chilling him. Fanning increases evaporation and cooling. Again, be careful not to cool the patient to the point of chilling. If the patient begins to shiver, stop fanning and perhaps cover the patient lightly.

5. *Treat for shock, if shock is suspected.* However, be careful not to cover the patient to the point of overheating him.

Symptoms should resolve with fluids, rest, and supine posturing with knees elevated. If they do not, consider that the symptoms may be due to an increased core body temperature, which is predictive of impending heatstroke and should be treated aggressively, as outlined in the following section. The decision to transport the patient should be based on local protocols. The range of heat exhaustion is wide, and some patients may respond quickly to cooling and fluids, requiring no additional treatment, while others progress rapidly to heatstroke despite aggressive measures.

Heatstroke

Heatstroke is a true environmental emergency that occurs when the body's hypothalamic temperature regulation is lost, causing uncompensated hyperthermia. This in turn causes cell death and damage to the brain, liver, and kidneys. There is no arbitrary core temperature at which heatstroke begins. However, heatstroke is generally characterized by a body temperature of at least 105°F (40.6°C), central nervous system disturbances, and usually the cessation of sweating.

Signs and Symptoms Sweating is thought to stop because of destruction of the sweat glands or when sensory overload

causes them to temporarily dysfunction. However, the patient's skin may be either dry or covered with sweat that is still present on the skin from earlier exertion. In either case, the skin will be hot.

The patient may present with the following signs and symptoms:

- Cessation of sweating
- Hot skin that is dry or moist
- Very high core temperature
- Deep respirations that become shallow, rapid at first but may later slow
- Rapid, full pulse, may slow later
- Hypotension with low or absent diastolic reading
- Confusion or disorientation or unconsciousness
- Central nervous system (CNS) symptoms such as headache, anxiety, paresthesia, impaired judgment, or psychosis
- Possible seizures

Classic heatstroke commonly presents in those with chronic illnesses, with the increased core body temperature caused by deficient thermoregulatory function. Predisposing conditions include age, diabetes, and other medical conditions. In this type of heatstroke hot, red, dry skin is common.

Exertional heatstroke commonly presents in those who are in good general health, with the increased core body temperature caused by overwhelming heat stress. There is excessive ambient temperature as well as excessive exertion with prolonged exposure and poor acclimatization. In this type of heatstroke you will find that, although sweating has ceased and the skin is hot, moisture from prior sweating may still be present.

If the patient develops heatstroke from exertion, he may go into severe metabolic acidosis caused by lactic acid accumulation. Hyperkalemia (excessive potassium in blood) may also develop because of the release of potassium from injured muscle cells, renal failure, or metabolic acidosis.

Treatment Prehospital management of the heatstroke patient is aimed at immediate cooling and replacement of fluids. Steps include:

1. *Remove the patient from the environment.* This first step is essential. If you do not remove the patient from the hot environment, any other measures will be only minimally useful. Move the patient to a cool environment, such as the air-conditioned ambulance.

2. *Initiate rapid active cooling.* Body temperature must be lowered to 102°F (39°C). A target of 102°F (39°C) is used to avoid an overshoot. This can be accomplished en route to the hospital. Remove the patient's clothing and cover the patient with sheets soaked in tepid water. Fanning

CONTENT REVIEW

► Heat Disorders

- Hyperthermia
- Heat cramps
- Heat exhaustion
- Heatstroke

► Heatstroke is a true environmental emergency.

and misting may also be used if necessary. Refrain from overcooling, as this may cause reflex hypothermia (low body temperature). This results in shivering, which can raise the core temperature again. Tepid water is used because ice packs and cold-water immersion may affect peripheral thermoreceptors, producing reflex vasoconstriction and shivering.

3. *Administer oxygen if the patient is hypoxic.* Administer supplemental oxygen as needed to correct hypoxia. If respirations are shallow, assist with a bag-valve-mask unit supplied with supplemental oxygen. Utilize pulse oximetry.

4. *Administer fluid therapy if the patient is alert and able to swallow.*

   ○ *Oral fluids.* If the patient can tolerate oral fluids, these may be administered initially. Sports drinks are preferred. Antiemetics, such as ondansetron, can be used to treat nausea and vomiting.

   ○ *Intravenous fluids.* Begin 1 to 2 IVs, using normal saline. Initially infuse them wide open.

5. *Monitor the ECG.* Cardiac arrhythmias may occur at any time. ST segment depression, nonspecific T wave changes with occasional PVCs, and supraventricular tachycardias are common.

6. *Avoid vasopressors and anticholinergic drugs.* These agents may potentiate heatstroke by inhibiting sweating. They can also produce a hypermetabolic state in the presence of high environmental temperatures and relatively high humidity.

7. *Monitor body temperature.* EMS systems operating in extremely warm climates should carry some device to record the body temperature, whether a simple rectal thermometer or a sophisticated electronic device. Simple glass thermometers generally do not measure above 106°F (41°C) or below 95°F (35°C). This may become significant during long transport when it is essential to detect changes in the patient's condition.

Role of Dehydration in Heat Disorders

Dehydration often goes hand in hand with heat disorders because it inhibits vasodilation and therefore thermolysis. Dehydration leads to orthostatic hypotension (increased pulse and decreased blood pressure on rising from a supine position) and the following symptoms that may occur along with the signs and symptoms of heatstroke:

- Nausea, vomiting, and abdominal distress
- Vision disturbances
- Decreased urine output
- Poor skin turgor
- Signs of hypovolemic shock

When these signs and symptoms are present, rehydration of the patient is critical. Oral fluids may be administered if the patient is alert and not nauseated. Administration of IV fluids may be necessary, especially if the patient has an altered mental status or is nauseated. It is not uncommon for the adult patient with moderate to severe dehydration to require 2–3 liters of IV fluids (occasionally more!).

Fever (Pyrexia)

A fever (**pyrexia**) is the elevation of the body temperature above the normal temperature for that person. (An individual person's normal temperature may be one or two degrees above or below 98.6°F, or 37°C.) The body develops a fever when pathogens enter and cause infection, which in turn stimulates the production of pyrogens.

Pyrogens are any substances that cause fever, such as viruses and bacteria or substances produced within the body in response to infection or inflammation. They reset the hypothalamic thermostat to a higher level. Metabolism is increased, which produces the elevation of temperature. The increased body temperature fights infection by making the body a less hospitable environment for the invading organism. The hypothalamic thermostat will reset to normal when pyrogen production stops or when pathogens end their attack on the body.

Fever is sometimes difficult to differentiate from heatstroke, and neurologic symptoms may present with either, but there is usually a history of infection or illness with a fever. While the heatstroke patient usually has a history of exertion and exposure to high ambient temperatures, this is not always the case. In some cases, heatstroke can be caused by impaired functioning of the hypothalamus without exertion or exposure to ambient heat. Treat for heatstroke if you are unsure which it is.

Although fever may be beneficial, it can be disconcerting to the parents of children with fever. In addition, fever can be uncomfortable for the patient. If the patient is uncomfortable, measures should be taken to treat the fever. Also, if a child has a history of febrile seizures, the fever should be treated. Parents will often have their febrile children wrapped in several layers of clothing or blankets because the child is "cold." These should be removed, leaving only the diaper or underclothes, exposing the child to the ambient air. This will allow a controlled cooling.

Sponge baths and cool-water immersion should not be used. These cause a rapid drop in the body core temperature and result in shivering. This again elevates the core temperature, which complicates the process. Several medications are good antipyretics (that is, they lower body temperature in fever). These include acetaminophen (Tylenol) and ibuprofen (Motrin). Many EMS systems will utilize an antipyretic in the treatment of fever, particularly in pediatric patients. Liquid acetaminophen and ibuprofen are easy to administer and effective. Acetaminophen is also available in a suppository form for patients with active vomiting. These antipyretics are typically dosed based on the patient's weight:

- *Acetaminophen*—15 mg/kg for pediatric patients; adult dose is typically 650–1,000 mg
- *Ibuprofen*—10 mg/kg for pediatric patients; adult dose is typically 600–800 mg

These liquid medications should be dosed with syringes as teaspoons are inaccurate measuring devices. EMS services with prolonged transport times should consider the use of antipyretics for patient comfort as well as for the prevention of febrile seizures.

COLD DISORDERS

Disruption of the body's normal thermoregulation may produce cold-related disorders such as hypothermia, frostbite, and trench foot.

Hypothermia

Hypothermia is a state of low body temperature, specifically low core temperature. When the core temperature of the body drops below 95°F (35°C), an individual is considered to be hypothermic. Hypothermia can be attributed to inadequate thermogenesis, excessive cold stress, or a combination of both. It is now a common practice to initiate induced therapeutic hypothermia (ITH) following resuscitation of cardiac arrest victims. Because of this, it is important to differentiate ITH from accidental hypothermia. While much of this discussion relates to both, we will primarily address accidental hypothermia.

Mechanisms of Heat Conservation and Loss

Exposure to cold normally triggers compensatory mechanisms designed to conserve and generate heat in order to maintain a normal body temperature. One such mechanism is piloerection (hair standing on end, "goose bumps") to impede airflow across the skin. Shivering and increased muscle tone occur, resulting in increased metabolism. There is peripheral vasoconstriction with an increase in cardiac output and respiratory rate. When these mechanisms can no longer adequately compensate for heat lost from the body surface, the body temperature falls. As the body temperature falls, so do the metabolic rate and cardiac output.

As discussed, major mechanisms of body heat loss are conduction, convection, radiation, evaporation, and respiration. Heat loss can be increased by the removal of clothing (decreased insulation, increased radiation), the wetting of clothing by rain or snow (increased conduction and evaporation), air movement around the body (increased convection), or contact with a cold surface or cold-water immersion (increased conduction).

Predisposing Factors

Several factors can contribute to the risk of developing hypothermia. They also contribute to the severity of damage if cold injury occurs. Risk factors that increase the danger of developing hypothermia include:

- *Age of the patient*—Pediatric or geriatric patients cannot tolerate cold environments and have less responsive heat-generating mechanisms to combat cold exposure. Elderly persons often become hypothermic in environments that seem only mildly cool to others.
- *Health of the patient*—Hypothyroidism suppresses metabolism, preventing patients from responding appropriately to cold stress. Malnutrition, diabetes, Parkinson's disease, fatigue, and other medical conditions can interfere with the body's ability to combat cold exposure.
- *Medications*—Some drugs interfere with proper heat-generating mechanisms. These include narcotics, alcohol, phenothiazines, barbiturates, antiseizure medications, antihistamines and other allergy medications, antipsychotics, sedatives, antidepressants, and various pain medications such as aspirin, acetaminophen, and NSAIDs.
- *Prolonged or intense exposure*—The length and severity of cold exposure have a direct effect on morbidity and mortality (Figure 4 ●).
- *Coexisting weather conditions*—High humidity, brisk winds, or accompanying rain can all magnify the effect of cold exposure on the human body by accelerating the loss of heat from skin surfaces.

Preventive Measures

Certain precautions can decrease the risk of morbidity related to cold injury.

- Dress warmly.
- Get plenty of rest to maximize the ability of heat-generating mechanisms to replenish energy supplies.
- Eat appropriately and at regular intervals to support metabolism.
- Limit exposure to cold environments.

Degrees of Hypothermia

There are several hypothermia classification schemes. The two-tiered hypothermia classification system classifies the patient as having mild or severe hypothermia, as follows:

- *Mild hypothermia*—a core temperature greater than 90°F (32°C) with signs and symptoms of hypothermia
- *Severe hypothermia*—a core temperature less than 90°F (32°C) with signs and symptoms of hypothermia

The three-tiered hypothermia classification system classifies the patient as having mild, moderate, or severe hypothermia, as follows:

- *Mild hypothermia*—a core temperature between 90°F and 95°F (32°C to 35°C) with signs and symptoms of hypothermia:
  ○ Tachycardia
  ○ Shivering

NWS Windchill Chart

Wind (mph) \ Temperature (°F)	Calm	40	35	30	25	20	15	10	5	0	-5	-10	-15	-20	-25	-30	-35	-40	-45
5		36	31	25	19	13	7	1	-5	-11	-16	-22	-28	-34	-40	-46	-52	-57	-63
10		34	27	21	15	9	3	-4	-10	-16	-22	-28	-35	-41	-47	-53	-59	-66	-72
15		32	25	19	13	6	0	-7	-13	-19	-26	-32	-39	-45	-51	-58	-64	-71	-77
20		30	24	17	11	4	-2	-9	-15	-22	-29	-35	-42	-48	-55	-61	-68	-74	-81
25		29	23	16	9	3	-4	-11	-17	-24	-31	-37	-44	-51	-58	-64	-71	-78	-84
30		28	22	15	8	1	-5	-12	-19	-26	-33	-39	-46	-53	-60	-67	-73	-80	-87
35		28	21	14	7	0	-7	-14	-21	-27	-34	-41	-48	-55	-62	-69	-76	-82	-89
40		27	20	13	6	-1	-8	-15	-22	-29	-36	-43	-50	-57	-64	-71	-78	-84	-91
45		26	19	12	5	-2	-9	-16	-23	-30	-37	-44	-51	-58	-65	-72	-79	-86	-93
50		26	19	12	4	-3	-10	-17	-24	-31	-38	-45	-52	-60	-67	-74	-81	-88	-95
55		25	18	11	4	-3	-11	-18	-25	-32	-39	-46	-54	-61	-68	-75	-82	-89	-97
60		25	17	10	3	-4	-11	-19	-26	-33	-40	-48	-55	-62	-69	-76	-84	-91	-98

Frostbite Times: 30 minutes | 10 minutes | 5 minutes

$$\text{Wind Chill (°F)} = 35.74 + 0.6215T - 35.75(V^{0.16}) + 0.4275T(V^{0.16})$$

Where, T= Air Temperature (°F) V= Wind Speed (mph)

Effective 11/01/01

● **Figure 4**   The Wind Chill Index. The Wind Chill Index factors in temperature and wind to determine the cooling effect on individuals.

○ Vasoconstriction

○ Tachypnea

○ Fatigue

○ Impaired judgment

● *Moderate hypothermia*—a core temperature between 82°F and 90°F (28°C to 32°C) with signs and symptoms of hypothermia:

○ Cold-induced arrhythmia (bradycardia, Osborn wave)

○ Hypotension

○ Respiratory depression

○ Altered mental status

○ Loss of shivering

● *Severe hypothermia*—a core temperature less than 82°F (28°C) with signs and symptoms of hypothermia:

○ Coma

○ Apnea

○ Ventricular arrhythmias or asystole

Initially some patients may exhibit *compensated* hypothermia. In this case, signs and symptoms of hypothermia will be present but with a normal core body temperature, temporarily maintained by thermogenesis. As energy stores from the liver and muscle glycogen are exhausted, the core body temperature will drop.

The onset of symptoms may be *acute,* as occurs when a person suddenly falls through ice into a frigid lake. *Subacute*

exposure can occur in situations such as when mountain climbers are trapped in a snowy, cold environment. Finally, *chronic* exposure to cold is a growing problem in our inner cities where homeless people endure frequent and prolonged cold stress without shelter.

In some cases cold exposure is the primary cause of hypothermia, but in others, hypothermia may develop secondary to other problems, such as medical problems. For example, hypothyroidism depresses the body's heat-producing mechanisms. Brain tumors or head trauma can depress the hypothalamic temperature control center, causing hypothermia. Other conditions such as myocardial infarction, diabetes, hypoglycemia, drugs, poor nutrition, sepsis, or old age can also contribute to metabolic and circulatory disorders that predispose to hypothermia. Any patient thought to have hypothermia, but with no history of exposure to a cold environment, should be assessed for any predisposing factors. Evaluate the patient for level of consciousness, cool skin, and shivering. Also, evaluate the rectal temperature. A rectal temperature of less than 95°F (35°C) indicates hypothermia. Key findings at different degrees of hypothermia are summarized in Table 1.

Patients who experience body temperatures above 86°F (30°C) will usually have a favorable prognosis. Those with temperatures below 86°F (30°C) show a significant increase in mortality rate. Remember that most thermometers used in medicine do not register below 95°F (35°C). EMS systems in colder areas should carry special thermometers for recording subnormal temperature readings because there is no reliable correlation between signs and symptoms and actual core body temperature.

TABLE 1 | Key Findings at Different Degrees of Hypothermia

C°	F°	Clinical Findings
37.6	99.6	Normal rectal temperature
37	98.6	Normal oral temperature
36	96.8	Metabolic rate increased
35	95	Maximum shivering seen
		Impaired judgment
34	93.2	Amnesia
		Slurred speech
33	91.4	Severe clouding of consciousness/apathy
		Uncoordinated movement
32	89.6	Most shivering ceases
		Pupils dilate
31	87.8	Blood pressure may no longer be obtainable
30	86	Atrial fibrillation/other arrhythmias develop
		Pulse and cardiac output decreased by 33 percent
29	84.2	Progressive decrease in pulse and breathing
		Progressive decrease in level of consciousness
28	82.4	Pulse and oxygen consumption decreased by 50 percent
		Severe slowing of respiration
		Increased muscle rigidity
		Loss of consciousness
		High risk of ventricular fibrillation
27	80.6	Loss of reflexes and voluntary movement
		Patients appear clinically dead
26	78.8	No reflexes or response to painful stimuli
25	77	Cerebral blood flow decreased by 66 percent
24	75.2	Marked hypotension
22	71.6	Maximum risk for ventricular fibrillation
19	66.2	Flat electroencephalogram (EEG)
18	64.4	Asystole
16	60.8	Lowest reported adult survival from accidental exposure
15.2	59.2	Lowest reported infant survival from accidental exposure
10	50	Oxygen consumption 8 percent of normal
9	48.2	Lowest reported survivor from therapeutic exposure

Assessment and Management of Hypothermia

Signs and Symptoms

Signs and symptoms of hypothermia are summarized in Table 2. Patients experiencing mild hypothermia (core temperature >90°F or 32°C) will generally exhibit shivering. The patient may be lethargic and somewhat dulled mentally. (In some cases, however, the patient may be fully oriented.) Muscles may be stiff and uncoordinated, causing the patient to walk with a stumbling, staggering gait.

Patients experiencing severe hypothermia (core temperature <90°F or 32°C) may be disoriented and confused. As their temperatures continue to fall, they will proceed into stupor and complete coma. Shivering will usually stop, and physical activity will become uncoordinated. Muscles may be stiff and rigid. Continuous cardiac monitoring is indicated for anyone experiencing hypothermia. The ECG will frequently show pathognomonic (indicative of a disease) J waves, also called Osborn waves, associated with the QRS complexes (Figure 5 ●), but these are not useful diagnostically. Atrial fibrillation is the most common presenting arrhythmia seen in hypothermia. As the body cools, however, the myocardium becomes progressively more irritable and may develop a variety of arrhythmias. In severe hypothermia, bradycardia is inevitable.

Ventricular fibrillation becomes more probable as the body's core temperature falls below 86°F (30°C). The severely hypothermic patient requires assessment of pulse and respirations for at least 30 seconds every 1 to 2 minutes.

Treatment

All victims of hypothermia should have the following care (Figure 6 ●):

1. *Remove wet garments.*
2. *Protect against further heat loss and wind chill.* Use *passive external warming* methods such as application of blankets, insulating materials, and moisture barriers.
3. *Maintain the patient in a horizontal position.*
4. *Avoid rough handling,* which can trigger arrhythmias.
5. *Monitor the core temperature.*
6. *Monitor the cardiac rhythm.*

Active Rewarming   Victims of mild hypothermia may also be rewarmed, using *active external methods.* This includes the use of warmed blankets and/or heat packs placed over areas of high heat transfer with the core: the base of the neck, the axilla, and the groin. Be sure to insulate between the heat packs and the skin to prevent burning. Intravenous fluid heaters can be used to heat the IV fluid to 95°F to 100°F (35°C to 38°C). If not available, use warmed IV fluids. Heat guns and lights may also be used, but this will most likely take place in the emergency department. Warm-water immersion in water between 102°F and 104°F (39°C to 40°C) may be used but can induce rewarming shock (see the next section), so this method also has little application in an out-of-hospital setting.

Active rewarming of the severely hypothermic patient is best carried out in the hospital using a prearranged protocol. Most patients who die during rewarming die from ventricular fibrillation, the risk of which is related to both the depth and the duration of hypothermia. Rough handling of the hypothermic patient may also induce ventricular fibrillation (Figure 7 ●). Active rewarming should not be attempted in the field unless travel to the emergency department will take more than 15 minutes.

If such is the case, *active internal rewarming* methods may also be used, including the use of warmed (102°F to 104°F or 39°C to 40°C) humidified oxygen and administration of warmed IV fluids (also warmed to 102°F to 104°F or 39°C to 40°C). This is crucial to prevent further heat loss, but actual heat transferred is minimal, so there is limited contribution to the rewarming effort.

Rewarming Shock   While application of warmed blankets is a safe and effective means of rewarming the hypothermic patient, application of external heat, as with heat packs, is usually not recommended in the prehospital setting. For effective rewarming, more heat transference is generally required than is possible with prehospital methods. Additionally, application of external heat may result in *rewarming shock* by causing reflex peripheral vasodilation. This reflex vasodilation causes the return of cool blood and acids from the extremities to the core. This may cause a paradoxical "afterdrop" core temperature decrease and further worsen core hypothermia. This, in turn,

TABLE 2	Hypothermia: Signs and Symptoms	
Mild	**Severe**
Lethargy	No shivering
Shivering	Arrhythmias, asystole
Lack of coordination	Loss of voluntary muscle control
Pale, cold, dry skin	Hypotension
Early rise in blood pressure, heart, and respiratory rates	Undetectable pulse and respirations

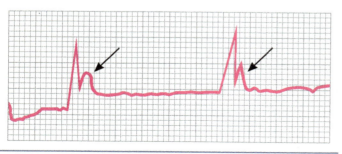

● **Figure 5**   ECG tracing showing J wave following the QRS complex as seen in hypothermia.

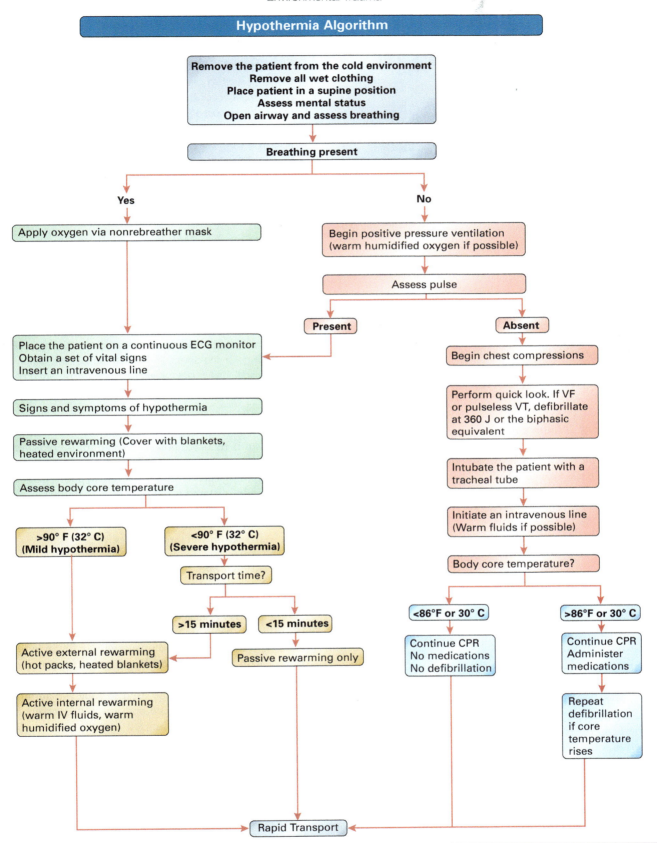

Hypothermia Algorithm

Remove the patient from the cold environment
Remove all wet clothing
Place patient in a supine position
Assess mental status
Open airway and assess breathing

Breathing present

Yes

Apply oxygen via nonrebreather mask

Place the patient on a continuous ECG monitor
Obtain a set of vital signs
Insert an intravenous line

Signs and symptoms of hypothermia

Passive rewarming (Cover with blankets, heated environment)

Assess body core temperature

>90° F (32° C) (Mild hypothermia)

<90° F (32° C) (Severe hypothermia)

Transport time?

>15 minutes **<15 minutes**

Active external rewarming (hot packs, heated blankets)

Passive rewarming only

Active internal rewarming (warm IV fluids, warm humidified oxygen)

No

Begin positive pressure ventilation (warm humidified oxygen if possible)

Assess pulse

Present **Absent**

Begin chest compressions

Perform quick look. If VF or pulseless VT, defibrillate at 360 J or the biphasic equivalent

Intubate the patient with a tracheal tube

Initiate an intravenous line (Warm fluids if possible)

Body core temperature?

<86°F or 30° C **>86°F or 30° C**

Continue CPR
No medications
No defibrillation

Continue CPR
Administer medications

Repeat defibrillation if core temperature rises

Rapid Transport

● **Figure 6** Algorithm for treatment of hypothermia.

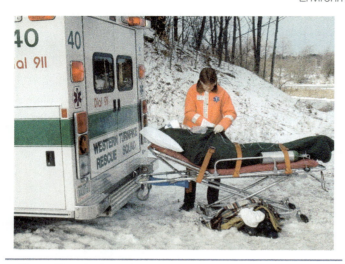

● **Figure 7**   The hypothermia patient should be handled gently because of myocardial irritability.

may cause the blood pressure to fall, especially when there is also volume depletion.

If active rewarming is necessary in the prehospital setting (e.g., when transport is delayed), administration of warmed IV fluids during rewarming can prevent the onset of rewarming shock.

Cold Diuresis   Volume depletion can occur as a result of *cold diuresis.* Core vasoconstriction causes increased blood volume and blood pressure, so the kidneys remove excess fluid to reduce the pressure, thus causing diuresis. A warmed IV volume expander (e.g., normal saline) should be used both to prevent rewarming shock and to replace fluid lost from cold diuresis.[2]

The conscious patient who is able to manage his airway may be given warmed, sweetened fluids. Alcohol and caffeine should be avoided.

Resuscitation

There are certain resuscitation considerations when handling cardiac arrest victims with core temperatures below 86°F (30°C).

Basic Cardiac Life Support   BLS providers should start cardiopulmonary resuscitation (CPR) immediately, although pulse and respirations may need to be checked for longer periods to detect minimal cardiopulmonary efforts. Use normal chest compression and ventilation rates and ventilate with warmed, humidified oxygen. If an AED is available and ventricular fibrillation is detected, a single shock at 360 joules (or the biphasic equivalent) may be given. Further shocks should be avoided until after rewarming to above 86°F. CPR, rewarming, and rapid transport should immediately follow the three defibrillation attempts.

Advanced Cardiac Life Support   Since there is no increased risk of inducing ventricular fibrillation from orotracheal or nasotracheal intubation, ALS providers may intubate the patient and ventilate with warmed, humidified oxygen. Drug

Some Cautions about Rewarming

It is important to remember that rewarming of a hypothermic patient must occur in conjunction with resuscitation. In addition, rewarming is most effective if active internal warming techniques are used (warmed IV fluids; warmed, humidified oxygen). It is virtually impossible to rewarm a hypothermic patient in the prehospital setting using external rewarming techniques alone.

During rewarming, as the patient's external surfaces (skin) begin to warm, blood vessels within the skin and extremities dilate. When this occurs, cool blood from the skin and extremities is shunted toward the core of the body. In addition, metabolic acids, such as lactic acid and pyruvic acid, which may have accumulated in the skin and extremities as a result of poor perfusion, are also shunted to the body's core structures. The influx of cool blood from the extremities can activate temperature sensors in the core and cause the hypothalamus to attempt to warm the body. This can lead to "rewarming shock" and can actually make the patient worse.

So if you do not have the capability of providing active internal rewarming for the severely hypothermic patient, simply try to prevent additional heat loss and transport the patient emergently to a facility where effective rewarming can take place.[3]

metabolism is reduced, however, so administered medications such as epinephrine and amiodarone may accumulate to toxic levels if used repeatedly in the severely hypothermic patient. In addition, administered drugs may remain in the peripheral circulation. When the patient is rewarmed and perfusion resumes, large, toxic boluses of these medications may be delivered to the central circulation and target tissues.

The American Heart Association recommends that, if the patient fails to respond to initial defibrillation attempts or initial drug therapy, subsequent defibrillations or boluses of medication should be avoided until the core temperature is about 86°F (30°C). This is because it is generally impossible to electrically defibrillate a heart that is colder than 86°F. Active core rewarming techniques are the primary modality in hypothermia patients who are either in cardiac arrest or unconscious with a slow heart rate.

Techniques that may be used include the administration of heated, humidified oxygen and warmed intravenous fluids, preferably normal saline, infused centrally at rates of 150 to 200 mL/hour to avoid overhydration. Peritoneal lavage with warmed potassium-free fluid administered 2 L at a time may be used, as may extracorporeal blood warming with partial cardiac bypass. Obviously some of these techniques may only be carried out in a hospital setting.

Transportation

When transporting a hypothermic patient, remember that gentle transportation is necessary because of myocardial irritability and that the patient should be kept level or slightly inclined with head down. Contact the receiving hospital for general rewarming options. When determining your destination, consider the availability of cardiac bypass rewarming.

Frostbite

Frostbite is environmentally induced freezing of body tissues (Figure 8 ●). As the tissues freeze, ice crystals form within and water is drawn out of the cells into the extracellular space. These ice crystals expand, causing the destruction of cells. During this process, intracellular electrolyte concentrations increase, further destroying cells. Damage to blood vessels from ice crystal formation causes loss of vascular integrity, resulting in tissue swelling and loss of distal nutritional flow.

Superficial and Deep Frostbite

Generally, there are two types of frostbite: superficial and deep. **Superficial frostbite** (frostnip) exhibits some freezing of epidermal tissue, resulting in initial redness, followed by blanching. There will also be diminished sensation. **Deep frostbite** affects the epidermal and subcutaneous layers. There is a white appearance and the area feels hard (frozen) to palpation. There is also loss of sensation in deep frostbite.

Frostbite mainly occurs in the extremities and in areas of the head and face exposed to the environment. Subfreezing temperatures are required for frostbite to occur, although they are not necessary to produce hypothermia. Many patients who have frostbite will also have hypothermia.

There can be tremendous variation in how an individual can present with frostbite. For example, some patients feel little pain at onset. Others will report severe pain. A certain degree of compliance may be felt beneath the frozen layer in superficial frostbite, but in deep frostbite, the frozen part will be hard and noncompliant.

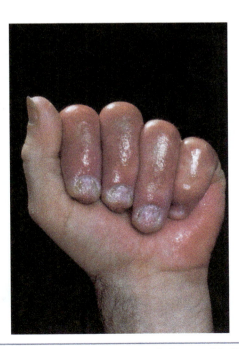

● **Figure 8** Frostbite. *(© SIU BioMed/Custom Medical Stock Photo)*

Treatment

In treating frostbite, take the following recommended steps:

- Do not thaw the affected area if there is any possibility of refreezing.
- Do not massage the frozen area or rub with snow. Rubbing the affected area may cause ice crystals within the tissues to damage the already injured tissues more seriously.
- Administer analgesia prior to thawing.
- Transport to the hospital for rewarming by immersion. If transport will be delayed, thaw the frozen part by immersion in a 102°F–104°F (39°C–40°C) water bath. Water temperature will fall rapidly, requiring additions of warm water throughout the process.
- Cover the thawed part with loosely applied dry, sterile dressings.
- Elevate and immobilize the thawed part.
- Do not puncture or drain blisters.
- Do not rewarm frozen feet if they are required for walking out of a hazardous situation.

Trench Foot

Trench foot (immersion foot) is similar to frostbite, but it occurs at temperatures above freezing. It is rarely seen in the civilian population. It received its name in World War I, when troops confined to trenches with standing, cold water developed progressive symptoms over days. Symptoms are similar to frostbite, but there may be pain. Blisters may form on spontaneous rewarming.

Treatment

Treatment of trench foot requires early recognition of developing symptoms and immediate steps to warm, dry, aerate, and elevate the feet. Measures to prevent trench foot are most effective, such as avoiding prolonged exposure to standing water, changing wet socks frequently, and never sleeping in wet boots or socks.

DROWNING

Drowning is defined as the *process* of experiencing respiratory impairment as the result of submersion or immersion in a liquid. There are three possible outcomes from a drowning incident:

- Mortality (death),
- Morbidity (having medical problems), or
- No morbidity (no problems).

Before 2002, there were many different definitions and terms related to "drowning." These varied definitions created confusion about the best techniques for prevention, rescue, and treatment. When the new definition was adopted in 2005 by the World Health Organization (WHO), American Heart Association (AHA), and other agencies, they recommended abandoning previous definitions and outdated terms. These outdated terms include "near drowning," "dry drowning," and "wet drowning." The next paragraph briefly discusses these terms in their historical context.[4]

"Near-drowning" was loosely used to identify persons who survived the initial drowning incident—yet who later either survived or died. "Dry drowning" and "wet drowning" were used to describe whether or not the patient experienced laryngospasm during the drowning process. We now understand that this phenomenon is not clinically relevant.

It is estimated that annually over 4,500 persons in the United States die from drowning. However, it is difficult to know the actual number of persons who die each year from drowning in the United States, because disaster-related drowning deaths (e.g., from floods or hurricanes) are considered natural-disaster deaths. Similarly, drowning incidents that occur from boats are counted as boating injuries. Additionally, for every drowning death in the United States, two people drown and survive with no morbidity while an additional two people survive with some morbidity (usually severe neurologic impairment).

Altogether, these make drowning the third most frequent cause of accidental death in the United States. Approximately 40 percent of these deaths occur in children under five years of age, making it the leading cause of death in this age group. There is a second peak incidence in teenagers, usually occurring during summer months and in a recreational setting. Finally, a third peak is noted in the elderly as a result of accidental bathtub drownings. Approximately 85 percent of drowning victims are male, two-thirds of whom did not know how to swim. Most commonly, these drownings result from freshwater submersion—especially in swimming pools. Commonly, alcohol use by the victim or momentary lapses in attention by the supervising adult are associated with this type of accident.

It is important to note that other emergency conditions are often associated with drowning. If the cause of the submersion is unknown, consider the possibility of trauma and treat the patient accordingly.

In some instances the submersion occurs in cold water, causing hypothermia. Hypothermia slows the body's metabolic processes, thereby decreasing the need for oxygen. If the water is near freezing, this can have a protective effect on organs and tissues that become hypoxic (low in oxygen). If it is just cold, it can complicate the resuscitation.

Pathophysiology of Drowning

As a paramedic, you need to understand the sequence of events that occur in drowning. Following submersion, if the patient is conscious, there will be an initial struggle, with attempted breath holding. This panicked struggle may include stereotypical loud splashing, such as with a teen caught in a river current, or the silent submersion of a three-year-old whose water-wing floats have slipped off. During this stage the patient makes violent inspiratory and swallowing efforts, often allowing water to enter the mouth, posterior oropharynx, and stomach. If the patient is unconscious when he reaches the water, he will become apneic from an involuntary reflex. During this time, blood is

shunted to the heart and brain because of the mammalian diving reflex, which is described later in this chapter.

Thus, with either mechanism (conscious or unconscious) the patient is apneic and not taking in oxygen. When the patient is apneic, the $PaCO_2$ in the blood rises to greater than 50 mmHg. Meanwhile, the PaO_2 of the blood falls, often below 50 mmHg. The stimulus from the hypoxia ultimately overrides the sedative effects of the hypercarbia, resulting in central nervous system stimulation. This, in turn, triggers the patient to gasp. Water in the hypopharynx, either from water in the mouth during the struggle or from the final gasp before unconsciousness, often causes reflexive laryngospasm and resultant bronchospasm (Figure 9 ●). Because of these mechanisms, usually less than 30 mL of water actually enters the lungs.

The laryngospasm that keeps water out of the lungs further aggravates the hypoxia, ultimately resulting in coma. Persistent anoxia results in a deepening of the coma. Following unresponsiveness, reflex swallowing continues, resulting in gastric distention and increased risk of vomiting and aspiration. If untreated, hypotension, bradycardia, and death result in a short period. The water that enters the lungs—either before laryngospasm or after laryngeal relaxation—can cause respiratory problems through mechanisms that are critical to understanding the appropriate treatment of drowned persons. First, the presence of water blocks gas exchange at the alveolar level. Secondly, even a small amount of fluid washes away the surfactant, causing atelectasis (alveolar collapse).

Surfactant is the substance in alveoli that is responsible for keeping the alveoli open. In drowning, some surfactant is lost when the capillaries of the alveoli are damaged. Plasma proteins then leak back into the alveoli, resulting in the accumulation of fluid in the small airways. This in turn leads to multiple areas of atelectasis—areas of alveolar collapse. Atelectasis causes shunting,

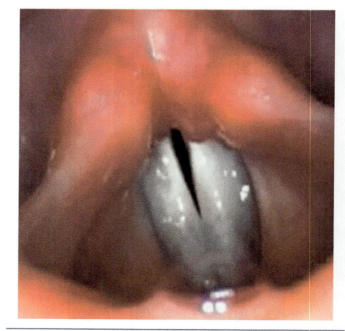

● **Figure 9** Laryngospasm as seen in drowning.
(© *Dr. Bryan E. Bledsoe*)

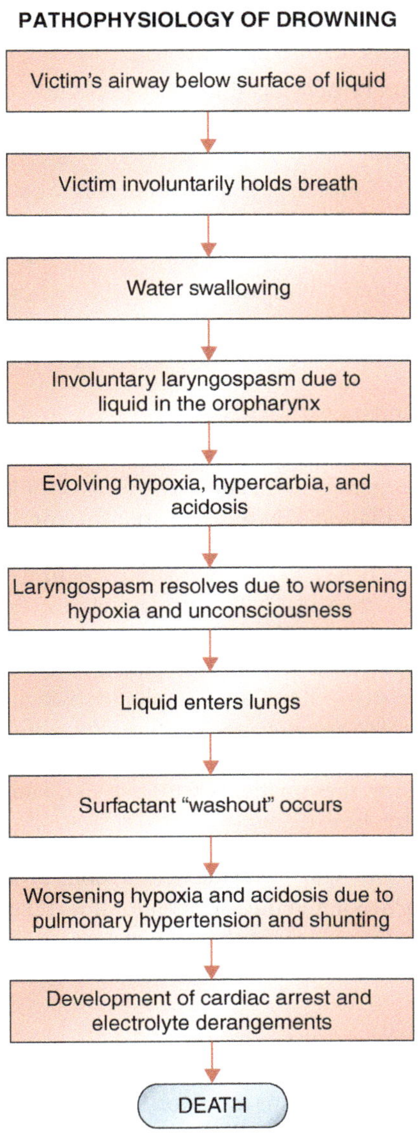

PATHOPHYSIOLOGY OF DROWNING

Victim's airway below surface of liquid

↓

Victim involuntarily holds breath

↓

Water swallowing

↓

Involuntary laryngospasm due to liquid in the oropharynx

↓

Evolving hypoxia, hypercarbia, and acidosis

↓

Laryngospasm resolves due to worsening hypoxia and unconsciousness

↓

Liquid enters lungs

↓

Surfactant "washout" occurs

↓

Worsening hypoxia and acidosis due to pulmonary hypertension and shunting

↓

Development of cardiac arrest and electrolyte derangements

↓

DEATH

● **Figure 10**   The pathophysiology of drowning.

which is the return of deoxygenated blood from the damaged alveoli to the bloodstream. In other words, blood is traveling through the lungs without being oxygenated. The result is hypoxemia (inadequate oxygenation of the blood) (Figure 10 ●).

Drowning morbidity and mortality are primarily due to anoxic brain injury caused by airway obstruction from laryngospasm or aspirated water. If the drowning process is interrupted at any time and does not end in death, the lungs are resilient and generally recover. The patient's outcome is determined by the amount of anoxia that the brain has suffered, and treatment should be directed at reversing anoxia.[5]

Freshwater versus Saltwater Drowning

Based on studies of dogs in the 1960s, it was previously believed that the type of water aspirated would cause different physiologic responses. These studies used massive amounts of water (up to 22 mL/kg), which would be the equivalent of 1,850 mL in a 185-pound adult or 330 mL in a 33-pound child.

But, as previously discussed, the amount of water that actually enters the lungs is a low volume (<30 mL) and does not cause hemodilution, electrolyte shifts, or metabolic abnormalities.[6] The prehospital treatment for all drowning persons is the same, regardless of the type of water.

Factors Affecting Survival

A number of factors have an impact on drowning and drowning survival rates. These include the cleanliness of the water, the length of time submerged, and the age and general health of the patient. Children have a longer survival time and a greater probability of a successful resuscitation. The most important factor affecting survival is immediate initiation of bystander CPR. This is why many organizations emphasize pool owners and other persons around water learn CPR.

There are numerous case reports of adults and children being successfully resuscitated after prolonged (30–60 minutes) periods in cold or near-freezing water. If the patient falls into water that is near freezing (≤10°C/34°F), there may be some protective effect from the mammalian diving reflex. The concept of developing brain death after 4 to 6 minutes without oxygen is not applicable in cases of drowning in near-freezing water. Some patients in cold water (below 68°F) can be resuscitated after 30 minutes or more in cardiac arrest. However, the slower induction of hypothermia generally does not trigger the mammalian diving reflex and leads to a worse outcome. Unfortunately, it is not possible for prehospital providers to predict the outcome, and all persons submerged for less than 60 minutes should be resuscitated. Persons underwater for 60 minutes or longer usually cannot be resuscitated.

A possible contribution to survival in near-freezing water may be the **mammalian diving reflex**. When a person dives into cold water, he reacts to the submersion of the face. Breathing is inhibited, the heart rate becomes bradycardic, and vasoconstriction develops in tissues relatively resistant to hypoxia. Meanwhile, cerebral and cardiac blood flow is maintained. In this way, oxygen is sent and used only where it is immediately needed to sustain life. The colder the water, the more oxygen is diverted to the heart and brain. A common saying in emergency medicine is, "The cold-water drowning patient is not dead until he is warm and dead." In other words, a person who has been submerged in cold water may only seem to be dead, but because of the continued supply of oxygen to the heart and brain that person may indeed still be alive.

Treatment for Drowning

The primary insult of drowning is anoxic brain injury, and treatment should be directed at reversing it. Your approach to a drowning patient should be directed toward reversing his profound hypoxia. Think about your "usual" arrest situation—an adult patient with coronary artery disease who has a sudden myocardial infarction resulting in ventricular fibrillation and unconsciousness. Though this patient has poor health, he still has circulating oxygen and will respond to chest compressions and defibrillation. Now think about a drowning patient—an otherwise healthy child or young adult unable to oxygenate or ventilate. The heart continues circulating blood to the brain until nearly all of the oxygen has been extracted, then cardiac arrest occurs. The person's blood is now depleted of oxygen and full of waste products (carbon dioxide and metabolic acids). Take the following steps to correct the hypoxia:

- Remove the patient from the water as soon as possible. This should be performed **ONLY** by a trained rescue swimmer.

- If possible, initiate ventilation while the patient is still in the water. Rescue personnel should wear protective clothing if water temperature is less than 70°F. In moving or open water, it is essential to use personnel specifically trained for this type of rescue.

- Position the patient. Many drowning resuscitations begin on sloped beaches, riverbanks, or boat ramps. The patient should be placed on a flat surface parallel to the water (perpendicular to the slope), so that blood does not pool at the head or the feet (Figure 11 ●).

- Administer oxygen at a 100 percent concentration.

- Examine the patient for airway patency, breathing, and pulse. If indicated, begin CPR and defibrillation.

- Manage the airway using proper suctioning and airway adjuncts.

- Anticipate vomitus and laryngospasm. Based on your protocols, use suction for vomitus and positive-pressure ventilation, jaw thrust, or RSI (rapid sequence induction) for laryngospasm. Of note: Many drowning patients will have significant foaming from the mouth and nose. Though copious secretions should be cleared, focus on oxygenation and ventilation rather than suctioning foam.

- Routine C-spine immobilization is unnecessary unless you suspect a significant mechanism of injury. Suspect a head and neck injury if the patient experienced a fall or was diving. Rapidly place the patient on a long backboard before removing him from the water and use C-spine precautions throughout care.

- Protect the patient from heat loss. Avoid laying the patient on a cold surface. Remove wet clothing and cover the body to the extent possible.

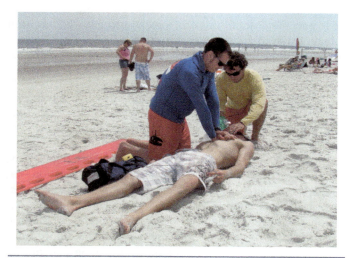

● **Figure 11** Proper positioning of the drowning victim parallel to the water and perpendicular to any detected slope. (© *Lifeguards Without Borders*)

- Use respiratory rewarming, if available, and if transport time is longer than 15 minutes.

- Establish an IV of lactated Ringer's or normal saline for venous access and run at 75 mL/hr. If indicated, carry out defibrillation.

- Follow ACLS protocols if the patient is normothermic. If the patient is hypothermic, treat him according to the hypothermia protocol presented earlier in the chapter.

- Resuscitation is not indicated if immersion has been extremely prolonged (unless hypothermia is present) or if there is evidence of putrefaction (decomposition).

Special Considerations

Compression-Only CPR
As previously discussed, drowning causes a hypoxic arrest, and the priority should be oxygenation and ventilation. There is no role for compression-only CPR in drowning resuscitation.

Airway Management
The drowning process inherently makes airway management difficult for BLS and ALS providers. In addition to vomitus and laryngospasm, atelectasis and bronchospasm decrease pulmonary compliance, which translates to more resistance to air entering the lungs. You should anticipate that you will need increased positive pressure (PEEP or CPAP) while ventilating these patients with a BVM, supraglottic airway, or endotracheal airway.

Heimlich Maneuver
Previous discussions on drowning resuscitation incorporated the use of abdominal thrusts to "clear" water from the airway. This should never be done. Abdominal thrusts delay oxygenation and ventilation while increasing the risk of aspiration.

Adult Respiratory Distress Syndrome

All drowning patients with respiratory symptoms (cough, foam, crackles [rales] and/or rhonchi) should be transported to the hospital for observation, since some complications may not appear for 24 hours.

Adult respiratory distress syndrome (ARDS) is one of the more severe postresuscitation complications, with a high rate of mortality. The physiologic stress of drowning causes the lungs to leak fluid into the alveoli. This fluid is loaded with chemical factors that cause severe inflammation of the tissues and subsequent failure of the respiratory system. In addition, some of these patients have problems with pulmonary parenchymal injury, destruction of surfactant, aspiration pneumonitis, or pneumothorax. A number require an extended hospital stay because of renal failure, hypoxia, hypercarbia, and mixed metabolic and respiratory acidosis. The resultant effects of cerebral hypoxia are often profound and require treatment throughout hospitalization and beyond.

DIVING EMERGENCIES

Scuba diving has become an extremely popular recreational sport. Divers wear portable equipment containing compressed air, which allows the diver to breathe underwater. Although scuba diving accidents are fairly uncommon, inexperienced divers have a higher rate of injury. Scuba diving emergencies can occur on the surface, in 3 feet of water, or at any depth. The more serious emergencies usually occur following a dive. To better assess and care for diving injuries, it is important to understand a few principles of pressure.

The Effects of Air Pressure on Gases

Water is an incompressible liquid. Freshwater has a density, or weight per unit of volume, of 62.4 pounds per cubic foot. Saltwater has a density of 64 pounds per cubic foot. This density can be equated to pressure, which is defined as the weight or force acting on a unit area. Thus, a cubic foot of freshwater exerts a pressure ("weight") of 62.4 pounds over an area of 1 square foot. This measurement is typically stated in pounds per square inch (psi).

Humans at sea level live in an atmosphere of air, which is a mixture of gases. These gases weigh and exert a pressure of 14.7 pounds per square inch (760 mmHg). This pressure, however, may vary within the environment. For example, ascending to an altitude of 1 mile will decrease the atmospheric pressure by 17 percent to approximately 12.2 pounds.

To understand how air pressure affects diving accidents, we look at three physical laws: Boyle's law, Dalton's law, and Henry's law.

Boyle's Law

Boyle's law states that the volume of a gas is inversely proportional to its pressure if the temperature is kept constant. As you increase pressure, the gas is compressed into a smaller space. For example, doubling the pressure of a gas mixture will decrease its volume by one-half. The pressure of air at sea level is 14.7 lb/in^2 or 760 mmHg. This pressure is called 1 "atmosphere absolute" or 1 "ata." Two ata occur at a depth of 33 feet of water, 3 ata occur at a depth of 66 feet of water, and so on. Therefore, 1 L of air at the surface is compressed to 500 mL at 33 feet. At 66 feet, 1 L of air would be compressed to 250 mL.

Dalton's Law

Dalton's law states that the total pressure of a mixture of gases is equal to the sum of the partial pressures of the individual gases. The air we breathe is a mixture of nitrogen (about 78 percent), oxygen (about 21 percent), and carbon dioxide plus traces of argon, helium, and other rare gases (about 1 percent). Since the pressure of air at sea level is 760 mmHg, the pressure of nitrogen is about 593 mmHg, the pressure of oxygen is about 160 mmHg, and the pressure of carbon dioxide is somewhat less than 4 mmHg—each gas exerting its proportion of the total pressure of the mixture.

At different altitudes above sea level or depths below sea level, the pressure of air will change (less at higher altitudes, more at greater depths), but the component gases will still account for the same proportion of whatever the total pressure is at that level: nitrogen 78 percent, oxygen 21 percent, and carbon dioxide less than 1 percent.

Henry's Law

Henry's law states that the amount of gas dissolved in a given volume of fluid is proportional to the pressure of the gas above it. When we descend below sea level, and the pressure bearing down on us increases, the gases that make up the air we breathe tend to dissolve in the liquids (mainly blood plasma) and tissues of the body.

Let us compare what happens to the two chief components of the air we breathe—oxygen and nitrogen—when a person descends to greater and greater depths below sea level. Much of the oxygen is used up in the normal metabolism of the cells, leaving only a small amount to be dissolved in the blood and tissues. Nitrogen, however, is an inert gas and, as such, is not used by the body. Therefore, a far greater quantity of nitrogen is available to dissolve in the blood and tissues as a person descends below sea level. In brief, at depths below sea level, oxygen metabolizes but nitrogen dissolves.

When the person ascends toward sea level again, the gases that are dissolved in the blood and tissues, being under less and less pressure, come out of the blood and tissues and, if the ascent is too rapid, form bubbles. To understand this phenomenon, compare the human body to a bottled carbonated soft drink—that is, a liquid in which carbon dioxide gas is dissolved. The gas is kept dissolved in the liquid by the cap on the bottle and a high-pressure gas under the cap, on top of the liquid. When the cap is removed and the pressure is released, the gas bubbles out of the liquid, causing a fizz that will sometimes rise completely out of the bottle.

In the following sections, we will discuss how the phenomena of gases and pressure can cause serious problems for divers.

Pathophysiology of Diving Emergencies

As noted, gases are dissolved in the diver's blood and tissues under pressure. As the diver goes deeper into the water, pressure increases, causing more gas to dissolve in the blood (Henry's law). According to Boyle's law, these gases will have a smaller volume because of the increased ambient pressure. During *controlled* ascent, with decreasing pressure, dissolved gases come out of the blood and tissues slowly, escaping gradually through respiration.

If ascent is *too rapid,* however, the dissolved gases, mostly nitrogen, come out of solution and expand quickly, forming bubbles in the blood, brain, spinal cord, skin, inner ear, muscles, and joints. Once bubbles of nitrogen have formed in various tissues, it is difficult for the body to remove them. The ascending diver who comes to the surface too rapidly, not adhering to safety measures, is at risk of becoming a veritable living bottle of soda.

Classification of Diving Injuries

Scuba diving injuries are the result of barotrauma, pulmonary overpressure, arterial gas embolism, decompression sickness, cold, panic, or a combination of these. Accidents generally occur at one of the following four stages of a dive:

- On the surface
- During descent
- On the bottom
- During ascent

Injuries on the Surface

Surface injuries can involve any of several factors. One such factor can be entanglement of lines or entanglement in kelp fields while swimming to the area of the dive. Divers in these situations may panic, become fatigued, and even drown. Another factor may be cold water that produces shivering and blackout. Boats in the area are another potential source of injury to the diver. To prevent such accidents, divers will usually mark the area of their dive with a flag. Maritime rules require boat operators to stay clear of a flagged area.

Injuries during Descent

Barotrauma means injuries caused by changes in pressure. Barotrauma during descent is commonly called "the squeeze." It can occur if the diver cannot equilibrate the pressure between the nasopharynx and the middle ear through the eustachian tube. The diver can experience middle ear pain, ringing in the ears, dizziness, and hearing loss. In severe cases, rupture of the eardrum can occur. A diver who has an upper respiratory infection, and who therefore cannot clear the middle ear through the eustachian tube, should not dive. A similar lack of equilibration can occur in the sinuses, producing severe frontal headaches or pain beneath the eye in the maxillary sinuses.

Injuries on the Bottom

Major diving emergencies while at the bottom of the dive often involve nitrogen narcosis (a state of stupor), commonly called "raptures of the deep." This is due to the effect on cerebral function of nitrogen or any gas in high concentration (similar to the altered mental status that high carbon dioxide causes in asthmatics). The diver may appear to be intoxicated and may take unnecessary risks. Other emergencies occur when a diver runs low on or out of air. The diver who panics will use more energy and exacerbate this situation by consuming even more oxygen and producing even more carbon dioxide.

Injuries during Ascent

Serious and life-threatening emergencies, many involving barotrauma, can occur during the ascent. For example, as during descent, an ascending diver may be unable to equilibrate inner ear and nasopharyngeal pressure.

Dives below 33 feet may require staged ascent to prevent decompression sickness, also called the bends or dysbarism. This condition develops in divers subjected to rapid reduction of air pressure while ascending to the surface following exposure to compressed air, with formation of expanding nitrogen bubbles causing severe pain, especially in the abdomen and the joints.

The most serious barotrauma that occurs during ascent is injury to the lung from pulmonary overpressure. This can occur with a deep dive, or it can occur with a dive of as little as 3 feet below the surface. The injury results from the diver holding his breath during the ascent. As the diver ascends, the air in the lung, which has been compressed, expands. If it is not exhaled, the alveoli may rupture. If this occurs, the result will be structural damage to the lung and, possibly, arterial gas embolism (AGE), an air bubble or air embolism that enters the circulatory system from the damaged lung. Another result may be pneumomediastinum, the release of gas (air) through the visceral pleura into the mediastinum and pericardial sac around the heart as well as into the tissues of the neck. Pneumothorax is possible if the alveoli rupture into the pleural cavity. Air embolism can occur if the air ruptures into the pulmonary veins or arteries and returns to the left atrium and finally into the left ventricle and out into the systemic circulation.

General Assessment of Diving Emergencies

In the early assessment of diving accidents, all symptoms of air embolism and decompression sickness are considered together. Early assessment and treatment of a diving injury is of more importance than trying to distinguish the exact problem. One of your most important tasks in a diving-related injury is elicitation of a diving history or profile.[7] The essential factors to consider are as follows:

- Time at which the signs and symptoms occurred
- Type of breathing apparatus utilized
- Type of hypothermia protective garment worn
- Parameters of the dive:
  - Depth of dive(s)
  - Number of dives
  - Duration of dive(s)
- Aircraft travel following a dive (in a pressurized cabin)
- Rate of ascent
- Associated panic forcing rapid ascent
- Experience of the diver, for example, student, inexperienced, or "pro"
- Properly functioning depth gauge
- Previous medical diseases
- Old injuries
- Previous episodes of decompression sickness
- Use of medications
- Use of alcohol

From a quick assessment of the patient's diving profile, you can rapidly determine if the diver is a likely candidate for a pressure disorder.

Pressure Disorders

Injuries caused by pressure, as noted earlier, are known as *barotrauma*. In the case of diving accidents, most barotrauma results from a pressure imbalance between the external environment and gases within the body. The following sections describe some of the most common forms of barotrauma involved in diving accidents.

Decompression Sickness (Dysbarism)

Decompression sickness develops in divers subjected to rapid reduction of air pressure after ascending to the surface following exposure to compressed air. A number of general and individual factors can contribute to the development of decompression sickness, or the bends (Table 3). Decompression sickness results as nitrogen bubbles come out of solution in the blood and tissues, causing increased pressure in various body structures and occluding circulation in the small blood vessels. This occurs in joints, tendons, the spinal cord, skin, brain, and inner ear. Symptoms develop when a diver rapidly ascends after being exposed to a depth of 33 feet or more for a time sufficient to allow the body's tissues to be saturated with nitrogen.

Signs and Symptoms

Decompression sickness is commonly classified as Type I or Type II. The signs and symptoms of the two classes of decompression sickness are detailed in Table 4. The principal signs and symptoms of decompression sicknesses are joint and abdominal pain, fatigue, paresthesias, and CNS disturbances. A rash is sometimes seen (Figure 12 ●). The most common symptom is joint pain and the most concerning is ataxia or any other CNS disturbance. The nitrogen bubbles produced by rapid decompression are thought to produce obstruction of blood flow, which leads to local ischemia, subjecting tissues to anoxic stress. In some cases, this stress may lead to tissue damage.

Treatment   Initial treatment includes oxygen. Patients with decompression sickness usually seek medical treatment within 12 hours of ascent from a dive. Some patients may not seek treatment for as long as 24 hours after the last dive. It is generally safe to assume that signs or symptoms developing more than 36 hours after a dive cannot reasonably be attributed to decompression sickness.

CONTENT REVIEW

▶ Pressure Disorders

- Hypothermia
- Pulmonary Overpressure
- Arterial Gas Embolism
- Pneumomediastinum
- Nitrogen Narcosis

TABLE 3 | Factors Related to the Development of Decompression Sickness

General Factors	Individual Factors
Cold-water dives	Age—older individuals
Diving in rough water	Obesity
Strenuous diving conditions	Fatigue—lack of sleep prior to dive
History of previous decompression dive incident	Alcohol—consumption before or after dive
Overstaying time at given dive depth	History of medical problems
Dive at 80 ft or greater	
Rapid ascent—panic, inexperience, unfamiliarity with equipment	
Heavy exercise before or after dive to the point of muscle soreness	
Flying after diving (24-hour wait is recommended)	
Driving to high altitude after dive	

TABLE 4 | Signs and Symptoms of Decompression Sickness

Type	Signs and Symptoms
I	<ul><li>Musculoskeletal symptoms:</li><li>Joint pain ("bends")</li><li>Myalgias</li></ul><ul><li>Dermatologic symptoms:</li><li>Rash (*cutis marmorata*)</li></ul><ul><li>Lymphatic symptoms:</li><li>Swollen or painful lymph nodes</li></ul>
II	<ul><li>Neurologic symptoms:</li><li>Numbness</li><li>Paresthesias</li><li>Mental status change</li></ul><ul><li>Inner ear symptoms ("staggers"):</li><li>Tinnitus (ears ringing)</li><li>Hearing loss</li><li>Vertigo</li><li>Dizziness</li><li>Ataxia</li><li>Nausea/vomiting</li></ul><ul><li>Cardiopulmonary symptoms ("chokes"):</li><li>Chest pain (worse with inspiration)</li><li>Cough</li><li>Tachypnea</li><li>Pulmonary congestion</li><li>Circulatory collapse</li></ul>

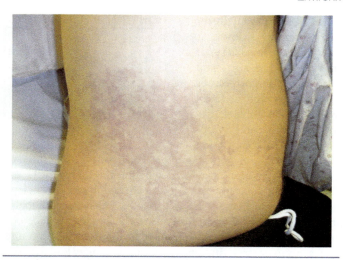

● **Figure 12**   Rash sometimes seen with decompression sickness (dysbarism). *(© Dr. Bryan E. Bledsoe)*

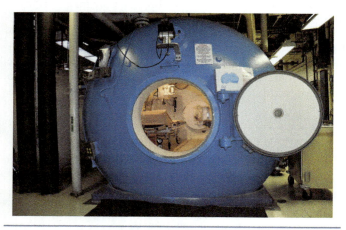

● **Figure 13**   Hyperbaric oxygen chamber used in the treatment of decompression illness. *(© Edward T. Dickinson, MD)*

Decompression sickness may require urgent definitive care through recompression. This can be accomplished by placing the patient in a hyperbaric oxygen chamber (Figure 13 ●). There the patient is subjected to oxygen under greater-than-atmospheric pressure to force the nitrogen in the body to re-dissolve, then gradually decompressed to allow the nitrogen to escape without forming bubbles. However, prompt stabilization at the nearest emergency department should be accomplished before transportation to a recompression chamber.[8]

Early oxygen therapy may reduce symptoms of decompression sickness substantially. Divers who are administered high-concentration oxygen have a considerably better treatment outcome. Many diving emergencies occur a significant distance from definitive care. Prehospital providers should administer high-concentration oxygen until their supplies are exhausted. Do not attempt to "ration" oxygen by maintaining a lower flow rate. The following list outlines some of the steps in the prehospital management of decompression sicknesses:

● Primary assessment.

● Check for, and treat, pneumothorax.

● Administer CPR, if required.

● Administer oxygen at 100 percent concentration with a nonrebreather mask (consider CPAP if no pneumothorax). An unconscious diver should be intubated.

● Consider contacting DAN (Divers Alert Network).

● Keep the patient in the supine position.

● Protect the patient from excessive heat, cold, wetness, or noxious fumes.

● Give the conscious, alert patient nonalcoholic liquids such as fruit juices or sports drinks.

● Evaluate and stabilize the patient at the nearest emergency department prior to transport to a recompression chamber. Begin IV fluid replacement with electrolyte solutions for unconscious or seriously injured patients. You may use lactated Ringer's or normal saline. Do not use 5 percent dextrose in water.

● If there is evidence of CNS involvement, consider dexamethasone, heparin, or diazepam if ordered by medical direction.

● If air evacuation is used, do not expose the patient to decreased barometric pressure. Cabin pressure must be maintained at sea level, or fly at the lowest possible safe altitude.

Send the patient's diving equipment with the patient for examination. If that is impossible, arrange for local examination and gas analysis.

Pulmonary Overpressure Accidents

Lung overinflation caused by rapid ascent is the common cause of a number of emergencies, particularly at shallow depths of less than 6 feet. Air can become trapped in the lungs by mucous plugs, bronchospasm, or simple breath holding. With rapid ascent, ambient pressure drops quickly, causing the trapped air to expand. Air expansion can rupture the alveolar membranes. This can result in hemorrhage, reduced oxygen and carbon dioxide transport, and capillary and alveolar inflammation. Air can also escape from the lung into other nearby tissues and cause pneumothorax and tension pneumothorax, subcutaneous emphysema, or pneumomediastinum.

Signs and Symptoms   Divers with this type of condition will complain of substernal chest pain. Respiratory distress and diminished breath sounds are common findings on examination.

Treatment   Treatment for this condition is the same as for pneumothorax caused by any other mechanism.

Arterial Gas Embolism

As described, a pressure buildup in the lung can damage and rupture alveoli. This can allow air in the form of a large bubble to escape into the circulation. This air embolism, or arterial gas embolism (AGE), can travel to the left atrium and ventricle of the heart and out into various parts of the body where it may lodge and obstruct blood flow, causing ischemia and possibly infarct. Such obstruction of blood flow can have devastating effects triggered by cardiac, pulmonary, and cerebral compromise.

Signs and Symptoms   Signs and symptoms of air embolism include onset within 2 to 10 minutes of ascent; a rapid and dramatic onset of sharp, tearing pain; and other symptoms related to the organ system affected by blocked blood flow. The most common presentation mimics a stroke with confusion, vertigo, visual disturbances, and loss of consciousness. Although rare, you may also encounter paralysis on one side of the body (hemiplegia), as well as cardiac and pulmonary collapse. If any person using scuba equipment presents with neurologic deficits during or immediately after ascent, an air embolism should be suspected. Prompt medical treatment is crucial because death or serious disability can result.

Treatment   Management of air embolism includes the following steps:

- Primary assessment.
- Check for, and treat, pneumothorax.
- Administer oxygen by nonrebreather mask at 100 percent (consider CPAP, if no pneumothorax).
- Consider contacting DAN (Divers Alert Network).
- Place the patient in a supine position.
- Monitor vital signs frequently.
- Place saline lock.
- Administer a corticosteroid agent, if ordered by medical direction.
- Transport to a recompression chamber as rapidly as possible. If air transport is utilized, it is very important to use a pressurized aircraft or to fly at a low altitude.

Pneumomediastinum

As noted earlier, a pneumomediastinum is the release of gas (air) through the visceral pleura into the mediastinum and pericardial sac around the heart. It can result from a pulmonary overpressure accident during rapid ascent from a dive.

Signs and Symptoms   Signs and symptoms of a pneumomediastinum include substernal chest pain, irregular pulse, abnormal heart sounds, reduced blood pressure and narrow pulse pressure, and a change in voice. There may or may not be evidence of cyanosis.

Treatment   The field management of pneumomediastinum includes:

- Administer high-concentration oxygen via nonrebreather mask.
- Check for, and treat, pneumothorax.
- Consider contacting DAN (Divers Alert Network).
- Start an IV lactated Ringer's or normal saline per medical direction.
- Transport to the emergency department.

Treatment generally ranges from observation to recompression for relief of acute symptoms. The patient should be observed for 24 hours for any other signs of lung overpressure. He should not be recompressed unless air embolism or decompression sickness is also present.

Nitrogen Narcosis

Nitrogen narcosis develops during deep dives and contributes to major diving emergencies while the diver is at the bottom. With an elevated partial pressure, more nitrogen dissolves in the bloodstream. With higher concentrations of nitrogen in the body, including the brain, the result is intoxication and altered levels of consciousness similar to the effects of alcohol or narcotic use. Between 70 and 100 feet these effects become apparent in most divers, but at 200 feet most divers become so impaired that they cannot do any useful work. At 300 to 350 feet unconsciousness occurs. The main concern with nitrogen narcosis is the same as with any person who is intoxicated while in a situation requiring alertness and common sense. Impaired judgment during a deep dive can cause accidents and unnecessary risk taking.

Signs and Symptoms   Signs and symptoms include altered levels of consciousness and impaired judgment.

Treatment   Treatment simply requires a return to a shallow depth since this condition is self-resolving on ascent. To avoid this problem altogether in deep dives, oxygen mixed with helium is used, since helium does not have the anesthetic effect of nitrogen.

Other Diving-Related Illnesses

There are less frequent problems that can occur as a result of scuba diving. For example, oxygen toxicity caused by prolonged exposure to high partial pressures of oxygen can cause lung damage or even convulsions. Hyperventilation caused by excitement or panic may lead to a decreased level of consciousness or muscle cramps and spasm. This will impair the diver's ability to function properly, possibly leading to injury. Inadequate breathing or faulty equipment may lead to increased CO_2 levels, or *hypercapnia*. This also may cause unconsciousness. Finally, poorly prepared air tanks may be contaminated with other gases, which can increase the risk of hypoxia, narcosis, and accidental injury.

Hyperbaric Chambers

Though many diving emergencies are treated in a hyperbaric chamber, many of these patients first require emergent stabilization at the closest appropriate emergency department. Recompression often does not take place immediately on arrival to the emergency department and the patient can usually be stabilized, then transferred to a hyperbaric center. Understand your local transport protocols with regard to special transport considerations in diving-related emergencies.

Divers Alert Network

Clearly, scuba diving has a unique set of potential problems. With the popularity of this activity rising so dramatically, it is important for EMS personnel in popular diving areas to become familiar with recognition and treatment of these problems. If assistance is needed, the Divers Alert Network (DAN) operates a nonprofit consultation and referral service in affiliation with Duke University Medical Center. For all emergency and non-emergency consultations, contact (919) 684-9111. DAN has a worldwide presence and can be consulted for any and all diving emergencies. Think of them as the Poison Control Center for dive emergencies. Consultations are free, and they always have a physician trained in dive medicine available 24 hours a day. You can call them collect or from anywhere in the world, and it is better to involve them sooner rather than later.

HIGH ALTITUDE ILLNESS

In contrast to illnesses related to diving and high atmospheric pressure, high altitude illnesses are caused by a decrease in ambient pressure. Essentially, high altitude is a low-oxygen environment. As noted in the discussion of Dalton's law, oxygen concentration in the atmosphere remains constant at 21 percent. Therefore, as you go higher and barometric pressure decreases, the partial pressure of oxygen also decreases (is 21 percent of a lower total pressure). Oxygen becomes less available, triggering a number of related illnesses as well as aggravating preexisting conditions such as angina, congestive heart failure, chronic obstructive pulmonary disease, and hypertension.

Even in healthy individuals, ascent to high altitude, especially if it is very rapid, can cause illness. It is difficult to predict who will be affected and to what degree. The only predictor is the hypoxic ventilatory response.

Every year millions of visitors to mountains expose themselves to altitudes greater than 2,400 m (8,000 ft), the altitude at which high altitude illnesses start to become manifest. For reference purposes, Denver, Colorado, is at 1,610 m where there is 17 percent less oxygen than at sea level. Aspen at 2,438 m has 26 percent less oxygen, and at the top of Mount Everest (8,848 m or 29,028 ft) there is 66 percent less oxygen than at sea level. At *high altitude* (4,900 to 11,500 ft) the hypoxic environment causes decreased exercise performance, although without major disruption of normal oxygen transport in the body. However, if ascent is very rapid, altitude illness will commonly occur at 8,000 ft and beyond. *Very high altitude* (11,500 to 18,000 ft) will result in extreme hypoxia during exercise or sleep. It is important to ascend to these altitudes slowly allowing for acclimatization to the environment. *Extreme altitude* beyond 18,000 ft will cause severe illness in almost everyone.

Some of the signs and symptoms of altitude illness are malaise, anorexia, headache, sleep disturbances, and respiratory distress that increases with exertion.

Prevention

Acclimatization, exertion, sleep, diet, and medication are key considerations in preventing or limiting high altitude medical emergencies.[9] A description of each follows.

Gradual Ascent

To avoid developing high altitude medical problems, it is important to allow a period of acclimatization. Slow, gradual ascent

over days to weeks gives the body a chance to adjust to the hypoxic state caused by high altitudes. A person who would normally become short of breath, dizzy, and confused by a rapid drop in oxygen can function quite well if the oxygen level is decreased to the same level gradually over a long period of time. Acclimatization occurs through several mechanisms. They are:

- *Ventilatory changes.* The *hypoxic ventilatory response (HVR)* is triggered by decreased oxygen. When oxygen is decreased, ventilation increases. This hyperventilation causes a decrease in CO_2, but the kidneys compensate by eliminating more bicarbonate from the body. In essence, the body resets its normal ventilation and operating level of CO_2. The process takes four to seven days at a given altitude.

- *Cardiovascular changes.* The heart rate increases at high altitude, allowing more oxygen to be delivered to the tissues. In addition, peripheral veins constrict, increasing the central blood volume. In response, the central receptors, which sense blood volume, induce a diuresis, which causes concentration of the blood. Unfortunately, pulmonary circulation also constricts in a hypoxic environment. This causes or exacerbates preexisting hypertension and predisposes to developing high altitude pulmonary edema.

- *Blood changes.* Within 2 hours of ascent to high altitude, the body begins making more red blood cells to carry oxygen. Over time, this mechanism will significantly compensate for the hypoxic environment. It is this mechanism that fostered the idea of "blood-doping" during athletic competition, especially at high altitudes. Athletes donate their own blood long in advance of a competition at high altitude. This allows them time to rebuild their red blood cells. Just before the competition they receive a transfusion of their own blood to increase their oxygen-carrying capacity. Most athletic governing bodies frown on this practice.

Limited Exertion

Clearly, one of the easiest ways to avoid some effects of high altitude is to limit the amount of exertion. By limiting the body's need for oxygen, the effects of oxygen deprivation will be minimized.

Sleeping Altitude

Sleep is often disrupted by high altitude. Hypoxia causes abnormal breathing patterns and frequent awakenings in the middle of the night. Descending to a lower altitude for sleep improves rest and allows the body to recover from hypoxia. This practice will, however, interfere with the process of acclimatization.

High Carbohydrate Diet

Carbohydrates are converted by the body into glucose and rapidly released into the bloodstream, providing quick energy. The theory that this is helpful in acclimatizing to high altitude is controversial.

Medications

Two medications will limit or prevent the development of medical conditions related to high altitude. They are:

Acetazolamide. Acetazolamide (Diamox) acts as a diuretic. It forces bicarbonate out of the body, which greatly enhances the process of acclimatization as discussed earlier. The hypoxic ventilatory response reaches a new set point more quickly. This improves ventilation and oxygen transport with less alkalosis. In addition, the periodic breathing that occurs at high altitude is resolved, thereby preventing sudden drops in oxygen.

Nifedipine. Nifedipine (Procardia, Adalat) is a medication used to treat high blood pressure. It causes blood vessels to dilate, preventing the increase in pulmonary pressure that often causes pulmonary edema.

Other treatments are currently under evaluation. Phenytoin (Dilantin), for example, is being studied because of its membrane stabilization effects. Steroids are commonly used but their efficacy is still controversial.

Types of High Altitude Illness

A variety of symptoms occur when the average person ascends rapidly to high altitude. These may range from fatigue and decreased exercise tolerance to headache, sleep disturbance, and respiratory distress. The following section will deal with some of the specific syndromes that will occur (Table 5).

Acute Mountain Sickness

Acute mountain sickness (AMS) usually manifests in an unacclimatized person who ascends rapidly to an altitude of 2,000 m (6,600 ft) or greater.

Signs and Symptoms The mild form of acute mountain sickness presents with the following symptoms:

- Light-headedness
- Breathlessness
- Weakness
- Headache
- Nausea and vomiting

CONTENT REVIEW
► Types of High Altitude Illness
- Acute Mountain Sickness
- High Altitude Pulmonary Edema
- High Altitude Cerebral Edema

TABLE 5 | Definitions of Altitude Illness (Lake Louise Consensus)

Disease	Criteria
Acute Mountain Sickness (AMS)	In the setting of a recent increase in altitude, the presence of a headache and at least one of the following symptoms: • Gastrointestinal problems (anorexia, nausea, or vomiting). • Fatigue or weakness. • Dizziness or light-headedness. • Difficulty sleeping.
High Altitude Cerebral Edema (HACE)	*Can be considered "end-stage" or severe AMS.* In the setting of a recent increase in altitude, either: • The presence of a change in mental status and/or ataxia in a person with AMS. *OR* • The presence of both mental status changes *and* ataxia in a person without AMS.
High Altitude Pulmonary edema (HAPE)	In the setting of a recent increase in altitude, the presence of the following: **Symptoms** (at least 2 of): • Dyspnea at rest. • Cough. • Weakness or decreased exercise performance. • Chest tightness or congestion. **Signs** (at least 2 of): • Crackles or wheezing in at least one lung field. • Central cyanosis. • Tachypnea. • Tachycardia.

These symptoms can develop from 6 to 24 hours after ascent. More severe cases can develop especially if the person continues to ascend to higher altitudes. These symptoms include:

- Weakness (requiring assistance to eat and dress)
- Severe vomiting
- Decreased urine output
- Shortness of breath
- Altered level of consciousness

Mild AMS is self-limiting and will often improve within one to two days if no further ascent occurs.

Treatment   Treatment of AMS consists of halting ascent, possibly lowering altitude, using acetazolamide (Diamox) and antinauseants such as ondansetron (Zofran) as necessary. It is not usually necessary to descend to sea level. Supplemental oxygen will relieve symptoms but is usually used only in severe cases. In severe cases oxygen, if available, will help. In addition, immediate descent is the definitive treatment. For very severe cases, hyperbaric oxygen may be necessary.

High Altitude Pulmonary Edema

High altitude pulmonary edema (HAPE) develops as a result of increased pulmonary pressure and hypertension caused by changes in blood flow at high altitude. Children are most susceptible, and men are more susceptible than women.

Signs and Symptoms   Initially, symptoms include dry cough, mild shortness of breath on exertion, and slight crackles in the lungs. As the condition progresses, so will the symptoms. Dyspnea can become quite severe and cause cyanosis. Coughing may be productive of frothy sputum, and weakness may progress to coma and death.

Treatment   In the early stages, HAPE is completely and easily reversible with descent and the administration of oxygen. It is

therefore critical to recognize the illness early and initiate appropriate treatment. If immediate descent is not possible, supplemental oxygen can completely reverse HAPE but requires 36 to 72 hours. Such a supply of oxygen is rarely available to mountain climbers. In this situation the portable hyperbaric bag can be very useful. This is a sealed bag that can be inflated to 2 psi, which simulates a descent of approximately 5,000 feet. Acetazolamide can be used to decrease symptoms. Medications such as morphine, nifedipine (Procardia), and furosemide (Lasix) have been used with some success, but they carry complications such as hypotension and dehydration and should be used with caution.

High Altitude Cerebral Edema

The exact cause of high altitude cerebral edema (HACE) is not known. It usually manifests as progressive neurologic deterioration in a patient with AMS or HAPE. The increased fluid in the brain tissue causes a rise in intracranial pressure.

Signs and Symptoms   The symptoms of high altitude cerebral edema include:

- Altered mental status
- Ataxia (poor coordination)
- Decreased level of consciousness
- Coma

Headache, nausea, and vomiting are less common. Occasionally actual focal neurologic changes may occur.

Treatment   As in all altitude illnesses, definitive treatment is descent to lower altitude. Oxygen and steroids may also help to improve recovery. The phosphodiesterase inhibitor sildenafil (Viagra) has shown some benefit in selected patients. In most cases the use of oxygen with steroids (dexamethasone) and a hyperbaric bag may be sufficient, although often unavailable. If coma develops, it may persist for days after descent to sea level but usually resolves, although sometimes leaving residual disability.

CHAPTER REVIEW

SUMMARY

Our environment provides us with all that we need to survive and prosper. The extremes of our environment, however, can have significant impact on human metabolism. Our bodies will, of course, compensate for these extremes, but sometimes it is not enough. Sometimes the heat gain or loss is too much. Sometimes the pressure change is too much. As a result, medical illnesses and emergencies arise. These can range from abnormal core body temperatures to decompensation, shock, and even death.

Basic knowledge of common environmental, recreational, and exposure emergencies is necessary in order for you to administer prompt and proper treatment in the prehospital setting. It is not easy to remember this type of information since these problems are not usually encountered on a daily basis. Remember the general principles involved. Remove the environmental influence causing the problem. Support the patient's own attempt to compensate. Finally, select a definitive care location and transport the patient as rapidly as possible.

In every case, remember that you must maintain your own safety. There are too many cases in which paramedics have lost their lives as a result of attempting a rescue for which they were not properly trained. Rapid action is always necessary when performing an environmental rescue; however, common sense must prevail.

YOU MAKE THE CALL

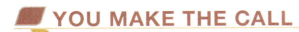

You and your partner, Christina, are paramedics stationed at Mike Leigh General Hospital in Lake Dulce, Colorado. You have enjoyed working at this beautiful mountain ski resort (elevation 8,815 ft) for the past year. This morning you are expecting a busy day since this is the first day of Spring Break and hundreds of visitors have been arriving daily for their weeklong romp in the snow.

Shortly after 10 A.M. a call comes in from the first-alert ski patrol. A skier on Mount Guilio is in unspecified distress. You and Christina hasten to your snowmobiles and proceed immediately to the slope. On arrival you find a 25-year-old man crouched in the snow, surrounded by curious onlookers. The ski patrol informs you that he is a scuba diving expert, Biff Western. Biff arrived yesterday with his wife Muffy to try skiing for the first time. Biff did not sleep well last night despite taking one sleeping pill he had brought with him. This morning he felt very tired, a condition that was aggravated by a dry cough he seemed to have developed. Now on his second run down the slope, the exertion has exhausted him. The ski patrol thinks he is becoming confused and disoriented. He is short of breath, weak, dizzy, and his cough has become productive of white frothy sputum.

On examination you find that Biff is breathing very rapidly. His heart is racing and his lips are tinged blue. Listening to the chest you note coarse diffuse crackles on inspiration. You and Christina share a momentary knowing glance then spring into action.

1. What illness are you probably dealing with?

2. What predisposing factors lead to this illness?

3. What is the definitive treatment for this condition?

4. If definitive treatment is not possible, what other measures can be used?

See Suggested Responses at the back of this chapter.

REVIEW QUESTIONS

1. The type of thermogenesis that results from exercise is _____.
a. metabolic
c. work induced
b. diet induced
d. thermoregulatory

2. Through the mechanism called evaporation, water evaporates from the skin and lungs at approximately _____ mL/day.
a. 200
c. 600
b. 400
d. 800

3. It is important in any heat-related or cold-related emergency to obtain a core temperature reading such as from the _____.
a. ear
c. rectum
b. mouth
d. axillae

4. Factors that may contribute to a susceptibility to hyperthermia include _____.
a. medications
b. age of the patient
c. health of the patient
d. all of the above

5. Treatment of the patient with heat cramps includes all of the following except _____.
a. administer salt tablets
b. administer an oral saline solution
c. place the patient in a cool environment
d. if the patient is unable to take fluids orally, consider an IV of normal saline

6. When the core temperature of the body drops below _____ an individual is considered to be hypothermic.
a. 95°F
c. 97°F
b. 96°F
d. 98°F

7. _____ is the most common presenting arrhythmia seen in hypothermia.
a. Atrial flutter
b. Sinus bradycardia
c. Atrial fibrillation
d. Ventricular fibrillation

8. The third most common cause of accidental death in the United States is _____.
a. stroke
c. drowning
b. trauma
d. heart disease

9. The return of unoxygenated blood from the damaged alveoli to the bloodstream is called _____.
a. shunting
c. atelectasis
b. pneumonitis
d. hemodilution

10. All symptomatic drowning patients should be transported to the hospital for observation since complications may not appear for _____ hours.
a. 10
c. 20
b. 16
d. 24

11. _____ law states that the volume of a gas is inversely proportional to its pressure if the temperature is kept constant.
   a. Henry's
   b. Boyle's
   c. Dalton's
   d. Starling's

12. _____ is the condition that develops in divers subjected to rapid reduction of air pressure while ascending to the surface following exposure to compressed air, with formation of nitrogen bubbles causing severe pain, especially in the abdomen and the joints.
   a. Nitrogen narcosis
   b. Arterial gas embolism
   c. Decompression sickness
   d. Pulmonary overpressure

13. _____ develops as a result of increased pulmonary pressure and hypertension caused by changes in blood flow at high altitude.
   a. AMS
   b. HACE
   c. HAPE
   d. AGE

14. If any person using scuba equipment presents with neurologic deficits during or immediately after ascent, _____ should be suspected.
   a. nitrogen narcosis
   b. air embolism
   c. decompression sickness
   d. pulmonary overpressure

See Answers to Review Questions at the back of this chapter.

REFERENCES

1. Becker, J. A. and L. K. Stewart. "Heat-Related Illness." *Am Fam Physician* 83 (2011): 1325–1330.

2. Polderman, K. H. "Mechanisms of Action, Physiological Effects, and Complications of Hypothermia." *Crit Care Med* 37 (7Suppl) (2009): S186–S202.

3. Imray, C., A. Grieve, and S. Dhillon. "Cold Damage to the Extremities: Frostbite and Non-Freezing Injuries." *Postgrad Med J* 85 (2009): 481–488.

4. Idris, A. H., R. Berg, J. Bierens, L. Bossaert, C. Branche, A. Gabrielli, S. A. Graves, J. Handley, R. Hoelle, P. Morley, et al. "Recommended Guidelines for Uniform Reporting of Data from Drowning: The "Utstein Style."" *Circulation* 108 (2003): 2565–2574.

5. Layon, A. J. and J. H. Modell. "Drowning: Update 2009." *Anesthesiology* 110 (2009): 1390–1401.

6. Modell, J. H., M. Gaub, F. Moya, B. Vestal, and H. Swarz. "Physiologic Effects of Near-Drowning with Chlorinated Freshwater, Distilled Water, and Isotonic Saline." *Anesthesiology* 27 (1966): 33–41.

7. Salahuddin, M., L. A. James, and E. Bass. "SCUBA Medicine: A First Responder's Guide to Diving Injuries." *Curr Sports Med Rep* 10 (2011): 134–139.

8. Vann, R. D., F. K. Butler, F. J. Mitchell, and R. E. Moon. "Decompression Illness." *Lancet* 377 (2011): 153–164.

9. Luks, A. M., S. E. McIntosh, C. K. Grissom, et al. "Wilderness Medical Society Consensus Guidelines for the Prevention and Treatment of Acute Altitude Illness." *Wilderness Environ Med* 21 (2010): 146–155.

FURTHER READING

Auerbach, P. S., ed. *Wilderness Medicine*. 6th ed. St. Louis: Mosby Year Book, 2011.

Bierens, J. L., ed. *Handbook on Drowning*. 2nd ed. New York: Springer, 2012.

Bledsoe, B. E. and D. E. Clayden. *Prehospital Emergency Pharmacology*. 7th ed. Upper Saddle River, NJ: Pearson/Prentice Hall, 2012.

Guyton, A. C., and J. E. Hall. *Textbook of Medical Physiology*. 12th ed. Philadelphia: Saunders, 2010.

Sutton, J. R., G. Coates, and C. S. Houston, eds. "The Lake Louise Consensus on the Definition and Quantification of Altitude Illness." *Hypoxia and Mountain Medicine*. Burlington, VT: Queen City Printers, 1992.

Tintinalli, J. E., et al., eds. "Environmental Injuries," in *Emergency Medicine: A Comprehensive Study Guide*. 7th ed. New York: McGraw-Hill, 2011.

SUGGESTED RESPONSES TO "YOU MAKE THE CALL"

The following are suggested responses to the "You Make the Call" scenarios presented in this chapter. Each represents an acceptable response to the scenario but should not be interpreted as the only correct response.

1. *What illness are you probably dealing with?*
   High altitude pulmonary edema (HAPE).

2. *What predisposing factors lead to this illness?*
   The victim, being a SCUBA instructor, had recently flown to a dramatically different, higher altitude.

3. *What is the definitive treatment for this condition?*
   Oxygen administration and descent to lower altitudes.

4. *If definitive treatment is not possible, what other measures can be used?*
   Oxygenation over 36 to 72 hours or a hyperbaric treatment with a portable hyberbaric bag that can simulate a descent of approximately 5,000 feet can be used. Additionally, acetazolamide can be used to decrease symptoms. Morphine, nifedipine, and furosemide are sometimes used but carry complications such as hypotension and dehydration, so they should be used with caution.

ANSWERS TO REVIEW QUESTIONS

1. c
2. c
3. c
4. d
5. a
6. a
7. c
8. c
9. a
10. d
11. b
12. c
13. c
14. b

GLOSSARY

absolute zero   the temperature at which all molecular motion stops (−273°C or −459°F).

acclimatization   the reversible changes in body structure and function by which the body becomes adjusted to a change in environment.

arterial gas embolism (AGE)   an air bubble, or air embolism, that enters the circulatory system from a damaged lung.

autonomic neuropathy   condition that damages the autonomic nervous system, which usually senses changes in core temperature and controls vasodilation and perspiration to dissipate heat.

barotrauma   injuries caused by changes in pressure. Barotrauma that occurs from increasing pressure during a diving descent is commonly called "the squeeze."

basal metabolic rate (BMR)   rate at which the body consumes energy just to maintain stability; the basic metabolic rate (measured by the rate of oxygen consumption) of an awake, relaxed person 12 to 14 hours after eating and at a comfortable temperature.

conduction   moving electrons, ions, heat, or sound waves through a conductor or conducting medium.

convection   transfer of heat via currents in liquids or gases.

core temperature   the body temperature of the deep tissues, which usually does not vary more than a degree or so from its normal 37°C (98.6°F).

decompression sickness   development of nitrogen bubbles within the tissues due to a rapid reduction of air pressure when a diver returns to the surface; also called "the bends" or dysbarism.

deep frostbite   freezing involving epidermal and subcutaneous tissues resulting in a white appearance, hard (frozen) feeling on palpation, and loss of sensation.

drowning   the process of experiencing respiratory impairment as the result of submersion or immersion in liquid.

environmental emergency   a medical condition caused or exacerbated by the weather, terrain, atmospheric pressure, or other local factors.

evaporation   change from liquid to a gaseous state.

exertional metabolic rate   rate at which the body consumes energy during activity. It is faster than the basal metabolic rate.

frostbite   environmentally induced freezing of body tissues causing destruction of cells.

heat cramps   acute painful spasms of the voluntary muscles following strenuous activity in a hot environment without adequate fluid or salt intake.

heat exhaustion   a mild heat illness; an acute reaction to heat exposure.

heat-related illness   increased core body temperature due to inadequate thermolysis.

heatstroke   acute, dangerous reaction to heat exposure, characterized by a body temperature usually above 105°F (40.6°C) and central nervous system disturbances. The body usually ceases to perspire.

homeostasis   the natural tendency of the body to maintain a stable, steady, and normal internal environment.

hyperbaric oxygen chamber   recompression chamber used to treat patients suffering from barotrauma.

hyperthermia   unusually high core body temperature.

hypothalamus   portion of the diencephalon producing neurosecretions important in the control of certain metabolic activities, including body temperature regulation.

hypothermia   state of low body temperature, particularly low core body temperature.

J waves   ECG deflections found at the junction of QRS complexes and the ST segments. They are associated with hypothermia and seen at core temperatures below 32°C, most commonly in leads II and V_6; also called Osborn waves.

mammalian diving reflex   a complex cardiovascular reflex, resulting from submersion of the face and nose in water, that constricts blood flow everywhere except to the brain.

negative feedback   homeostatic mechanism in which a change in a variable ultimately inhibits the process that led to the shift.

nitrogen narcosis   a state of stupor that develops during deep dives due to nitrogen's effect on cerebral function; also called "raptures of the deep."

pneumomediastinum   the presence of air in the mediastinum.

pneumothorax   a collection of air in the pleural space. Air may enter the pleural space through an injury to the chest wall or through an injury to the lungs. In a tension pneumothorax, pressure builds because there is no way for the air to escape, causing lung collapse.

pulmonary overpressure   expansion of air held in the lungs during ascent. If not exhaled, the expanded air may cause injury to the lungs and surrounding structures.

pyrexia   fever, or above-normal body temperature.

pyrogens   any substances causing a fever, such as viruses and bacteria or substances produced within the body in response to infection or inflammation.

radiation   transfer of energy through space or matter.

recompression   resubmission of a person to a greater pressure so that gradual decompression can be achieved; often used in the treatment of diving emergencies.

respiration   the exchange of gases between a living organism and its environment.

scuba   acronym for self-contained underwater breathing apparatus. Portable apparatus that contains compressed air that allows the diver to breathe underwater.

superficial frostbite   freezing involving only epidermal tissues resulting in redness followed by blanching and diminished sensation; also called frostnip.

surfactant   a compound secreted by cells in the lungs that regulates the surface tension of the fluid that lines the alveoli, which is important in keeping the alveoli open for gas exchange.

thermal gradient   the difference in temperature between the environment and the body.

thermogenesis   the production of heat, especially within the body.

thermolysis   the loss of heat, especially from the body.

thermoregulation   the maintenance or regulation of a particular temperature of the body.

trench foot   a painful foot disorder resembling frostbite and resulting from exposure to cold and wet, which can eventually result in tissue sloughing or gangrene; also called immersion foot.

references followed by "f" indicate illustrated
s or photographs; followed by "t" indicates a

egree log roll, 289

gree log roll, 289

s, 8, 147, 173, 371
men
rteries of, 135
etailed physical exam, 29-31
jury management, 25
ediatric patients, 39
hysical examination, 31, 252
apid trauma assessment, 18, 25, 29-31, 43,
        107-108, 141, 147, 174, 212-213,
        239-240, 278, 280, 363
oft-tissue injury, 39, 107, 128, 150, 212
ominal aorta, 150, 202, 204, 208, 223, 340
ominal cavity, 101, 114, 197, 199-200, 202-203,
        205-209, 212-213, 216, 219, 224, 339-340,
        372
ominal evisceration, 207, 216, 372
ominal injuries, 23, 197-199, 210-211
ominal pain
rehospital care, 213-214
ominal quadrants, 340
ominal thrusts, 398
ominal trauma, 197-219, 374
ucens nerve, 58, 258
uction, 62, 75, 156, 160, 166, 187, 193, 258
asion, 2, 29, 92, 123, 126, 129, 142, 151, 153
asions, 2, 39, 107, 124, 128-129, 132, 151, 212,
        272, 294, 364
uptio placentae, 42-43, 197, 210, 214, 219
se
alcohol, 125
child, 38, 189, 313
drug, 125, 189
geriatric, 38, 313, 384
physical, 313, 384
celeration, 39, 55, 63, 65, 332-333, 349, 351-353,
        360, 363, 372, 376
cident scene, 10
cidental Death and Disability: The Neglected
        Disease of Modern Society, 4
climatization, 380, 384, 387, 404-405, 409
etabulum, 156, 162-163, 183, 186, 193
hilles tendon, 164, 167
idosis, 37, 66, 99, 103, 129, 137, 148, 226, 231,
        373, 387, 397-398
tions, 6, 17, 19, 22, 37, 48, 50, 93, 102-103, 112,
        114, 119-120, 126, 182, 293
tive rewarming, 392, 394
cute mountain sickness (AMS), 405
dalat, 405
duction, 75, 156, 160, 166, 193
denosine, 99
dolescents, 39
drenal cortex, 102, 118
drenal gland, 381
drenal glands, 150, 202
drenal medulla, 71, 101, 119-120
drenaline, 37
dult respiratory distress syndrome (ARDS), 99, 398
dvanced airway
    BURP maneuver, 283
    Combitube, 283
    endotracheal intubation, 73, 112, 243, 277,
            282-283
    LMA, 283

orotracheal intubation, 277, 283
AED, 394
Aerobic metabolism, 57, 88, 99, 118, 120
Affinity, 309
Afterload, 88, 90, 100-101, 118, 120
Aggregate, 88, 93-94, 118
Air bags, 5-6, 18, 23, 53, 199, 253, 349, 356-357,
        359-361, 374
Air splint, 136, 178, 180, 184-188
Air splints, 180, 187
Airway
    anatomy, 17, 39, 54, 149, 223, 253, 255-256, 258,
            299, 301, 326, 358, 363
    BVM, 246, 398
    complications, 43, 78, 149, 243, 299, 321, 371, 398
    nasal cannula, 292-293
    no suspected spinal injury, 285
    nonrebreather mask, 73, 78, 88, 292, 300, 393
    physiology, 17, 39, 42, 54, 223, 253, 255, 258, 299,
            301, 309, 326
    suctioning, 145, 149, 277, 282, 285, 398
    supplemental oxygen, 27, 35, 42-43, 78, 116, 239,
            243-244, 278, 292, 300
    suspected spinal injury, 285-286
    thermal burn, 309, 318, 321
    trauma assessment, 10, 14, 17-18, 25, 28, 30-32,
            35, 37, 43, 48, 76, 78, 106-107, 109, 123,
            141, 147, 177, 212, 239-240, 274,
            278-281, 300, 315, 321, 349, 363
    ventilating the patient, 35, 73, 106
Airway management
    breathing, 282, 321, 398
    opening, 282
    shock, 49, 79, 83, 321
    ventilation, 17, 83, 246, 282, 398
Airway obstruction, 27, 37, 39, 67, 79, 106, 147, 149,
        284, 309, 397
Airway techniques, 283
Alarm, 75
Alcohol use, 281, 363, 396
Alkalosis, 375, 405
Allergic reaction
    treatment, 189
Allergy, 389
Alpha particles, 306
Alpha radiation, 300, 306-307, 325, 327
ALS, 18-19, 376, 394, 398
Alveolar collapse, 229, 396
Alveolar/capillary membrane, 234
Alveoli, 92, 99, 224-225, 230, 244, 247, 284, 309, 337,
        339, 352, 358, 371, 396-398, 400, 402, 407,
        410
Ambulance
    parking, 3
Ambulances, 8, 24
American Heart Association (AHA), 395
Amiodarone, 245, 394
Amniotic fluid, 42, 209-210
Amniotic sac, 203, 210
Ampere, 300, 327
Amphiarthroses, 156, 159, 193
Ampule, 320
Amputation, 123, 131, 134, 148, 153
Amputations, 95, 123-124, 128-129, 131-132, 143,
        146, 188
AMS, 405-406, 408
Anaerobic, 88, 95, 99, 103, 117-118, 120, 134-135,
        137, 148, 151, 153, 373
Anaerobic metabolism, 88, 99, 103, 118, 137, 373
Analgesia, 317, 319, 395
Analgesics, 31, 80, 144, 188, 243
Anaphylactic shock, 88, 105, 118
Anastomosis, 100
Anatomy
    bone, 39, 60, 155, 158-159, 192, 203, 255-257,
            259, 353, 374
    cardiovascular, 39, 50, 87, 221, 248

ear, 255-256
eye, 251, 255, 257-258, 302, 310, 357
heart, 38-39, 149, 223, 302, 363, 374
infants and children, 38-39, 357
kidneys, 374
lower airway, 256, 258
upper airway, 149
Anemia, 42, 88, 97, 99, 118, 134, 204, 216
Ankle injury, 187
Ankles
    bandaging, 179
Anoxia, 305, 396-397
Antagonist, 80, 189
Anterior, 2, 29, 53, 55, 58-60, 62, 68-69, 84, 86,
        107-108, 128, 135-136, 145, 162-163, 165,
        175, 177, 183-187, 199-200, 203, 205-208,
        210, 212, 223-226, 229, 234-236, 239, 244,
        246, 254-260, 262-266, 270-273, 279,
        283-284, 287-288, 294, 296, 310-312, 315,
        331, 349, 353, 366
Anterior hip dislocation, 186
Antibodies, 135, 151
Antibody, 133, 154
Antidepressants, 389
Antihistamines, 384, 389
Anxiety, 28, 35, 37, 45, 65, 73-75, 79-81, 97-98, 104,
        106, 108-109, 188-189, 212, 214, 245, 275,
        281, 286, 292-293, 304, 324, 331, 371,
        386-387
Aortic dissection, 221, 237, 243, 245, 247
Aortic rupture, 223, 228, 237, 247
Apnea, 68, 85, 319, 390
Apneustic center, 82, 225
Appendicular skeleton, 156, 161, 193
Aqueous humor, 252, 257, 296
Arachnoid membrane, 53, 55, 60, 84, 86
Arm, 2, 18, 62, 68, 70-71, 123-124, 127, 129, 135,
        137, 144-145, 161, 167-170, 179, 181, 185,
        187, 258, 289, 304, 312, 325, 327, 358, 367,
        376
Arrhythmia, 144, 249, 390, 392, 407
Arrhythmias, 43-44, 108, 137, 143, 148-149, 234-235,
        239, 246, 309, 312-313, 321, 373, 375, 388,
        390-392
Arterial bleeding, 93, 95, 132, 141, 278
Arterial gas embolism (AGE), 380, 400, 402, 409
Arterial hemorrhage, 24, 92-93, 95, 105, 110, 173
Arterial system, 99, 104, 204
Arteries
    abdominal, 204, 207-208, 210, 224-225, 236-237,
            247, 249, 340, 372
Arterioles, 69, 90-91, 93, 99-100, 103-105, 107, 116,
        118-120, 126, 129, 132
Articulates, 162-163, 195, 256, 262, 264, 295
Artificial ventilation, 44, 106
Ascending reticular activating system, 53, 56, 58, 67,
        84
Ascites, 67
Aspiration, 31, 73, 96, 107, 112, 138, 145, 149, 209,
        216, 244, 270, 277, 282, 285, 293, 396, 398
Aspirin, 31, 78, 94, 98, 109, 135, 141, 144, 157, 389
Assault, 42, 97, 206, 208, 231, 264, 332, 335-336
Assault rifle, 336
Assessment
    abruptio placentae, 42-43, 197, 210
    angina, 82
    asthma, 240
    blast injuries, 180, 350, 367, 371, 373, 375
    blunt trauma, 1, 3, 23, 28, 38, 42-43, 107, 210-213,
            239, 241, 247, 267-268, 275, 285, 332,
            348-350, 354, 362-364, 367, 371, 373,
            375
    cardiac arrest, 10, 28, 42-43, 106, 112, 309, 313,
            321, 375
    cardiogenic shock, 88, 105, 108, 116, 241
    circulation, 10, 25, 27-29, 35, 42-43, 47-48, 74, 88,
            95, 105-107, 109, 112, 141-143, 147,

151, 167-168, 175-177, 182, 190, 212,
216, 239, 246, 267-268, 275, 278,
285-286, 292, 314, 318, 363, 371, 373,
375, 400, 402
congestive heart failure, 240
diving emergencies, 379, 400, 402-403
emphysema, 29-30, 44, 107, 142, 213, 240-242,
246, 279, 341, 402
focused, 9-10, 14, 20, 25, 28-32, 35, 37, 43, 72,
107-109, 123-124, 140-142, 157,
173-174, 176, 210, 274, 278, 281, 288,
313, 315, 317
headaches, 78, 400
heart failure, 240-241
hemorrhage, 3-4, 10, 14, 17, 19, 24, 26-31, 35, 37,
39, 42-44, 47, 53, 74, 87-89, 95-96,
105-109, 112, 116, 122, 129, 141-143,
150-151, 167, 173-174, 176-177, 180,
182, 190, 210-213, 216, 239-240, 246,
253, 268, 278, 280-281, 285, 293, 331,
338, 342, 350, 371, 373, 402
increased intracranial pressure, 39
injuries, 1-4, 6, 8-11, 13-14, 20, 22-25, 27-32, 34,
36-37, 39, 42, 44-45, 48, 52, 72-75, 78,
95-96, 106-109, 112, 122-124, 129,
140-143, 147, 150-151, 155-158,
167-168, 173-177, 180, 182, 190,
197-198, 210-213, 221, 239, 241, 246,
251, 253, 267-268, 274-276, 278-279,
281, 285, 287-288, 293, 299, 301,
308-309, 313-314, 317, 320-321,
324-325, 331-332, 338, 341-342, 345,
348-350, 354, 362-364, 367, 371, 373,
375, 379, 400
mental status, 13, 25-26, 76, 106, 108-109, 112,
143, 173, 239, 276, 375, 400
myocardial infarction, 105, 241, 371
penetrating trauma, 1, 3, 23, 32, 38, 54, 72, 95,
107, 141, 143, 150, 167, 198, 211-213,
217, 239-241, 245, 247, 251, 267, 301,
330-332, 338, 341-342, 345, 350, 371
penetrating wound, 241-242, 276, 342
pulmonary embolism, 106
pupils, 54, 74, 108, 124
radiation burns, 324
syncope, 109, 309
tension pneumothorax, 27, 29-30, 36-37, 39, 44,
107, 112, 150, 216, 221-222, 239,
241-242, 245-247, 342, 402
thoracic trauma, 221-222, 239-242, 245-247
toxic inhalation, 308, 314-315
trauma patient, 4, 6, 8, 10-11, 13-14, 17, 20, 26, 28,
31-32, 35, 37, 42, 44-45, 47, 105-106,
109, 116, 147, 173, 177, 210, 213, 242,
276, 278, 286, 313, 317, 350, 364
upper respiratory infection, 400
Asystole, 28, 321, 390-392
Atelectasis, 222, 225, 229-232, 234, 243, 249, 396,
398, 407
Atria, 101, 119-120
Atrial fibrillation, 391-392, 407
Atrial flutter, 235, 407
Atropine
spinal injury, 80
Attempted suicide, 31, 265
Auscultation
physical exam, 28-30
Autonomic nervous system, 37, 63, 71, 100-101, 166,
384, 409
Autoregulation, 53, 57, 66, 85
AV junction, 67
AVPU, 26
Avulsion, 123, 130-131, 134, 153, 183, 268, 272, 292
Avulsions, 124, 128-130, 151, 292
Axial loading, 26, 72, 265-267, 275, 287, 294-295,
349, 358, 367, 376
Axial skeleton
structures, 193

B

Back injuries, 125
Bag of waters, 210
Ballistics, 330, 333, 343-345
Bandages
applying, 111, 144-146, 148
roller, 139, 144-145
triangular, 139-140
Bandaging
objectives, 122, 143, 177

Barbiturates, 389
Barotrauma, 380-381, 400-401, 409-410
Basal metabolic rate (BMR), 380, 383, 409
Base, 26, 57-60, 64, 162, 203, 225, 254-255, 260,
268, 270, 285, 290-291, 296, 334, 383, 392
Baseline vital signs, 28, 108, 141-142, 213, 281, 315
Basilar skull, 30, 65, 268-271, 279, 282, 294, 296-297
Battery, 9, 362
Battle's sign, 30, 269, 279, 294, 297
Beck's triad, 236, 242
Benadryl, 189
Beta particles, 306
Beta radiation, 300, 306-307, 325, 327
Biaxial joints, 160, 191
Bicarbonate, 118, 148, 246, 321, 373, 404-405
Bicycle helmet, 2
Bilateral, 18, 30, 54, 74-75, 174-175, 187, 190, 222,
227, 252, 269, 279-280, 284, 296, 358, 364
Bilateral periorbital ecchymosis, 30, 252, 269, 279,
296
Bipolar traction splint, 181
Bladder, 31, 69-71, 83, 85, 150, 166, 183, 199-200,
202-203, 205, 207-209, 211, 213, 217, 252,
288, 338-339, 352, 356, 374
Blanching, 395, 410
Blast wind, 349, 368-370, 376
Bleeding
arterial, 29, 64, 85, 87, 92-93, 95, 106, 109-110,
116-117, 131-132, 141, 143, 168, 176,
274, 278
blood loss, 28, 42-43, 64, 92-95, 97-98, 106-112,
117-118, 124, 131-132, 135, 141, 143,
150, 152, 190, 207, 210, 214, 216, 233,
278-279, 285
capillary, 28-29, 35, 64, 79, 85, 87, 92-93, 95, 108,
112, 118-119, 124, 131-132, 135, 141,
144, 146, 168, 176, 190, 214, 233, 350
controlling, 94, 111, 141, 143-145, 285
direct pressure, 35, 95, 107, 110-111, 118-119, 124,
137-138, 143, 145-147, 149, 214, 278,
284-285
elevation, 79, 110, 144
evaluating, 78, 106, 143, 176, 191
external, 4, 35, 79, 87, 92, 94-95, 98, 106-108, 112,
117, 119, 141, 147, 176, 214, 271, 278,
285, 350, 373
internal, 4, 28, 87, 93-95, 98, 106-109, 112,
116-117, 119-120, 124, 129, 137, 141,
146, 149-150, 168, 176, 190, 207, 214,
216, 233, 271, 340, 373, 375
pressure points, 110, 145
venous, 29, 43, 64, 87, 92-93, 95, 97, 107, 109,
111, 117, 119, 131-132, 141, 143-144,
146, 152, 168, 222, 233, 274, 278, 285
Blisters, 309-310, 316, 395
Blood
clot formation, 94, 113, 135, 138-139
fluid replacement, 387
plasma, 29, 35-36, 42, 92, 97, 99-100, 102, 105,
117, 120, 154, 304, 311, 396, 399
red blood cells, 19, 42, 47, 90, 92, 94, 99-100,
102-103, 110, 113, 119-120, 158, 172,
217, 222, 292, 404
Blood clotting, 37, 113, 120
Blood glucose, 52, 75, 80, 200
Blood loss, 5-6, 9, 28, 31, 36, 39, 41-43, 47, 64-65, 68,
74, 76, 89, 92-98, 102-114, 117-118, 124,
128, 130-132, 135, 141, 143, 150, 152, 157,
174, 182-184, 190, 192, 207-210, 213-214,
216-217, 226, 233-234, 239, 243, 268-269,
278-280, 285, 313, 343, 356, 376
Blood pressure
diastolic, 76, 85, 91, 97, 100, 103, 105, 109, 120,
214
measuring, 388
shock and, 48, 74, 81, 89, 97, 113, 120, 237, 394
systolic, 32, 34, 36, 40, 47-48, 66-67, 74, 76,
78-80, 85, 89, 91, 95, 98, 100, 102-103,
109-111, 113, 120, 144, 183, 214, 224,
236-237, 243-245, 250, 280, 294
Blood tubing, 35, 113, 331
Blood vessels
great vessels, 223, 226, 258, 339, 352
of the neck, 58, 107, 258, 265, 273
Blood volume, 36, 39, 42-43, 57, 63, 66, 83, 90-92, 95,
97-100, 102-104, 109, 113, 116, 118-119,
202, 209-210, 212-213, 216, 233, 273, 282,
385, 394, 404
Bloodborne pathogens, 173, 195

Blood-brain barrier, 53, 55, 57, 63, 68-69, 85
BLS, 18, 349, 394, 398
BLS ambulance, 18
Blunt abdominal trauma, 210, 213
Blunt force trauma, 282
Blunt trauma
automobile crashes, 237
chest wall injuries, 228
crush injuries, 3, 128, 226, 348, 354, 366, 368-
371, 373, 375
falls, 3, 38, 42, 187, 237, 241, 264-265, 267, 2?,
332, 354, 366-367, 373-374
kinetics of, 332, 348, 350, 352, 360
motorcycle crashes, 264, 364-365
sports injuries, 3, 354, 372-374
BMR, 380, 383, 409
Body, 3-4, 9-10, 15-16, 23-26, 28-31, 35-40, 43-44
50, 54, 56-60, 62-63, 66-71, 73-77, 79-80,
82-86, 87, 89-109, 112-114, 116, 118-120,
124-127, 129-130, 132-148, 150-151,
153-154, 157-163, 166-168, 177, 181-183,
185-187, 191, 193-194, 198-200, 202, 20?,
208, 211, 213-215, 217, 223-226, 229,
233-234, 247-248, 250, 253, 255-256,
258-267, 269-270, 272, 274-277, 280,
285-289, 291, 293, 295-297, 299-306, 30?,
310-321, 323-325, 327-328, 330, 333-34?,
348, 350-358, 360, 363-369, 371, 373-37?,
379, 381-390, 392-396, 398-399, 401-407,
409-410
Body armor, 234, 335, 339
Body cavities, 96, 146, 198, 374
Body collision, 354-355
Body fluids, 23-24, 95, 105, 120, 140, 146, 302, 31?
Body surface area, 38, 138, 215, 299-300, 304,
310-311, 313, 315, 318, 324-325, 327-328
Body surface area (BSA), 300, 310, 315, 327
Body temperature, 36-37, 50, 56, 67-68, 70, 76, 85,
94, 114, 118, 126-127, 158, 167, 302, 318,
323, 379, 381, 383-390, 409-410
Bolus, 19, 40, 80, 100, 113, 189, 214, 222, 244, 256,
319, 326, 350
Bone, 29-30, 37, 39, 48, 55, 60, 68-69, 72, 96,
130-131, 137, 153, 155-156, 158-163,
166-167, 169-172, 174-178, 180-182,
184-189, 191-195, 202-203, 207-208,
229-230, 247, 254-257, 259-261, 266-269,
271, 279, 284, 294, 296-297, 303, 305-306,
308, 338-339, 341, 343-344, 352-353, 356,
367, 374-375
Bone aging, 163
Bone marrow, 156, 159, 195, 306, 308
Bone structure, 158, 163, 171, 191
Bones, 39, 44, 55, 64, 72, 124, 129-130, 133, 135,
142-143, 154, 156-163, 166, 169, 171-172,
177-178, 182, 184, 187-188, 190-191,
193-194, 228, 254-257, 259, 263-264, 268,
271, 279, 285, 297, 302, 310, 339, 353, 36?,
372-373
Bounding pulse, 74, 76
Bowel obstruction, 206
Boyle's law, 399
BP cuff, 19
Bradycardia, 71, 73-74, 82, 85, 116, 241, 390, 392,
396, 407
Brain
damage, 63-69, 74, 79, 81, 85, 97, 111, 253-254,
256, 264-265, 267-269, 271, 273, 277,
282, 338-340, 342, 352, 369, 371-372,
383, 387, 401, 403
Brain death, 57, 397
Brain injury, 26, 32, 52, 54, 57, 63-64, 66-68, 72-74,
76, 78-79, 81, 83, 85, 110, 113, 268,
276-278, 281-282, 285, 292, 369, 397
Brainstem, 53, 55-58, 63-68, 76, 82, 85-86, 280
Branch, 57, 59, 61, 226, 234-235, 264, 350, 376
Breath sounds, 18-19, 27, 29, 40, 44, 48, 54, 89, 107,
198, 222, 228, 230-235, 240-242, 244, 247,
249, 277, 283-284, 301, 319, 331, 342, 349,
371, 402
Breathing
adequate, 35, 43, 48, 73, 81, 99, 109, 112, 116,
123, 147, 149-150, 239, 243-244, 278,
284-285, 300, 315, 410
expiration, 112, 240, 284, 294
inadequate, 35, 50, 112, 120, 397, 403, 410
inspiration, 107, 112, 228, 240, 270, 273, 285, 309,
407
rescue, 147, 300, 363, 398

piratory cycle, 112
ning patterns, 73, 404
ning rate, 19, 112
hi, 149, 223-226, 238, 249-250, 258
hioles, 166, 224, 358
300, 310-311, 315, 317-319, 325-328
e fractures, 171
y taping, 188
dressings, 146, 293, 318, 343
njuries
ie, 301, 313, 317
rcumferential burns, 313
s
dy surface area, 138, 299-300, 304, 310-311,
 313, 315, 318, 324-325, 327-328
emical, 299, 301-303, 305-306, 308-309, 314,
 317, 319-325
assification of, 310
epth of, 309, 318, 324, 341
ectrical, 105, 299, 301-305, 312-314, 317,
 320-321, 323-324, 326, 328, 371
ndotracheal intubation and, 319
ll-thickness, 370
ghtning, 321
adiation, 299-300, 302-303, 306, 308, 310, 320,
 322-325, 327-328, 371
everity, 3, 5, 39, 300, 304-305, 308-311, 314,
 316-317, 319, 324-325, 327, 341
everity of, 3, 309, 311, 314
uperficial, 29, 300, 309-310, 316-317, 319-320,
 325, 328, 368, 370
ystemic complications, 105, 299, 311
hermal, 299-305, 308-314, 316, 318-322, 326, 328
sae, 161, 172
ock, 31, 207

caneus, 156, 163, 193, 367
cium, 148, 158, 171-172, 191, 194, 258, 279, 322
ber, 23, 211, 222-223, 239, 274, 330-333,
 339-342, 344-345
ncer
prevention, 3, 14
nnulation, 36, 318, 325
pillaries, 57, 67, 85, 90-93, 96-97, 99-100, 103,
 120, 126-127, 129, 132-133, 136, 153-154,
 176, 238, 304, 309, 328, 371, 396
pillary bleeding, 64, 87
pillary hemorrhage, 92
pillary refill, 2, 18, 27-29, 31, 35, 38, 47-48, 53, 79,
 103, 108, 124, 141-142, 144, 146, 157,
 168-169, 174-176, 179, 185, 187, 190, 212,
 214, 253, 300, 350
pillary washout, 88, 103, 119
pnography, 27, 54, 66, 73-74, 78-79, 106-107, 109,
 112, 149, 239, 242-243, 277-278, 282-285,
 293, 315, 342, 350
psules, 302
arbon dioxide, 27, 42, 52, 55, 66, 73-74, 78, 92,
 98-99, 101, 103, 112, 119, 126, 158, 167,
 223, 230-231, 258, 278, 284-285, 398-400,
 402
arbon dioxide concentrations, 66
arbon monoxide, 8, 14, 20, 99, 299, 308-309,
 314-315, 319-320, 326
arbon monoxide poisoning
 assessment and management, 314
 burns and, 319
arboxyhemoglobin, 309, 315
ardiac conduction system, 90
ardiac contusion, 234, 241
ardiac cycle, 236
ardiac monitoring, 235, 324-325, 392
ardiac muscle, 101, 118, 137, 166, 234
ardiac output, 39, 42-43, 57, 63, 71, 90, 100-105,
 119, 200, 204, 219, 225, 232, 234-236, 245,
 250, 385, 389, 391
ardiac physiology, 118
ardiac resuscitation, 383
ardiac tamponade, 223, 235
ardiogenic shock, 88, 105, 108, 114, 116, 119, 234,
 241
ardiovascular injuries, 221, 234
ardiovascular system
 arterial system, 99, 104
 blood, 35, 43, 50, 66, 76, 80, 90, 98-105, 243
 blood flow, 36, 76, 90, 92, 100-103
 cardiac conduction system, 90
 perfusion, 50, 66, 76, 80, 98, 101-104

venous system, 44, 90, 100, 102, 104
Carina, 224, 238, 258
Carotid artery, 255-256, 258
Carotid pulse, 27, 112, 222
Carpal bones, 156, 160, 162, 194
Carpals, 159, 161
Cartilage, 38-39, 72, 133, 156-161, 163, 167, 169,
 171-173, 187, 191, 194, 223-224, 226,
 255-258, 271, 277, 279, 282-284
Cataracts, 308
Catecholamines, 98, 103, 116, 304
Cell, 2, 5-6, 42, 55, 59, 65-66, 90, 92, 99-100, 103,
 119-120, 126-127, 133-134, 137, 154,
 167-168, 183, 194, 200, 301-306, 308, 315,
 325, 337-338, 353, 383, 387
Cellular environment
 hydration, 98
Cellular ischemia, 102
Celsius, 382
Centers for Disease Control and Prevention (CDC), 32
Central nervous system, 52, 54-57, 59, 66, 68, 72, 74,
 76, 78-79, 81, 83, 85-86, 98, 105, 119-120,
 126, 161, 167, 253, 264, 274-275, 278, 280,
 292-294, 387, 396, 410
Cerebellum, 53-56, 63, 66, 82, 85-86
Cerebral contusion, 64
Cerebral perfusion pressure (CPP), 53, 57, 85
Cerebrospinal fluid, 30, 53, 55, 57, 60-61, 64-66, 68,
 83, 85, 97, 111, 145, 269, 271, 278, 295-296
Cerebrospinal fluid (CSF), 53, 85
Cerebrum, 53, 55-56, 58, 63-64, 66-67, 78, 80, 82,
 85-86
Cervical collar, 2, 18, 27, 54, 82, 106-107, 276-277,
 285, 287-288, 290, 349
Cervical collars, 295
Cervical immobilization, 46, 157, 252, 274-275, 277,
 286-291, 295, 300, 349, 373
Cervical immobilization device (CID), 291, 373
Cervical region, 60, 71, 260, 262, 266-267, 273
Cervical spine, 4, 14, 27, 44, 48, 54, 69, 71-72, 78, 83,
 85, 99, 260-262, 266-267, 273-274, 277-278,
 280, 282, 286-288, 290-291, 295, 344, 358,
 360, 367, 373, 376
Cervical vertebra, 59, 62, 71-72, 160, 253, 260-261,
 360
Cervical vertebrae, 62, 252, 259-261, 296
Charring, 310
CHART, 311-312, 390
Chemical burns
 dry lime, 322
 eyes and, 308
Chemical name, 321
Chemical reactions, 94, 119, 381
Chemoreceptors, 58, 101-103, 116
Chest cavity, 43, 231, 371
Chest pain
 care for, 108, 331
Chest wall
 musculature of, 228
Chest wall contusion, 228-229, 247
Chest wall injuries, 221, 228-229
Cheyne-Stokes respirations, 53, 68, 85
Chief complaint, 10, 109, 142, 157, 176
Children
 assessment of, 39, 72, 210, 274
 blood pressure, 39-40, 73, 98, 108, 113, 189, 210,
 244, 253, 274, 285, 388
 blood volume, 39, 98, 113, 210
 burn, 29, 301, 304
 death and, 20, 38, 253
 extremities, 29, 38, 108, 365
 head and neck, 72, 274, 287
 injury prevention, 15, 20
 pulse rate, 73, 210, 253, 274
 respiratory rate, 73, 98, 253
 spinal injuries, 287
Chloride, 118, 137, 148
Chronic alcoholism, 65, 80
Chronic exposure, 390
Chronotropy, 101
Chyme, 197, 200, 207, 219
Circle of Willis, 57
Circulation
 fetal, 42-43, 209, 212, 216
 peripheral, 57, 59, 74, 88, 98, 100, 103-104,
 106-107, 114, 119, 147, 167, 246, 267,
 383, 394, 404
Circulatory system, 42, 57, 87, 90, 102, 168, 200, 204,
 244, 328, 400, 409

Circumduction, 156, 160, 162, 166, 194
Circumferential burns, 300, 313, 316, 319
Clavicles, 229, 258, 340
Clavicular fracture, 185
Closed injuries, 124-125, 135
Closed pneumothorax, 227, 230, 244
Clot formation, 94, 113, 135, 138-139
Clotting, 31, 37, 47, 88, 92, 94-98, 110-111, 113-114,
 119-120, 128, 132, 135, 138, 142, 144, 200,
 215, 243
Clues, 74, 309
CNS, 57, 59, 72, 309, 387, 401-402
Coagulation
 zone of, 300, 303-304, 328
Coccygeal spine, 260, 264
Coccyx, 183, 252, 259-260, 264, 267, 296-297
Cold disorders, 381, 389
Cold diuresis, 394
Cold-water drowning, 397
Colles' fracture, 185, 188
Collision, 2-3, 5-7, 9, 11, 13-15, 18, 22, 24, 45, 48, 54,
 71-72, 116, 192, 216, 226, 241, 247,
 265-266, 335, 348-349, 351-352, 354-358,
 360-368, 373-374
Colon, 109, 199-201, 204-205, 207-208, 211, 217
Coma, 2, 9-11, 26, 32, 34-35, 41, 45, 49, 53-54, 58,
 67, 73-74, 76-78, 81-86, 96, 108-109,
 112-113, 141, 174, 243, 274-275, 280-281,
 309, 315, 390, 392, 396, 406
Combative patients, 14
Command, 23-25, 41, 63, 76-77, 101, 140, 173, 314,
 371
Common pathway, 93
Communications
 medical, 45, 54
Comorbidity, 229
Compartment syndrome, 71, 122-123, 135-136,
 147-148, 153, 167-169, 176-177, 182, 184,
 188, 192, 285, 348, 373, 375
Compensated shock, 88, 103-104, 116, 119
Competency, 1, 17, 52, 87, 122, 155, 197, 221, 251,
 299, 330, 348, 379
Competent, 79
Compression injury, 266-267, 353, 367
Concentration, 19, 27, 54, 99, 106, 109, 112, 189, 214,
 231, 243-244, 246, 293, 303-305, 308,
 314-315, 319-320, 326, 369, 371-372, 384,
 398, 400, 402-404
Concussion, 19, 53, 64-65, 68, 85
Concussions, 64-65
Conduction, 68, 90, 234, 245, 380, 382, 389, 409
Conduction system, 90, 234
Condyloid joint, 160
Confined space rescue, 147
Confined spaces, 106, 369
Congenital, 231
Congestive heart failure, 234, 240, 404
Conjunctiva, 29, 252, 257, 279, 296
Consciousness
 level of, 9-11, 19, 26, 28, 30, 35-36, 41, 65, 67,
 72-74, 76-77, 79, 81, 89, 103, 113, 141,
 176, 183, 210, 212, 214, 216, 222, 243,
 246, 274-275, 280-281, 284-285, 293,
 300-301, 314, 371, 384, 390-391, 403,
 406
Consent
 informed, 44
Contact lenses, 279, 293, 322
Contamination, 130, 134, 137-138, 142, 144, 146,
 175, 213, 279, 292, 306, 312, 314, 318,
 321-323, 325, 336-337, 369, 371
Continuous positive airway pressure (CPAP), 244
Contraindications, 52, 180, 286
Contrecoup injuries, 64
Contusion
 chest wall, 228-230, 233-234, 244, 247
 myocardial, 108, 234, 241-242
 pulmonary, 29, 107-108, 228-230, 233-234,
 240-244, 247, 359-360
Contusions, 43, 64, 95, 107-108, 124, 128-129, 142,
 148-149, 167, 182, 188, 211-212, 214, 228,
 233-234, 241, 335, 349-350, 356-358, 365
Convection, 167, 380, 382, 389, 409
Convulsions, 305, 403
COPD, 47, 229, 240, 309
Core body temperature, 50, 384, 387, 390, 410
Core temperature, 36, 114, 253, 311, 380, 383-384,
 387-390, 392-394, 407, 409
Cornea, 252, 257, 272, 293, 296, 310

Coronary arteries, 103, 225, 236
Coronary artery disease, 234, 397
Cortex, 54-55, 65, 67, 102, 118, 269
Costal cartilage, 223
Coughing, 234, 249, 300, 314, 322, 376, 406
Coumadin, 31, 78, 95, 135
CPR
    carotid pulse, 112
    chest compressions, 393, 397
    circulation and, 394
    effective, 394
    rib fractures, 43, 112
Crackles, 29, 36, 44, 80, 234, 240-243, 331, 371, 398, 405-407
Cranial bones, 55, 254, 268, 285
Cranial region, 267
Cranial vault, 56-57, 111, 254
Cranium, 39, 44, 54-57, 60, 64-66, 68, 72, 85, 159, 161, 252-255, 267-269, 271, 278, 282, 292, 294, 296-297, 340, 367
Cravat, 95, 118, 185, 289
Cravats, 109, 140, 179-181, 185, 187, 291
Crepitus, 2, 30, 53, 142, 149, 157, 174-175, 193, 212, 228-229, 240-241, 270, 279, 341, 349
Cricoid cartilage, 38, 258, 279, 284
Cricoid pressure, 282
Cricothyroid membrane, 283-284, 301
Crime scene, 341
Cross-contamination, 321
Crowing, 309
Crumple zone, 349, 358, 360, 376
Crumple zones, 5-6, 360, 362-363, 366
Crush injuries
    hemorrhage control, 111, 143
Crush injury, 89, 111, 123, 129, 134, 136-137, 140, 143, 147-148, 151, 153, 226, 246, 373
Crying, 41, 77
Crystalloid solutions, 48, 113
Crystalloids, 113
CSF, 53, 57, 85
C-Spine, 350, 398
Current, 7, 9-10, 19, 23, 31, 80, 83, 94, 113, 146, 180, 210, 288, 292, 295, 300, 304-305, 318, 320-321, 327-328, 331, 362, 381, 385, 396
Cushing's reflex, 53, 67, 82, 85
Cushing's triad, 47, 53, 67-68, 74, 76, 78, 82, 85, 280, 294
Cyanide poisoning, 99, 299, 315, 319
Cyanosis, 232-233, 236, 238, 246, 403, 405-406
Cyanotic, 29, 103, 106, 142, 175, 214, 239-240
Cytoplasm, 92, 99, 120

D
Dalton's law, 399, 404
Data collection, 1, 7
Dead space, 231
Death
    clinical, 4, 11, 49, 104, 223, 232, 246, 248
Deceleration, 31, 39, 55, 63, 65, 199, 206, 208, 226, 233, 237, 247, 255, 332-333, 349, 351-356, 358-360, 363, 367, 372, 376
Decerebrate, 26, 41, 54, 65, 68, 73-74, 76-77
Decerebrate posturing, 26, 54, 77
Decompensated shock, 88, 103-104, 116-117, 119
Decompression sickness, 380, 400-403, 408-409
Decontamination, 143, 323-324, 326
Decorticate, 26, 41, 65, 67-68, 73-74, 76-77
Decorticate posturing, 26, 65, 67-68, 77
Deep frostbite, 380, 395, 410
Defecation, 200
Degloving injury, 123, 130-131, 153
Dehydration
    results from, 67, 384
Delivery
    abnormal, 9, 100
    field, 308
    normal, 42, 72, 267
Denature, 133, 300, 303-305, 327
Depression
    patients with, 80, 107, 388
    symptoms of, 80, 388, 390
Depth of breathing, 150
Dermatome, 53, 71, 75, 85
Dermis, 123, 125-126, 129, 132, 151, 153-154, 301-303, 309-310, 328
Descending aorta, 237
Devascularization, 156, 158, 194
Dextrose
    injury, 80, 292

Diabetes, 43, 80, 172, 387, 389-390
Diamox, 405-406
Diaphoresis, 232, 384
Diaphoretic, 98, 236
Diaphragm, 62, 101, 149-150, 199-202, 204-205, 207-208, 212, 215, 221, 223-226, 230-232, 237, 245, 247, 252, 294, 340, 342, 358, 360, 374
Diaphysis, 156, 158-159, 163, 171-172, 194
Diarrhea, 105, 308, 324, 386-387
Diarthroses, 156, 159-160, 194
Diastole, 120, 225, 227
Diastolic blood pressure, 85, 91, 103, 105, 109
Diastolic pressure, 76, 85, 90, 97
Diazepam, 78-81, 188-189, 292, 402
Diazepam (Valium), 78-79
Diet-induced thermogenesis, 381
Diffuse axonal injury, 53, 64-65, 85
Digestive system, 63, 96, 200-201, 219
Digestive tract, 102, 166, 197, 200-201, 205, 219, 256, 270, 306
Digital intubation, 283
Diphenhydramine, 189
Diphenhydramine (Benadryl), 189
Direct force, 184
Direct pathway, 337
Direct pressure, 35, 88, 95, 107, 110-111, 118-119, 124, 130, 137-138, 143, 145-147, 149, 214-215, 278, 284-285, 293
Dirty bomb, 369
Diseases
    effects of, 172, 313
Dislocation
    ankle, 156, 177, 184, 186-187, 190-191, 194
    elbow, 156, 177-178, 185, 187-188
    finger, 178, 182, 188, 190
    foot, 156, 175, 184-187, 191, 194
    hip, 156, 176, 184-186, 190, 358
    knee, 156, 169, 177, 184-187, 190-191, 358
    shoulder, 156, 169, 177, 185, 187, 190-191, 194, 229, 243, 265-266, 273, 358
    sternal, 229, 240
Dislocations, 142, 172-175, 178-179, 181, 183-184, 186-188, 228-229, 270, 356-358
Dispatch, 5-6, 9, 18, 20, 22, 24, 50, 156, 190, 322, 331, 380
Dispatcher, 2, 18, 349
Distal, 29, 31, 35, 38, 47, 53-54, 59, 68, 75, 92, 95, 105, 108, 124, 130, 134-135, 142-144, 146-148, 151-153, 162-163, 167-169, 172, 174-182, 184-188, 190-191, 193-194, 242, 274, 281, 284, 300, 312, 314, 316-320, 325, 342, 395
Distal pulse, 29, 31, 35, 53, 108, 124, 144, 168, 178-179, 182
Distributive shock, 114
Diuresis, 147, 394, 404
Diuretic, 80, 148, 405
Diuretics, 148, 292, 384
Divers alert network (DAN), 404
Diverticulosis, 96
Diving emergencies, 379, 381, 398-400, 402-404, 410
Diving injury immobilization, 291
Division, 63, 219, 328
Dizziness, 108-109, 157, 212, 309, 386, 400-401, 405
Documentation
    importance, 13
    special considerations, 34, 37
Doll's eyes, 74
Dopamine, 80, 114
Dorsal, 60-62, 135, 167
Dose, 80, 189, 308, 319, 321, 323-324, 327-328, 388
Dosimeter, 308
DOT, 20
Down-and-under pathway, 358-359
Drag, 272, 289, 330, 333, 336, 343-345
Dressings
    bulky, 124, 145-146, 150, 215, 292-293, 318, 343
    occlusive, 30, 138-139, 145, 149, 215, 278-279, 281, 285, 296, 331, 342
    pressure, 30, 109-110, 124, 135, 138, 140, 144-146, 149, 152, 188, 215, 278, 281, 284-285, 292-293, 296, 312, 318-319, 323, 331, 342-343
Dressings and bandages, 110, 135, 138, 281
Dromotropy, 101
Drug overdose, 136
Drug use, 172
Drugs

musculoskeletal injuries, 189
    spinal cord injury, 74
Dry drowning, 396
Duodenum, 200-201, 205, 207-208, 212
Dura mater, 53-56, 60, 64, 82, 85-86, 269, 271
Dyspnea, 27, 36-37, 42, 81, 107, 228, 231-234, 2_, 238-244, 275, 300, 309, 315, 319, 331, 3_, 349, 371-372, 376, 405-406

E
Ear, 58, 111, 145, 255-256, 265, 269-271, 278-279, 288, 292, 297, 369, 371-372, 399-401, 4_
Ear injuries, 271, 371-372
Ecchymosis, 29-30, 109, 123, 128, 142, 153, 167, 175, 206, 212, 217, 228, 252, 269, 279, 2_, 296-297
Ectopic beats, 245
Ectopic pregnancy, 97
Edema
    cerebral, 56-57, 65-67, 80, 149, 285, 405-406
    laryngeal, 277
Education
    continuing education, 13
    initial, 6
    public, 1, 6-7, 13, 20
Efficacy, 113, 326, 405
Elbow, 62, 70, 124, 128, 143, 145-146, 156, 159, 1_, 172, 177-178, 180-181, 185, 187-188, 33_, 367
Elbow injuries, 187
Elderly, 10, 27, 29, 44, 65, 78, 87, 98, 125, 134-135, 172, 176, 229, 253, 276, 279, 293, 309, 3_, 366-367, 389, 396
Elderly patients, 98, 172
Electrical alternans, 222, 236, 249
Electrical burn, 321, 324
Electrical burns, 299, 304, 312, 314, 317, 321, 323
Electrocution, 9, 106, 267, 326, 362, 369
Electrodes, 239
Electrons, 304, 328, 409
Elevation, 79, 110, 144, 148, 181, 185, 189, 241, 36_, 388, 407
ELM, 282-283
Emboli, 95, 103, 107, 138, 143, 149, 170, 172, 349, 371-372, 375-376
Embolism, 30, 79, 106, 170, 172, 226, 273, 278, 285, 294, 340, 380, 400-403, 408-409
Embolus, 272, 296
Embryo, 163
Emergency care
    chest pain, 48
    closed wounds, 142
    eye injuries, 137
    heat cramps, 385-386
    heat exhaustion, 385-386
    impaled objects, 142
    internal bleeding, 375
    neck wounds, 138, 281
    open wounds, 138, 142, 190
    soft-tissue injuries, 137, 189-190, 281
    spine injuries, 295
Emergency medical care, 1, 37
Emergency Response Guidebook, 23
Emphysema, 29-30, 44, 107, 134, 142, 149, 213, 232, 238, 240-242, 246, 273, 279, 284, 294, 341, 402
EMS operations
    hazards, 371
EMS systems
    components, 32, 120
    protocols and, 28, 46
    purpose, 142
Endocrine system, 202, 258, 381
Endotracheal intubation
    procedures, 11, 36, 277
    proper placement, 112, 283
Endotracheal tube, 35, 40, 79, 106-107, 112, 149, 277, 282-283, 315, 320, 340, 342
End-tidal CO2 (ETCO2), 106
Energy, 3, 5-6, 9, 11, 23, 36-37, 39, 45, 57, 99, 103, 118-120, 124, 128, 158-159, 163, 167-170, 172-173, 177-178, 183-184, 191, 205-207, 226-228, 230, 233-234, 236-237, 239-241, 253, 259, 265-266, 269, 278, 301, 303-306, 309-311, 313, 320-321, 327, 330, 332-341, 345, 348-356, 358, 360-361, 364-371, 374, 376, 381, 383, 389-390, 400, 404, 409-410
Enhanced, 230, 269, 271
Environmental emergencies

ld disorders, 381
owning, 379, 381
at gain and loss, 381
eatstroke, 381
omeostasis, 379, 381
onmental hazards, 9
ardium, 222, 225, 249
ermis, 123, 125-126, 129, 132, 153, 301-303,
306-307, 309-310, 328
dymis, 203
ural hematoma, 53-54, 64-65, 85
ottitis, 273
epsy, 108
ephrine, 63, 71, 88, 97, 100-102, 119-120, 202,
381, 394
hysis, 156, 158-159, 171-172, 194
taxis (nosebleed), 271
ipment
esuscitation, 20, 28, 43, 47, 147, 312, 398
hema, 29-30, 107, 109, 123, 128, 133-134, 142,
153, 167, 175, 206, 212, 228, 240, 294, 303,
308-310, 312, 322
hrocyte, 88, 119, 216, 306
hrocytes, 29, 92, 97, 99, 103, 119, 132, 159, 191,
195, 200, 204, 269
hropoietin, 102-103
har, 300, 311-312, 315-316, 319, 327
phageal rupture, 238
phageal varices, 88, 96, 119
phagus, 38, 96, 149, 200-201, 219, 221, 223-226,
229, 237-240, 256, 258, 265, 273, 282, 285,
340, 352
tube, 149, 296
C, 317
moid bone, 254-255
acuation, 15, 49, 166, 180, 323, 402
aporation, 126, 167, 301-302, 380, 382, 385, 387,
389, 407, 410
sceration, 197, 206-207, 215-217, 219, 372
scerations, 138, 150, 212, 214
amination, 18, 28-31, 50, 84, 108, 117, 124, 134,
142, 149, 152, 173, 192, 198, 218, 223, 248,
252, 278, 295, 321, 326, 341, 372, 402, 407
cretion, 200
ercise, 168, 188, 282, 381, 401, 404-405, 407
ertional metabolic rate, 380, 383, 410
halation, 27, 112, 224-225, 229, 231
haustion, 380, 383-387, 410
it wound, 198, 213, 231, 241, 269, 305, 320, 337,
340-341, 344
plosions, 72, 95, 264-265, 271, 354, 367-369,
371-372, 375
sanguination, 107, 217, 245, 294, 349, 367, 374,
376
tension, 26, 41, 62, 65, 68-69, 72, 75-77, 85, 145,
157, 159-160, 166, 176, 178, 186, 194, 261,
265-266, 277, 280, 286-287, 290-291, 295,
357
tension (decerebrate) posturing, 68
tension injury, 69, 266
ternal hemorrhage, 4, 14, 17, 35, 37, 79, 81, 87, 89,
94-95, 106-108, 112-113, 117, 125, 214
ternal jugular vein, 147, 240, 258, 273, 285
ternal laryngeal manipulation (ELM), 282
travasation, 83, 217
travascular, 300, 304, 327
travascular space, 300, 304, 327
tremities
examination of, 18, 31, 252
fracture care, 181
injuries to, 2, 69, 135, 157, 163, 183, 190, 213,
264, 266, 273, 342, 356, 363
Extremity injuries
angle, 360
mechanisms of, 32, 157
Extrinsic pathway, 88, 93-94, 119
Eye, 24, 30, 32, 34, 41, 48, 53, 58, 74, 76-77, 81, 85,
106, 110-111, 137, 251, 255, 257-258, 269,
271-272, 274, 279-280, 288, 292-294,
296-297, 302, 310, 322, 357, 400
Eye injuries, 137, 251, 293, 357
Eye protection, 24, 106, 274, 288
Eyes
anatomy of, 256-257
anatomy of the, 256-257
Eyewear, 173

F

Face, 18, 29, 53, 74, 76, 87, 123, 134, 145, 148-149,

152, 161, 239, 251-297, 316-317, 330, 338,
340, 342, 357, 395, 397, 410
Face shield, 239, 252
Facial bones, 159, 254-255, 257, 279
Facial injuries
ears, 111, 269
eyes, 269
soft-tissue, 149, 270, 358
Facial lacerations, 357
Fallopian tubes, 200, 202-203
Falls
fractures in the elderly, 367
Fascia, 88, 95, 119, 135-136, 148, 153, 158, 164, 167,
176, 253, 258, 268, 273, 302
Fasciculus, 59
Fasciotomy, 136, 148
FDA, 110, 138
Fear, 37, 74, 106
Febrile seizures, 388-389
Femoral pulse, 41
Femur, 18, 49, 95, 107-108, 148, 152, 155-156, 158,
161-163, 169-170, 172, 174, 177-178,
180-181, 183-186, 190, 192, 194-195, 356,
358, 360-361, 363-365, 367, 376
Femur fractures, 18, 95, 148, 152, 177, 180-181,
183-184, 190
Fertilization, 203
Fertilizers, 306
Fetal circulation, 42-43
Fetal development, 163
Fetus, 19, 41-43, 59, 98, 203-204, 209-210, 213-214,
216, 219, 309
Fever, 134, 173, 195, 383-384, 388, 410
Fever (pyrexia), 388
Fibers, 55, 59, 65, 70, 74, 85, 93-94, 119, 126-127,
133, 135, 158-159, 166-168, 172, 191,
194-195, 226, 237, 302, 353
fibrillation, 148, 235, 305, 321, 380, 391-392, 394,
397, 407
Fibrin, 88, 93-94, 119, 132, 135, 153
Fibula, 95, 107-108, 136, 155-156, 159, 161, 163, 178,
184, 194, 365
"Fight-or-flight" response, 27, 176, 275
Filtration, 92
First Responder, 22, 408
First-degree burn, 309, 328
Flail chest, 27, 32, 112, 221-222, 228-230, 240-241,
243, 249, 358
Flail segment, 27, 230, 243, 246-247, 249
Flank, 198-199, 202, 207, 211-212, 217
Flanks, 30, 202, 206-207, 212
Flechettes, 349, 369, 376
Flexion, 18, 26, 41, 62, 68-69, 72, 75-77, 136, 145,
157, 160, 166-167, 173, 175, 177-178, 186,
194, 252, 261, 265-266, 280, 286-287, 290,
295
Flexion injury, 177
Floating ribs, 223-224, 263
Floods, 271, 396
Flow regulator, 322
Fluid resuscitation
in trauma, 17, 27, 35-36, 43, 47-49, 98, 113
Flushed, 71, 175
Focused assessment, 25, 32, 109, 124, 174, 281
Focused physical exam, 28, 157
Focused trauma assessment, 9-10, 14, 20, 28-32, 35,
37, 43, 72, 107-109, 123, 140-142, 157,
173-174, 176, 210, 274, 278, 281, 313, 315,
317
Fontanelles, 39, 68
Force, 3, 16, 23, 30, 44, 63, 65, 68, 117, 120, 127,
129-131, 142-143, 147, 157, 167-170, 173,
176, 184, 189, 191, 206-207, 226, 228-229,
231, 238, 246-247, 265-268, 280, 282,
286-287, 330, 332-333, 335, 338, 345, 348,
350-358, 360, 367, 369, 376, 399, 402
Forearm, 2, 9, 36, 62, 71, 75, 116, 135, 137, 143, 158,
161-162, 167, 169, 174, 176-177, 185,
187-188, 194-195, 300, 325, 327, 363, 367,
373
Foreign body, 134, 146, 153, 270, 272, 293
Formable splints, 179
Fracture
femur, 18, 49, 108, 148, 156, 162-163, 169-170,
172, 174, 177-178, 181, 183-186, 192,
194-195, 356, 360, 364-365, 367
rib, 18, 30, 39, 43, 70, 208, 210, 226, 228-231,
233-234, 237, 240-241, 247, 350, 356
skull, 30, 32, 39, 65, 110-111, 145, 159, 253-255,

268-271, 277-279, 282, 294, 296-297,
360, 365
sternum, 135, 159, 162, 185, 191, 194, 199,
228-229, 234, 247, 356, 367
Fractures
bend, 185, 188, 229, 266, 285
buckle, 171
clavicle, 155, 169, 185, 187, 229, 243, 356, 361,
367
greenstick, 170-171, 189
hemorrhage in, 95
humerus, 95, 108, 155, 159, 177-178, 181, 185,
187, 361, 367
radius/ulna, 155, 178, 185
tibia/fibula, 95, 108, 155, 178, 184
wrist/hand, 188
Frontal bone, 254, 279
Frontal impact, 18, 45, 53, 211, 226, 245, 266, 352,
357-360, 364
Frontal impacts, 359, 363, 374
Frontal lobe, 64, 67
Frostbite, 380, 389-390, 395, 408, 410
Frostnip, 395, 410
Full-thickness burns, 370
Furosemide, 148, 292, 406, 409
Furosemide (Lasix), 406

G

Gag reflex, 149, 282
Galea aponeurotica, 252, 296
Gallbladder, 199-201, 207, 217
Gamma radiation, 300, 306-307, 325, 327-328
Gamma rays, 306
Gangrene, 123, 134, 151, 153, 410
Gases, 234, 303, 306, 308-309, 314, 333, 335, 341,
356, 368-370, 399, 401, 403, 409-410
Gastric distention, 396
Gauze pads, 372
Geiger counter, 308
Geriatric patients
caring for, 44
Gestation, 42, 209-210
Glasgow Coma Scale, 9, 11, 32, 34-35, 41, 45, 49,
53-54, 73-74, 76-78, 81-86, 96, 108-109,
112-113, 141, 243, 274-275, 280-281, 315
Glasgow Coma Scale (GCS), 32, 76, 280
Glottic opening, 282
Glottis, 39, 226, 229, 231, 247, 309, 358
Glucagon, 200, 217
Glucocorticoids, 116
Glucose, 37, 52, 55, 57, 75, 80, 99, 114, 118-119, 200,
404
Glycolysis, 88, 99, 117-120
Golden Hour, 10
Gown, 106, 173, 239, 321, 323
Gowns, 24
GPS, 6, 18
Granules, 139
Granulocytes, 123, 133, 151, 153
Gray matter, 55, 59-60
Great vessels, 149, 222-223, 225-227, 229, 237,
239-241, 249, 258, 339, 342, 352
Greenstick fractures, 189
Grey-Turner's sign, 212
Ground transport, 2, 10-11, 46, 48
Group, 20, 36, 48, 62, 90, 120, 172, 280, 309, 396
Growth plate, 159, 171, 189, 194
Grunting, 229
Guarding, 29-30, 107, 197, 208, 212, 216, 219
Gunshot wounds, 3, 6, 23, 95, 111, 149, 206-207, 209,
211, 239, 253, 265, 332, 342-344
Gurgling, 27, 294

H

Hair, 125-126, 133, 253, 287, 301-302, 309, 323, 389
Half-life, 80, 314, 319
Hand injuries, 168
Haversian canals, 156, 158, 191, 194
Hazard identification, 23
Hazards
fire, 9, 20, 23-24, 106, 308, 314, 323, 332, 362, 369
hazardous materials, 23
oxygen, 43, 106, 308, 314, 323, 371, 376
Head
structures of, 39, 59, 255, 258, 271, 363
Head and spinal injuries, 269
Head injuries
concussion, 64-65, 85

contusion, 64-65, 268
  epidural hematoma, 64-65, 85
  intracranial pressure, 64-66, 85, 111
  skull fracture, 65, 111, 268
  subdural hematoma, 64-65, 86
Head trauma, 39, 52, 65, 68, 74, 76, 79, 107, 129, 265, 271, 277, 364, 390
Headache, 65, 71, 85, 173, 309, 386-387, 404-406
Head-on collision, 45
Head-to-toe examination, 278
Heart
  chambers of, 97
  valves, 90, 101, 225, 236-237
Heart attack, 94, 108, 363
Heart failure, 234, 237, 240-241, 404
Heart sounds, 29-30, 241-242, 403
Heat cramps, 380, 384-387, 407, 410
Heat disorders, 384, 386-388
Heat exhaustion, 380, 383-387, 410
Heat loss, 37, 69, 114, 302, 311, 317-318, 366, 379, 382, 384, 389, 392, 394, 398
Heatstroke, 380-381, 383-388, 410
Heimlich maneuver, 398
Helmet, 2, 252, 274, 277, 288, 365-366, 373
Helmets
  motorcycle, 20, 274, 288, 365
  removal, 288
Hematemesis, 88, 96, 119, 197, 207, 219
Hematochezia, 88, 97, 109, 119, 197, 207, 219
Hematocrit, 88, 92, 102, 119
Hematoma, 29, 53-54, 57, 64-65, 85-86, 88, 95, 119, 123, 129, 142, 145, 151, 153, 167, 172, 234, 268, 273, 285, 340
Hematomas, 95, 108, 124, 128-129, 149, 167, 182, 188
Hematuria, 197, 207, 219
Hemoglobin, 88, 92, 99, 114, 118-119, 128, 292, 309, 314-315, 319-320
Hemopneumothorax, 222, 227, 233, 249
Hemoptysis, 88, 96, 222, 234, 238, 241, 249, 349, 371, 376
Hemorrhage
  clotting, 31, 37, 47, 88, 92, 94-98, 110-111, 113-114, 119-120, 132, 135, 138, 142, 144, 200, 215, 243
  control, 4, 10, 14, 24, 27-28, 30, 35, 56, 66, 68-70, 74, 81, 85, 87, 90-91, 93-97, 99, 101, 104-114, 116-120, 131, 135, 137-138, 141, 143-146, 152, 167, 178, 182-183, 185, 190, 214, 268, 270-271, 277-278, 280, 284-285, 296, 340, 373
  stages of, 28-29, 43, 92-93, 103-104, 132
Hemorrhagic shock, 89, 98, 105, 108-109, 296
Hemorrhoids, 96
Hemostasis, 87-88, 93, 113, 119-120, 122-123, 132-133, 135, 152-153
Hemothorax
  chest trauma, 221, 227, 229, 233, 237, 241-243
Henry's law, 399
Herniation, 47, 57, 67-68, 73-74, 80, 82, 84, 163, 237-238, 285
High altitude, 379, 381, 401, 404-406, 408-409
High altitude cerebral edema (HACE), 405-406
High altitude illness, 379, 381, 404-405
High altitude pulmonary edema (HAPE), 405-406, 409
Hilum, 61, 222, 224, 249
Hinge joints, 160
Hip dislocation, 186, 358
Hip joint, 157, 186
History
  comprehensive, 30, 50, 84, 117, 142, 152, 192, 218, 248, 295, 326
  questioning, 28, 30, 54, 78, 108-109, 142, 240, 252, 278, 280-281
Hoarseness, 300, 309, 314
Hormone, 88, 101-103, 116, 118-120, 133
Hormones, 57, 63, 71, 100-102, 200, 202, 209, 381
How to, 5, 11, 46, 90, 141, 396
Human body
  cavities, 150
  regions, 90, 324
  systems, 90, 99, 101, 150, 158, 191, 301, 381
Humerus, 95, 107-108, 155-156, 158-159, 161-163, 166, 177-178, 181, 185, 187, 194, 360-361, 367
Humidified oxygen, 392-394
Humidity, 175, 381, 384-385, 388-389
Humoral immunity, 154
Hydration, 98, 104, 385

Hydraulic, 137
Hydrochloric acid, 200
Hydrogen sulfide, 308, 314
Hydrostatic pressure, 88, 90, 92, 100, 103, 119-120
Hyoid, 161, 256, 284
Hyoid bone, 256, 284
Hyperbaric chamber, 403
Hyperbaric oxygen chamber, 380, 402, 410
Hypercarbia, 66, 277, 283, 396-398
Hyperextension injury, 266
Hyperglycemia, 75, 80
Hypermetabolic phase, 300, 304-305, 325, 328
Hypertension, 43, 66, 71, 79-80, 82-83, 85, 96, 116, 217, 234, 237, 280, 304, 397, 404, 406, 408
Hyperthermia, 107, 380, 384, 387, 407, 410
Hypertonic, 48, 83, 113
Hypertonic solutions, 113
Hypertrophy, 43
Hyperventilation, 66, 68, 76, 79, 83, 107, 280, 285, 375, 403-404
Hypoglycemia, 75, 80, 390
Hypoperfusion, 18, 35, 49-50, 66, 212-213, 216
Hypopharynx, 396
Hypotension, 18, 31, 35, 42-43, 49-50, 66, 69-70, 76, 79-80, 82, 88, 94, 108-109, 113, 116, 120, 183, 189, 204, 209, 213, 216, 218, 232, 234-239, 241-242, 245, 247, 280, 285, 309, 320, 387-388, 390-392, 396, 406, 409
Hypothermia
  generalized, 29
  key findings at different degrees of, 390-391
  mild, 383, 389, 392-393, 410
Hypothermia algorithm, 393
Hypovolemia, 18, 26-27, 29-31, 35, 38-40, 42-44, 47-50, 68, 71, 74, 76, 79-80, 96, 103-109, 112, 114, 116-118, 120, 124, 129, 137, 142-143, 167, 174, 177, 182-183, 188-190, 209, 212-213, 216, 231-235, 237, 239-243, 246, 268, 270, 273, 280, 285, 311, 313, 318-319
Hypovolemic shock, 88, 98-99, 105, 120, 388
Hypoxemia, 231-234, 238, 241, 243-244, 305, 319, 397
Hypoxic, 78, 103-105, 136, 143, 168, 238, 243, 246, 272, 292, 388, 396, 398, 404-405

I

ICP, 53, 57, 65-68, 76, 80, 85, 252, 254, 269, 277, 280, 282, 285, 296
Iliac crest, 156, 183, 194
Ilium, 156, 159, 163, 194
Illustration, 61
Immersion foot, 395, 410
Immobilization
  diving injury, 291
  musculoskeletal trauma, 157, 190
Impaled object, 123, 130, 146-147, 150, 153, 211, 215, 268-269, 277, 293, 372
Incendiary, 349, 370, 376
Incident, 5, 9-10, 14, 22-25, 31, 45, 67, 72, 78, 97, 106, 140-141, 173, 175-176, 190, 211, 274, 290-292, 300, 306, 314, 322, 363, 366, 371, 373, 395-396, 401
Incision, 123, 130, 134, 136, 153, 319
Incontinence, 69-70
Increased ICP, 65, 67
Index of suspicion, 1, 9, 16, 22, 25, 31, 43, 81, 106, 108, 174, 176, 190, 206, 211-212, 216, 245, 275, 309, 343, 350, 354, 356, 360, 363, 371, 374-375
Indication, 30, 75, 140, 142, 212, 267, 274, 284-285
Inertia, 330, 348-350, 352-354, 357-358, 374, 376
Infant, 20, 38-39, 71, 79, 98, 107, 159, 274, 277, 291, 310-311, 313, 357, 391
Infants
  growth and development, 39
  respiration, 40
  ventilation and, 226
Infarction, 69, 105, 135, 234-236, 241, 264, 371, 390, 397
Inferior, 42-43, 56, 101, 127, 150, 187, 199, 202-205, 207-209, 219, 223-226, 245, 249, 254-256, 258-263, 269, 271-272, 286, 340
Inferior vena cava, 42-43, 101, 127, 150, 204-205, 209, 219, 224-225, 249, 340
Inflammatory process, 133, 142
Informed consent, 44
Infusion, 36, 44, 47-48, 89, 113, 214-215, 244, 246, 319

Inguinal region, 184
Inhalation
  carbon monoxide, 299, 308-309, 314-315, 319, 326
  toxic, 147, 308-309, 314-315, 319
Inhalation injuries, 309, 317, 325
Inhalation injury, 299, 308-309, 314, 317, 319, 325
Injection
  subcutaneous, 137
Injury, 1-6, 8-11, 13-16, 17, 19-20, 22-32, 34-50, 52-54, 57-76, 78-86, 89, 92-94, 96-99, 1, 105-114, 116, 119, 122-125, 128-138, 140-154, 155, 157-159, 161, 167-193, 1, 197-200, 202, 205-218, 221, 223, 225-2, 251-253, 256-258, 260, 264-296, 299, 302-323, 325-327, 330-333, 335-345, 3, 350-354, 356-373, 375, 377, 381, 389, 397-400, 403, 410
Injury prevention, 1, 3, 6, 11, 15, 17, 19-20, 48-49, 157, 375
Injury risk, 210, 360
Inotropy, 101
Inspection, 9, 20-21, 28-30, 123-124, 142, 146, 19, 281
Inspiration, 79, 107, 112, 205, 224-225, 228-233, 2, 240, 242, 270, 273, 277, 285, 309, 401, 4
Insulin, 37, 200
Integrity, 108, 111, 126, 158, 168, 241, 271-273, 27, 339, 395
Integumentary system, 123-124, 151, 153, 301
Interatrial septum, 236
Internal bleeding
  seriousness, 216
  signs, 4, 146, 149-150, 216
Internal hemorrhage, 7, 28, 30, 37, 47, 87, 93-96, 106-109, 112, 114, 117, 178, 180, 182, 18, 208, 212-214, 216, 233, 239, 244, 246, 336-337, 340, 342, 352
Interneurons, 63
Interstitial fluid, 29, 99, 102, 148, 306
Interventions, 6, 16, 17, 20, 45-46, 49, 52, 101, 103, 107, 109, 114, 143, 239, 246, 384
Interventricular septum, 236
Intoxication
  patients and, 98
Intracerebral hemorrhage, 53, 64-65, 85
Intracranial hemorrhage, 39, 64, 68, 253, 293
Intracranial pressure, 39, 53, 56-57, 64-68, 76, 78-8, 85, 111, 145, 252-254, 269, 277, 280, 282, 292, 294, 296, 406
Intracranial pressure (ICP), 53, 57, 85, 252, 254, 296
Intrathoracic pressure, 224, 228, 230-232, 236, 239, 244, 273, 285
Intravenous fluids, 114, 147, 388, 394
Intrinsic pathway, 88, 93-94, 120
Intubation, 11, 27, 30, 35-36, 39-40, 48-49, 73-74, 76-77, 79, 83-84, 99, 106-107, 112, 117, 149, 216, 243, 277, 282-283, 292, 295, 300-301, 314-315, 319, 321, 325, 342, 350, 394
Investigation, 157, 176, 280, 341, 352
Ion, 102
Ionization, 300, 306, 308, 328
Ionize, 306
Ions, 328, 409
Irreversible shock, 28, 39, 44, 87-88, 103-105, 116, 120
Ischemia, 69, 85, 88, 102-103, 120, 143, 146, 148-149, 153-154, 168, 176, 208, 226, 236, 267, 309, 319, 401, 403
Ischium, 156, 162-163, 183, 194
Isotonic, 35-36, 47, 49, 79, 113, 408
Isotonic solutions, 47
Isthmus, 237, 249
IV fluids, 108, 113-114, 210, 245, 247, 388, 392-394

J

Jackson's theory of thermal wounds, 300, 303-304, 328
Jaw-thrust maneuver, 149
Joint
  structure of, 161, 260
Joint capsule, 156, 161, 168-169, 173, 181, 194-195
Joint structure, 159, 171, 182, 260
Joule's law, 300, 304, 328
JVD, 232, 236, 238, 240

K

139, 180
..y, 29, 56, 80, 99, 101-103, 137, 199, 202, 211,
    313, 373, 375
. energy, 5-6, 23, 169, 173, 226-227, 253, 269,
    330, 332-335, 337-338, 340-341, 348-355,
    366, 368, 376
...s, 330, 332, 343, 348-350, 352, 360, 376
  139, 180
  injuries, 186
  injury, 186, 363
  joint, 146, 163, 186
..s, 227, 267, 332, 335-336, 338
.. cycle, 88, 99, 119-120
..naul's sign, 236, 242
..sis, 252, 279, 296

..r, 210
..ration, 9, 20, 29, 68-69, 123, 128-130, 144, 153,
    167, 206, 208, 223, 227, 229, 233-234,
    272-273, 358
..rations, 3, 53, 69, 108, 124, 128-130, 132, 149,
    151-152, 168, 227, 270, 272, 294, 349,
    356-357, 364
..mal bone, 254-255
..mal fluid, 252, 257, 272, 293, 296
..ated Ringer's, 113-114, 318, 322, 398, 402-403
..ated Ringer's solution, 113-114
.. acid, 88, 95, 99, 103, 117, 119-120, 129, 137,
    168, 387, 394
..inae, 259, 263, 265-266, 295
.. intestine, 201, 205
..ngeal manipulation, 277, 282
..ngeal mask airway (LMA), 283
..ngopharynx, 283
..ngoscope, 283-284, 342
..nx, 39, 67, 110-111, 201, 225, 256, 258, 265, 273,
    282-283, 340, 342
..ix, 406
..eral, 23, 26, 30, 43, 59-61, 72, 75, 94, 107, 128,
    135-136, 158, 161-163, 166, 168-169, 175,
    184-187, 193-194, 200, 202, 205, 208,
    213-214, 216, 224, 229, 236-237, 239-241,
    244, 246-247, 254-255, 258-267, 269, 277,
    279, 286-287, 289-291, 294, 297, 337,
    353-354, 357-358, 360-361, 363, 365, 372,
    374, 376
..eral impact, 237, 239, 266, 357-358, 360-361, 374
..eral malleolus, 163
..eral recumbent, 43, 213-214, 216, 277, 372
..eral recumbent position, 43, 213-214, 216, 277,
    372
..teral rotation, 168
.. of conservation of energy, 332
..ying the bike down, 364
..adership, 7, 20
..ft, 18-19, 43, 53-54, 56, 59, 78, 89, 100, 123, 134,
    146, 150, 168, 186, 198-200, 202, 204,
    207-208, 210-211, 213-214, 216-218,
    222-226, 229, 236-238, 246-247, 249, 255,
    257-258, 260, 262, 268, 272, 277, 279,
    293-294, 300, 312, 323, 331, 354, 360, 372,
    400, 402
..ft atrium, 225, 400, 402
..ft lower quadrant, 199, 217
..ft upper quadrant, 198-200, 202, 216-217
..sion, 56-57, 74-76, 80, 254, 293, 324
..eukocyte, 306
..eukocytes, 151
..evel of consciousness, 9-11, 26, 28, 30, 35-36, 41,
    65, 67, 72-74, 76-77, 79, 81, 89, 103, 113,
    141, 176, 183, 210, 212, 214, 216, 222, 243,
    246, 274-275, 280-281, 284-285, 293,
    300-301, 314, 371, 384, 390-391, 403, 406
..ife-threatening problems, 4, 116, 278
..igament, 60, 160, 168-169, 177, 182, 188, 203, 208,
    260-262, 266, 352, 354, 357, 365, 373
..igaments, 72, 126, 129, 150, 156-157, 160-161,
    167-169, 172, 177-178, 182, 186, 188,
    190-191, 194, 200, 260, 265-267, 272, 338,
    353, 360, 372-373
..igamentum arteriosum, 222, 226, 237, 249, 367
..ightning strikes, 321
..istening, 27, 241, 371, 407
..iters, 2, 47, 88-89, 97, 100, 174, 183, 200, 212, 240,
    292, 331, 385, 388
..iver injury, 208, 360
..obes, 55, 224, 240-241
..og roll, 31, 212, 277, 286, 288-289

Long backboard, 295, 398
Long board, 192, 246, 291
Long bones, 39, 158-159, 161, 172, 178, 191, 194,
    339, 372
Long spine board, 27, 37, 54, 79, 96, 136, 181,
    184-187, 190, 274, 276-277, 285-292, 349,
    373
Lorazepam (ativan), 78, 80
Lower airway, 256, 258, 282-283, 309, 328, 342
Lower extremities, 18, 47, 59, 69-70, 74-75, 77, 88-89,
    114, 120, 135, 161-163, 170, 174, 181, 183,
    190, 194, 204, 209, 237, 252, 259, 264, 266,
    312, 356, 363, 365
Lower leg, 192, 194-195, 312, 365, 375
Lubricant, 225
Lumbar region, 263
Lumbar spine, 61, 83, 163, 171, 183, 199, 202, 260,
    263, 266, 273, 280, 289, 291, 295, 358, 367
Lumbar vertebrae, 252, 259, 263, 273, 297
Lumen, 90, 93-94, 113, 120, 123, 126, 132, 153, 166,
    200, 208, 237, 283, 286, 309, 315
Lung, 2, 27, 30, 36, 43-44, 53, 67, 149, 169, 185,
    204-205, 224-227, 229-234, 238-245,
    249-250, 308, 318-319, 337, 339-340, 342,
    350, 352, 358, 371-372, 375, 377, 400,
    402-403, 405, 409-410
Lung parenchyma, 239
Lung sounds, 53, 318, 350
Lungs, 67, 80, 92, 96, 100, 102, 149, 223-226, 228,
    231, 233, 239-240, 247, 249, 270, 284, 302,
    338-340, 352, 368-369, 371, 374, 377, 382,
    396-398, 402, 406-407, 410
Lymphatic system, 127
Lymphocytes, 126, 133

M

Mainstem bronchi, 224, 238, 258
Malnutrition, 389
Malpractice insurance, 8
Management
    abdominal injury, 213-214, 216
    amputations, 123, 143, 146
    carbon monoxide poisoning, 8, 314, 326
    crush syndrome, 122-123, 146-147
    musculoskeletal injury, 155, 173, 177
    tachycardia, 39, 82, 109
    uterine rupture, 42, 214
Mandible, 252, 254-256, 258, 271, 277, 279, 286-287,
    291, 297, 367
Manual stabilization, 252, 276, 295
Manual traction, 184
Manubrium, 162, 223-224, 229, 247
Mask, 2, 19, 24, 27, 35, 44, 46, 54, 73, 78, 80, 88-89,
    105, 112, 117, 173, 240, 243-244, 246,
    282-284, 288, 292, 300-301, 309, 315,
    319-321, 323, 331, 350, 388, 393, 402-403
Masks, 3, 24, 363
Mass-casualty incident, 290
MAST, 114, 126, 133, 151
Mastoid process, 254, 256, 297
Maxilla, 252, 255, 270-271, 279, 285, 297, 367
Maxillary arteries, 255
Maxillary bone, 254-255, 271
Mechanism of injury
    explosions, 72, 369, 371
Mechanisms of injury, 11, 22, 32, 37, 40, 136, 140,
    157, 251, 264, 266, 276, 287, 293, 313-314,
    330, 348, 350, 354, 364, 368
Medial, 2, 59, 62, 128, 162-163, 175-176, 184-187,
    200, 224, 249, 257, 285-286, 291-292
Medial malleolus, 163
Mediastinal shift, 230, 232
Mediastinum, 39, 225-226, 230-232, 237-239, 242,
    249, 273, 400, 403, 410
Medical, 1-11, 14, 19-20, 23-24, 28-29, 31-32, 34,
    36-38, 44-46, 49-50, 53-54, 71, 76, 79-81,
    85, 89, 108-110, 113-114, 124-125, 134, 140,
    144, 147-148, 150, 157, 172, 176, 182, 186,
    189-190, 192, 222, 228, 236, 238, 252,
    275-276, 280, 284, 288, 291-292, 301,
    313-315, 317-319, 321-322, 324-325,
    330-331, 341, 349-350, 363, 367, 373, 381,
    387, 389-390, 395, 400-404, 406, 408, 410
Medical anti-shock trouser (MAST), 114
Medical direction
    on-line, 54, 81, 148, 150, 315, 317
Medical director, 28, 32, 79-80, 110, 113, 288
Medical emergencies
    heat and, 381

Medical history, 31, 45, 108-109, 172, 176, 252, 280,
    331
Medications
    administration, 40, 78-80, 148, 157, 292, 373, 388,
        394, 406
    prescription, 31, 381
Medulla, 53-54, 56, 59, 67, 71, 82, 85-86, 101-102,
    116, 119-120, 231
Medulla oblongata, 53-54, 56, 59, 67, 82, 85-86,
    101-102, 116
Medullary canal, 156, 158-159, 169-170, 194
Meninges, 53-54, 60, 64, 82-86, 97, 111, 253, 265,
    268-269
Meningitis, 111
Menopause, 171
Menstruation, 97
Mental status
    altered, 108, 232, 276, 319, 375, 388, 390, 400,
        406
    examination, 108, 173
Mesentery, 197, 205-206, 208, 219
Metabolic acidosis, 99, 103, 129, 387
Metabolic rate, 57, 63, 119, 258, 380, 383, 389, 391,
    409-410
Metabolism, 37, 57, 79, 88, 99-100, 103, 117-120,
    133, 137, 158, 171, 173, 191, 200, 223, 320,
    328, 368, 373, 381, 383-384, 388-389, 394,
    399, 406
Metacarpals, 159-162, 367
Metaphysis, 156, 158-159, 194
Metatarsals, 159, 161, 163, 187
Meters, 332, 338
Midaxillary, 19, 224, 244
Midaxillary line, 19, 224, 244
Midazolam (Versed), 78
Midbrain, 53, 56, 58, 67, 85-86
Midclavicular, 36, 112, 222, 224, 244-245, 331
Midclavicular line, 36, 112, 222, 224, 244-245, 331
Midline, 27, 30, 73, 160, 193, 222-223, 235, 246, 252,
    266-267, 279, 284
Mild hypothermia, 383, 389, 392-393
Minor burns, 318
Minute volume, 42-43, 73, 240, 243
Miscarriage, 97
Mitochondria, 99
MOI, 1, 9, 11, 16, 19, 25, 32, 73, 96, 106-108, 274,
    293
Monaxial joints, 160
Motion, 2, 30, 42, 58, 65, 69, 71, 78, 81, 128, 133,
    144, 158, 160-163, 166-170, 175, 177-178,
    181, 185, 188, 191, 193, 195, 206, 208, 215,
    219, 226, 228, 240-241, 249, 256, 258,
    260-261, 266-267, 269, 271, 273-274, 276,
    278-279, 286-291, 293-294, 297, 300,
    332-333, 337-338, 345, 349-354, 356-358,
    360, 368, 376-377, 381, 409
Motor function, 38, 60, 71, 84, 124, 147, 174, 176,
    178-180, 182, 184, 186-188, 190, 193, 281
Motor vehicle collisions, 6, 42, 354
Motorcycle crashes, 264, 364-365
Mottled skin, 107, 310
Mucous membrane, 296, 322
Mucus, 24, 106, 200
Muscle tissue, 135, 137, 166-169, 234, 253, 305, 321,
    337, 352
Musculoskeletal injuries
    dislocation, 156, 173-174, 176-178, 188-189
    dislocations, 172-174, 178-179, 181, 188
    fracture, 156-157, 172-174, 176-178, 181, 188-189
    fractures, 155, 172-174, 177-179, 181, 188-189
    mechanism of, 140, 157, 173-174, 176, 189
    sprains, 172, 177-178, 188-189
    strain, 156, 177-178
    strains, 177-178, 189
Musculoskeletal system
    functions, 158
        muscles, 158, 172, 188
        skeletal tissue and structure, 158
        skeleton, 158
Musculoskeletal trauma
    femur fractures, 190
    splinting devices, 179
Mutual aid, 88
Myocardial contusion, 108
Myocardium, 102, 166, 226, 235-236, 309, 392
Myotome, 53, 71, 75, 86

N

Nails, 126, 332, 338, 369

Naloxone, 80, 189
Napalm, 370
Narcan, 80, 189
Narcotics, 80, 389
Nasal bone, 254-255, 271
Nasal cannula, 292-293
Nasal cavity, 96, 254-256, 269, 271, 282, 285
Nasal passage, 39, 277
Nasopharyngeal airways
Nasopharynx, 400
National Highway Traffic Safety Administration, 375
Natural gas, 367-368
Nausea and vomiting, 80, 96, 108, 189, 324, 388, 405
Near-drowning, 396, 408
Neck
   stabilizing, 2, 183, 251, 283
Neck wounds, 107, 111, 138, 145, 149, 278, 281, 285
Necrosis, 123, 137, 143, 148, 154, 176, 208, 234, 236, 238, 300, 306, 325, 327-328
Needle, 19, 27, 112, 148-149, 153, 224, 233, 244-245, 247-248, 318, 342-343, 345
Neisseria gonorrhoeae, 173
Nerve tissue, 304
Nerves, 53-54, 56-59, 61-63, 68, 71, 74, 82, 86, 95, 124-127, 129-131, 135, 142, 150, 153, 157, 159, 167, 169, 172, 174, 176, 178, 182, 184, 187-188, 194, 205, 225-226, 245, 255-259, 268, 272, 302, 305, 320, 356
Nervous system
   autonomic, 37, 53, 63, 69-71, 85, 90, 100-101, 166, 191, 384, 409
   dysfunction, 65, 71, 85, 98, 387
Net filtration, 92
Neuron, 85
Neutron radiation, 300, 306, 325, 328
Newborn, 38
Newton's second law of motion, 351
Nipple, 62, 205-206, 222, 237
Nitrogen narcosis, 380, 400-401, 403, 408, 410
Nonrebreather mask, 2, 19, 73, 78, 88-89, 292, 300, 331, 393, 402-403
Normal pulse, 73
Normal saline solution, 144, 198
Normal sinus rhythm, 198, 253
Nose, 30, 39, 53, 82, 108, 111, 119, 255, 257, 269, 277, 284-286, 288, 290-291, 293, 314, 334, 398, 410
Nosebleed, 96, 119, 271
Nostrils, 96, 255, 297
Nuclear detonation, 367
Nuclear radiation, 307, 327
Nucleus, 259-260, 306
Nutrition, 135, 390

O
Oblique, 156, 161, 165, 170-171, 191, 194, 199, 338, 349, 354, 358, 360-361, 364, 374, 377
Occipital bone, 254, 260
Occipital region, 56, 64, 67, 286
Occlusive dressing, 107, 111, 145, 149, 215, 244, 247, 285, 342
Occupational Safety and Health Administration (OSHA), 20, 157
Oculomotor nerve, 56, 58, 68, 74, 258
Ohm's law, 300, 304, 328
Old age, 390
Olecranon, 156, 162, 164, 172, 194
Ongoing assessments, 45
On-line medical direction, 81, 150, 315, 317
Onset of action, 80, 189
Open injuries, 124-125, 188
Open pneumothorax, 138, 149, 221, 227, 230-233, 240-241, 243-244, 339, 342-343
Open soft-tissue injury, 365
Open wounds
   abrasions, 124, 128-129, 151, 212, 294, 364
   avulsions, 124, 128-129, 151
   lacerations, 124, 128-129, 151, 294, 364
   punctures, 124, 128-129
Operations
   ambulance, 37
OPQRST, 142
Oral intubation, 282-283, 350
Orbit, 252, 255, 257, 272, 297
Organ, 16, 43, 66-67, 74, 82, 100, 103-104, 119, 124, 126, 140, 197, 200, 202-203, 205-208, 216-217, 226-227, 256, 258, 278, 302, 312-313, 337-340, 342, 352-356, 358, 371, 374-375, 403

Organ collision, 354-355
Organ system, 67, 403
Organism, 99, 101, 104, 120, 381, 388, 410
Organophosphates, 321
Oropharynx, 396-397
Orotracheal intubation, 277, 283
Orthopedic stretcher, 37, 141, 157, 184, 277, 285, 287-289
Orthostatic hypotension, 88, 109, 116, 120, 388
OSHA, 20, 157
Osmosis, 311
Osmotic pressure, 65, 98, 101
Osteoarthritis, 156, 173, 192, 194
Osteoblasts, 158-159, 172
Osteoclast, 156, 172, 194
Osteocytes, 158, 169
Osteoporosis, 156, 163, 171-172, 194, 279
Ovaries, 200, 202-203
Ovary, 203
Overdose, 136
Overdrive respiration, 88, 112, 120
Overhydration, 44, 94, 394
Overpressure, 65, 349, 368-370, 372, 375, 377, 380, 400-403, 408, 410
Oxidizer, 349, 367, 377
Oxygen
   administering, 214, 243, 319, 350, 372
   brain and, 54-55, 57, 66, 79
   cylinders, 158
   delivery system, 100
   therapy, 78-79, 94, 117-118, 216, 218, 231, 243-245, 319-320, 326, 376, 388, 394, 402
   use of, 42, 44, 78, 134, 157-158, 231, 239, 243, 284, 292, 308, 319, 392, 398, 400, 406
Oxygen saturation, 19, 27, 35, 42-43, 54, 73, 78, 89, 106, 198, 214, 234, 239, 242-243, 278, 282, 284-285, 292-293, 300-301, 315, 350, 371
Oxygen saturation (SpO2), 292, 315
Oxygen therapy, 118, 402
Oxygen transport, 79, 87, 92, 99, 309, 404-405
Oxygenation, 8, 14, 17, 27, 35-36, 66, 73-74, 81, 112, 134, 148, 150, 214, 239, 242-243, 245-246, 272, 277, 284, 397-398, 409

P
PaCO2, 396
Pain
   referred, 184, 207, 213, 218, 350
   response to, 26, 28, 31, 44, 63, 71, 73-74, 76-77, 84, 98, 103, 150, 152, 190, 193, 208, 213-214, 217-218, 229, 280, 296, 304, 327
   somatic, 191
   visceral, 207, 400, 403
Pale, 18, 27, 29, 71, 98, 103, 106-108, 123-124, 134-135, 142, 175, 222, 331, 392
Palmar, 311, 328
Palpation, 18-19, 28-30, 89, 124, 137, 142, 168, 175, 208, 211-214, 219, 222, 229, 252, 279, 281, 350, 395, 410
Pancreas, 103, 150, 199-201, 204-207, 212, 217, 338-340, 342, 352, 356, 374
Pancreatitis, 105
PaO2, 396
Paradoxical motion, 228, 240-241
Paradoxical movement, 230
Paramedic, 1-4, 8, 13-14, 17-18, 23, 32, 36, 48, 51, 83, 87-88, 90, 105, 121, 125, 128, 146, 148, 155, 157, 176, 180, 191-192, 197-198, 221, 246, 249, 251, 253, 269, 274, 299, 302, 309, 325, 329, 331, 344, 347, 349, 354, 364, 371, 375, 379, 381, 396
Paramedics, 1, 11, 13-14, 28, 45, 49, 53, 79, 89, 93-94, 123-124, 131, 150, 156-157, 198, 217, 222, 246-247, 252-253, 300, 335, 406-407
Parasympathetic nervous system, 58, 63, 90
Parathyroid glands, 258, 273
Parenchyma, 239
Parietal bone, 254
Parietal pleura, 224, 241, 245
Parking, 3
Parkland formula, 319, 325
Partial airway obstruction, 27
Partial pressure, 99, 112, 244, 403-404
PASG, 47, 88-89, 113-115, 117, 120, 136, 174, 178, 183-184, 190, 192, 216, 247

Passive rewarming, 393
Past medical history, 31, 109, 172, 176, 280
Patella, 159, 161, 163, 172, 186
Patent airway, 112, 147, 246, 282
Pathogens
   bloodborne, 173, 195
Pathophysiology
   heat and cold disorders, 381
Patient assessment
   scene safety and, 9, 173
Patient management, 26, 43, 45, 87, 112, 146, 177, 213-214, 243, 285
Patient positioning, 78, 283, 288, 290
Patient priority, 10-11, 278
Patient transport
   hemorrhage and, 107, 172, 182, 239
   indicators for immediate, 11
Patients
   approaching, 173, 274, 286, 314, 317
   chief complaint and, 109
   moving, 6, 9, 23, 28, 30, 73, 85, 95, 98, 112, 145, 172-173, 177, 188, 211-212, 215, 226, 228, 233, 238, 251, 256, 285-290, 293, 323, 343, 350, 367, 398
   transfer of, 410
Pediatric patients
   burn injuries, 313
   physical abuse, 313
Pedicles, 259, 263, 265-266, 352
PEEP, 99, 112, 229, 244, 398
Pelvic cavity, 42, 264, 339
Pelvic fractures, 42-43, 95, 108, 180, 183, 192
Pelvic space, 183, 197, 199, 208, 219
Pelvis, 4, 25, 29-31, 39, 59, 88-89, 96, 107-108, 114, 141, 155-156, 159, 161-163, 174, 180-181, 183-184, 186, 190-191, 193-194, 199, 203-204, 211-213, 259, 263-264, 266, 273, 285-286, 289-291, 296, 349-350, 360-361, 363-365, 367, 376
Penetrating trauma
   entrance and exit wounds, 213, 330, 341-342
   open pneumothorax, 227, 230, 233, 240-241, 339, 342-343
   tissue/organ injuries, 338
   wound assessment, 342
Penis, 82, 203
Perforating canals, 156, 158-159, 191, 194
Pericardial tamponade, 29-30, 99, 107-108, 112, 149, 221-223, 225, 227, 229, 234-237, 239, 241-245, 247, 249-250, 330, 339, 342-343, 345
Pericardium, 222, 225, 235-236, 249
Perineum, 70, 317
Periorbital ecchymosis, 30, 252, 269, 279, 294, 296
Periosteum, 55, 156, 158-159, 169, 171-172, 194, 294
Peripheral circulation, 100, 394
Peripheral nervous system, 54
Peripheral vascular resistance, 57-58, 63, 71, 86, 88, 90, 98, 100-104, 114, 118-120
Peristalsis, 197, 219
Peritoneal space, 150, 197, 199, 205-206, 208, 219, 340
Peritoneum, 150, 197, 200, 202, 205-208, 219
Peritonitis, 31, 197, 205, 208, 211-212, 214, 219, 372
Personal protective equipment (PPE)
   gloves, 24
Personal safety, 332, 345
Personnel, 8, 16, 20, 24, 36, 45-47, 111, 118, 141, 146-147, 214, 216, 275, 282, 290, 313-315, 317, 319-323, 332, 341, 356-357, 362-363, 366, 368-371, 373, 385, 398, 403
Perspiration, 382, 384, 387, 409
Phagocytosis, 123, 133, 154
Phalanges, 131, 156, 159, 161-163, 187-188, 194
Pharmacological interventions, 114
Pharynx, 39, 58, 149, 201, 256, 270, 277, 283-285
Phosphate, 137, 158
Physical abuse, 313
Physical exam
   abdomen, 29-31, 252, 278
   detailed, 29-31, 109, 140, 142, 173, 176, 313
   lower back, 157
   neck, 29-31, 74, 157, 252, 278
   rapid, 28-31, 74, 109, 140, 142, 173, 176, 278, 313, 349
Physical examination
   back, 31, 117, 152, 192, 295, 326
   neck injuries, 149
   techniques, 31

ater, 53-55, 60, 65, 82, 86
 splint, 187
, 252, 256, 271, 292, 297, 372
 joint, 160
nta previa, 97
, 136, 160, 274, 286, 288, 290-291
ar, 75, 175, 187, 252
na, 29, 35-36, 42, 92, 97, 99-100, 102, 105, 117, 120, 154, 247, 304, 311, 396, 399
na losses, 105
et phase, 88, 93, 119-120, 132, 153
lets, 36-37, 93-95, 113, 119-120, 132, 152-153, 324
ra, 149, 205, 224-226, 238, 241, 245, 400, 403
al space, 27, 29, 149, 230-233, 244-245, 249, 340, 372, 377, 410
us, 58, 62, 258, 271
matic anti-shock garment (PASG), 47, 88, 114, 120, 174
matic splints, 110
motaxic center, 225
mothorax
 simple, 99, 107, 149-150, 223, 227, 230-233, 241, 244-245, 402
 ension, 27, 29-30, 36-37, 39, 44, 99, 107, 112, 149-150, 216, 221-224, 227, 230-233, 238-239, 241-250, 273, 294, 339-340, 342-343, 377, 402, 410
, 92
son control center, 404
s, 53, 56, 58, 67, 82, 85-86, 225
liteal artery, 186
ition of function, 145, 178, 182, 185-186, 188, 190, 193, 286
itive end expiratory pressure (PEEP), 99, 229, 244
sterior, 29, 39, 56-62, 68, 79, 86, 96, 101, 119, 135-136, 141, 150, 157, 161-164, 167, 175, 183, 185-187, 194, 199-200, 202, 205-206, 210, 219, 224, 226, 228-229, 233, 236, 243-244, 252, 254-260, 262-264, 266-267, 269, 271-272, 278-279, 282, 285-286, 297, 300, 310-312, 315, 331, 352-353, 396
sterior hip dislocation, 186
sterior tibial pulse, 157
sture, 26, 59, 73
sturing, 26, 54, 60, 65, 67-69, 74, 77, 81, 387
tassium, 95, 103, 118-119, 129, 137, 148, 312-313, 387, 394
wder burns, 344
ecordium, 222, 235-236, 249
eload, 31, 44, 63, 71, 80, 88, 90, 92, 100, 102-104, 120, 189, 204
eschooler, 107
eschoolers, 39
essure dressing, 135
essure points, 110, 145
essure wave, 226, 233, 336-339, 341, 343, 349, 368-371, 377
evention
 cancer, 3, 14
evention strategies, 157
iapism, 69-71, 78, 82-83
rimary blast injuries, 370-371
riority determination, 10
rocardia, 405-406
rojectiles
 injury process, 206, 265, 340
rone, 39-40, 44, 48, 78, 98, 125, 148, 167, 172, 207-209, 216, 239, 254-255, 269, 271, 286-288, 290, 292, 309, 334, 363, 367, 372
rone position, 288, 290
rostate gland, 202-203
rotective equipment
 personal, 24, 28, 173, 314
rotective eyewear, 173
rotective gear, 158, 274, 323, 373
rotocol, 13, 23, 72, 81, 190, 251, 275-277, 281, 285, 297, 319, 380, 392, 398
rotocols
 communication, 373
roximal, 110-111, 143, 152, 162-163, 171, 178, 180, 182, 184-188, 193-194, 207, 213, 318
sychosis, 387
Pubis, 150, 156, 162-163, 174, 183, 194, 203, 212
Pulmonary artery, 225-226, 233, 237, 249
Pulmonary circulation, 100, 107, 170, 225, 371, 404
Pulmonary contusion, 29, 229-230, 233-234, 240-244, 247, 359-360
Pulmonary edema

high altitude, 404-406, 409
Pulmonary embolism, 106, 172
Pulmonary hilum, 222, 224, 249
Pulmonary injuries
 hemothorax, 221, 230
 simple pneumothorax, 230
Pulmonary vein, 225
Pulmonary veins, 224-225, 400
Pulse
 brachial, 187, 247
 carotid, 27, 41, 107, 112, 116, 222
 distal, 29, 31, 35, 38, 53-54, 68, 108, 124, 144, 168-169, 176, 178-180, 182, 187, 190, 193, 242, 274, 281, 284, 300, 318-319
 irregular, 67-68, 73-74, 76, 85, 214, 235, 280, 285, 294, 326, 403
 posterior tibial, 157
 radial, 2, 18, 26-27, 187, 222, 247, 350
Pulse oximeter, 27, 53-54, 89, 106, 145, 149-150, 157, 179, 239, 253, 292, 319, 331, 350
Pulse oximetry, 19, 52, 73, 78, 214, 222, 240, 242-243, 277-278, 283-285, 315, 319, 388
Pulse pressure, 31, 35-36, 68, 76, 78, 85, 88, 90-91, 97-98, 103, 106-107, 109, 112, 114, 120, 212, 214, 232, 235-236, 239, 280, 403
Pulse rate, 19, 31, 35-36, 42, 67-68, 73-74, 76, 88-89, 97, 103-104, 109, 112, 118, 120, 123, 210, 212, 214, 216, 253, 274, 278, 280-281
Pulsus paradoxus, 222, 236, 242, 250
Puncture, 61, 123, 130, 134, 138, 152, 154, 342, 344, 395
Pupils, 54, 56, 67-68, 74, 81, 108, 124, 391
Pyrexia, 380, 388, 410
Pyrogens, 380, 388, 410
Pyruvic acid, 99, 118, 120, 394

Q

QRS complex, 68, 148, 392
Quality improvement (QI), 13
Quality management (QM), 13
Quiet, 18, 212, 225

R

Raccoon eyes, 30, 269, 279, 294, 296
Rad, 300, 308, 324, 328
Radial pulse, 2, 18, 26-27, 350
Radiation, 23, 126, 167, 172, 240, 299-300, 302-303, 306-308, 310, 320, 322-325, 327-328, 371, 380, 382, 389, 410
Radiation burns, 322, 324
Radioactive contamination, 369, 371
Radioactive materials, 306
Radius, 155-156, 159, 161-162, 178, 185, 194, 367
Rapid extrication, 18, 246, 288, 290
Rapid trauma assessment
 general examination, 28
Reabsorption, 65, 118, 148
Rear-end impact, 360, 374
Reassessment, 10-11, 25, 35, 46, 54, 78, 109, 143, 148, 176, 198, 214, 222, 239, 242, 281, 318, 323
Rebound tenderness, 29-30, 197, 208, 216, 219
Receptor, 101
Recompression, 380, 402-403, 410
Recovery position, 73, 79, 96
Rectum, 71, 97, 108-109, 183, 199-202, 204-205, 207-208, 217, 384, 407
Recumbent, 43, 213-214, 216, 277, 372
Red blood cells, 19, 42, 47, 90, 92, 94, 99-100, 102-103, 110, 113, 119-120, 158, 172, 217, 222, 292, 404
Red bone marrow, 156, 195
Reduction, 6, 8, 35, 44, 66, 105, 118, 156, 171, 176-177, 182, 186-190, 192, 195, 227, 243, 282, 309, 335, 400-401, 408-409
Referred pain, 207, 218
Renal artery and vein, 202
Renin, 102, 118
Research
 trauma registry, 11
Resiliency, 231, 330, 338-339, 345
Resistance, 43-44, 57-58, 63, 66, 71, 75, 86, 88, 90, 96, 98, 100-104, 113-114, 118-120, 167, 178, 182, 193, 275, 286, 300, 304-305, 328, 333, 369, 398
Resolution phase, 300, 304-305, 325, 328
Respect, 1, 36, 38, 72, 187
Respiration

diaphragm and, 207, 224
 overdrive, 27, 88, 112, 120, 240
Respiratory acidosis, 398
Respiratory arrest, 305, 309, 315, 319, 321
Respiratory cycle, 112, 236
Respiratory distress
 abnormal breathing patterns, 404
Respiratory failure, 233-234
Respiratory rates, 38-39, 392
Respiratory sounds, 232
Respiratory system
 of infants and children, 39
Response
 primary, 2, 10-11, 24, 26-28, 30, 32, 48, 63, 65, 68, 74, 140-141, 153, 174, 190, 210, 275, 281, 313, 331, 368
 secondary, 10-11, 26, 28, 36, 65-66, 68, 73-74, 97, 141, 174, 176, 229, 305, 366, 368
Response time, 10
Restraint, 5, 9, 11, 125, 157, 355-360, 362-363, 366
Retina, 58, 252, 257, 272, 297
Retraction, 29
Retractions, 30, 239-241, 247
Retroauricular ecchymosis, 30, 252, 269, 279, 294, 297
Retrograde, 53, 65, 67, 72, 78, 81-82, 86, 183, 283
Retroperitoneal, 150, 183, 197, 199-200, 205, 207-208, 212-213, 219, 340
Retroperitoneal space, 150, 197, 199-200, 205, 219, 340
Revised trauma score, 32, 34, 48
Rewarming, 37, 392-395, 398
Rewarming shock, 392, 394
Rhonchi, 398
Rib fracture, 208, 226, 228-231, 233-234, 240-241, 247, 350
Rib fractures, 18, 43-44, 112, 213, 221, 226, 228-229, 233, 241, 243, 335, 358
Rib injuries, 81
Ribs, 18, 30, 129, 159, 161, 163, 199, 207, 223-224, 228-230, 240-241, 245, 262-263, 295, 340, 350, 352, 360, 376
Rifle, 23, 169, 211, 231, 271, 332-338, 340-341, 343-345
Right, 2-3, 5-6, 18-19, 34, 39-40, 48, 56, 59, 61, 124, 150, 157, 160, 176, 186, 191, 199-200, 202, 204, 207-208, 210-211, 216-218, 222-226, 229, 234-238, 255, 258-263, 279, 283, 300, 312, 352, 354, 360
Right lower quadrant, 199, 217
Right mainstem bronchus, 39-40
Right time, 176
Right upper quadrant, 199-200, 217
Rigid splints, 179, 181, 184, 186-187, 192
Ring-type degloving injury, 131
Riot control agents, 322
Roller bandage, 139, 144
Rollover, 6, 23, 247, 354, 358, 360, 362-363, 366, 374
Rotation, 26, 72, 160, 162-163, 166, 168, 176, 178, 183, 187, 260-261, 266, 277, 286-287, 290, 334, 357, 360, 372
Rotation injury, 266
Rouleaux, 88, 103, 119-120
Route, 2, 11, 14, 18-19, 23-24, 46, 54, 109, 141, 143, 174, 176, 198, 214, 222, 243, 245, 247, 265, 268-269, 283, 285, 300, 318, 331, 341-342, 349-350, 380, 386-387
Rule of nines, 300, 310-311, 315, 328
Rule of palms, 300, 310-311, 315, 328
Rupture of the aorta, 237, 247

S

Sacral region, 63
Sacral spine, 43, 260, 264, 273
Sacrum, 60, 159, 161-163, 183, 193, 252, 259-260, 264, 266, 296-297
Saddle joint, 160
Safety
 aircraft and, 11
 roadway, 5
 scene, 4-6, 9, 11, 20, 23, 25, 28, 106, 125, 147, 156, 173, 290, 313, 320, 332, 345, 357
Safety seats, 356-357
Saline lock, 113, 239, 403
Salivary glands, 256
Scalp, 54, 107, 110-111, 130, 134, 144-145, 251, 253-254, 265, 267-268, 292
Scan

cervical collar, 54
Scapula, 156, 161-162, 187, 194-195, 223, 227-228, 367
Scene safety
 ensuring, 125, 147, 290
Scene size-up
 mechanism of injury and, 2, 140, 176, 211
 number of patients, 14, 24, 28, 371
School-age children, 39, 125
Sclera, 252, 257, 279, 297
Scoop (orthopedic) stretcher, 107
Scoop stretcher, 289, 295
Scoop stretchers, 295
Scrotum, 203
Scuba, 8, 14, 380, 398-400, 403, 407-410
Seat belts, 5-6, 20, 23, 42, 199, 211, 253, 349, 355-357, 362, 374
Sebaceous glands, 123, 126, 151, 154, 301
Sebum, 123, 126, 154, 301
Secondary blast injuries, 371
Secondary collisions, 354-356, 364
Secondary impacts, 333, 335
Second-degree burn, 310, 328
Secretion, 102, 154, 302
Sedatives, 79, 81, 188, 292, 315, 389
Seizure, 78
Sellick maneuver, 282
Semicircular canals, 252, 256, 271, 297, 372
Sensation, 2, 28-30, 35, 38, 58-59, 69-71, 74-75, 78, 81-82, 84-85, 108, 124, 142, 147, 159, 169, 174-180, 182, 184-188, 190, 193, 213, 229, 247, 252, 255-256, 271-272, 280-281, 293, 301-302, 315-316, 318, 320, 324, 395, 410
Sensory nerves, 59, 68
Septic shock, 88, 105, 116, 120
Septum, 225, 236, 255, 271
Sesamoid bone, 156, 159, 195
Shock
 airway and breathing management, 112
 anaphylactic, 88, 105, 108, 118
 cardiogenic, 88, 105, 108, 114, 116, 119, 234, 241
 case study, 53, 88, 380
 classifying, 104
 compensated, 28, 87-88, 103-105, 116, 119
 decompensated, 87-88, 103-105, 116-117, 119
 development of, 6, 36, 39, 42, 112, 150-151, 280, 296
 fluid resuscitation, 27, 35-36, 43, 47-49, 79-80, 94, 98, 113-114, 116, 144, 147-148, 174, 204, 208, 214, 216, 318
 hemorrhagic, 89, 98, 105, 108-109, 296
 hypovolemic, 28, 47, 74, 80, 88, 92, 98-100, 105, 114, 120, 137, 148, 214, 240, 388
 neurogenic, 35, 53, 70-71, 80-81, 85-86, 88, 99, 105, 108, 116, 120, 253
 patterns, 5, 70-71
 pharmacological intervention, 114
 preventing, 5, 36, 148, 150, 239, 247, 318
 septic, 88, 105, 108, 116, 120, 173
 temperature control, 38, 70, 114
 tilt test, 88, 109, 116, 120
Short bones, 159
Short spine board, 277, 288-289
Shotgun, 23, 206, 210-211, 227, 231, 241, 271, 283, 336, 339-343
Shoulder girdle, 161, 187, 193
Shoulder injuries, 187
Shunt, 384
Side effect, 135, 308
Side effects, 80, 189
Side impact, 199, 211, 229
Sign, 11, 29-31, 34, 39, 49, 65, 67-68, 75-76, 78, 89, 96, 103, 106-109, 112, 128, 148-149, 157, 174-176, 188, 207-208, 212, 214, 218, 236, 241-242, 267, 269, 274, 279, 285, 294-295, 297, 351, 371
Signs and symptoms
 respiratory difficulty, 233
Simple pneumothorax, 149, 230-231, 233, 241, 244
Sinus, 53, 56-57, 65, 119, 157, 198, 235, 253, 271-272, 407
Sinus bradycardia, 407
Sinus tachycardia, 235
Skeletal injuries, 72, 267
Skeletal muscle, 37, 123, 127, 129, 137, 148, 154, 166, 172, 188, 250
Skeletal organization, 161
Skeleton
 bones of the, 39, 161, 193

Skin
 color, 18, 29, 31, 35, 48, 59, 72, 107-108, 133, 141-142, 144, 153, 179, 185, 187, 222, 239-240, 242-243, 284, 292, 310, 316, 331
 condition, 19, 27, 29-31, 35, 54, 71, 97-98, 106-109, 130, 137, 141-142, 167, 176, 179, 194, 214, 229, 232, 238, 279, 285, 313, 324, 331, 338, 372, 384-385, 388, 407
 lesions, 69
 of the scalp, 54, 292
 temperature, 29, 31, 35, 44, 59, 69-70, 76, 114, 118-119, 126-127, 133, 141-142, 144, 158, 167, 169, 179, 187, 253, 301-303, 309, 311, 318, 338, 382-385, 387-390, 392, 394, 399, 407
 turgor, 388
Skin temperature, 29, 31, 179, 187, 253, 302, 384
Skull
 bones of the human, 254
Skull fractures, 256, 268, 374
Sling and swathe, 181, 185, 187-188
Slings, 140, 180
Small intestine, 201, 204-205, 219
Smoke inhalation, 326
Smooth muscle, 93-94, 101, 119, 127, 166, 258
Snoring, 18, 27
Sodium, 80, 102, 118, 137, 148, 202, 246, 312, 319-322, 373, 384-385
Sodium bicarbonate, 148, 246, 321, 373
Soft palate, 255, 277
Soft splints, 180
Soft tissue trauma, 152
Soft-tissue injuries
 closed injuries, 124-125
 dressings and bandages, 281
 eviscerations, 150
 open injuries, 124-125
Soft-tissue trauma
 face and neck, 123, 148-149
Somatic nervous system, 166
Spalding effect, 234
Sperm, 203, 308
Sphenoid bone, 254
Sphygmomanometer, 144
Spinal canal, 59-60, 70, 252, 259-260, 262, 266, 273, 295, 297
Spinal column, 31, 54-55, 59-61, 70, 72, 74-76, 81, 85, 204, 206-207, 227, 251, 253, 255, 259-261, 263-267, 270, 273-282, 285-286, 292-294, 297, 340, 357, 372
Spinal curvature, 171
Spinal injuries
 alignment, 287
Spinal meninges, 53, 60, 86
Spinal nerves, 53, 61-63, 82, 86
Spinal trauma
 final patient positioning, 288, 290
 helmet removal, 288
 log roll, 277, 286, 288-289
 standing takedown, 287
 vest-type immobilization device, 274, 287, 289-290
Spine
 curvature of the, 163, 279, 296
Spinous process, 59, 259-263, 295
Spleen, 150, 198-202, 204-207, 210-211, 217-218, 229, 247, 337-340, 342, 344, 352, 356, 374
Splint, 18, 112, 136, 144-145, 148, 175-188, 190-193, 212, 243, 291, 295
Splinting
 ankle and foot injuries, 180
 materials, 110, 343
 position of function, 178, 182, 185, 190, 193
Splinting devices, 178-179, 182
Splints, 45, 49, 110, 140, 148, 179-181, 184, 186-188, 192, 230
SpO2, 27, 239, 292, 315
Sports helmets, 288
Sports injuries, 3, 6, 72, 135, 157-158, 276, 354, 372-374
Sprain, 156, 168-169, 177-178, 190-191, 195, 353
Sprains, 168, 170, 172, 175, 177-178, 187-190
ST segment, 235, 388
S-T segment, 68, 148
Stabbing, 3, 341
Standard of care, 106, 180
Standard precautions, 9, 22-24, 105, 141, 173, 211, 239, 274, 312, 325

Standing takedown, 287
Staphylococcus aureus, 133
Starling's law of the heart, 102
Sterile, 107, 111, 124, 134-135, 138-139, 149, 161, 177, 215, 244, 284, 292-293, 312, 318, 326, 372, 395
Sterile dressing, 124, 138, 177, 215, 292-293, 326, 372
Sternoclavicular dislocation, 221, 243
Sternum, 129, 135, 159-162, 185, 191, 194, 199, 222-224, 228-229, 234, 243, 245, 247, 249-250, 258, 340, 356, 367
Stomach, 31, 96, 108, 150, 198-202, 204-205, 207-209, 211-213, 219, 256, 258, 339, 374, 385, 387, 396
Stored energy, 57
Strain, 156, 167-168, 177-178, 190, 195
Strains, 175, 177-178, 189-190
Stress
 response, 34, 37, 44, 63, 102, 150, 304
Stretch receptors, 63
Striated muscle, 166
Stridor, 27, 229, 309, 314
Stroke volume, 37, 39, 44, 88, 90, 102, 120
Structural collapse, 314, 368-371, 373
Stylet, 283
Styloid process, 254
Subarachnoid space, 55, 60, 64-65
Subcutaneous emphysema, 29-30, 107, 134, 142, 149, 213, 232, 238, 240-242, 246, 273, 284, 294, 341, 402
Subcutaneous fatty tissue, 302
Subcutaneous layer, 126
Subcutaneous tissue, 123-126, 154, 158, 169, 255, 284, 301-303, 310, 353
Subdural hematoma, 53, 64-65, 86
Subglottic, 300, 309, 328
Sucking chest wound, 227, 231, 339-340
Suction, 73, 79, 112, 149, 180, 277, 282-283, 285, 293, 337, 398
Sudden death, 137, 235, 241
Sudoriferous glands, 123, 126, 151, 154, 301
Sugar, 185
Suicide, 4-5, 31, 265, 271, 340, 363, 369
Summation, 9
Superficial burn, 300, 309-310, 328
Superficial burns, 328
Superficial frostbite, 380, 395, 410
Superficial frostbite (frostnip), 395
Superior, 56-57, 65, 127, 162, 202, 204, 208, 211, 224-225, 238, 249, 254, 259-264, 282, 285, 294, 296
Superior vena cava, 57, 127, 225, 238, 249
Supine, 30, 39, 42-43, 96, 107, 109, 120, 185-186, 197, 204, 207, 209, 212, 219, 222, 233, 243-244, 270, 282, 284, 286-291, 293, 300, 320, 386-388, 393, 402-403
Supine hypotensive syndrome, 197, 204, 219
Supine position, 243, 286-287, 289-291, 293, 386-388, 393, 402-403
Supplemental oxygen, 27, 35, 42-43, 50, 78, 116-117, 239, 243-245, 278, 292, 300, 386, 388, 406
Supplemental restraint systems (SRS), 356, 359
Supraglottic, 74, 79, 283, 300, 309, 328, 398
Surfactant, 380, 396-398, 410
Survival, 10-11, 13, 15, 19, 47, 49, 97-98, 116-117, 152, 235, 246, 282, 321, 338, 383, 391, 397
Swathe, 181, 185, 187-188
Swathes, 140
Sweat glands, 387
Sweating, 59, 70-71, 85, 102, 105, 383-385, 387-388
Swelling, 27, 30, 67-69, 71, 79, 108, 126, 129, 133, 135, 140, 142, 144-146, 148, 150-152, 167-168, 170, 172-175, 177, 179, 182, 187-188, 191, 193, 198, 206, 208, 240, 254, 258, 262, 267, 270-271, 273, 277-279, 281, 314, 318-319, 340, 395
Sympathetic nervous system, 63, 69, 90, 101, 114
Symphysis pubis, 150, 162-163, 174, 183, 203, 212
Symptom, 31, 107-108, 148, 174, 228, 233, 238, 274, 279, 371, 401
Symptoms
 acute mountain sickness, 405
 arterial gas embolism, 400-402, 409
 cardiac disease, 44
 cyanide poisoning, 319
 dehydration, 67, 101, 137, 147, 385, 388, 406, 409
 heat (muscle) cramps, 385
 high altitude cerebral edema, 405-406

h altitude pulmonary edema, 404-406, 409
ogen narcosis, 400-401, 403
eumomediastinum, 241, 400-403
pe, 109, 309
ial capsule, 161
ial fluid, 156, 161, 167, 193-195
ial joint, 156, 173, 194-195
ges, 388
mic, 43, 57, 63, 66, 85, 94, 98, 102, 105, 129,
    133, 137-138, 142, 147, 153, 173, 178,
    224-225, 232, 236-237, 258, 299, 311, 318,
    400
le, 118
lic blood pressure, 32, 34, 36, 48, 66-67, 74, 76,
    78-80, 89, 91, 95, 98, 102-103, 109-111, 113,
    120, 144, 183, 214, 224, 236, 243-245, 250,
    280, 294
lic pressure, 85, 107, 236

ve, 388
ts, 385, 387, 407
ycardia
ctopic, 97
nus, 235
ypnea, 85, 97-98, 103, 106, 231, 304, 309, 390,
    401, 405
e, 140, 145-146, 179, 244, 291, 318
als, 159, 161, 163
chable moment, 5-6
perature
ore body, 50, 383-384, 387, 390, 410
perature regulation, 36, 44, 85, 302, 383, 387, 410
poral bone, 254, 256, 268
poromandibular joint, 256, 270
derness, 27, 29-31, 69, 107-108, 134, 142, 157,
    172, 175-176, 197, 208, 214, 216, 219, 252,
    275-276, 279
don, 29, 161, 163-164, 166-169, 172, 175, 177,
    182, 188, 195, 225
dons, 59, 123-127, 129-131, 133, 150, 154,
    156-157, 159, 161-163, 166-169, 172,
    177-178, 188, 190-191, 265, 267, 302, 338,
    372, 401
sion pneumothorax, 27, 29-30, 36-37, 39, 44, 99,
    107, 112, 149-150, 216, 221-224, 227,
    230-233, 238-239, 241-250, 273, 294,
    339-340, 342-343, 377, 402, 410
m, 42-43, 56-57, 65, 71, 78, 129, 158, 177, 185,
    188, 209, 216, 253, 274, 292, 301, 308
tiary blast injuries, 371
stes, 203
stis, 203
tanus vaccine, 135
alamus, 53, 56, 86
ermal gradient, 380-381, 410
ermogenesis, 380-381, 389-390, 407, 410
ermolysis, 380, 382, 384, 387-388, 410
ermometers, 383, 388, 390
ermoreceptors, 383, 388
ermoregulation, 379-380, 383-384, 389, 410
ermoregulatory thermogenesis, 381
niamine
chronic alcoholism, 80
high, 2, 62, 129, 135, 144, 157-158, 162, 167-169,
    174, 186, 290, 304, 312, 373
Third space" losses, 105
hird-degree burn, 303, 310, 327
horacic cavity, 101, 207, 215, 223-226, 230, 237,
    239, 244, 340, 358
horacic duct, 239, 247
horacic skeleton, 223
horacic trauma
    aortic rupture, 223, 228, 237, 247
    cardiovascular injuries, 221, 234
    chest wall contusion, 228-229, 247
    penetrating injury, 226, 233, 235, 238-239, 241,
        244
    pericardial tamponade, 221-223, 225, 227, 229,
        234-237, 239, 241-245, 247, 249-250
    pulmonary contusion, 229-230, 233-234, 240-244,
        247
    pulmonary injuries, 221, 230
    rib fracture, 226, 228-231, 233-234, 240-241, 247
    tracheobronchial injury, 221, 238, 241, 243, 246
    traumatic asphyxia, 221, 226, 238-241, 243,
        246-247
Thoracic vertebrae, 252, 259, 262-263, 297
Thorax, 18, 43, 53, 123, 145, 147-149, 161-162, 183,

187, 193, 205-207, 212-213, 221, 223-226,
    228, 230-234, 238, 240, 244, 250, 263, 266,
    285-287, 297, 300, 316, 339-340, 342, 360,
    363, 367
Thready pulse, 27, 79, 236
Throat, 271, 280
Thyroid, 258, 273, 279, 282-284, 342, 345, 381
Thyroid cartilage, 258, 279, 282-284
Thyroid gland, 258, 284, 381
Tibia, 40, 89, 95, 107-108, 136, 155-156, 159, 161,
    163, 169, 171, 177-178, 184, 186, 195, 365,
    367
Tidal volume, 27, 42-43, 204, 230, 233, 312, 315
Tilt test, 88, 109, 116, 120
Tinnitus, 401
Tissue
    connective, 54-55, 92, 124, 126, 130, 133, 153,
        155, 159-160, 166-168, 173, 175, 182,
        184, 188, 190-191, 194-195, 253-255,
        265, 267, 294, 296, 302, 338, 353, 356,
        360, 372-373
    epithelial, 132-133, 153
    muscle, 29, 39, 59, 69, 71, 74-75, 79, 86, 94-95,
        100, 119-120, 123-127, 129-130, 132,
        135, 137, 141-142, 144, 148, 152-154,
        155, 163, 166-169, 171-176, 182, 184,
        188, 191, 193-195, 206, 208, 226,
        229-230, 234, 240, 253-255, 258, 271,
        279, 302, 305, 310, 314, 321, 327,
        337-340, 352-353, 372-373, 401
    nerve, 54, 57, 59, 63-65, 67-69, 71, 74-75, 85-86,
        102, 119, 125-126, 147, 159, 167-169,
        172, 182, 225, 229, 239, 255-258, 265,
        267, 273, 279, 301-302, 304, 310
Toddler, 40
Toddlers, 39
Tolerance, 28, 44, 61, 405
Torso, 72, 111, 145, 187, 213, 252-253, 266, 289-290,
    295, 357, 362
Total blood volume, 90, 98, 100, 119, 233
Touching, 142, 175, 321, 382
Tourniquet, 35, 87-88, 95, 111-112, 117-118, 120, 124,
    143-144, 146, 148-149, 152, 318
Tourniquets, 95, 111, 144
Toxic inhalation, 308, 314-315, 319
Toxin, 135
Toxins
    cardiac drugs, 148
Trachea, 30, 38-40, 110-112, 145, 201, 222-226, 229,
    231, 235, 239-241, 243, 246, 250, 258, 265,
    273, 277, 279, 282-284, 287, 296, 340,
    342-343
Tracheobronchial injury, 221, 238, 241, 243, 246
Tracheostomy, 41
Traction splint, 178, 180-181, 184, 192
Traction splints, 49, 180, 184, 192
Tractors, 321
Trajectory, 244, 330, 333, 343-345, 364
Transport, 2-4, 7-11, 13-15, 17, 19-20, 23, 25, 28-29,
    31-32, 34, 36-39, 41, 46-49, 54, 71, 73-74,
    76, 78-79, 84, 87-88, 92, 95-96, 99, 103,
    105-113, 117, 119, 123-124, 132, 140-148,
    150, 156-158, 172-174, 176-179, 181-184,
    186-187, 189-190, 192-193, 198, 200,
    210-216, 218, 239, 243-247, 253, 267, 274,
    277-281, 285-287, 290-293, 300-301, 306,
    309, 313-315, 317-323, 325-326, 331, 336,
    342-343, 350, 367, 371-373, 376, 387-389,
    393-395, 398, 402-406
Transport protocols, 403
Transverse process, 259-263, 295
Trauma
    penetrating, 1, 3, 7, 16, 23, 32, 38, 41, 47, 54, 63,
        69-72, 79, 81, 95, 99, 107, 111, 114, 117,
        124, 128, 130, 137, 141, 143, 149-150,
        157, 166-168, 187, 197-199, 205-209,
        211-213, 215-218, 221, 223-224,
        226-228, 230-231, 233-242, 244-247,
        251, 264-267, 270, 272-273, 276-277,
        295, 301, 306-307, 327-328, 329-345,
        350, 352-353, 356, 369, 371-372, 374
Trauma Care Systems Planning and Development Act
    of 1990, 7
Trauma center
    specialty centers, 8
Trauma registry, 1, 11, 16, 83
Trauma triage criteria, 1-2, 4, 8, 11, 13, 16, 24-25,
    28-29, 32, 37, 140
Traumatic asphyxia, 30, 221, 226, 238-241, 243,

246-247
Treatment
    trench foot, 395, 410
Treatment protocols, 192
Trench foot (immersion foot), 395
Trendelenburg position, 79
Trending, 35, 37, 47
Triage protocols, 8, 13
Trial, 83, 217
Triangular bandages, 140
Triaxial joints, 160
Trimester, 18, 42, 203-204, 210, 213, 216
Trochlear nerve, 58, 258
Tuberculosis, 96
Turbinates, 255
Turgor, 388
Turnout gear, 300

U

Ulna, 155-156, 159, 161-162, 178, 185, 194-195, 367
Unit, 24, 45, 53-54, 79, 112, 177, 181, 224, 288, 301,
    327-328, 349, 366, 388, 399
Units, 18, 97, 189, 300, 308-309, 357, 383
Up-and-over pathway, 358-359
Upper airway, 149, 277, 282-284, 309, 328
Upper extremities
    bones, 135, 157, 161-162, 263, 367
Upper respiratory infection, 400
Ureter, 202
Ureters, 150, 200, 202, 208
Urethra, 97, 183, 200, 202-203, 208
Urinary bladder, 150, 183, 199-200, 202-203, 205,
    207, 217, 338-339, 352, 356
Urinary system, 200, 202
Uterine rupture, 42, 209-210, 214
Uterus, 19, 42-43, 200, 202-205, 207-210, 213-214,
    216, 219

V

Vaccinations, 45, 151-152
Vacuum splints, 180
Vagina, 108, 200, 202-203, 208
Vagus nerve, 58, 63, 67, 225, 239, 258, 273
Valium, 78-79, 188
Vas deferens, 203
Vascular phase, 88, 93, 119-120, 132, 153
Vasopressin, 101
Vein, 35, 88, 91, 107-108, 113, 120, 125, 127, 132,
    138, 145, 147, 153, 159, 189, 202, 225, 236,
    240-242, 244, 246, 255, 257-258, 273, 281,
    285, 302, 340
Veins, 18, 30, 36, 40, 44, 57, 71, 90-92, 95, 97,
    107-108, 119, 126-127, 129, 132, 147, 169,
    183, 208, 222, 224-226, 232-233, 235-236,
    238-241, 249, 254, 258, 268, 273, 328, 340,
    383-384, 400, 404
Velocity, 23, 95, 170, 205-206, 211, 223, 227, 231,
    233-234, 241, 247, 330, 332-338, 343, 349,
    351-354, 366, 369, 376-377
Vena cava, 42-43, 57, 101, 119, 127, 150, 204-205,
    208-209, 213, 216, 219, 224-225, 230, 232,
    237-238, 249, 340
Venae cavae, 237, 352, 367
Venous bleeding, 95, 274
Venous hemorrhage, 92-93, 117, 209, 278
Venous system, 44, 90, 100, 102, 104, 113, 170, 172,
    258
Ventilating the patient, 35, 73, 106
Ventral, 60, 62
Ventricles, 55, 57, 60, 97, 102, 120
Ventricular fibrillation, 148, 235, 305, 321, 380,
    391-392, 394, 397, 407
Venules, 90-91, 93, 102, 119-120, 126, 129
Versed, 78
Vertebrae, 59, 62, 71-72, 159, 252, 259-267, 273, 279,
    294, 296-297, 353, 360, 367
Vertebral body, 59, 259, 261-262, 265-266, 295
Vertebral column
    divisions of the, 260
Vertigo, 256, 271, 401, 403
Very high altitude, 404
Vessels, 47, 55, 57-58, 63-66, 80, 90, 92-93, 95-96,
    98, 100, 103, 105, 107, 110, 119-120, 124,
    126-134, 136-137, 142-144, 149-150,
    152-153, 157-159, 166-167, 169-170, 172,
    174, 178, 182-184, 186-188, 191, 194, 205,
    208-209, 222-223, 225-227, 229, 237-241,
    245, 249, 253-255, 257-258, 260, 265,

267-268, 271, 273, 278-279, 287, 294, 296,
301-302, 305-306, 311, 316, 318, 320, 328,
335-340, 342, 352-353, 356, 368, 371, 373,
376, 383, 394-395, 401, 405
Vest-type immobilization device, 107, 274, 287,
289-290
VF, 393
Vial, 189
Vials, 189
Violence, 3, 9, 16, 22-23, 42, 49, 72, 106, 157, 199,
239, 264-265, 270, 341
Violent patients, 9
Viruses, 173, 388, 410
Visceral pericardium, 225, 249
Visceral pleura, 224, 400, 403
Vital signs
baseline, 28-29, 31, 35, 108, 124, 141-142, 174,
213, 281, 315
measurement of, 176
pulse oximetry and, 242
Vitreous humor, 252, 257, 272, 297
Vocal cords, 58
Voltage, 300, 304, 314, 317, 321, 328, 362
Voluntary muscle, 392

W

Warfarin, 31, 78, 94-95, 98, 109, 135, 141
Warfarin (Coumadin), 31, 78, 95
Washout, 88, 103, 119, 397
Wet drowning, 396
Wheezing, 27, 405
White blood cells, 126, 133-134, 151, 153, 324
White matter, 55, 59, 85
Wind chill index, 390
Withdrawal, 41, 77
Witnesses, 36
Work-induced thermogenesis, 381
Wound dressing, 143
Wounds
exit, 211, 213, 222, 224, 231, 240, 267, 304-305,
320-321, 326, 330, 337, 339-342, 344
immediate transport, 321
Wrist injuries, 188

X

Xiphisternal joint, 222, 224, 247, 250
Xiphoid process, 199-200, 223-224, 247, 250

Y

Yaw, 330, 333-335, 344-345
Yellow bone marrow, 156, 159, 195

Z

Zygoma, 252, 255-257, 271, 279, 297
Zygomatic arch, 254-255, 258, 271
Zygomatic bone, 254-255

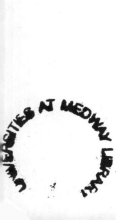

Pearson New International Edition

Paramedic Care
Principles & Practice, Volume 5, Trauma
Bledsoe Porter Cherry
Fourth Edition

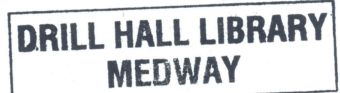
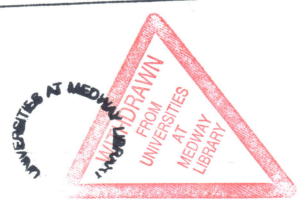
PEARSON

Pearson Education Limited
Edinburgh Gate
Harlow
Essex CM20 2JE
England and Associated Companies throughout the world

Visit us on the World Wide Web at: www.pearsoned.co.uk

© Pearson Education Limited 2014

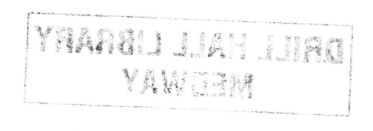

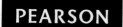 ISBN 10: 1-292-02164-0
ISBN 13: 978-1-292-02164-5

British Library Cataloguing-in-Publication Data
A catalogue record for this book is available from the British Library

Printed in the United States of America

Table of Contents

1. Trauma and Trauma Systems
Bryan E. Bledsoe/Robert S. Porter/Richard A. Cherry   **1**

2. Special Considerations in Trauma
Bryan E. Bledsoe/Robert S. Porter/Richard A. Cherry   **17**

3. Nervous System Trauma
Bryan E. Bledsoe/Robert S. Porter/Richard A. Cherry   **51**

4. Hemorrhage and Shock
Bryan E. Bledsoe/Robert S. Porter/Richard A. Cherry   **87**

5. Soft-Tissue Trauma
Bryan E. Bledsoe/Robert S. Porter/Richard A. Cherry   **121**

6. Orthopedic Trauma
Bryan E. Bledsoe/Robert S. Porter/Richard A. Cherry   **155**

7. Abdominal Trauma
Bryan E. Bledsoe/Robert S. Porter/Richard A. Cherry   **197**

8. Thoracic Trauma
Bryan E. Bledsoe/Robert S. Porter/Richard A. Cherry   **221**

9. Head, Face, Neck, and Spinal Trauma
Bryan E. Bledsoe/Robert S. Porter/Richard A. Cherry   **251**

10. Burn Trauma
Bryan E. Bledsoe/Robert S. Porter/Richard A. Cherry   **299**

11. Penetrating Trauma
Bryan E. Bledsoe/Robert S. Porter/Richard A. Cherry   **329**

12. Blunt Trauma
Bryan E. Bledsoe/Robert S. Porter/Richard A. Cherry   **347**

13. Environmental Trauma
Bryan E. Bledsoe/Robert S. Porter/Richard A. Cherry   **379**